TARGETS IN GENE THERAPY

Edited by **Yongping You**

Targets in Gene Therapy
Edited by Yongping You

Published by InTech
Janeza Trdine 9, 51000 Rijeka, Croatia

Technical Editor Sonja Mujacic

Cover Designer InTech Design Team

Additional hard copies can be obtained from orders@intechopen.com

Targets in Gene Therapy,
Edited by Yongping You
p. cm.
ISBN 978-953-307-540-2

For EU product safety concerns:
IN TECH d.o.o., Prolaz Marije Krucifikse Kozulić 3, 51000 Rijeka, Croatia,
info@intechopen.com or visit our website at intechopen.com.

Meet the editor

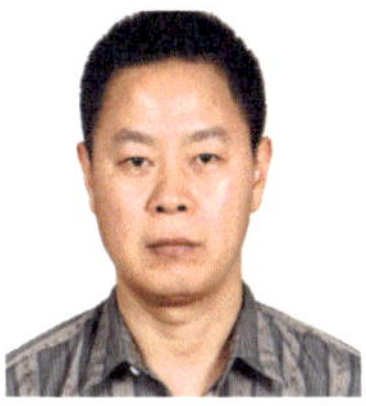

Dr. Yongping You is Professor and Chief Physician at Department of Neurosurgery, The First Affiliated Hospital of Nanjing Medical University, P. R. China. He is a member of many professional societies, including American Association for Cancer Research, Chinese Neurosurgical Society. Dr. You received his bachelor degree in Medicine from Second Military Medical University, Shanghai, P. R. China in 1990 and his Ph.D. in neurosurgery from Tianjin Medical University General Hospital, Tianjin, P. R. China in 2001. He specializes in surgery and chemotherapy of brain tumor, and basic and applied research in neuro-oncology, especially glioma. His research interests mainly involve optimal strategy of gene therapy in glioma, target and marker screen in brain tumor, miRNA, pathway and transcription regulation in glioma. His research has received sustained funding from the Chinese Natural Science Foundation, Jiangsu Province's Natural Science Foundation and other foundations. Dr. You has supervised the research efforts of over 30 postdoctoral associates, doctoral candidates and master's level graduate students in the past 10 years.

Contents

Preface

Up to now, major diseases often attempted to be treated by gene therapy include cancer, cardiovascular disease and monogenic diseases. Despite many decades of gene therapy research on these fatal diseases, most of the products fail to make it to market. One urgent problem is to identify the key targets for specific drugs.

The aim of our book is to cover key aspects of existing problems in the emerging field of targets in gene therapy. With the contribution of leading experts and pioneers in various disciplines of gene therapy, this book brings together major approaches:

1. Target Strategy in Gene Therapy,

2. Gene Therapy of Cancer,

3. Gene Therapy of Other Diseases.

The publication of this book was made possible by the efforts and collaboration of many individuals. We thank the contributors and section editors for generously sharing their expertise and scientific skills.

We hope that this book will provide a realistic image of the huge potential, perspective and challenges facing the field of gene therapy in its quest to cure disease and prolong life.

Yongping You
Professor and Chief Physician
Department of Neurosurgery
The First Affiliated Hospital of Nanjing Medical University
China

Part 1

Target Strategy in Gene Therapy

1

Choosing Targets for Gene Therapy

Karina J. Matissek, Ruben R. Bender,
James R. Davis and Carol S. Lim
University of Utah
USA

1. Introduction

Gene therapy is often attempted in fatal diseases with no known cure, or after standard therapies have failed. Targeting gene defects includes addressing a single mutation, multiple mutations in several genes, or even addressing missing or extra copies in a particular disease. A defect in one specific gene may impair normal function of the corresponding expressed protein. For example, in X-linked severe combined immunodeficiency (X-SCID), there is a mutation in the IL2 receptor γ gene. Another classic example occurs in thalassemia propagated by a defect in the β-globulin gene. Some diseases are caused by multiple mutations in several genes. For example, some cardiovascular diseases may manifest due to mutations in different chromosomes which are a result of inherited or environmental factors. Before approaching a disease using gene therapy, the key protein(s) and pathways involved in the disease should first be identified. However, in some cases an abnormal gene is formed that results in disease; such is the case for the Bcr-Abl gene. The oncogenic Bcr-Abl protein is the causative agent of chronic myelogenous leukemia (CML) which could be blocked for CML treatment. Genomic sequencing information, microarrays, and biochemical assays can be used to determine up- or down-regulated proteins involved in disease, and will help determine the function of these proteins. In the case of some cancers, the signal transduction pathways for oncogenesis have been mapped out, allowing hub proteins to be identified. Hub proteins are essential proteins that interact with multiple other proteins in signaling cascades. If selected properly, adding back a tumor-suppressing hub protein (such as p53), or blocking an oncogenic hub protein (such as survivin) could halt cancer or alter disease progression. Gene mutations can result in mislocalization of these key proteins which can cause cancer; this mislocalization can be exploited with gene therapy approaches. Further, new types of gene therapy are being developed in our lab to direct proteins to other cellular compartments where their function is altered. This chapter will summarize these and other known targets and also focus on choosing newer targets for gene therapy.

2. Known targets for gene therapy

The general aim of gene therapy is to introduce a well-defined DNA sequence into specific cells. Almost any disease can be targeted with gene therapy by replacing defective genes or imparting a new function. In fact, 85% of clinical trials in gene therapy have been conducted for cancer, cardiovascular diseases and for inherited monogenic diseases. In addition, 6.5%

of clinical trials have been conducted for infectious diseases (mainly HIV). Cancer, cardiovascular diseases and HIV are ideal gene therapy targets because of their enormous prevalence and the associated fatal consequences of these diseases, whereas monogenic disorders reflect the original idea of gene therapy which is replacement of a defective gene. Gene therapy offers a unique opportunity to cure patients with monogenic disorders. One third of clinical trials for monogenic disorders are for cystic fibrosis while about 20% are for SCID (Edelstein et al. 2004). This section highlights the advantages of gene therapy for multifactorial diseases such as cancer, vascular diseases, and HIV and describes the utility of gene therapy for monogenic diseases such as cystic fibrosis, SCID and β-thalassemia.

2.1 Cancer

Cancer was responsible for 7.6 million deaths in 2008 (WHO 2011) and is the largest target for gene therapy clinical trials. The complexity of cancer may make it difficult to bring a product to the market due to the number of genes involved compared to monogenetic disorders. However, gene therapeutics are not designed to correct these mutations by adding an enormous amount of DNA to the cells. Instead, they target critical proteins involved in signaling cascades such as the tumor suppressor p53. For example, the first gene therapy product was Gendicine™, an adenovirus containing the tumor suppressor p53.

The tumor suppressor p53 is mutated in 40% of many types of cancers, and malfunction of p53 is the major contributor for chemotherapy resistance (Goh et al. 2011). Apoptosis can be triggered by transcriptionally active p53 in the nucleus (Taha et al. 2004) as well as by p53-mediated transcriptionally independent mechanisms in the mitochondria (Vaseva et al. 2009). Various animal studies have shown that p53 induces apoptosis even in advanced tumors such as lymphoma and hepatocellular carcinoma (Ventura et al. 2007; Palacios & Moll 2006; Xue et al. 2007).

The first p53 based gene therapy in humans was conducted in 1996. This trial used a retroviral vector containing wild type p53 with an actin promoter for the treatment of non-small cell lung carcinoma. In this study three patients showed tumor regression and three other patients showed tumor growth stabilization (Roth et al. 1996). China was the first country which approved a p53 adenovirus for gene therapy, Gendicine™ SiBiono, in combination with radiotherapy for head and neck squamous cell cancer in 2004 (Shi & Zheng 2009). Gendicine™ is a recombinant serotype 5 adenovirus with the E1 region replaced by the p53 expressing cassette (with a Rous sarcoma virus promoter). The adenovirus particles infect tumor target cells carrying therapeutic p53 (Peng 2005). Clinical trials for Gendicine™ showed that in combination with radiation therapy it caused partial or complete tumor regression (Peng 2005; Xin 2006). There were also some clinical trials for Gendicine™ in advanced liver cancer, lung cancer and other advanced solid tumors (Peng 2005). It should be kept in mind that China's State Food and Drug Administration (SFDA) has different standards for the approval of a cancer drug compared to the U.S. FDA and the European Medicine Agency (EMA). Gendicine™ was approved in China on the basis of tumor shrinkage. The U.S. FDA and the EMA require novel cancer drugs to extend the lifetime of the treated patients (Guo & Xin 2006).

Another p53 product is Oncorine™ from Shanghai SunwayBiotech, an oncolytic virus. Oncorine™ was approved for the treatment of head and neck cancer in China in 2006 (Yu & Fang 2007). It is a replicative adenovirus 2/adenovirus 5 hybrid with deletion in E1B55K and E3B (Raty et al. 2008). This oncolytic virus was expected to infect and lyse cancer cells only and not affect normal cells (Guo et al. 2008). Even though clinical studies showed that it was not specific for cancer cells, it did, however, kill tumor cells preferentially (Garber 2006). Phase I/II trials showed little dose-limiting toxicity (Lockley et al. 2006) and the combination of Oncorine™ with chemotherapy showed greater tumor shrinkage in patients with head and neck cancer, compared to chemotherapy alone. It should be kept in mind that like Gendicine™, Oncorine™ was also approved by the SFDA based on objective response rate, not on survival (Garber 2006). Nevertheless, all the available data concerning p53 and its proven function as tumor suppressor qualifies it as an adjuvant treatment with radiotherapy or chemotherapy.

Another approach to cancer gene therapy is gene-directed enzyme prodrug therapy (GDEPT). GDEPT transfers an activating transgene into tumor cells followed by systemic treatment with a non-toxic drug which becomes activated only in cells expressing the transgene. Cerepro® is an adenovirus containing a herpes simplex type-1 thymidine kinase transgene under the cytomegalovirus promoter. Cerepro® is under phase I, II and III clinical trials in Europe for malignant glioma, a fatal form of brain cancer. In these clinical trials Cerepro® was injected multiple times into healthy brain tissues of patients following surgical removal of the solid tumor mass. Then the patients were treated with the prodrug ganciclovir, which is converted to its toxic form, deoxyguanosine, by thymidine kinase. This toxic metabolite affects newly dividing cells, thus it prevents new tumors from growing. In phase I and II trials, patients given Cerepro® showed a significant increase in survival. However, after phase III studies, the EMA rejected the marketing application for Cerepro® due to inadequate efficacy (van Putten et al. 2010; Cerepro 2009; Mitchell 2010; Raty et al. 2008). Despite this particular failure, systemic side effects are avoided with the GDEPT concept. The general goal of GDEPT is the improvement of chemotherapy in terms of safety and efficiency using concomitant gene therapy (Edelstein et al. 2004).

2.2 Cardiovascular diseases

Cardiovascular diseases (CVD) encompass disorders of the heart and blood vessels and include hypertension, coronary heart disease, cerebrovascular disease, peripheral vascular disease, heart failure, rheumatic heart disease, congenital heart disease and cardiomyopathies (Chiuve et al. 2006). Cardiovascular diseases are the largest health problem worldwide, claiming 17.1 million lives per year. Despite the complexity of cardiovascular disease, there is great potential for gene therapy especially in ischemia, angiogenesis, hypertension and hypercholesterolemia. Currently there is no gene therapy product on the market for CVD. Nevertheless, several clinical trials have been conducted (Edelstein et al. 2004; Edelstein et al. 2007). Most gene therapies for CVD aim to increase angiogenesis which is a mechanism to overcome ischemia. Ischemia is a condition in which the flow of blood is restricted to parts of the body. The response of the body is to form new blood vessels around the blockage, called angiogenesis, and is triggered by angiogenic proteins such as vascular endothelial growth factor (VEGF), fibroblast growth factor (FGF) and hepatocyte growth factor (HGF) (Abo-Auda & Benza 2003; Kass et al. 1992). The goal of introducing genes coding for these growth factors is to increase the local concentration of these factors to stimulate angiogenesis (Edelstein et al. 2004). Two companies are conducting phase III clinical trials using FGF. Bayer Schering Pharm AG has developed alferminogene tadenovec, which is a replication-deficient human adenovirus serotype 5 which encodes human FGF4. Since myocardial ischemia is linked to coronary artery disease, the therapeutic goal is to improve the reperfusion of ischemic myocardium. Phase IIb/III clinical trials showed that it is well-tolerated; a phase III trial is ongoing to prove its efficacy (Flynn &

O'Brien 2008; CardioVascular BioTherapeutics). Sanofi-Aventis is developing a FGF gene therapy product called riferminogene pecaplasmide or NV1FGF (Riferminogene pecaplasmide 2010). It is a novel pCOR (conditional origin of replication) plasmid-based gene delivery system (Maulik 2009). NV1FGF is injected into muscle cells, and expresses FGF-1. The therapeutic goal is to treat chronic/critical limb ischemia since limb ischemia is linked to peripheral artery disease (Baumgartner et al. 2009). Phase III clinical trials are ongoing in 32 countries (Riferminogene pecaplasmide 2010).

Another gene therapy approach to treat limb ischemia uses HGF. There are several animal studies showing that HGF can trigger formation of new blood vessels (Shigematsu et al. 2010). The injection of the naked HGF gene is well-tolerated as shown in the first clinical trial conducted in Japan (Morishita et al. 2004). Another clinical trial in the U.S. showed that HGF injection increased tissue perfusion compared to placebo (Powell et al. 2008). Lastly, there is also a clinical trial to prove efficacy of HGF gene therapy, using reduction of ulcer size and decrease in rest pain (pain occurring during sleep) as objectives (Shigematsu et al. 2010).

2.3 HIV

The human immunodeficiency virus (HIV) causes acquired immunodeficiency syndrome (AIDS), a severe disease characterized by profound negative effects on the immune system leading to life-threatening opportunistic infections. Although antiretroviral drugs have decreased the morbidity and mortality of HIV infected patients, currently there is no cure. However, new developments in gene therapy have focused on introducing genes encoding RNA or proteins which are capable of interfering with intracellular replication of HIV, so-called intracellular immunization. So far, the approaches range from protein-based strategies such as fusion inhibitors or zinc finger nucleases to RNA-based approaches such as ribozymes, antisense or short hairpin RNA. Currently, a promising target is the chemokine receptor 5 (CCR5) which is needed for fusion of HIV with immune cells. Studies have shown that patients with mutated CCR5 have a higher long-term survival and slower progression of the disease. A homozygous defect in the CCR5 gene, a Δ32 deletion, resulting in a lack of functional CCR5 protein and confers resistance to HIV infection (Liu et al. 1996). An allogeneic stem-cell transplantation of CCR5 defective cells in a patient with HIV infection and acute myeloid leukemia resulted in both a negative HIV plasma viral load and no detection of HIV proviral DNA for more than 3.5 years after treatment (without the use of antiviral drugs). This result has been classified as a cure of HIV (Kitchen et al. 2011, and references therein; Symonds et al. 2010, and references therein).

2.4 Monogenic diseases

Monogenic diseases are prime targets for gene therapy due to their simple single gene mutations. Their disease causing mechanisms are easier to elucidate which is advantageous for choosing a target for gene therapy. In addition, the execution of therapy is more straightforward, since it is easier to transfer single genes into cells instead of several genes. Other important factors are the location and the type of cell in which the gene has to be transferred. Is the cell reachable with existing delivery systems? Is the cell already differentiated or is it a still dividing stem cell? Does gene transfer need to be repeated or is a one-time transfer sufficient? All these questions have to be considered in order to choose the right target for gene therapy, and it must be noted that not every disease caused by single gene mutations can be targeted. Three examples of well-studied diseases and attempts to treat these diseases using gene therapy will be discussed.

2.4.1 Cystic fibrosis

Cystic fibrosis (CF) is a complex inherited disease affecting the lungs and digestive system. The cause of this disease is a defect in the cystic fibrosis transmembrane conductance regulator (CFTR), which is a chloride channel on the apical membrane of respiratory epithelia. This leads to reduced Cl^- and increased Na^+ permeability (Boucher et al. 1988). CF is caused by several different mutations in the CFTR gene located on chromosome 7 (Knowlton et al. 1985). Of the hundreds of mutations that cause CF, the most common mutation, which occurs in approximately 70% of all cases, is the deletion of a phenylalanine residue at amino acid position 508 (ΔF508) (Kerem et al. 1989). CF results in decreased production of pancreatic enzymes leading to malnutrition, and also blocks the lung with unusually viscous mucus leading to life-threatening infections (Cystic Fibrosis Foundation; Wood 1997). It is possible to treat symptoms of CF to improve quality of life but there is no current cure for this disease. Mainstays for symptomatic treatment include enzymatic therapies (pancreatic enzymes and DNAse I) (McPhail et al. 2008), airway clearance and hypertonic saline for improved lung function, use of drugs that enhance Cl^- secretion in airway epithelium (Cloutier et al. 1990) and anti-inflammatories involving ibuprofen or corticosteroids (Flume et al. 2010, and references therein). Despite a clear understanding of genetic links, gene therapy is not yet a standard treatment for CF, as recent attempts to cure patients with CF have not been successful. Moss et al. showed improvement in pulmonary function in a phase II clinical trial with 42 CF patients, of whom 20 received at least one dose of aerosolized adeno-associated serotype 2 virus carrying the CFTR gene. A significant enhancement in FEV_1 (forced expiratory volume per second) was noted after 30 days compared to placebo. Furthermore, this study showed no adverse events demonstrating the safety of adeno-associated vectors (Moss et al. 2004). However, when this same group performed a second, larger phase IIb trial with 102 subjects, there was no significant improvement in FEV1 seen after 30 days compared with placebo (Moss et al. 2007). Expression of CFTR was noted in airway epithelium of 7 individuals with CF after the first administration but the effect lasted only 30 days. The second administration showed decreased expression. Finally, at the third administration, the expression fell to zero (Harvey et al. 1999). In conclusion, there is some indication that gene therapy could be used to cure CF, but no method has shown to be universally applicable. Further research is needed to find the right vector with repeatable administration and subsequent high expression while simultaneously being safe. Gene therapy for CF targets epithelial cells which have a limited life span and do not divide. Because of that, the gene has to be transferred repeatedly into new growing cells, which is problematic since repeated transfections have been ineffective.

2.4.2 Severe combined immunodeficiency

Severe combined immunodeficiency (SCID) is a rare, fatal syndrome with an incidence of 24.3 cases per million live births (Ryser et al. 1988). The disease is characterized clinically by defects in humoral and cellular immunity due to profound deficiencies of T-and B-cell function, and if left untreated usually leads to death in infancy (Buckley et al. 1997). Mutations leading to SCID appear in various genes including Jak-3, adenosine deaminase, IL-7 receptor (Puel et al. 1998), tyrosine phosphatase CD45 (Kung et al. 2000), the interleukin-2 (IL-2) receptor γ chain (IL2-Rγ), the Artemis gene (Kobayashi et al. 2003) and recombinase activating genes 1 or 2 (Schwarz et al. 1996; Buckley et al. 1997, and references therein). The most frequently diagnosed form of SCID is X-SCID, which is characterized by a mutation in the IL2-Rγ gene located on the X chromosome. This disease shows a male

predominance, with a mean age of diagnosis of 6.6 months. The IL2-Rγ chain is a critical component of many cytokine receptors including those for IL-2, -4, -7, -9, -15 and 21, where defects may result in greatly decreased numbers of T and NK cells. The number of B cells is generally normal but their activity is abnormal (Buckley et al. 1997). After maternal antibodies have vanished, the extreme susceptibility to infection due to opportunistic microbes, persistent diarrhea and failure to thrive usually lead to death in the first year of life unless immunologic reconstruction can be achieved.
Hematopoietic stem cell transplantation is the standard of care for all genetic types of SCID with a survival rate of nearly 80% with HLA-identical parental marrow (Antoine et al. 2003). Even with a matched donor, stem cell transplantation may lead to long-term clinical complications (De Ravin & Malech 2009). Thus, other treatments for SCID are needed. An ex vivo gene therapy trial with two X-SCID patients, aged 8 and 11 months, demonstrated that gene therapy has curative potential. Administration of a retroviral vector containing the correct IL2-Rγ gene resulted in T cell counts similar to that of age-matched controls after 105 days. Furthermore, the immune system responded to tetanus toxin and polioviruses within the normal range after primary vaccination. Both patients later showed normal growth and psychomotor development (Cavazzana-Calvo et al. 2000). Other studies confirmed these results (Hacein-Bey-Abina et al. 2002; Thrasher et al. 2005). A separate study of gene therapy for X-SCID with children aged 2.5, 4 and 8 years old showed mixed results. Only the youngest patient experienced benefit from the treatment (Chinen et al. 2007). Another trial with two patients, aged 15 and 20 years old also failed (Thrasher et al. 2005). Despite the variable outcome from these studies, gene therapy may still potentially cure X-SCID and other SCIDs, in particular for younger patients. It is already possible to cure newborn children with this modern technique, if traditional methods like BMT fail. If the safety of gene therapy vectors can be improved to lower the risk of insertional mutagenesis, gene therapy will likely become first-line therapy for to the treatment of X-SCID. In contrast to CF, the presence of accessible stem cells in which the functional gene could be transferred would allow continuous expression of this gene, making X-SCID a good candidate for gene therapy.

2.4.3 β–thalassemia

β-thalassemia syndromes are a group of inherited blood disorders. Thalassemia major is the only transfusion-dependent type of β-thalassemia and manifests itself clinically between 6 and 24 months of life by paleness and failure to thrive. It is marked by reduced (β^+) or absent (β^0) beta globin chain synthesis caused by several different single gene mutations, resulting in reduced hemoglobin in red blood cells (Weatherall 1976). If left untreated, this disease results in growth retardation, pallor, jaundice, poorly developed musculature, skeletal changes and other consequences leading to death during infancy (Cao & Galanello 2010). Blood transfusion is the current standard therapy for β-thalassamia and aims to correct the anemia from reduced hemoglobin (Cao & Galanello 2010). This treatment, however, carries the risk of infection from blood borne diseases such as HIV and hepatitis and as well as the serious side effect of transfusional iron overload which is fatal if untreated. Currently, BMT offers the best chance for curing β-thalassemia in both in children and adults if a HLA identical donor is found, but is limited by complications like graft-versus-host disease or finding suitable donors (Lucarelli & Gaziev 2008).

Gene therapy of human β-thalassemia is still in its infancy and requires the development of efficient, safe and high level gene transfer into target hematopoietic stem cells. It also requires regulation of erythroid lineage-specific expression and therapeutic levels of β-globin expression (Malik & Arumugam 2005). Meeting these requirements may be difficult, but a successful gene therapy trial was achieved in 2007 when an 18 year-old patient was effectively treated using a β-globin-expressing lentiviral vector. The vector was transfected ex vivo into harvested $CD34^+$ cells and then transplanted back into the patient's bone marrow. The patient, who had no HLA-matched donors (making BMT impossible), was treated with high dose chemotherapy with intravenous busulfan to eliminate defective hematopoetic stem cells (HSC) prior to transplantation. This step was critical for the success of this treatment to prevent the defective HSC from diluting the corrected HSC. Three years post-transplant this patient no longer required blood transfusions and showed stable hemoglobin levels. However, mild anemia, compensatory expansion of red-blood-cell precursors in bone marrow, and other safety concerns have been raised (including development of cancers) (Cavazzana-Calvo et al. 2010). Although the long-term prognosis and outcome of gene therapy for β-thalassemia is currently unclear, it still has the same advantage of the presence of accessible stem cells as X-SCID. With this in mind, targeting stem cells may be more successful than differentiated cells, and may be sufficient to cure the disease.

3. Identifying novel targets for gene therapy

Before targeting a disease with gene therapy, the genetic basis of that disease should be identified. Strategies for finding disease genes have greatly improved in the last few years due to the Human Genome Project and the Hap Map Project. The Hap Map Project identifies and catalogs genetic similarities and differences in humans (Human Genome Project; The International Hap Map Consortium 2003) and supplies computerized databases to search through and identify new gene therapy targets (Hap Map Project 2003). To find genes the two most common options are candidate-gene studies and genome-wide studies. Candidate-gene association studies are based on prior biological knowledge of gene function or on significant findings in linkage studies. This method is based on a single polymorphism and haplotypes and compares allele or haplotype frequencies between the case and the control group. Genome-wide studies can be divided into linkage mapping and genome-wide association studies. Genetic linkage mapping studies are used to discover and identify new genes by using genetic and phenotypic data from families. The analysis is conducted without any prior knowledge about genetic basis of disease. Linkage analysis functions by comparing genotype polymorphic markers at known locations in the genome. Genome-wide association studies are the most recent technology. They search the whole genome for single nucleotide polymorphisms (SNPs). Each study can look at hundreds or thousands of SNPs at the same time (for an excellent review see (Hirschhorn & Daly 2005)). The results are plotted into biostatistics algorithms (Nakamura 2009; Hirschhorn & Daly 2005). The proteins identified by genomic methods can be further characterized by standard molecular and biochemical assays. In addition, protein targets have been identified by individual labs using standard molecular and biochemical methods without a priori use of genomic information. With the growing understanding of genes associated with many diseases the future for new gene therapeutics shows promise.

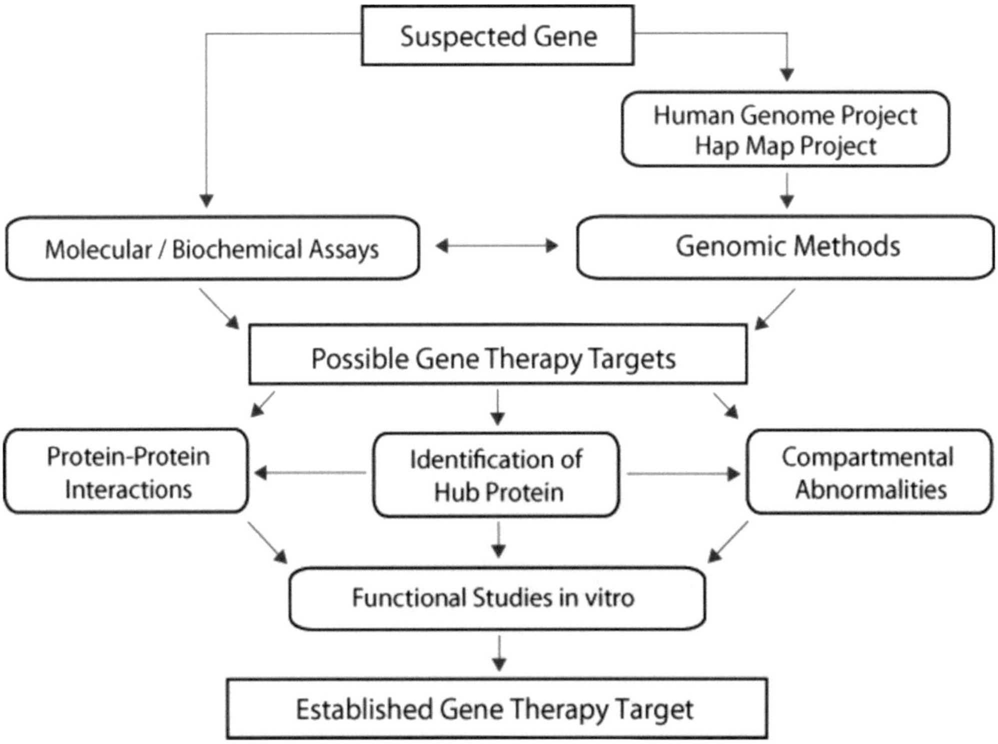

Fig. 1. Finding Novel Gene Therapy Targets. Integration of standard and modern technologies for disease-causing targets for gene therapy.

3.1 Methods to find gene therapy targets

Microarrays lay the groundwork for the methods mentioned above. The two most important advantages of microarrays are their small scale (multi-well plate formats) and ability to detect thousands of different immobilized genes simultaneously (Duggan et al. 1999; Siegmund et al. 2003; NCBI 2007). There are three types of microarray technologies: comparative genomic hybridization, expression analysis and mutation/polymorphism analysis, though the principle remains the same for all. First, the DNA chip corresponding to the DNA of interest is selected. Then, isolated messenger RNA (mRNA) is used as a template to generate complementary DNA (cDNA), with a fluorescent tag. This mixture is incubated with the DNA chip. During this incubation, tagged cDNA can specifically bind to the complementary DNA template on the chip. Afterwards, the hybridized cDNA can be detected with lasers specific to different fluorophores followed by analysis using computational methods (NCBI 2007).

The Human Genome Project and the HapMap project have provided the foundation for candidate gene and genome-wide studies. Using these methods may allow us to draw conclusions between gene abnormalities and diseases. For example, many different studies have been conducted to determine the genes associated with cardiovascular diseases. In fact many CVDs are linked to mutated genes. For example, there is evidence based on genetic linkage analysis that chromosomes 1, 2, 3, 13, 14, 16 and X are involved in myocardial infarction, which is the major killer world-wide. Additionally, myocardial infarction and stroke are associated with mutations in chromosome 13q12-13 containing the ALOX5AP gene encoding arachidonate 5-lipoxygenase-activating protein. Furthermore, high LDL, low HDL and high triglycerides values are high risk factors for cardiovascular disease, with linkage results located in all autosomes except for 2 and 14 (Arnett et al. 2007, and references therein).

Finding disease-causing genes may not only help to better understand the pathophysiology of the disease, but may improve the diagnosis of the disease by discovery of disease-specific marker genes. Importantly, identification of disease-causing genes will lead to new targets for improved therapeutics. Genome-wide association studies which scan markers across the entire genome can find single mutations causing monogenic disorders as well as different mutations in several genes, which may lead to more gene therapy-based cures for these diseases.

3.2 Hub proteins

Genomic sequencing information, microarrays, and molecular/biochemical assays are tools that can help determine which proteins are responsible for disease. This information can be analyzed to identify hub proteins involved in disease progression. Hub proteins are key proteins that signal to multiple other proteins in transduction cascades. They are highly connected to other proteins with multiple interaction partners. Hub proteins bind with several distinct binding sites to other proteins. Studying the binding interface of cancer-related proteins maybe useful for better understanding of cellular function and biological processes (Keskin & Nussinov 2007; Kim et al. 2006).

3.2.1 Tumor suppressor hub proteins

3.2.1.1 p53

The tumor suppressor p53 is an example of a hub protein involved in cancer which loses the ability to bind different other proteins due to mutations (Shiraishi et al. 2004). It induces transactivation of target genes which are responsible for cell cycle arrest, DNA repair and apoptosis. p53 is mutated in 40% of cancers (Goh et al. 2010). In normal, healthy cells p53 is rapidly degraded via the MDM2 pathway, but when stress signals occur, p53 accumulates dramatically in the cell, allowing it to accomplish its apoptotic functions. p53 stimulates multiple signaling mechanisms which lead to apoptosis: the extrinsic pathway through death receptors and the intrinsic pathway through the mitochondria (Haupt et al. 2003). As a transcription factor it binds to p53-responsive genes, and the expressed proteins trigger apoptosis, G1 arrest, as well as DNA repair through different mechanisms. In addition, p53 translocates to the mitochondria and induces a rapid apoptotic response (Erster et al. 2004; Haupt et al. 2003). Consequently, p53 fulfills the requirements for an ideal hub protein for gene therapy. Indeed, p53 adenovirus has been used for cancer therapy, and was the first gene therapeutic on the market.

3.2.1.2 BRCA1 and BRCA2

Breast cancer susceptibility protein (BRCA)1 and BRCA2 are highly associated with breast and ovarian cancer. The lifetime risk of developing breast cancer for a person carrying mutations in both genes is 82%; mutations in BRCA1 account for 52% and BRCA2 for 23% of all cases. Furthermore, the risk for ovarian cancer is dramatically increased due to mutations in BRCA1 and/or BRCA2. Thus, it is important to identify patients with a probability of having mutations in these proteins. BRCA1 and BRCA2 regulate cell cycle progression, DNA repair and gene transcription (Metcalfe et al. 2005). Their export into the cytoplasm is associated with apoptosis. In cooperation with cellular partner BARD1 (BRCA1-associated RING domain protein), BRCA1 is able to enter the nucleus and accomplish its role in DNA repair, centrosome regulation and RNA processing (Henderson 2005; Rodriguez et al. 2004). When the sensitive balance between BARD1 and BRCA1 is defective due to cancer-promoting mutations in both, they remain as a dimer which results in nuclear compartmentalization leading to dramatic reduction of their apoptotic activity (Davis et al. 2007; Rodriguez et al. 2004). Silencing BRCA1 expression using RNA-mediated interference, results in increased cytoplasmic levels of BARD1 and causes apoptosis in breast cancer cell lines (Rodriguez et al. 2004). BARD1 translocates to the mitochondria and causes oligomerization of Bax which results in apoptosis (Tembe & Henderson 2007). Therefore, targeting BRCA1 is a viable gene therapy-based approach.

3.2.2 Hub proteins that promote cancer

3.2.2.1 Survivin

In addition to adding back hub tumor suppressors for gene therapy, oncogenic hub proteins can be blocked as well. The oncogene survivin is nearly universally expressed in various types of cancer and is almost undetectable in most adult tissue. Survivin is a unique member of the inhibitor of apoptosis protein (IAP) family and plays a major role as a mitotic regulator (Altieri 2001, and references therein). It is involved in multiple cancer-promoting mechanisms, particularly inhibition of apoptosis. Various parallel pathways, such as intervention in mitochondrial function, inhibition of caspases, and influence on gene expression are responsible for survivin's anti-apoptotic function (Altieri 2008, and references therein). For example, survivin and its binding partners act to prevent caspase activation; activated caspase 9 is required to activate effector caspase 3 and caspase 7, which execute mitochondrial-induced apoptosis (Li & Yuan 2008). Also, a splice variant of survivin, survivin ΔEx-3, translocates to the mitochondria where it interacts with proteins from the Bcl-2 family. These proteins are inhibitors of permeabilization of the mitochondrial outer membrane which is essential for cytochrome c release. Stabilization of Bcl-2 proteins prevents cytochrome c release, thus resulting in the inhibition of caspase 9 and caspase 3 (Altieri 2008, and references therein). Furthermore, survivin's role as a mitotic regulator is related to its inhibition of apoptosis. Survivin expression is upregulated at the G2/M phase to localize to the mitotic apparatus and is downregulated in interphase via ubiquitin-dependent destruction (Li, Ambrosini, et al. 1998; Zhao et al. 2000). High survivin expression was detected in various types of cancers including breast, lung, colon, stomach, esophagus, pancreas, uterus, ovary and liver (Altieri 2008, and references therein). Dramatic overexpression of survivin correlates with more aggressive and invasive clinical phenotypes which means a poor prognosis compared to survivin-negative tumors, an increased rate of recurrence and chemotherapy resistance (Kato et al. 2001; Grossman & Altieri 2001). The differential expression and function of survivin make it an excellent target for cancer therapy (Altieri 2003). There are many gene-based strategies to inhibit survivin in cancer cells, with some in phase I and II clinical trials. One gene-based method uses survivin antisense oligonucleotides to prevent expression in cancer cells. Two phase II trials and one phase I trial by Eli Lilly and Co. are ongoing for relapsed or refractory acute myeloid leukemia, hormone refractory prostate cancer and advanced hepatocellular carcinoma (Ryan et al. 2009). Furthermore, Alteri et al. created a replication-deficient adenovirus containing a dominant negative survivin mutant where threonine 34 is mutated to alanine. This mutation abrogates phosphorylation of threonine which impairs survivin's ability act as a mitotic regulator, as only phosphorylated survivin is able to localize to the mitotic apparatus (O'Connor et al. 2000). Injection of adenovirus containing survivin mutant triggers apoptosis by cytochrome c release which leads to caspase 3 activation. Alteri et al. demonstrated in several cancer cell lines that this mutant causes apoptosis and confirmed these results in three xenograft breast cancer mice models. Interestingly, this survivin mutant was not able to cause apoptosis in proliferating normal human cells (Mesri et al. 2001).

3.2.2.2 Ras

The RAS supergene family is divided into six subfamilies RAS, RHO, RAB, ARF, RAN and RAD which code for more than 50 structurally related proteins. Their main function is to transmit signals from cell-surface receptors to the cell interior. All proteins have a guanosine triphosphate (GTP) binding motif in common and participate in signaling cascades. The RAS subfamily functions in proliferation and differentiation which makes it a prime target for anti-cancer therapy. The localization of Ras on the cell membrane, and binding to GTP are essential for its function. When Ras binds to GTP, it initiates the signaling pathway for cell proliferation and differentiation. However, when Ras-GTP is hydrolyzed to Ras-GDP by GTPase-activating proteins (GAPs), it is unable to activate its signal transduction pathway. This sensitive regulation process is out of balance in cancer cells due to different mutations in the RAS gene. Most of these mutations occur in the Ras gene itself and in the regulatory proteins of the Ras pathway. These mutations cause Ras to stay in the active Ras-GTP form and prevent conversion into the inactive Ras-GDP form. Mutated Ras protein is hyperactive and triggers cancer development. Hyperactive Ras is associated with different types of solid tumors such as pancreatic, cervical, thyroid, colon, skin, and lung tumors as well as with hematopoietic malignancies such as chronic myelomonocytic leukemia, acute myelogenous leukemia and multiple myeloma to list a few. Ras is an excellent gene therapy target due to its involvement in various cancers (Beaupre & Kurzrock 1999, and references therein). Recently it has been shown that knocking out Ras with an anti-Ras mRNA plasmid-mediated short-hairpin RNA in combination with clinical drug vincristine resulted in inhibition of the growth of human hepatoma HepG2 in vivo (Sun et al. 2009). This illustrates once again that the combination of gene therapy with standard chemotherapy is a promising approach for treatment of cancer.

3.2.2.3 AKT

AKT, a serine/threonine kinase, plays an essential role in oncogenesis. The AKT family consists of three cellular homologues AKT1, AKT2 and AKT3. The encoded proteins have a similar structure consisting of an amino-terminal pleckstrin homology domain, a short α-helical linker and a carboxy-terminal kinase domain. Tissues have different expression levels of the three homologues AKT1, AKT2 and AKT3, which is why it is not surprising that the three different variants of AKT are overexpressed in different types of cancers. For example, AKT1 is overexpressed in gastric cancer and is associated with poor prognosis in breast and prostate cancer; AKT2 is overexpressed in ovarian and pancreatic cancer. AKT3 is overexpressed in estrogen receptor-deficient breast cancer and in androgen-insensitive prostate cancer which implies that AKT3 contributes to aggressive steroid hormone-insensitive cancer. AKT acquires growth signal autonomy and inhibits apoptosis in cancer cells. It promotes cell survival through its phosphorylation of MDM2, which enhances nuclear accumulation of MDM2. MDM2 inhibits the transcriptional activity of p53 and promotes its degradation by the proteasome (Testa & Bellacosa 2001). AKT gene therapy has been conducted with an aerosol delivery system consisting of nano-sized glucosylated polyethylenimine (GPEI). It has been shown that this aerosol is capable of delivering AKT wild-type and kinase deficient genes into the lung of mice (Tehrani et al. 2007). Dominant negative alleles of AKT directly injected into lung carcinoma cells have also been shown to block cell survival and proliferation (Li, Simpson, et al. 1998).

3.3 Protein-protein interactions

A protein dimer or oligomer is a macromolecular structure formed by two (dimer) or several (oligomer) proteins of either same origin (homo-oligomers) or different origins (hetero-oligomers). For several proteins the formation of oligomers or dimers is essential in order to form functional systems. Both Bcr-Abl and p53 proteins function in the homo-oligomeric form. On the other hand, hemoglobin forms hetero-oligomers consisting of two α and two β subunits to form a functional structure. If one of these subunits is defective or missing, the protein cannot master its tasks leading to diseases such as the previously described β-thalassemia. Mutations in the oligomerization domain can lead to loss of function. Dimer or oligomer formation is governed by non-covalent interactions, including salt bridges, hydrogen bonds and hydrophobic interactions. A common structural motif for dimerization is a coiled coil consisting of usually two to five α-helices that wind around one another like strands of a rope, meshed together like "knobs-into-holes." They contain a characteristic seven-residue sequence repeat (Mason & Arndt 2004; Crick 1952). Coiled coil motifs play an important role in the function of several different proteins ranging from transcription factors such as Jun and Fos which are responsible for cell growth and proliferation (Glover & Harrison 1995) to the oncoprotein Bcr-Abl which leads to cancer (McWhirter et al. 1993). A subgroup of the coiled coil motif is represented by the "leucine zipper", an unusually long α-helix with protruding leucine residues in periodic repetition. The leucine residues from one peptide interact with leucine residues from a second peptide, forming a molecular zipper (Landschulz et al. 1988). Another important dimerization interface for proteins is the helix-loop-helix (HLH) motif. Characterized by two α-helices connected by a short loop, this structure is highly conserved in many diverse organisms. Proteins containing this structure are transcription factors that are only functional as homo- or hetero-dimers (Murre et al. 1994, and references therein). Important HLH family members are myc proteins which play an essential role in cell proliferation, differentiation, cell growth, and apoptosis, but are also involved in development of numerous kinds of cancer (Vita & Henriksson 2006). Finally, another interaction motif is the zinc finger motif, containing several subgroups such as C2H2, Gag knuckle, treble clef, zinc ribbon, Zn2/Cys6, TAZ2 domain like, zinc binding loops and metallothionein (Krishna et al. 2003). The C2H2 zinc finger represents the most prevalent motif and contains a zinc ion coordinated by cysteines and histidines (Wolfe et al. 2000). Although most C2H2 fingers apparently contribute to protein-DNA or protein-RNA interactions, examples for protein-protein interactions also exist. One example is Ikaros, a transcription factor participating in gene silencing and activation in hematopoietic cells. In this protein, dimerization is important for its activity and affinity to DNA (McCarty et al. 2003, and references therein). In addition, more complex oligomerization structures exist. For example, p53 forms a dimer with an antiparallel β-sheet and an antiparallel helix-helix interface. Two dimers associate as a parallel helix-helix to form a tetramer (Jeffrey et al. 1995).

Gene therapy may be used to enhance or inhibit dimerization interfaces. Currently, small molecule drugs are unable to re-establish the ability of proteins to form dimers with the aim of restoring their natural function. In contrast, gene therapy can supply dimerization-capable and functional proteins. On the other hand, if the formation of a dimer is unwanted, it is possible to disrupt the dimerization interface of a disease-causing protein by introducing proteins into the cell which compete for dimerization. Normal dimerization of the disease-causing protein is then blocked, hence stopping the disease.

3.3.1 Homo-oligomerization for apoptotic activity

The classic example of a protein that is only functional as a homo-oligomer is p53. The protein p53 is 393 amino acids long and contains a transactivation domain (amino acids 1-43) and a proline-rich domain (amino acids 61-94), a DNA-binding domain (amino acids 110-286), a tetramerization domain (amino acids 326-355) and a regulatory region (amino acids 363-393) (Chene 2001). As already mentioned, mutations of TP53, the gene encoding for p53, occur in a large proportion of human cancers. Some of these mutations may prevent the formation of tetramers, which lead to loss of p53 function (Vogelstein et al. 2000). Not only does the site-specific binding to DNA depend on oligomerization , but so do a number of post-translational modifications of p53 which are believed to be important regulators of p53 activity (Chene 2001, and references therein). Reintroducing tetramerization-capable p53 using gene therapy may allow treatment of cancers which are caused by mutations in this region of TP53. So far 49 mutations in the tetramerization domain of p53 have been described, even though not all mutations prevent dimerization or tetramerization. Most of these occurring mutants still form tetrameric structures like wild-type p53 but with reduced stability (Kamada et al. 2011).

Another example where protein oligomerization yields functionality occurs with DJ-1. This protein bears cytoprotective functions within cells and protects neurons from stressful stimulants. A L166P mutation in the DJ-1 gene may prevent its ability to homodimerize, and it has been speculated that this can lead to neurodegeneration in autosomal recessive early onset Parkinsonism (Gorner et al. 2007, and references therein). Re-introduction of dimerization-capable DJ-1 with gene therapy is therefore a possible treatment option.

3.3.2 Disruption of disease-causing homo-oligomerization

Like p53, Bcr-Abl is also a protein that functions as a homo-oligomer (dimer of dimers). However, Bcr-Abl derives oncogenic function rather than tumor suppression from oligomerization. Bcr-Abl results from the fusion of the breakpoint cluster region (Bcr) gene on chromosome 22 and the Abelson leukemia oncogene (Abl) on chromosome 9. This results in an abnormal shortened chromosome called the Philadelphia chromosome. Bcr-Abl functions as an oncoprotein leading to increased cell proliferation and inhibition of apoptosis due to the constitutive activation of tyrosine kinase activity and causes 95% of all cases of chronic myeloid leukemia (CML) (Sawyers 1999, and references therein). The oligomerization of Bcr-Abl is essential for the activation of the tyrosine kinase activity of Bcr-Abl (McWhirter et al. 1993). Destroying the ability of Bcr-Abl to form tetramers or using the dimerization domain to disrupt Bcr-Abl activity would be a possible gene therapy approach for CML (Dixon et al. 2009).

Finally, serpins (serine protease inhibitors) such as serpin α1-antitrypsin function aberrantly as oligomers/polymers (Silverman et al. 2001; Lomas & Mahadeva 2002). In fact, the polymerization of serpin α1-antitrypsin is known to cause hepatocellular carcinoma and liver cirrhosis due to accumulation in the endoplasmatic reticulum of the liver (Lomas & Mahadeva 2002). Disruption of polymerization could also be targeted for gene therapy, using an exogenously added polymerization domain that could compete for binding to serpin α1-antitrypsin.

3.4 Cell compartments

Targeting a gene therapy product to a specific subcellular compartment is another way to overcome disease. There are many diseases associated with protein malfunction in different organelles of the cell (Davis et al. 2007). For example, certain cancers can arise when a protein localizes to the wrong compartment. The typical example is cytoplasmically mislocalized p53. When p53 is in the cytoplasm, it cannot act as tumor suppressor since it is a transcription factor that needs to be in the nucleus in order to function (Kau et al. 2004; Wurzer et al. 2001). In addition to mislocation from the nucleus, the incorrect localization of proteins normally destined for lysosomes, peroxisomes, Golgi apparatus, endoplasmic reticulum (ER) or mitochondria can also lead to disease. Directing gene therapy products to specific subcellular compartments represents not only novel targets but a new way to approach gene therapy (Mossalam et al. 2010).

3.4.1 Lysosomes

Lysosomes degrade unused cellular constituents, receptors and release active enzymes extracellularly and are involved in post-translational maturation of proteins. Dysfunction of lysosomal hydrolases leads to loss of cell growth control and results in chemotherapy resistance as well as high metastatic potential (Castino et al. 2003). Furthermore, lysosome and lysosome-related organelles are associated with Lysosomal Storage Disease (LSD), Alzheimer's disease and development of several types of tumors. LSD is collective term for 40 genetic disorders due to single or multi enzyme deficiency which results in neurodegenerative disorders. Therapy options are limited to BMT and enzyme replacement. The disadvantages of BMT are morbidity and mortality as well as incomplete response to therapy. Enzyme replacement fails because of fast degradation of the enzyme from bloodstream. Due to these limitations, gene therapy represents a potential alternative. Currently, gene therapy is focused on using cargo proteins that deliver proteins to the lysosome. Since clathrin-dependent receptor-mediated endocytosis (RME) is the main transport mechanism for delivery to the lysosome, it is thought that all forms of LSDs can be treated with gene therapy (Bareford & Swaan 2007, and references therein).

3.4.2 Peroxisomes

Peroxisomes are multifunctional organelles which are involved in biochemical and metabolic processes such as oxidation of fatty acids, plasmalogen biosynthesis and glyoxylate detoxification. Malfunction of or defects in peroxisomes are associated with a variety of diseases which can be classified as Zellweger spectrum peroxisome biogenesis disorders or rhizomelic chondrodysplasia punctate. Defects in peroxisome biogenesis proteins (peroxins, encoded by PEX genes) can lead to eye anomalies, extreme hypotension, and hepatomegaly (to name a few), and usually are fatal by age 1-2. In general deficiencies in a single peroxisomal enzyme (PEX) are associated with a variety of diseases. The therapy approaches are focused on protein therapeutics, peroxisomal enzymes and gene therapy.

One possible gene therapy target is the antioxidant enzyme, catalase. A modified catalase molecule was transduced into hypocatalasemic fibroblasts and reduced hydrogen peroxide levels dramatically. This resulted in the restoration of oxidative balance, which may have cytoprotective effects (Terlecky & Koepke 2007). The cytoprotective role of catalase makes it an excellent gene therapy target, because many diseases such as cardiovascular diseases are linked to high hydrogen peroxide levels (Gong et al. 2010).

3.4.3 Proteasome

Targeting the proteasome, the cell's degradation machinery, represents another possible target for gene therapy. The general inhibition of the proteasome is already used for treatment of inflammatory disease and cancer (Nalepa et al. 2006) while the activation of the proteasome can be used for neurodegenerative diseases and cardiac diseases (Dahlmann 2007). Targeting disease-specific components of the ubiquitin-proteasome system provides the possibility for directed therapy approaches (Nalepa et al. 2006). The E3 ubiqitin ligases are important for specificity of proteasomal degradation because they recognize the proteins which should be destroyed (Nalepa et al. 2006). More classical drug targets are the ubiquitin-activation and the actual degradation step which occurs in the proteasome. A new approach suggested by our lab involves capturing oncogenic proteins such as survivin and sending them to the proteasome for degradation. This could be achieved by including a gene therapy construct that has a survivin dimerization domain and a proteasomal degradation domain, capable of capturing endogenous survivin and sending it to the proteasome (Mossalam et al. 2010).

3.4.4 Mitochondria

Mitochondria are essential for production of cellular ATP. The mitochondria consist of the outer membrane, the inner membrane, intermembrane space, cristae and mitochondrial DNA. Mutations in mitochondrial DNA are associated with muscle and central nervous system dysfunction, but only if most of the DNA is mutated. An interesting gene therapy approach is to tag mitochondria targeting signals to endonucleases which are able to degrade the mutated mitochondrial DNA. This mutant DNA contains the T8399G mutation which creates a unique restriction site and allows the restriction enzyme to distinguish between normal DNA and mutated DNA. It provides new therapy options for neuropathy, ataxia and retinitis pigmentosa (Srivastava & Moraes 2001). In addition, the mitochondrion is also essential in cellular apoptosis. Proteins such as p53 can be sent to the mitochondria, eventually resulting in cytochrome c release and apoptosis. Indeed, p53 targeted to the mitochondria has shown to cause apoptosis in different cancer cell lines (Palacios & Moll 2006).

3.4.5 Endoplasmic reticulum

The endoplasmic reticulum (ER) produces almost all cellular lipids, and the majority of proteins are synthesized on the cytosolic surface of the ER. A wide range of diseases occur due to mistakes in protein folding/assembly in the ER such as CF and neurodegenerative diseases. CF is a classic gene therapy target with one single mutation which can be targeted by replacing the defect gene. Unfortunately, all gene therapy approaches for CF have failed thus far. Certain neurodegenerative diseases are affected by mutations in proteins involved in ER assembly. Mutations in Parkin, which is an E3 ligase responsible for ubiquitinylation and regulation of proteasomal degradation, is associated with juvenile Parkinsonism. The Parkin proteasomal pathway normally degrades Pael-R in dopaminergic neurons. Pael-R accumulates in brain cells when Parkin is mutated (Aridor et al. 2004, and references therein). Adding back functional Parkin would then be a possible gene therapy approach for juvenile Parkinsonism.

3.4.6 Golgi apparatus

In addition to the synthesis of carbohydrates, the Golgi apparatus (GA) sorts as well as dispatch proteins to the ER. SPCA1 is a protein found in the trans-Golgi. When mutations occur in the gene (ATP2C1) encoding SPCA1, a genetic disorder results called Hailey-Hailey disease. These various mutations result in skin lesions which are usually benign and lead only in a few cases into squamous cell carcinoma (Pizzo et al. 2011). Replacing mutated SPCA1 would be a possible gene therapy approach to treat Hailey-Hailey disease.

3.4.7 Nucleus

Many diseases are associated with problems in nuclear import and export. For example, various types of cancers are associated with p53 and FOXO mislocalization in the cytoplasm, while their normal localization is the nucleus. There are several examples of proteins that when mislocalized to different compartments lose their function or may become oncogenic. The control of compartmentalization of key proteins can be used to overcome disease. Besides, tumor suppressors such as p53, cell cycle inhibitors, G-protein coupled receptors and transcription factors can also lose their function when mislocalized (Chinen et al. 2007). $p21^{WAF-1}$ is localized in the nucleus where it accomplishes its function as cell cycle inhibitor. When moved to the cytoplasm, it is associated with tumor progression (Davis et al. 2007; Keeshan et al. 2003). G-protein coupled receptors like rhodopsin, vasopressin V_2, LDL and CFTR all require proper localization for function. For example, rhodopsin is found in the membrane sacs within the rods, and when mislocalized it is confined in the plasma membrane of photoreceptor cell body and causes retinitis pigmentosa (Edwards et al. 2000). Additional transcription factors such as NF-κB and FOXO are both associated with various types of cancer when mislocalized to different compartments. NF-κB is located in the cytoplasm of normal cells whereas nuclear accumulation causes cancer. In contrast FOXO is found in the nucleus of normal cells and cytoplasmic localization results in cancer (Davis et al. 2007, and references therein).

There are several different gene therapy approaches for targeting mislocalized proteins. The standard method is to add back the protein which contains functional localization signals, such as the adenoviral p53 vectors Gendicine™ and Oncorine™. On the other hand, blocking general nuclear import or export machinery has been attempted, but due to the non-specific blockage of import/export, these methods suffer from toxicity. Instead of general inhibition of import/export, the protein itself can be modified. Adding nuclear localization signals (NLS) or nuclear export signals (NES) to the genes encoding mislocalized proteins allows targeting of proteins directly to the desired compartments.

The localization of proteins can be changed by using a protein switch developed in our laboratory (Kakar et al. 2007; Davis et al. 2007). The protein switch is a plasmid encoding a NES, a NLS and a ligand binding domain (LBD) from steroid hormone receptor. The LBD serves as a ligand-inducible nuclear localization switch. The protein switch is cytoplasm in the absence of ligand and translocates to the nucleus when ligand is added. The protein switch has also been designed to contain dimerization domain that allows capture of an endogenous protein of interest. Upon ligand addition, the protein switch-endogenous protein complex will then translocate to the nucleus. Removal of the endogenous protein from the cytoplasm can result in decrease cytoplasmic signaling or increased apoptotic signaling in the nucleus, with potential use in cancer therapy (Kakar et al. 2007).

4. Conclusions

Some of the major diseases currently targeted by gene therapy include cancer, cardiovascular disease, HIV, and monogenic diseases. Despite many decades of gene therapy research on these diseases, there currently are very few products that have made it to market. The search for new gene therapy targets and improved methods are therefore warranted. The integration of new and standard technologies (genome sequencing, microarrays, improved analysis, and linkage to molecular and biochemical assays) recently have yielded methods to uncover new drivers of cancer (Akavia et al. 2010). In 2008, the NIH started its Undiagnosed Diseases Program. These NIH investigators first try to diagnose an illness by first looking at known genetic markers, followed by standard molecular and biochemical assays. If no candidate genes are revealed, they then use state-of-the-art genetic analyses that can sequence the entire exome (all exons in the human genome) of a patient and their family; high resolution microarrays can genotype the rest of the genome to "bring genomics to the clinic." After comparison to family data and a reference sequence (from the Human Genome Project), the gene causing a particular rare disease may be discovered (Maxmen 2011). Currently patients enrolled in this program are not cured; the candidate gene and corresponding protein are only identified. Small molecule inhibitors of these proteins can take years or decades to screen, therefore making replacement of these defective or mutant genes prime candidates for gene therapy treatment in patients with a rare disease.

Further analysis of the protein can uncover the molecular basis of the disease. Is this protein a hub protein which interacts with many other proteins? What are the protein-protein interactions that govern its activity? Are there any cell compartmentalization abnormalities that promote disease? With this information in mind, more modern gene therapy approaches can be developed. In our laboratory, we have designed a protein switch designed to capture and change location of a harmful protein in a cell. This altered location could be exploited for disease therapy. For example, the Bcr-Abl protein is oncogenic in the cytoplasm, but causes apoptosis when moved to the nucleus (Dixon et al. 2009). A protein switch against Bcr-Abl is being developed in our laboratory that can dimerize to wild type (wt) Bcr-Abl by virtue of a coiled-coil dimerization domain (Mossalam et al. 2010). The protein switch also contains a ligand-inducible domain that can move the protein from the cytoplasm to the nucleus upon the addition of ligand (Kakar et al. 2007). Therefore, after capture, wt Bcr-Abl is dragged to the nucleus, where apoptosis ensues. Understanding the molecular mechanisms that govern protein activity can therefore be used as the next phase in gene therapy, where altered protein location can completely change the function of a protein. Other emerging modern gene therapy-based approaches including anti-gene therapies (antisense, siRNA, ribozymes) and immunotherapy are desired to have a significant impact on disease treatment.

5. References

Abo-Auda, W., and R. L. Benza. 2003. Therapeutic angiogenesis: review of current concepts and future directions. *J Heart Lung Transplant* 22 (4):370-82.

Akavia, U. D., O. Litvin, J. Kim, F. Sanchez-Garcia, D. Kotliar, H. C. Causton, P. Pochanard, E. Mozes, L. A. Garraway, and D. Pe'er. 2010. An integrated approach to uncover drivers of cancer. *Cell* 143 (6):1005-17.

Altieri, D. C. 2001. The molecular basis and potential role of survivin in cancer diagnosis and therapy. *Trends Mol Med* 7 (12):542-7.

Altieri, D. C. 2003. Validating survivin as a cancer therapeutic target. *Nat Rev Cancer* 3 (1):46-54.

Altieri, D. C. 2008. Survivin, cancer networks and pathway-directed drug discovery. *Nat Rev Cancer* 8 (1):61-70.

Antoine, C., S. Muller, A. Cant, M. Cavazzana-Calvo, P. Veys, J. Vossen, A. Fasth, C. Heilmann, N. Wulffraat, R. Seger, S. Blanche, W. Friedrich, M. Abinun, G. Davies, R. Bredius, A. Schulz, P. Landais, and A. Fischer. 2003. Long-term survival and transplantation of haemopoietic stem cells for immunodeficiencies: report of the European experience 1968-99. *Lancet* 361 (9357):553-60.

Aridor, M., A. K. Guzik, A. Bielli, and K. N. Fish. 2004. Endoplasmic reticulum export site formation and function in dendrites. *J Neurosci* 24 (15):3770-6.

Arnett, D. K., A. E. Baird, R. A. Barkley, C. T. Basson, E. Boerwinkle, S. K. Ganesh, D. M. Herrington, Y. Hong, C. Jaquish, D. A. McDermott, and C. J. O'Donnell. 2007. Relevance of genetics and genomics for prevention and treatment of cardiovascular disease: a scientific statement from the American Heart Association Council on Epidemiology and Prevention, the Stroke Council, and the Functional Genomics and Translational Biology Interdisciplinary Working Group. *Circulation* 115 (22):2878-901.

Bareford, L. M., and P. W. Swaan. 2007. Endocytic mechanisms for targeted drug delivery. *Adv Drug Deliv Rev* 59 (8):748-58.

Baumgartner, I., N. Chronos, A. Comerota, T. Henry, J. P. Pasquet, F. Finiels, A. Caron, J. F. Dedieu, R. Pilsudski, and P. Delaere. 2009. Local gene transfer and expression following intramuscular administration of FGF-1 plasmid DNA in patients with critical limb ischemia. *Mol Ther* 17 (5):914-21.

Beaupre, D. M., and R. Kurzrock. 1999. RAS and leukemia: from basic mechanisms to gene-directed therapy. *J Clin Oncol* 17 (3):1071-9.

Boucher, R. C., C. U. Cotton, J. T. Gatzy, M. R. Knowles, and J. R. Yankaskas. 1988. Evidence for reduced Cl- and increased Na+ permeability in cystic fibrosis human primary cell cultures. *J Physiol* 405:77-103.

Buckley, R. H., R. I. Schiff, S. E. Schiff, M. L. Markert, L. W. Williams, T. O. Harville, J. L. Roberts, and J. M. Puck. 1997. Human severe combined immunodeficiency: genetic, phenotypic, and functional diversity in one hundred eight infants. *J Pediatr* 130 (3):378-87.

Cao, A., and R. Galanello. 2010. Beta-thalassemia. *Genet Med* 12 (2):61-76.

CardioVascular BioTherapeutics, Inc. 2011. *Fibroblast Growth Factor-1 (FGF-1) for the Treatment of Coronary Heart Disease (ACORD)* [cited 03/2011 2011]. Available from http://www.clinicaltrials.gov/ct2/show/NCT00117936?term=henry+FGF&rank=1.

Castino, R., M. Demoz, and C. Isidoro. 2003. Destination 'lysosome': a target organelle for tumour cell killing? *J Mol Recognit* 16 (5):337-48.

Cavazzana-Calvo, M., S. Hacein-Bey, G. de Saint Basile, F. Gross, E. Yvon, P. Nusbaum, F. Selz, C. Hue, S. Certain, J. L. Casanova, P. Bousso, F. L. Deist, and A. Fischer. 2000. Gene therapy of human severe combined immunodeficiency (SCID)-X1 disease. *Science* 288 (5466):669-72.

Cavazzana-Calvo, M., E. Payen, O. Negre, G. Wang, K. Hehir, F. Fusil, J. Down, M. Denaro, T. Brady, K. Westerman, R. Cavallesco, B. Gillet-Legrand, L. Caccavelli, R. Sgarra, L. Maouche-Chretien, F. Bernaudin, R. Girot, R. Dorazio, G. J. Mulder, A. Polack, A. Bank, J. Soulier, J. Larghero, N. Kabbara, B. Dalle, B. Gourmel, G. Socie, S. Chretien, N. Cartier, P. Aubourg, A. Fischer, K. Cornetta, F. Galacteros, Y. Beuzard, E. Gluckman, F. Bushman, S. Hacein-Bey-Abina, and P. Leboulch. 2010. Transfusion independence and HMGA2 activation after gene therapy of human beta-thalassaemia. *Nature* 467 (7313):318-22.

Cerepro, EMEA recommendation on. 2009. European Medicines Agency recommendation on Cerepro.

Chene, P. 2001. The role of tetramerization in p53 function. *Oncogene* 20 (21):2611-7.

Chinen, J., J. Davis, S. S. De Ravin, B. N. Hay, A. P. Hsu, G. F. Linton, N. Naumann, E. Y. Nomicos, C. Silvin, J. Ulrick, N. L. Whiting-Theobald, H. L. Malech, and J. M. Puck. 2007. Gene therapy improves immune function in preadolescents with X-linked severe combined immunodeficiency. *Blood* 110 (1):67-73.

Chiuve, S. E., M. L. McCullough, F. M. Sacks, and E. B. Rimm. 2006. Healthy lifestyle factors in the primary prevention of coronary heart disease among men: benefits among users and nonusers of lipid-lowering and antihypertensive medications. *Circulation* 114 (2):160-7.

Cloutier, M. M., L. Guernsey, P. Mattes, and B. Koeppen. 1990. Duramycin enhances chloride secretion in airway epithelium. *Am J Physiol* 259 (3 Pt 1):C450-4.

Consortium, International HapMap. 2003. The International HapMap Project. *Nature* 426 (6968):789-96.

Crick, F. H. 1952. Is alpha-keratin a coiled coil? *Nature* 170 (4334):882-3.

Dahlmann, B. 2007. Role of proteasomes in disease. *BMC Biochem* 8 Suppl 1:S3.

Davis, J. R., M. Kakar, and C. S. Lim. 2007. Controlling protein compartmentalization to overcome disease. *Pharm Res* 24 (1):17-27.

De Ravin, S. S., and H. L. Malech. 2009. Partially corrected X-linked severe combined immunodeficiency: long-term problems and treatment options. *Immunol Res* 43 (1-3):223-42.

Dixon, A. S., M. Kakar, K. M. Schneider, J. E. Constance, B. C. Paullin, and C. S. Lim. 2009. Controlling subcellular localization to alter function: Sending oncogenic Bcr-Abl to the nucleus causes apoptosis. *J Control Release* 140 (3):245-9.

Duggan, D. J., M. Bittner, Y. Chen, P. Meltzer, and J. M. Trent. 1999. Expression profiling using cDNA microarrays. *Nat Genet* 21 (1 Suppl):10-4.

Edelstein, M. L., M. R. Abedi, and J. Wixon. 2007. Gene therapy clinical trials worldwide to 2007--an update. *J Gene Med* 9 (10):833-42.

Edelstein, M. L., M. R. Abedi, J. Wixon, and R. M. Edelstein. 2004. Gene therapy clinical trials worldwide 1989-2004-an overview. *J Gene Med* 6 (6):597-602.

Edwards, S. W., C. M. Tan, and L. E. Limbird. 2000. Localization of G-protein-coupled receptors in health and disease. *Trends Pharmacol Sci* 21 (8):304-8.

Erster, S., M. Mihara, R. H. Kim, O. Petrenko, and U. M. Moll. 2004. In vivo mitochondrial p53 translocation triggers a rapid first wave of cell death in response to DNA damage that can precede p53 target gene activation. *Mol Cell Biol* 24 (15):6728-41.

Flume, P. A., P. J. Mogayzel Jr, K. A. Robinson, R. L. Rosenblatt, L. Quittell, B. C. Marshall, and Committee Clinical Practice Guidelines For Pulmonary Therapies. 2010. Cystic Fibrosis Pulmonary Guidelines: Pulmonary Complications: Hemoptysis and Pneumothorax. *Am J Respir Crit Care Med.*

Flynn, A., and T. O'Brien. 2008. Alferminogene tadenovec, an angiogenic FGF4 gene therapy for coronary artery disease. *IDrugs* 11 (4):283-93.

Foundation, Cystic Fibrosis. 2011. *Cystic Fibrosis Foundation* 2011 [cited 01/18/2011 2011]. Available from http://www.cff.org/.

Garber, K. 2006. China approves world's first oncolytic virus therapy for cancer treatment. *J Natl Cancer Inst* 98 (5):298-300.

Glover, J. N., and S. C. Harrison. 1995. Crystal structure of the heterodimeric bZIP transcription factor c-Fos-c-Jun bound to DNA. *Nature* 373 (6511):257-61.

Goh, A. M., C. R. Coffill, and D. P. Lane. 2010. The role of mutant p53 in human cancer. *J Pathol.*

Goh, A. M., C. R. Coffill, and D. P. Lane. 2011. The role of mutant p53 in human cancer. *J Pathol* 223 (2):116-26.

Gong, G., Y. Qin, W. Huang, S. Zhou, X. Wu, X. Yang, Y. Zhao, and D. Li. 2010. Protective effects of diosgenin in the hyperlipidemic rat model and in human vascular endothelial cells against hydrogen peroxide-induced apoptosis. *Chem Biol Interact* 184 (3):366-75.

Gorner, K., E. Holtorf, J. Waak, T. T. Pham, D. M. Vogt-Weisenhorn, W. Wurst, C. Haass, and P. J. Kahle. 2007. Structural determinants of the C-terminal helix-kink-helix motif essential for protein stability and survival promoting activity of DJ-1. *J Biol Chem* 282 (18):13680-91.

Grossman, D., and D. C. Altieri. 2001. Drug resistance in melanoma: mechanisms, apoptosis, and new potential therapeutic targets. *Cancer Metastasis Rev* 20 (1-2):3-11.

Guo, J., and H. Xin. 2006. Chinese gene therapy. Splicing out the West? *Science* 314 (5803):1232-5.

Guo, Z. S., S. H. Thorne, and D. L. Bartlett. 2008. Oncolytic virotherapy: molecular targets in tumor-selective replication and carrier cell-mediated delivery of oncolytic viruses. *Biochim Biophys Acta* 1785 (2):217-31.

Hacein-Bey-Abina, S., F. Le Deist, F. Carlier, C. Bouneaud, C. Hue, J. P. De Villartay, A. J. Thrasher, N. Wulffraat, R. Sorensen, S. Dupuis-Girod, A. Fischer, E. G. Davies, W. Kuis, L. Leiva, and M. Cavazzana-Calvo. 2002. Sustained correction of X-linked severe combined immunodeficiency by ex vivo gene therapy. *N Engl J Med* 346 (16):1185-93.

Harvey, B. G., P. L. Leopold, N. R. Hackett, T. M. Grasso, P. M. Williams, A. L. Tucker, R. J. Kaner, B. Ferris, I. Gonda, T. D. Sweeney, R. Ramalingam, I. Kovesdi, S. Shak, and R. G. Crystal. 1999. Airway epithelial CFTR mRNA expression in cystic fibrosis patients after repetitive administration of a recombinant adenovirus. *J Clin Invest* 104 (9):1245-55.

Haupt, S., M. Berger, Z. Goldberg, and Y. Haupt. 2003. Apoptosis - the p53 network. *J Cell Sci* 116 (Pt 20):4077-85.

Henderson, B. R. 2005. Regulation of BRCA1, BRCA2 and BARD1 intracellular trafficking. *Bioessays* 27 (9):884-93.

Hirschhorn, J. N., and M. J. Daly. 2005. Genome-wide association studies for common diseases and complex traits. *Nat Rev Genet* 6 (2):95-108.

Jeffrey, P. D., S. Gorina, and N. P. Pavletich. 1995. Crystal structure of the tetramerization domain of the p53 tumor suppressor at 1.7 angstroms. *Science* 267 (5203):1498-502.

Kakar, M., J. R. Davis, S. E. Kern, and C. S. Lim. 2007. Optimizing the protein switch: altering nuclear import and export signals, and ligand binding domain. *J Control Release* 120 (3):220-32.

Kamada, R., T. Nomura, C. W. Anderson, and K. Sakaguchi. 2011. Cancer-associated p53 tetramerization domain mutants: quantitative analysis reveals a low threshold for tumor suppressor inactivation. *J Biol Chem* 286 (1):252-8.

Kass, R. W., M. N. Kotler, and S. Yazdanfar. 1992. Stimulation of coronary collateral growth: current developments in angiogenesis and future clinical applications. *Am Heart J* 123 (2):486-96.

Kato, J., Y. Kuwabara, M. Mitani, N. Shinoda, A. Sato, T. Toyama, A. Mitsui, T. Nishiwaki, S. Moriyama, J. Kudo, and Y. Fujii. 2001. Expression of survivin in esophageal cancer: correlation with the prognosis and response to chemotherapy. *Int J Cancer* 95 (2): 92-5.

Kau, T. R., J. C. Way, and P. A. Silver. 2004. Nuclear transport and cancer: from mechanism to intervention. *Nat Rev Cancer* 4 (2):106-17.

Keeshan, K., T. G. Cotter, and S. L. McKenna. 2003. Bcr-Abl upregulates cytosolic p21WAF-1/CIP-1 by a phosphoinositide-3-kinase (PI3K)-independent pathway. *Br J Haematol* 123 (1):34-44.

Kerem, B., J. M. Rommens, J. A. Buchanan, D. Markiewicz, T. K. Cox, A. Chakravarti, M. Buchwald, and L. C. Tsui. 1989. Identification of the cystic fibrosis gene: genetic analysis. *Science* 245 (4922):1073-80.

Keskin, O., and R. Nussinov. 2007. Similar binding sites and different partners: implications to shared proteins in cellular pathways. *Structure* 15 (3):341-54.

Kim, P. M., L. J. Lu, Y. Xia, and M. B. Gerstein. 2006. Relating three-dimensional structures to protein networks provides evolutionary insights. *Science* 314 (5807):1938-41.

Kitchen, S. G., S. Shimizu, and D. S. An. 2011. Stem cell-based anti-HIV gene therapy. *Virology* 411 (2):260-72.

Knowlton, R. G., O. Cohen-Haguenauer, N. Van Cong, J. Frezal, V. A. Brown, D. Barker, J. C. Braman, J. W. Schumm, L. C. Tsui, M. Buchwald, and et al. 1985. A polymorphic DNA marker linked to cystic fibrosis is located on chromosome 7. *Nature* 318 (6044):380-2.

Kobayashi, N., K. Agematsu, K. Sugita, M. Sako, S. Nonoyama, A. Yachie, S. Kumaki, S. Tsuchiya, H. D. Ochs, Y. Fukushima, and A. Komiyama. 2003. Novel Artemis gene mutations of radiosensitive severe combined immunodeficiency in Japanese families. *Hum Genet* 112 (4):348-52.

Krishna, S. S., I. Majumdar, and N. V. Grishin. 2003. Structural classification of zinc fingers: survey and summary. *Nucleic Acids Res* 31 (2):532-50.

Kung, C., J. T. Pingel, M. Heikinheimo, T. Klemola, K. Varkila, L. I. Yoo, K. Vuopala, M. Poyhonen, M. Uhari, M. Rogers, S. H. Speck, T. Chatila, and M. L. Thomas. 2000. Mutations in the tyrosine phosphatase CD45 gene in a child with severe combined immunodeficiency disease. *Nat Med* 6 (3):343-5.

Landschulz, W. H., P. F. Johnson, and S. L. McKnight. 1988. The leucine zipper: a hypothetical structure common to a new class of DNA binding proteins. *Science* 240 (4860):1759-64.

Li, F., G. Ambrosini, E. Y. Chu, J. Plescia, S. Tognin, P. C. Marchisio, and D. C. Altieri. 1998. Control of apoptosis and mitotic spindle checkpoint by survivin. *Nature* 396 (6711):580-4.

Li, J., L. Simpson, M. Takahashi, C. Miliaresis, M. P. Myers, N. Tonks, and R. Parsons. 1998. The PTEN/MMAC1 tumor suppressor induces cell death that is rescued by the AKT/protein kinase B oncogene. *Cancer Res* 58 (24):5667-72.

Li, J., and J. Yuan. 2008. Caspases in apoptosis and beyond. *Oncogene* 27 (48):6194-206.

Liu, R., W. A. Paxton, S. Choe, D. Ceradini, S. R. Martin, R. Horuk, M. E. MacDonald, H. Stuhlmann, R. A. Koup, and N. R. Landau. 1996. Homozygous defect in HIV-1 coreceptor accounts for resistance of some multiply-exposed individuals to HIV-1 infection. *Cell* 86 (3):367-77.

Lockley, M., M. Fernandez, Y. Wang, N. F. Li, S. Conroy, N. Lemoine, and I. McNeish. 2006. Activity of the adenoviral E1A deletion mutant dl922-947 in ovarian cancer: comparison with E1A wild-type viruses, bioluminescence monitoring, and intraperitoneal delivery in icodextrin. *Cancer Res* 66 (2):989-98.

Lomas, D. A., and R. Mahadeva. 2002. Alpha1-antitrypsin polymerization and the serpinopathies: pathobiology and prospects for therapy. *J Clin Invest* 110 (11):1585-90.

Lomas, David A., and Ravi Mahadeva. 2002. α1-Antitrypsin polymerization and the serpinopathies: pathobiology and prospects for therapy. *The Journal of Clinical Investigation* 110 (11):1585-1590.

Lucarelli, G., and J. Gaziev. 2008. Advances in the allogeneic transplantation for thalassemia. *Blood Rev* 22 (2):53-63.

Malik, P., and P. I. Arumugam. 2005. Gene Therapy for beta-thalassemia. *Hematology Am Soc Hematol Educ Program*:45-50.

Mason, J. M., and K. M. Arndt. 2004. Coiled coil domains: stability, specificity, and biological implications. *Chembiochem* 5 (2):170-6.

Maulik, N. 2009. NV1FGF, a pCOR plasmid-based angiogenic gene therapy for the treatment of intermittent claudication and critical limb ischemia. *Curr Opin Investig Drugs* 10 (3):259-68.

Maxmen, A. 2011. Exome sequencing deciphers rare diseases. *Cell* 144 (5):635-7.

McCarty, A. S., G. Kleiger, D. Eisenberg, and S. T. Smale. 2003. Selective dimerization of a C2H2 zinc finger subfamily. *Mol Cell* 11 (2):459-70.

McPhail, G. L., J. D. Acton, M. C. Fenchel, R. S. Amin, and M. Seid. 2008. Improvements in lung function outcomes in children with cystic fibrosis are associated with better nutrition, fewer chronic pseudomonas aeruginosa infections, and dornase alfa use. *J Pediatr* 153 (6):752-7.

McWhirter, J. R., D. L. Galasso, and J. Y. Wang. 1993. A coiled-coil oligomerization domain of Bcr is essential for the transforming function of Bcr-Abl oncoproteins. *Mol Cell Biol* 13 (12):7587-95.

Mesri, M., N. R. Wall, J. Li, R. W. Kim, and D. C. Altieri. 2001. Cancer gene therapy using a survivin mutant adenovirus. *J Clin Invest* 108 (7):981-90.

Metcalfe, K. A., H. T. Lynch, P. Ghadirian, N. Tung, I. A. Olivotto, W. D. Foulkes, E. Warner, O. Olopade, A. Eisen, B. Weber, J. McLennan, P. Sun, and S. A. Narod. 2005. The risk of ovarian cancer after breast cancer in BRCA1 and BRCA2 carriers. *Gynecol Oncol* 96 (1):222-6.

Mitchell, P. 2010. Ark's gene therapy stumbles at the finish line. *Nat Biotechnol* 28 (3):183-4.

Morishita, R., M. Aoki, N. Hashiya, H. Makino, K. Yamasaki, J. Azuma, Y. Sawa, H. Matsuda, Y. Kaneda, and T. Ogihara. 2004. Safety evaluation of clinical gene therapy using hepatocyte growth factor to treat peripheral arterial disease. *Hypertension* 44 (2):203-9.

Moss, R. B., C. Milla, J. Colombo, F. Accurso, P. L. Zeitlin, J. P. Clancy, L. T. Spencer, J. Pilewski, D. A. Waltz, H. L. Dorkin, T. Ferkol, M. Pian, B. Ramsey, B. J. Carter, D. B. Martin, and A. E. Heald. 2007. Repeated aerosolized AAV-CFTR for treatment of cystic fibrosis: a randomized placebo-controlled phase 2B trial. *Hum Gene Ther* 18 (8):726-32.

Moss, R. B., D. Rodman, L. T. Spencer, M. L. Aitken, P. L. Zeitlin, D. Waltz, C. Milla, A. S. Brody, J. P. Clancy, B. Ramsey, N. Hamblett, and A. E. Heald. 2004. Repeated adeno-associated virus serotype 2 aerosol-mediated cystic fibrosis transmembrane regulator gene transfer to the lungs of patients with cystic fibrosis: a multicenter, double-blind, placebo-controlled trial. *Chest* 125 (2):509-21.

Mossalam, M., A. S. Dixon, and C. S. Lim. 2010. Controlling subcellular delivery to optimize therapeutic effect. *Ther Deliv* 1 (1):169-193.

Murre, C., G. Bain, M. A. van Dijk, I. Engel, B. A. Furnari, M. E. Massari, J. R. Matthews, M. W. Quong, R. R. Rivera, and M. H. Stuiver. 1994. Structure and function of helix-loop-helix proteins. *Biochim Biophys Acta* 1218 (2):129-35.

Nakamura, Y. 2009. DNA variations in human and medical genetics: 25 years of my experience. *J Hum Genet* 54 (1):1-8.

Nalepa, G., M. Rolfe, and J. W. Harper. 2006. Drug discovery in the ubiquitin-proteasome system. *Nat Rev Drug Discov* 5 (7):596-613.

NCBI. 2011. *Microarrays: Chipping away at the Mysteries of science and medicine* 2007 [cited 03/2011 2011]. Available from http://www.ncbi.nlm.nih.gov/About/primer/microarrays.html.

O'Connor, D. S., D. Grossman, J. Plescia, F. Li, H. Zhang, A. Villa, S. Tognin, P. C. Marchisio, and D. C. Altieri. 2000. Regulation of apoptosis at cell division by p34cdc2 phosphorylation of survivin. *Proc Natl Acad Sci U S A* 97 (24):13103-7.

Palacios, G., and U. M. Moll. 2006. Mitochondrially targeted wild-type p53 suppresses growth of mutant p53 lymphomas in vivo. *Oncogene* 25 (45):6133-9.

Peng, Z. 2005. Current status of gendicine in China: recombinant human Ad-p53 agent for treatment of cancers. *Hum Gene Ther* 16 (9):1016-27.

Pizzo, P., V. Lissandron, P. Capitanio, and T. Pozzan. 2011. Ca(2+) signalling in the Golgi apparatus. *Cell Calcium*.

Powell, R. J., M. Simons, F. O. Mendelsohn, G. Daniel, T. D. Henry, M. Koga, R. Morishita, and B. H. Annex. 2008. Results of a double-blind, placebo-controlled study to assess the safety of intramuscular injection of hepatocyte growth factor plasmid to improve limb perfusion in patients with critical limb ischemia. *Circulation* 118 (1):58-65.

Project, Human Genome. 2011. *Human Genome Project* 2011]. Available from http://www.ornl.gov/sci/techresources/Human_Genome/home.shtml.

Project, The International HapMap. 426. *The International HapMap Project* (2003/12/20), Dec 18 2003 [cited 6968 426]. Available from http://www.ncbi.nlm.nih.gov/pubmed/14685227.

Puel, A., S. F. Ziegler, R. H. Buckley, and W. J. Leonard. 1998. Defective IL7R expression in T(-)B(+)NK(+) severe combined immunodeficiency. *Nat Genet* 20 (4):394-7.

Raty, J. K., J. T. Pikkarainen, T. Wirth, and S. Yla-Herttuala. 2008. Gene therapy: the first approved gene-based medicines, molecular mechanisms and clinical indications. *Curr Mol Pharmacol* 1 (1):13-23.

Riferminogene pecaplasmide. 2010. *Am J Cardiovasc Drugs* 10 (5):343-6.

Rodriguez, J. A., S. Schuchner, W. W. Au, M. Fabbro, and B. R. Henderson. 2004. Nuclear-cytoplasmic shuttling of BARD1 contributes to its proapoptotic activity and is regulated by dimerization with BRCA1. *Oncogene* 23 (10):1809-20.

Roth, J. A., D. Nguyen, D. D. Lawrence, B. L. Kemp, C. H. Carrasco, D. Z. Ferson, W. K. Hong, R. Komaki, J. J. Lee, J. C. Nesbitt, K. M. Pisters, J. B. Putnam, R. Schea, D. M. Shin, G. L. Walsh, M. M. Dolormente, C. I. Han, F. D. Martin, N. Yen, K. Xu, L. C. Stephens, T. J. McDonnell, T. Mukhopadhyay, and D. Cai. 1996. Retrovirus-mediated wild-type p53 gene transfer to tumors of patients with lung cancer. *Nat Med* 2 (9):985-91.

Ryan, B. M., N. O'Donovan, and M. J. Duffy. 2009. Survivin: a new target for anti-cancer therapy. *Cancer Treat Rev* 35 (7):553-62.

Ryser, O., A. Morell, and W. H. Hitzig. 1988. Primary immunodeficiencies in Switzerland: first report of the national registry in adults and children. *J Clin Immunol* 8 (6):479-85.

Sawyers, C. L. 1999. Chronic myeloid leukemia. *N Engl J Med* 340 (17):1330-40.

Schwarz, K., G. H. Gauss, L. Ludwig, U. Pannicke, Z. Li, D. Lindner, W. Friedrich, R. A. Seger, T. E. Hansen-Hagge, S. Desiderio, M. R. Lieber, and C. R. Bartram. 1996. RAG mutations in human B cell-negative SCID. *Science* 274 (5284):97-9.

Shi, J., and D. Zheng. 2009. An update on gene therapy in China. *Curr Opin Mol Ther* 11 (5):547-53.

Shigematsu, H., K. Yasuda, T. Iwai, T. Sasajima, S. Ishimaru, Y. Ohashi, T. Yamaguchi, T. Ogihara, and R. Morishita. 2010. Randomized, double-blind, placebo-controlled clinical trial of hepatocyte growth factor plasmid for critical limb ischemia. *Gene Ther* 17 (9):1152-61.

Shiraishi, K., S. Kato, S. Y. Han, W. Liu, K. Otsuka, M. Sakayori, T. Ishida, M. Takeda, R. Kanamaru, N. Ohuchi, and C. Ishioka. 2004. Isolation of temperature-sensitive p53 mutations from a comprehensive missense mutation library. *J Biol Chem* 279 (1):348-55.

Siegmund, K. H., U. E. Steiner, and C. Richert. 2003. ChipCheck--a program predicting total hybridization equilibria for DNA binding to small oligonucleotide microarrays. *J Chem Inf Comput Sci* 43 (6):2153-62.

Silverman, G. A., P. I. Bird, R. W. Carrell, F. C. Church, P. B. Coughlin, P. G. Gettins, J. A. Irving, D. A. Lomas, C. J. Luke, R. W. Moyer, P. A. Pemberton, E. Remold-O'Donnell, G. S. Salvesen, J. Travis, and J. C. Whisstock. 2001. The serpins are an expanding superfamily of structurally similar but functionally diverse proteins. Evolution, mechanism of inhibition, novel functions, and a revised nomenclature. *J Biol Chem* 276 (36):33293-6.

Srivastava, S., and C. T. Moraes. 2001. Manipulating mitochondrial DNA heteroplasmy by a mitochondrially targeted restriction endonuclease. *Hum Mol Genet* 10 (26):3093-9.

Sun, H. X., H. W. He, S. H. Zhang, T. G. Liu, K. H. Ren, Q. Y. He, and R. G. Shao. 2009. Suppression of N-Ras by shRNA-expressing plasmid increases sensitivity of HepG2 cells to vincristine-induced growth inhibition. *Cancer Gene Ther* 16 (9):693-702.

Symonds, G. P., H. A. Johnstone, M. L. Millington, M. P. Boyd, B. P. Burke, and L. R. Breton. 2010. The use of cell-delivered gene therapy for the treatment of HIV/AIDS. *Immunol Res* 48 (1-3):84-98.

Taha, T. A., W. Osta, L. Kozhaya, J. Bielawski, K. R. Johnson, W. E. Gillanders, G. S. Dbaibo, Y. A. Hannun, and L. M. Obeid. 2004. Down-regulation of sphingosine kinase-1 by DNA damage: dependence on proteases and p53. *J Biol Chem* 279 (19):20546-54.

Tehrani, A. M., S. K. Hwang, T. H. Kim, C. S. Cho, J. Hua, W. S. Nah, J. T. Kwon, J. S. Kim, S. H. Chang, K. N. Yu, S. J. Park, D. R. Bhandari, K. H. Lee, G. H. An, G. R. Beck, Jr., and M. H. Cho. 2007. Aerosol delivery of Akt controls protein translation in the lungs of dual luciferase reporter mice. *Gene Ther* 14 (5):451-8.

Tembe, V., and B. R. Henderson. 2007. BARD1 translocation to mitochondria correlates with Bax oligomerization, loss of mitochondrial membrane potential, and apoptosis. *J Biol Chem* 282 (28):20513-22.

Terlecky, S. R., and J. I. Koepke. 2007. Drug delivery to peroxisomes: employing unique trafficking mechanisms to target protein therapeutics. *Adv Drug Deliv Rev* 59 (8):739-47.

Testa, J. R., and A. Bellacosa. 2001. AKT plays a central role in tumorigenesis. *Proc Natl Acad Sci U S A* 98 (20):10983-5.

Thrasher, A. J., S. Hacein-Bey-Abina, H. B. Gaspar, S. Blanche, E. G. Davies, K. Parsley, K. Gilmour, D. King, S. Howe, J. Sinclair, C. Hue, F. Carlier, C. von Kalle, G. de Saint Basile, F. le Deist, A. Fischer, and M. Cavazzana-Calvo. 2005. Failure of SCID-X1 gene therapy in older patients. *Blood* 105 (11):4255-7.

van Putten, E. H., C. M. Dirven, M. J. van den Bent, and M. L. Lamfers. 2010. Sitimagene ceradenovec: a gene-based drug for the treatment of operable high-grade glioma. *Future Oncol* 6 (11):1691-710.

Vaseva, A. V., N. D. Marchenko, and U. M. Moll. 2009. The transcription-independent mitochondrial p53 program is a major contributor to nutlin-induced apoptosis in tumor cells. *Cell Cycle* 8 (11):1711-9.

Ventura, A., D. G. Kirsch, M. E. McLaughlin, D. A. Tuveson, J. Grimm, L. Lintault, J. Newman, E. E. Reczek, R. Weissleder, and T. Jacks. 2007. Restoration of p53 function leads to tumour regression in vivo. *Nature* 445 (7128):661-5.

Vita, M., and M. Henriksson. 2006. The Myc oncoprotein as a therapeutic target for human cancer. *Semin Cancer Biol* 16 (4):318-30.

Vogelstein, B., D. Lane, and A. J. Levine. 2000. Surfing the p53 network. *Nature* 408 (6810):307-10.

Weatherall, D. J. 1976. Molecular pathology of the thalassemia disorders. *West J Med* 124 (5):388-402.

WHO. 2011. *Cancer* 20112011]. Available from http://www.who.int/mediacentre/factsheets/fs297/en/.

Wolfe, S. A., L. Nekludova, and C. O. Pabo. 2000. DNA recognition by Cys2His2 zinc finger proteins. *Annu Rev Biophys Biomol Struct* 29:183-212.

Wood, B. P. 1997. Cystic fibrosis: 1997. *Radiology* 204 (1):1-10.

Wurzer, G., W. Mosgoeller, M. Chabicovsky, C. Cerni, and J. Wesierska-Gadek. 2001. Nuclear Ras: unexpected subcellular distribution of oncogenic forms. *J Cell Biochem Suppl* Suppl 36:1-11.

Xin, H. 2006. Chinese gene therapy. Gendicine's efficacy: hard to translate. *Science* 314 (5803):1233.

Xue, W., L. Zender, C. Miething, R. A. Dickins, E. Hernando, V. Krizhanovsky, C. Cordon-Cardo, and S. W. Lowe. 2007. Senescence and tumour clearance is triggered by p53 restoration in murine liver carcinomas. *Nature* 445 (7128):656-60.

Yu, W., and H. Fang. 2007. Clinical trials with oncolytic adenovirus in China. *Curr Cancer Drug Targets* 7 (2):141-8.

Zhao, J., T. Tenev, L. M. Martins, J. Downward, and N. R. Lemoine. 2000. The ubiquitin-proteasome pathway regulates survivin degradation in a cell cycle-dependent manner. *J Cell Sci* 113 Pt 23:4363-71

2

Gene Modulation by Peptide Nucleic Acids (PNAs) Targeting microRNAs (miRs)

Rosangela Marchelli et al.*
Department of Organic and Industrial Chemistry, University of Parma
Italy

1. Introduction

Since non-viral gene therapy was developed and employed in different *in vitro* and *in vivo* experimental systems as an effective way to control and modify gene expression, RNA has been considered as a molecular target of great relevance (Li &Huang, 2008, López-Fraga et al., 2008). In combination with standard chemotherapy, the siRNA therapy can reduce the chemoresistance of certain cancers, demonstrating its potential for treating many malignant diseases. Examples of RNA sequences to be targeted for therapeutic applications are mRNAs coding oncoproteins or RNA coding anti-apoptotic proteins for the development of anti-cancer therapy.

In the last years, progresses in molecular biology have allowed to identify many genes Coding for small non coding RNA molecules, microRNA (miRNAs or miRs), able to regulate gene expression at the translation level (Huang et al., 2008, Shrivastava & Shrivastava, 2008, Sahu et al. 2007, Orlacchio et al., 2007, Williams et al., 2008, Papagiannakopoulos & Kosik, 2008). Accordingly, an increasing number of reports associate the changed expression with specific phenotypes and even with pathological conditions (Garzon & Croce, 2008, Mascellani et al., 2008, Sontheimer & Carthew, 2005, Filipowicz et al., 2005, Alvarez-Garcia & Miska, 2005). Interestingly, microRNAs play a double role in cancer, behaving both as oncogenes or tumor suppressor genes. In general, miRs promoting cancer targets mRNA coding for tumor-suppression proteins, while microRNAs exhibiting tumor-suppression properties usually target mRNAs coding oncoproteins. MicroRNAs which have been demonstrated to play a crucial role in the initiation and progression of human cancer are defined as oncogenic miRNAs (oncomiRs) (Cho, 2007). The oncomiR expression profiling of human malignancies has also identified a number of diagnostic and prognostic cancer signals (Cho, 2007, Lowery et al., 2008). Moreover, microRNAs have been firmly demonstrated to be involved in cancer metastasis (metastamiRs).

Examples of metastasis-promoting microRNAs are, miR-10b (Calin et al., 2006), miR-373 and -520c (Woods et al., 2007), miR-21, -143 and -182 (Hayashita et al., 2005; Si et al., 2007; Zhu et al.,

---

* Roberto Corradini[1], Alex Manicardi[1], Stefano Sforza[1], Tullia Tedeschi[1], Enrica Fabbri[3], Monica Borgatti[3], Nicoletta Bianchi[3] and Roberto Gambari[2,3].
1 Department of Organic and Industrial Chemistry, University of Parma,Italy.
2 Laboratory for the Development of Pharmacological and Pharmacogenomic Therapy of Thalassaemia, Biotechnology Center, University of Ferrara,Italy
3 BioPharmaNet, Department of Biochemistry and Molecular Biology, University of Ferrara,Italy

2007). Reviews on metastamiR has been recently published Hurst et al. (Hurst et al. 2009, Edmonds et al. 2009). Reviews on metastamiRs has been recently published by Hurst et al. Table 1 shows examples of microRNAs involved in cancer onset and progression.

MicroRNAs	Tumor	Target mRNA	Reference(s)
miR-17-92	Lung cancer, lymphoma	E2F1	Woods et al., 2007
miR-21	Breast cancer, cholangiocarcinoma, head & neck cancer, leukemia, cervical cancer	tropomyosin 1	Iorio et al., 2005; Zhu et al., 2007
miR-155	Breast cancer, leukemia, pancreatic cancer, B-cell lymphoma	FOXO3a; SHIP1	Costinean et al., 2006; Kong et al., 2010; Pedersen et al., 2009
miR-221	Glioblastoma	PUMA	Ciafre et al., 2005; Zhang et al., 2010
miR-222	Thyroid carcinoma	$P27^{Kip1}$	Visone et al., 2007
miR-31	Lung cancer	LATS2	Liu et al., 2010

Table 1. Examples of microRNAs involved in cancer onset and their putative targets.

Thus, therapeutic strategies involving miRNA silencing could be proposed based on the roles of these small non-coding RNAs as oncogenes. For these reasons, the development of molecules able to specifically recognize microRNA target sequences is of particular interest, from both a diagnostic and a therapeutic point of view.

Indeed, miRNAs can be antagonized *in vivo* by highly-affine oligonucleotides (Lowery et al., 2008, Stenvang & Kauppinen, 2008). Up to now synthetic oligonucleotides have been used for targeting microRNAs, although with several problems, including delivery and stability. However, the use of oligonucleotide analogues has recently been proposed to be effective for the inhibition of miR expression and, accordingly, as a potent tool for the regulation of gene expression (Kota & Balasubramanian, 2010).

Peptide nucleic acids (PNAs) (figure 1) are DNA analogues in which the sugar-phosphate backbone is replaced by *N*-(2-aminoethyl)glycine units (Nielsen et al., 1991, Nielsen and Egholm, 1999, Lundin et al., 2006).

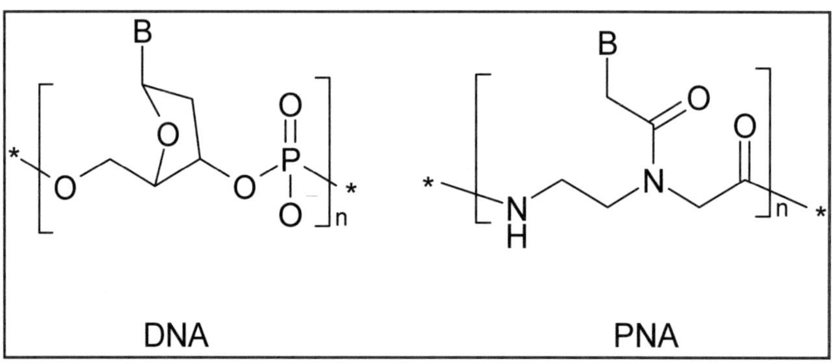

Fig. 1. Structure of DNA and PNA

These molecules efficiently hybridize with complementary DNA and RNA, forming Watson-Crick double helices. In addition, they can generate triple helix structures with double stranded DNA and perform strand invasion. Accordingly, they have been proposed for antisense and anti-gene therapy in a great number of studies (Larsen and Nielsen, 1996, Gambari, 2004, Nielsen 2005, 2006, Yin et al. 2008). PNAs are very promising for RNA recognition, since they have a higher affinity for RNA than for DNA, are more specific and are resistant to DNAses and proteases (Demidov et al 1994).

PNAs can be modified in order to achieve better performances in terms of cellular permeation, higher affinity, and specificity for the target DNA and RNA sequences (Corradini et al., 2004, 2007, Sforza et al., 2000, 2007, 2010, Tedeschi et al., 2005 a,b,c, Wojciechowski and Hudson, 2007, Dragulescu-Andrasi 2005, Rapireddy 2007).

In this chapter we will describe the recent results reported in the literature by using PNAs as anti-miR agents and the perspectives of this technology for future development.

2. MiR targeting: therapeutic significance

MicroRNAs are a family of small (19 to 25 nucleotide in length) noncoding RNAs that regulate gene expression by sequence-selective targeting of mRNAs, leading to a translational repression or mRNA degradation, depending on the degree of complementarity between miRNAs and the target sequences (Krol et al., 2010).

The expression pathway of these molecules consists in several steps as depicted in figure 2.

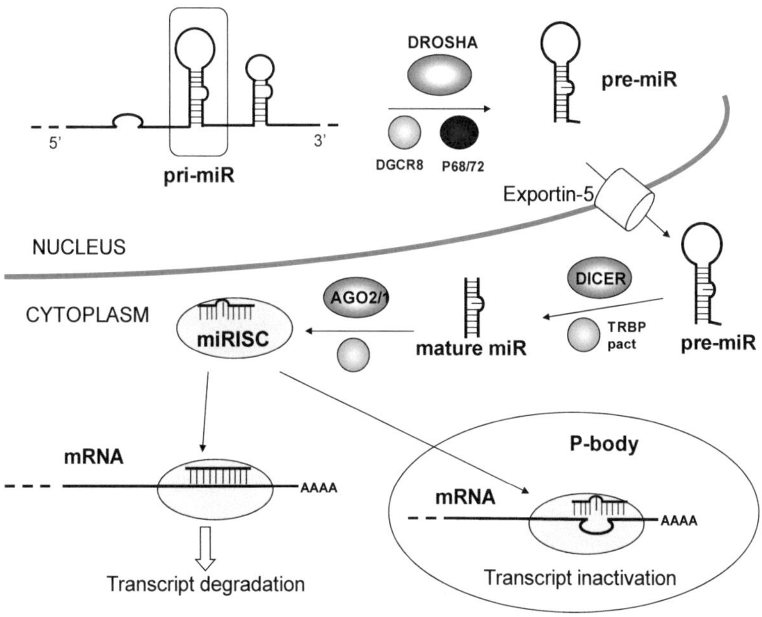

Fig. 2. Pathways of miR production and action. The primary transcript microRNA (pri-miR) is processed by DROSHA in combination with other factors such as DGCR8 to yield an hairpin structure called pre-miR, which is then exported by exportin 5 to the cytoplasm where it is cleaved by DICER in combination with other factors. The mature 21-23nt long dsRNA is processed by incorporation of the guiding strand into the miRISC complex, which act as inhibitor of translation, by either degradation of the mRNA bearing the target sequence or by incorporation of the miRISC-mRNA complex into the P-body, leading to inactivation.

Since their discovery and first characterization, the number of microRNA sequences deposited in the miRBase databases is significantly growing (Kozomara & Griffiths-Jones, 2010). On the other hand, considering that a single miRNA can target several mRNAs and a single mRNA might contain in the 3'UTR sequence several signals for miRNA recognition, it can be calculated that at least 10-40% of human mRNAs are targets for microRNAs (He & Hannon, 2004). Therefore, a great interest is concentrated on the identification of validated targets of microRNAs. This specific field of research has confirmed that the complex networks constituted by miRNAs and RNA targets coding for structural and regulatory proteins leads to the control of highly regulated biological functions, such as differentiation (Masaki et al., 2007), cell cycle (Wang & Blelloch, 2009) and apoptosis (Subramanian & Steer, 2010).

More in detail, and considering the role of microRNAs, a low expression of a given miR is expected to be linked with a potential accumulation of targets mRNAs; conversely, a high expression of miRNAs is expected to be responsible for a low expression of the target mRNAs.

However, since a single 3'UTR of a given mRNA contains signal sequences for several microRNAs, which microRNA should be targeted in order to achieve alteration of the expression of the gene should be experimentally evaluated. With respect to the possible effects of the expression of other mRNA targets, it should be clearly stated that alteration of a single microRNA might retain multiple effects. Finally, multiple targeting of several microRNAs might be considered for achieving strong biological effects. Whatever strategy is considered, several examples of biological effects of targeting microRNA involved in human pathologies are already available in the literature.

3. MiR targets relevant in gene therapy

The number of known microRNAs which regulate gene expression is continuously growing, with 1048 sequences present to date in the miRbase for humans (as available on march 30th, 2011 at http://www.mirbase.org/cgi-bin/mirna_summary.pl?org=hsa).

Although the discovery of new miRNA is presently carried out using massive sequencing technologies (Kozomara & Griffiths-Jones, 2010), the miR targets important in biochemical processes rely on comparison schemes. As a general rule, selection of the target miRNA can be achieved using the microarray approach by quantitative analyisis of the miR profile in a particular cellular state compared to a control lineage. MiR specific RT-PCR protocols can be used, followed by hybridization to specialized miR microarrays. This analysis has been used to identify miR targets which are over- or, more frequently, under-expressed under pathological conditions. Moreover, several very important miR targets have been addressed by many studies on account of the fact that they were able to act as critical points in the regulation of pathological states.

Chemically engineered oligonucleotides, termed 'antagomirs', are efficient and specific silencers of endogenous miRNAs in mice. Silencing of microRNAs in vivo with 'antagomirs' is a very interesting strategy, supporting studies on the involvement of miRs in gene expression and providing new tools for non-viral gene therapy (Czech, 2006).

MiR-155 is one of the first known miR to be overexpressed in cancers, especially in those occurring in B-cells; high level of this miR have been associated to several neoplastic states and to autoimmune diseases, since it leads to the suppression of a large number of genes involved in the control of cellular proliferation. Therefore miR-155 has been identified as possible target for gene therapy associated to lymphomas and chronic lymphocytic leukemias and colorectal cancer (Zhang et al., 2007, Kota & Balasubrasmanian, 2010). Furthermore, miR-155 was shown to control inflammatory response to microbes (Ceppia et al., 2009).

MiR-21 overexpression was shown to be associated to several solid tumours (lung, breast, colon, gastric and prostate carcinomas and endocrine pancreatic tumours) as well as to cholangiocarcinoma and glioblastoma, since it is correlated to inhibition of apoptosis (Calin & Croce, 2006, Papagiannakopoulos et al., 2008). Knock down of this miR by locked nucleic acids (LNA) oligonucleotides, associated with neural precursor cells (NPC) expressing a secretable variant of the cytotoxic agent tumor necrosis factor–related apoptosis inducing ligand (S-TRAIL), was shown to have high antitumor activity (Corsten et al., 2007).

MiR-122 is another very important target: it is a well characterized liver-specific microRNA exhibiting particular therapeutic interest, since it is related to cholesterol levels in plasma, and it has been shown not only to facilitate Hepatitis C RNA replication (Jopling et al., 2005) but also to be up-regulated in HIV-1 infected cells (Triboulet et al., 2007). Krützfeldt and coworkers (Krützfeldt et al., 2005) demonstrated that intravenous administration of antagomirs against several miRs, including miR-122, resulted in a marked reduction of the corresponding miRNA levels in liver, lung, kidney, heart, intestine, fat, skin, bone marrow, muscle, ovaries and adrenals. The silencing of endogenous miRNAs by this novel method is specific, efficient and long-lasting. The biological significance of silencing miRNAs with the use of antagomirs was studied with miR-122. Gene expression and bioinformatic analysis of messenger RNA from antagomir-treated animals revealed that the 3' untranslated regions of upregulated genes are strongly enriched in miR-122 recognition motifs, whereas down-regulated genes are depleted of these motifs. These findings show that antagomirs are powerful tools to silence specific miRNAs in vivo and may represent a therapeutic strategy for silencing miRNAs in disease. This was confirmed by Elmén et al. (Elmén et al., 2008a), who demonstrated that antagonism of microRNA-122 in mice, systemically treated with LNA-antimiR, leads to up-regulation of a large set of predicted target mRNAs in the liver. These results were also confirmed in non-human primates (Elmén et al.,2008b), showing that lowering of plasma cholesterol could be achieved without signs of toxicity.

That interest on this target has been recently boosted by a report which showed increased resistance to chronic hepatitis C virus (HCV) in primates was achieved by targeting miR122 with LNA, with long-lasting suppression of HCV viremia, with no evidence of viral resistance or side effects in the treated animals (Landfrod et al., 2010).

MiR-221 and mir-222 have been shown to be associated to the suppression of $p27^{Kip1}$, a cell cycle inhibitor and tumor suppressor; high levels of these miRs are present in glioblastoma (Le Sage et al 2007) and have been proposed as very important therapeutic targets.

More recently, miR-210 was identified as an highly expressed miR in the erythroid precursor cells from a patient exhibiting hereditary persistence of fetal haemoglobin (HPFH). When RT-PCR was performed on mithramycin-induced K562 cells and erythroid precursor cells, miR-210 was found to be induced in time-dependent and dose-dependent fashion, together with increased expression of the fetal γ-globin genes (Bianchi et al., 2009). Thus miR-210 plays a crucial role in the erythroid differentiation pathway, by limiting the expression of genes whose down-modulation might be associated with the progression of erythroid differentiation.

Other highly expressed miRs (such as miR-142-3p) are very important tools in gene therapy protocols since specific targets can be inserted in gene constructs in order to suppress toxicity associated to viral vectors or to inhibit immune response against a transgene, but they are not easily used as targets for specific inhibition of a pathological state (Brown & Naldini, 2009).

4. MiR targeting by PNAs

PNAs are very promising tools for RNA recognition, since they have a higher affinity for RNA than for DNA (Nielsen, 2004), are more specific and are resistant to DNases and proteases (Demidov et al 1994).

As far as their role in targeting mRNAs in the antisense strategy, it should be underlined that, unlike oligonucleotide (ON) molecules, PNAs do not activate the RNAse H mediated degradation (Bonham et al., 2005). However, since the RNAse H degradation was shown not to be effective in the inhibition of miR by oligonucleotides, the steric block mechanism, i.e. the base pairing of the therapeutic ON with one of the strands of the miR target, should be one of the possible mechanisms, although a degradation of the miR target by a still unknown mechanism has been proposed for some ON derivatives (Krutzfeldt et al., 2007).

The steric block mechanism is highly efficient when using PNAs, due to their high affinity for RNA, and the high stability to both chemical and enzymatic degradation (Demidov et al., 1994).

However, very few works have been reported so far concerning the use of PNAs as anti-miR agents, showing good performances (table 2). One of the reasons is the lack of cellular permeation by simple unmodified PNA, or segregation in lysosomes of some PNA-peptide conjugates, which can prevent the access to the target miRNA. However, these problems can be easily circumvented by using appropriate carriers, as shown by our own experience and by other examples reported in the next paragraph.

Ref.	targets	PNA modification	Cellular /animal system	Effect
Fabani et al., 2008	miR-122	K-PNA-K_3	human hepatocellular carcinoma cells primary rat hepatocytes	Decrease in miR-122 and mRNA of its target genes (Aldolase A)
Oh et al ., 2009	miR-16 miR-21 miR-24	Different cell penetrating peptides (CPP) Most effective: Tat-modified	HeLa cells	Upregulation of mRNA targets measured by luciferase assay
Fabani et al., 2010	miR-155	K-PNA-K_3	LPS-activated primary B cells and mice	Up-regulation of 724 transcripts
Fabbri et al., 2011	miR-210	R_8-PNA	K562 chronic myelogenous leukemia cells	Alteration of erythroid differentiation

Table 2. Works reporting PNA induced miR suppression.

The first example of targeting microRNAs using PNA-based molecules is provided by miR-122. Fabani and Gait demonstrated, using PNAs and PNA-peptide conjugates, that these oligonucleotide analogs, evaluated for the first time in microRNA inhibition, are more effective than standard 2'-O-methyl oligonucleotides in binding and inhibiting microRNA action (Fabani & Gait, 2009). In their experiments, PNAs were delivered by electroporation. Inhibition of miR-122 was evaluated by Northern blot and by the up-regulation effect upon both chemical and enzymatic degradation.

Interestingly, these authors showed that microRNA inhibition can be achieved without the need for transfection or electroporation, by conjugating the PNA to the cell-penetrating peptide R6-Penetratin, or merely by linkage to four Lys residues, highlighting the potential of PNAs for future therapeutic applications as well as for studying microRNA function. Both LNA/OMe and PNA oligomers were found to be much more effective than 2′-O-methyl RNA oligonucleotides usually used as anti-miR agents. The target miR disappeared from the Northen-blot analysis of the PNA-treated sample, suggesting a still unknown mechanism of degradation or segregation induced by PNA.

In a parallel work, Oh et al. described the effectiveness of miR targeting by PNA-peptide conjugates, using a series of cell penetrating peptides (CPP) as carriers, including R6 pen, Tat, a four Lys sequence, and transportan (Oh, et al., 2009). The best conditions were obtained with cationic peptides, and in particular with the Tat-modified peptide RRRQRRKKRR. In this study, cells were transfected with a plasmid containing a luciferase gene carrying a target site for each miR tested. Inhibition of the miR activity was monitored by expression of the luciferase gene. Inhibition of miR-16, which regulates Bcl-2 expression, and of miR-21 activity could be monitored in this way. PNAs were found to be more effective than LNAs and 2′-OMe oligonucleotides (Figure 3 A). Furthermore, PNAs showed no cytotoxicity at the concentration used, unlike LNAs which showed a reduction in cell viability (Figure 3 B). Furthermore PNAs were found to be more resistant to degradation than LNAs, even if stored at room temperature, suggesting better performances of the former class as candidate drugs.

More recently, a PNA targeted against miR-155 has been used in cellular systems and in mice (Fabani et al., 2010). In this study, the induction of miR-155 by bacterial lipopolysaccharide (LPS) was reduced by using a PNA matching the miR target and linked to four lysine residues. Mice challenged with sub-lethal dose of LPS were treated with 50 mg PNA/kg/day for 2 days and 24 h after the last injection (At which time the miR-155 expression is maximal) they were sacrified and their spleen tissue was analysed. Complete suppression of miR-155 induction was observed. Genome-wide analysis of gene expression revealed a profile of normal mice treated with LPS and then with anti-miR PNA similar to transgenic miR-155-deficient animals receiving control PBS buffer.

This study revealed important clues on the miR-155 regulation of B-cells and suggested a possible use of anti-miR PNA in the treatment of diffuse large B-cell lymphoma (DLBCL).

In a recent study we evaluated the activity of a PNA targeting microRNA-210, which is firmly associated to hypoxia and is modulated during erythroid differentiation, in leukemic K562 cells (Fabbri et al., 2010). The major conclusions of our study were that a PNA against miR-210 conjugated with a polyarginine peptide (R-pep-PNA-a210): (a) is efficiently internalized within the target cells; (b) strongly inhibits miR-210 activity; (c) deeply alters the expression of raptor and γ-globin genes. Unlike commercially available antagomiRs, which need continuous administrations, a single administration of R-pep-PNA-a210 was sufficient to obtain the biological effects.

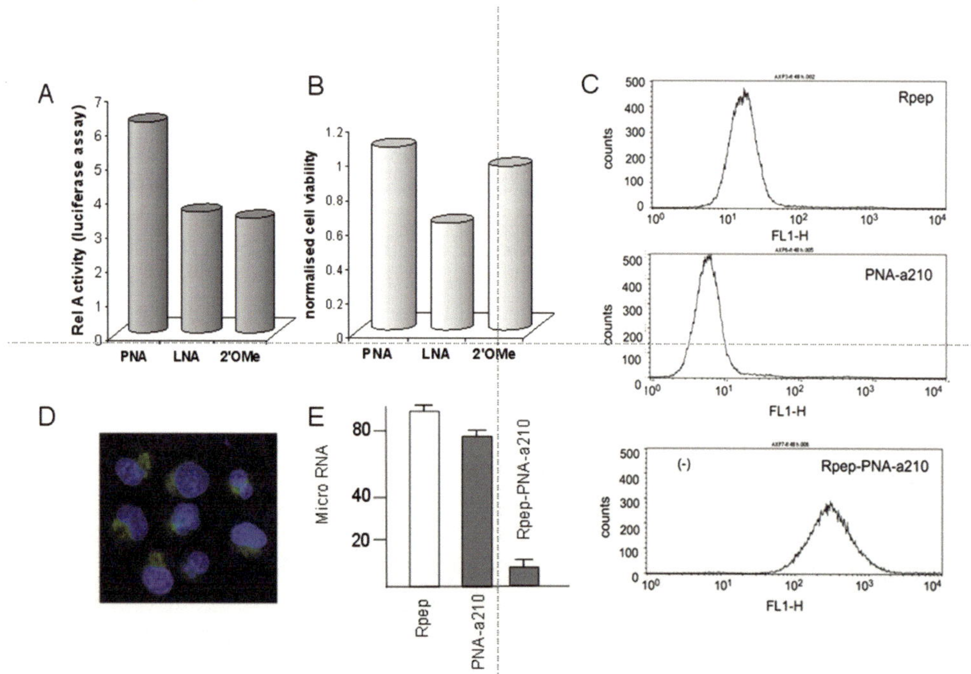

Fig. 3. A, B: Comparison of the PNA-based anti-miR activity and cellular toxicity with other oligonucleotide mimics as reported by Oh and coworkers (data from Oh et al., 2009). A) Effect of anti-miR on HeLa cells transfected with 200 nM of PNA, LNA-modified oligonucleotide, and a 2'-OMe-modified oligonucleotide (2'-OMe) specific for miR-24; a luciferase assay was performed to evaluate the effect anti-miR oligonucleotide mimics. B) Cell viability of HeLa cells after incubation with 200nm of PNA, LNA and 2'OMe oligonucleotides. (C-E) Cellular delivery and anti-miR210 activity of fluoresceinated R_8-PNA. C. FACS analysis showing the uptake of fluoresceinated R_8 peptide (R-pep), anti-miR-210 PNA (PNA-a210), and R_8-PNA (R-pep-PNA-a210) after 48 hours incubation of K562 cells at a 2 μM concentration. D. Intracellular distribution of K562 cells cultured for 48 hours with 2 μM of Fluoresceinated Rpep-PNA-a210 and then analyzed using a fluorescence microscope. The picture is the merged analysis of the fluorescence and of the staining of the same cell population with Hoechst 33258 (selectively staining nuclei). E. Effects of the treatment with Rpep, PNA-a210, Rpep-PNA-a210 on the miR-210 content in K562 cells.

Interestingly, cellular uptake was found to be crucial in order to obtain biological activity, since the PNA lacking of the polyarginine tail (PNA-a210), despite being able to hybridize to target nucleotide sequences, displayed very low activity on cells (Figure 3 C-E).

5. Modified PNAs can improve miR targeting

The major limit in the use of PNAs for the alteration of gene expression is the low uptake by eukaryotic cells (Rasmussen et al., 2006). In order to remove this drawback, several approaches have been considered, including the delivery of PNA analogues with liposomes and microspheres (Nastruzzi et al., 2000, Cortesi et al., 2004, Borgatti, 2002). One of the possible strategy is to link PNAs to polylysine (K) or a polyarginine (R) tails, based on the

observation that this cell-membrane penetrating oligopeptides are able to facilitate uptake of conjugated molecules (Abes et al., 2008).
Since their discovery, many modifications of the original PNA backbones have been proposed in order to improve performances in term of affinity and specificity.
Modification of the PNA backbone with positively charged groups (figure 4) has also been demonstrated to enhance cellular uptake and consequently PNA efficiency (Corradini et al., 2007, Zhou et al., 2003, 2006).

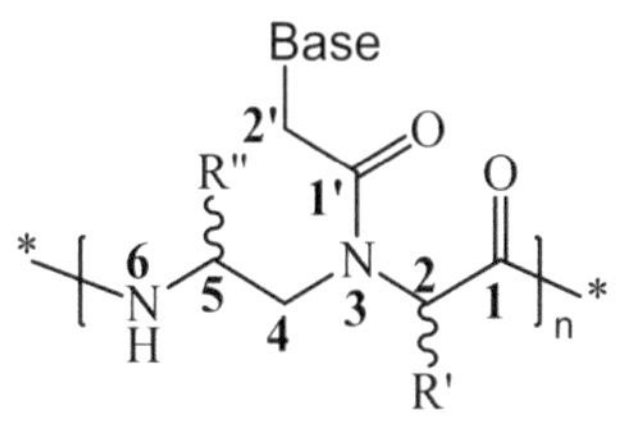

R' = R" = H : standard achiral PNA
R' = side chain, R" = H : acyclic chiral PNA substituted at position 2
R' = H, R" = side chain : acyclic chiral PNA substituted at position 5

Fig. 4. Structure of backbone modified PNA.

Although the steric requirements for binding RNA have not been extensively studied so far, the availability of different chemical strategies to design and synthesize PNA analogues is the basis for the development of new peptide nucleic acids (PNAs) specifically aimed at targeting RNA, to be used for miR targeting.
In the last few years several research groups have been involved in the synthesis and in the studies of the binding properties of PNAs with a chiral constrained backbone obtained by insertion of stereogenic centers either at the C2 (alpha) or C5 (gamma) position of the monomer.
The insertion of one chiral monomeric unit in a PNA strand has resulted in increased DNA binding affinity, when the side chain was positively charged (e.g. lysine or arginine). The PNA:DNA duplex stability was found to be dependent on stereochemistry: PNAs carrying a monomer with a stereocenter derived from a D-amino acid at the C2 position bound complementary antiparallel DNA strands with higher affinity than the corresponding PNA carrying a monomer with a stereocenter derived from an L-amino acid at the same position. Therefore, the affinity of chiral PNAs for complementary DNA emerged to be a contribution of different factors: electrostatic interactions, steric hindrance and, most interestingly, enantioselectivity with a preference for the D-configuration at the 2 position of the monomer. A PNA:DNA duplex, in which three adjacent chiral monomers based on 2D-lysine ("chiral box") were present in the middle of the PNA strand, was characterized by X-ray diffraction, and the results showed that the D-lysine-based chiral PNA-DNA heteroduplex adopts the so-called P-helix conformation, with helical parameters significantly different from those of the canonical DNA helical forms (Menchise et al., 2003). The P-helix is characterized by a small twist angle, a large x-displacement and a wide, deep major groove. The 2D-lysine "chiral box" PNA showed also an increased sequence selectivity, both in terms of direction control and of recognition of a single base mismatch (Sforza et al., 2000). Therefore, this type of structures was found ideal for targeting point mutations in genes of diagnostic interest (Corradini et al., 2004, Tedeschi et al., 2005a,b). Recently chiral PNAs with L- or D-stereocenters either at the 2- or the 5-positions of the monomer or with both stereocenters simultaneously present have also been synthesized and

studied (Sforza et al., 2007, Manicardi et al., 2010).[76] The strongest directing factor was found to be the L-stereogenic center at position 5 derived from L-lysine. This preference (L-configuration at position 5) and the former (D-configuration at position 2) are related to the ability to form a preferred right-handed helicity of PNA and therefore a preferential preorganization for binding right-handed DNA.

More recently, three consecutive different chiral monomers, respectively modified with 2D-Arg, with 5L,2D-Arg and with 5L-Arg, were used by our group in order to build an "extended chiral box" PNA. Such PNA, analogously to the above mentioned "chiral box" PNA, showed very good mismatch discrimination towards DNA, was even more specific in RNA recognition, showing that PNA modifications can also be used in order to tailor PNA recognition towards RNA (Calabretta et al., 2011).

Recently, Ly and co-workers reported the synthesis and uptake properties of γGPNA, in which the PNA backbone had a homo-arginine side chain at the 5-position (or γ position) (Sahu et al., 2009), showing an excellent cellular uptake.

Substitution at both C2 and C5 carbons of the PNA backbone with amino acid side chains leads to ambivalent structures having properties of DNA or RNA mimic on one side and peptide mimics on the other side, thus allowing recognition by specific receptors, as shown very recently by a short PNA mimicking the function of a nuclear localization peptide (NLS) (Sforza et al., 2010). Thus, and to obtain PNAs with both peptide properties and RNA binding ability. This strategy can be used to further improve the efficiency of PNAs for miR targeting. In fact, the use of peptides as carriers represents a "Achille's heel" of the potential PNA-based drug candidates, since the peptide part might be subjected to enzymatic degradation, whereas the incorporation of the peptide signal into the PNA backbone does not lead to enzymatic degradation, even in the presence of highly active proteases.

PNAs bearing modified nucleobases able to induce additional interactions providing high improvement in RNA and DNA binding affinities have also been described (Wojciechowski et al., 2009). Combination of modified nucleobases and backbone modification with C2 or C5 modified residues was found to be the best approach in order to achieve strand invasion into mixed DNA sequences (Ishizuka et al., 2008, 2009, Chenna et al., 2008), a strategy which could also be very fruitful in challenging double-stranded miRs.

6. Conclusions and perspectives

PNAs are very promising tools for the inhibition of miR activities, and this effect can be very important for obtaining gene modulation in a relatively simple way, with very important applications in gene therapy and in drug development.

The issue of the correct delivery of PNAs to their targets is still open, although efficient strategies have already been described, including conjugation with carrier peptides and backbone modification.

The very high affinity of PNAs for RNA and the very strong chemical and enzymatic stability of these compounds (especially the backbone-modified version) make them ideal candidates as miR inhibitors with long-lasting effect.

The first data available already indicate that this technology is likely to succeed, despite the limited number of targets studied so far. Apart from model systems, PNAs have the potentiality to perform like (and eventually outperform) other anti-miR agents such as 2'-OMe oligonucleotides and LNAs.

Furthermore, the possibility to introduce functional groups along the chain of the PNA strand by chemical synthesis allows to envisage strategies in which the PNA can be endowed of catalytic sites, thus leading to molecules not only capable of binding, but also of cleaving, leading to miR specific nuclease models.

7. Acknowledgment

This work was supported by a grant by MIUR (Italian Ministry of University and Research). RG is granted by Fondazione CARIPARO and Telethon GGP10124.

8. References

Abes, R.; Arzumanov, A.; Moulton, H.; Abes, S.; Ivanova, G.; Gait, M.J.; Iversen, P.& Lebleu, B. (2008) Arginine-rich cell penetrating peptides: design, structure-activity, and applications to alter pre-mRNA splicing by steric-block oligonucleotides. *Journal of Peptide Science*, Vol. 14, No. 4, pp.455-60. ISSN 1075-2617.

Alvarez-Garcia, I. & Miska, E.A. (2005). MicroRNA functions in animal development and human disease. *Development,* Vol. 132, No 21, pp. 4653–62. . ISSN 0950-1991.

Bianchi, N.; Zuccato, C.; Lampronti, I.; Borgatti, M. & Gambari, R. (2009) Expression of miR-210 during erythroid differentiation and induction of γ-globin gene expression. *BMB reports,* Vol. , No. 8, pp. 493-499. ISSN 1976-6696.

Bonham, M.A.; Brown, S.; Boyd, A.L.; Brown, P.H.; Bruckenstein, D.A.; Hanvey, J.C.; Thomson, S.A.; Pipe, A.; Hassman, F. Bisi, J.E.; Froehler, B.C.; Matteucci, M.D.; Wagner, R.W.; Noble, S.A. & Babiss, L. (1995) An assessment of the antisense properties of RNase H-competent and steric-blocking oligomers. *Nucleic Acids Research*, Vol. 23, No. 7, pp. 1197-1203. ISSN 0305-1048

Borgatti, M.; Breda, L.; Cortesi, R.; Nastruzzi, C.; Romanelli, A.; Saviano, M.; Bianchi, N.; Mischiati, C.; Pedone, C. & Gambari R. (2002) Cationic liposomes as delivery systems for double-stranded PNA-DNA chimeras exhibiting decoy activity against NF-kappaB transcription factors. *Biochemical Pharmacology,* Vol.64, No. 4, pp. 609-616. ISSN 0006-2952.

Brown, B.D. & Naldini, L. (2009) Exploiting and antagonizing microRNA regulation for therapeutic and experimental applications. *Nature Reviews Genetics* Vol. 10, No. 8, pp. 578-585. ISSN. 1471-0056.

Calabretta, A.; Tedeschi, T.; Corradini, R.; Marchelli, R. & Sforza, S. (2011) DNA and RNA binding properties of an arginine-based "Extended Chiral Box" Peptide Nucleic Acid. *Tetrahedron Letters,* Vol. 52, No. 2, pp. 300-304. ISSN 0040-4039.

Calin, G.A. & Croce C.M. (2006) MicroRNA signatures in human cancers. *Nature Reviews Cancer* Vol. 6, No. 11, pp. 857-866. ISSN 1474-175X.

Ceppi, M.; Pereira, P.M., Dunand-Sauthier, I.; Barras, E.; Reith, W.; Santos, M.A. & Pierre, P. (2009). MicroRNA-155 modulates the interleukin-1 signaling pathway in activated human monocyte-derived dendritic cells. *Proceedings of the National Academy of Sciences U.S.A.* Vol. 106, No. 8, pp. 2735–2740. ISSN 0027-8424.

Chenna, V.; Rapireddy, S.; Sahu, B.; Ausin, C.; Pedroso, E. & Ly, D.H. (2008) A Simple Cytosine to G-Clamp Nucleobase Substitution Enables Chiral □-PNAs to Invade

Mixed-Sequence Double-Helical B-form DNA. *ChemBioChem*, Vol. 9, No. 15 , pp. 2388 - 2391. ISSN 1439-4227.

Cho, W.C.S. (2007) OncomiRs: the discovery and progress of microRNAs in cancers. *Molecular Cancer*, Vol. 6, Art. No 60. ISSN 1476-4598.

Corradini, R.; Feriotto, G.; Sforza, S.; Marchelli, R. & Gambari, R. (2004) Enhanced recognition of cystic fibrosis W1282X DNA point mutation by chiral peptide nucleic acid probes by a surface plasmon resonance biosensor. *Journal of Molecular Recognition*, Vol. 17, No. 1, pp.76-84. . ISSN 0952-3499.

Corradini, R.; Sforza, S.; Tedeschi, T.; Totsingan, F. & Marchelli, R. (2007) Peptide Nucleic Acids with a Structurally Biased Backbone: Effects of Conformational Constraints and Stereochemistry. *Current Topics in Medicinal Chemistry*, Vol. 7, No. 7, pp. 681-694. ISSN 1568-0266.

Corsten, M.F.; Miranda, R.; Kasmieh, R.; Krichevsky, A. M.; Weissleder, R. & Shah, K. (2007) MicroRNA-21 Knockdown Disrupts Glioma Growth In vivo and Displays Synergistic Cytotoxicity with Neural Precursor Cell–Delivered S-TRAIL in Human Gliomas. *Cancer Research* Vol. 67, No. 19, pp. 8994-9000. ISSN 0008-5472.

Cortesi., R.; Mischiati, C.; Borgatti, M.; Breda, L.; Romanelli, A.; Saviano, M.; Pedone, C.; Gambari, R. & Nastruzzi, C. (2004) Formulations for natural and peptide nucleic acids based on cationic polymeric submicron particles. *AAPS Pharmsci*, Vol.6, No. 1, pp.10-21.ISSN 1522-1059.

Costinean, S.; Zanesi, N.; Pekarsky, Y.; Tili, E.; Volinia, S.; Heerema, N. & Croce, C.M. (2006) Pre-B cell proliferation and lymphoblastic leukemia/ high-grade lymphoma in E(mu)- *miR155* transgenic mice. *Proc Natl Acad Sci USA* Vol. 103, No. 18, pp. 7024-7029. .ISSN 0027-8424.

Czech, M.P. (2006) MicroRNAs as Therapeutic Targets. *New England Journal of Medicine* , Vol. 354, No. 11, pp. 1194-1195. ISSN.

Demidov, V.V.; Potaman, V.N.; Frank-Kamenetskii, M.D.; Egholm, M.; Buchard, O.; Sonnichsen, S.H. & Nielsen, P.E. (1994) Stability of peptide nucleic acids in human serum and cellular extracts. *Biochemical Pharmacology*, Vol. 48, No. 6, pp.1310-3. ISSN 0006-2952.

Dragulescu-Andrasi, A.; Zhou, P.; He, G. & Ly, D.H. (2005) Cell-permeable GPNA with appropriate backbone stereochemistry and spacing binds sequence-specifically to RNA *Chemical Communications*, No. 3, 244–246. ISSN 1359-7345.

Edmonds, M.D.; Hurst, D.R. & Welch, D.R. (2009) Linking metastasis suppression with metastamiR regulation. *Cell Cycle*. Vol. 8, No 17, pp.2673-5. ISSN 1538-4101

Elmén, J.; Lindow, M.; Silahtaroglu, A.; Bak, M.; Christensen, M. & Lind-Thomsen, A. (2008 a) Antagonism of microRNA-122 in mice by systemically administered LNA-antimiR leads to up-regulation of a large set of predicted target mRNAs in the liver. *Nucleic Acids Research* Vol.36, No. 4, pp. 1153-62. ISSN 0305-1048.

Elmén, J.; Lindow, M.; Schütz, S.; Lawrence, M.; Petri, A.; Obad S.; Lindholm M.; Hedtjärn, M.; Hansen, H.F.; Berger, U.; Gullans, S.; Kearney, P.; Sarnow, P.; Straarup, E.M. & Kauppinen, S. (2008 b) LNA-mediated microRNA silencing in non-human primates. *Nature*, Vol. 452, No. 7189, pp. 896-900. ISSN 0028-0836.

Fabani, M.M. & Gait, M.J. (2008) miR-122 targeting with LNA/2'-O-methyl oligonucleotide mixmers, peptide nucleic acids (PNA), and PNA-peptide conjugates. *RNA*. Vol. 14, No. 2 pp. 336-46. ISSN 1355-8382.

Fabani, M.M.; Abreu-Goodger, C.; Williams, D.; Lyons, P.A.; Torres, A.G.; Smith, K.G.C.; Enright, A.J., Gait, M.J. & Vigorito, E. (2010) Efficient inhibition of miR-155 function in vivo by peptide nucleic acids. *Nucleic Acids Research,* Vol. 38, No. 13, pp. 4466–4475. ISSN 0305-1048

Fabbri, E.; Bianchi, N.; Brognara, E.; Finotti, A.; Breveglieri, G.; Borgatti, M.; Manicardi, A.; Corradini, R.; Marchelli, R. & Gambari, R. (2010) Inhibition of micro RNA 210 biological activity with an anti-miR-210 peptide nucleic acid. *International Journal of Molecular Medicine,* Vol. 26, Suppl. 1., pp. S61-S61. ISSN 1107-3756.

Filipowicz, W.; Jaskiewicz, L.; Kolb, F.A. & Pillai, R.S. (2005). Post-transcriptional gene silencing by siRNAs and miRNAs. *Current Opinions in Structural Biology,* Vol. 15, No. 3 pp. 331–41. ISSN 0959-440X.

Gambari, R. (2004) Biological activity and delivery of peptide nucleic acids (PNA)-DNA chimeras for transcription factor decoy (TFD) pharmacotherapy. *Current Medicinal Chemistry,* Vol. 11, No.10, pp.1253-63. ISSN 0929-8673

Garzon, R. & Croce, C.M. (2008). MicroRNAs in normal and malignant hematopoiesis. *Current Opinions in Hematology,* Vol. 15 No. 4, pp. 352-8. ISSN 1065-6251.

Hayashita, Y.; Osada, H.; Tatematsu, Y.; Yamada, H.; Yanagisawa, K.; Tomida, S.; Yatabe, Y.; Kawahara, K.; Sekido, Y. & Takahashi, T. (2005) A polycistronic microRNA cluster, *miR-17-92*, is overexpressed in human lung cancers and enhances cell proliferation. *Cancer Research* Vol. 65, No. 21 , pp.9628-9632. ISSN 1078-0432

He, L. & Hannon, G.J. (2004) MicroRNAs: small RNAs with a big role in gene regulation. *Nature Reviews Genetics* Vol. 5,No. 7, pp. 522–531. ISSN 1471-0056.

Huang, C.; Li, M.; Chen, C. & Yao, Q. (2008). Small interfering RNA therapy in cancer: mechanism, potential targets, and clinical applications. *Expert Opinions in Therapeutic Targets,* Vol. 12, No. 5, pp. 637-45.ISSN 1472-8222.

Hurst, D.R.; Edmonds, M.D. & Welch, D.R.; (2009) Metastamir: the field of metastasis-regulatory microRNA is spreading. *Cancer Research.*Vol. 69, No.19, pp. 7495-8. ISSN 1078-0432

Iorio, M.V.; Ferracin, M.; Liu, C.G.; Veronese, A.; Spizzo, R.; Sabbioni, S.; Magri, E.; Pedriali, M.; Fabbri, M.; Campiglio, M.; Menard, S.; Palazzo, J.P.; Rosenberg, A.; Musiani, P.; Volinia, S.; Nenci, I.; Calin, G.A.; Querzoli, P.; Negrini, M. & Croce, C.M. (2005) MicroRNA gene expression deregulation in human breast cancer. *Cancer Research* Vol. 65, No. 16, pp. 7065-7070. ISSN 1078-0432

Ishizuka, T.; Tedeschi, T.; Corradini,R.; Komiyama, M.; Sforza, S. & Marchelli, R. (2009) SSB-Assisted Duplex Invasion of Preorganized PNA into Double-Stranded DNA. *ChemBioChem,* Vol. 10, No. 16 , pp. 2607 - 2612. ISSN 1439-4227.

Ishizuka, T.; Yoshida, J.; Yamamoto Y.; Sumaoka, J.; Tedeschi, T.; Corradini, R.; Sforza, S. & Komiyama, M. (2008) Chiral introduction of positive charges to PNA for double-duplex invasion to versatile sequences. *Nucleic Acid Research.,* Vol. 36, No. 5, pp. 1464-1471. ISSN 0305-1048.

Jopling,C.L., Yi,M., Lancaster,A.M., Lemon,S.M. & Sarnow,P. (2005) Modulation of hepatitis C virus RNA abundance by a liver-specific microRNA. *Science*, Vol. 309, No. 5740, pp. 1577–1581. ISSN 0036-8075.

Kong, W.; He, L.; Coppola, M.; Guo, J.; Esposito, N.N.; Coppola, D. & Cheng, J.Q. (2010) MicroRNA-155 regulates cell survival, growth, and chemosensitivity by targeting FOXO3a in breast cancer. *Journal of Biological Chemistry* Vol. 285, No. 23, pp.17869-79. ISSN 0021-9258

Kota, S.K. & Balasubramanian, S. (2010) Cancer therapy via modulation of micro RNA levels: a promising future. *Drug Discovery Today*. Vol. 15, No 17/18, pp. 733-740. ISSN 1359-6446.

Kozomara, A. & Griffiths-Jones, S. (2010) miRBase: integrating microRNA annotation and deep-sequencing data. *Nucleic Acids Research*, Vol. 39, Database issue, D152–D157. ISSN 0305-1048.

Krol. J.; Loedige, I. & Filipowicz, W. (2010) The widespread regulation of microRNA biogenesis, function and decay. *Nature Reviews Genetics*, Vol. 11, No. 9, pp. 597-610. ISSN 1471-0056.

Krutzfeldt, J.; Kuwajima, S.; Braich, R.; Rajeev, K.G.; Pena, J.; Tuschl, T.; Manoharan, M. & Stoffel, M. (2007) Specificity, duplex degradation and subcellular localization of antagomirs. *Nucleic Acids Research*, Vol. 35, No. 9, pp. 2885–2892. ISSN 0305-1048.

Krützfeldt, J.; Rajewsky, N.; Braich, R.; Rajeev, K.G.; Tuschl, T.; Manoharan, M. & Stoffel, M. (2005) Silencing of microRNAs in vivo with 'antagomirs'. *Nature*, Vol. 438, No. 7068, pp. 685-689. ISSN 0028-0836.

Lanford, R.E.; Hildebrandt-Eriksen, E.S.; Petri, A.; Persson, R.; Lindow, M.; Munk, M.E.; Kauppinen, S. & Ørum, H. (2010). Therapeutic Silencing of MicroRNA-122 in Primates with Chronic Hepatitis C Virus Infection. *Science*, Vol. 327, No. 5962, pp. 198-201. ISSN 0036-8075.

Larsen, H.J. &Nielsen PE. (1996) Transcription-mediated binding of peptide nucleic acid (PNA) to double-stranded DNA: sequence-specific suicide transcription. *Nucleic Acids Research*, Vol 24, No. 3, pp. 458-63. ISSN 0305-1048

Le Sage, C.; Nagel, R.; Egan, D.A.; Schrier, M.; Mesman, E.; Mangiola, A.; Anile, C.; Maira, G.; Mercatelli, N.; Ciafrè, S.A.; Farace, M.G. & Agami R. (2007) Regulation of the p27Kip1 tumor suppressor by miR-221 and miR-222 promotes cancer cell proliferation. *EMBO Journal* Vol. 26, No. 15, pp. 3699–3708. ISSN 0261-4189.

Li, S.D. & Huang, L. (2008). Targeted delivery of siRNA by nonviral vectors: lessons learned from recent advances. *Current Opinion in Investigational Drugs* , Vol 9, No. 12 pp. 1317-23. ISSN 1472-4472.

Liu, X.; Sempere, L.F.; Ouyang, H.; Memoli, V.A.; Andrew, A.S.; Luo, Y.; Demidenko, E.; Korc, M.; Shi, W.; Preis, M.; Dragnev K.H.; Li, H.; Direnzo, J.; Bak, M.; Freemantle, S.J.; Kauppinen, S. & Dmitrovsky, E. (2010) MicroRNA-31 functions as an oncogenic microRNA in mouse and human lung cancer cells by repressing specific tumor suppressors. *Journal of Clinical Investigations* Vol. 120, No. 4, pp. 1298-309.ISSN 0021-9738.

López-Fraga, M.; Wright, N. & Jiménez, A. (2008). RNA interference-based therapeutics: new strategies to fight infectious disease. *Infection Disorders-Drug Targets*, Vol 8, No. 4, pp. 262-73. ISSN 1871-5265.

Lowery, A.J.; Miller, N.; McNeill, R.E. & Kerin, M.J. (2008). MicroRNAs as prognostic indicators and therapeutic targets: potential effect on breast cancer management. *Clinical Cancer Research,* Vol. 14, No. 2, pp. 360-5. . ISSN 1078-0432

Lundin, K.E.; Good, L.; Strömberg, R.; Gräslund, A. & Smith, C.I. (2006) Biological activity and biotechnological aspects of peptide nucleic acid. *Advances in Genetics* Vol. 56, pp. 1-51. ISSN 0065-2660

Manicardi, A.; Calabretta, A.; Bencivenni, M.; Tedeschi, T.; Sforza, S.; Corradini, R. & Marchelli, R. (2010) Affinity and Selectivity of C2- and C5-Substituted "Chiral-Box" PNA in Solution and on Microarrays. *Chirality* Vol. 22, No.IE, pp. E161-E172. ISSN 0899-0042.

Masaki, S.; Ohtsuka, R.; Abe, Y.; Muta, K. & Umemura, T. (2007) Expression patterns of microRNAs 155 and 451 during normal human erythropoiesis. *Biochemical and Biophysical Research Communication* Vol. 364, No. 3, pp.509-514. ISSN 0006-291X.

Mascellani, N.; Tagliavini, L.; Gamberoni, G.; Rossi, S.; Marchesini, J.; Taccioli, C. Di Leva, G.; Negrini, M.; Croce, C. & Volinia, S. (2008) Using miRNA expression data for the study of human cancer. *Minerva Biotecnologica,* Vol. 20, No.1, pp. 23-30. ISSN 1120-4826.

Menchise, V.; De Simone, G.; Tedeschi, T.; Corradini, R.; Sforza, S.; Marchelli, R.; Capasso, D.; Saviano, M. & Pedone C. (2003) Insights into peptide nucleic acid (PNA) structural features: The crystal structure of a D-lysine-based chiral PNA–DNA duplex. *Proceedings of the National Academy of Sciences U.S.A.,* Vol. 100, No. 21, pp. 12021-12026. ISSN 0027-8424.

Nastruzzi, C.; Cortesi, R.; Esposito, E.; Gambari, R.; Borgatti, M.; Bianchi, N.; Feriotto, G. & Mischiati, C. (2000) Liposomes as carriers for DNA-PNA hybrids. *Journal of Controlled Release,* Vol. 68, No. 2, pp. 237-49.ISSN 0168-3659.

Nielsen PE (Ed.). (2004) *Peptide Nucleic Acids: Protocols and Applications, Second Edition,* Horizon Bioscience, ISBN 0-9545232-4-5, Norfolk (UK).

Nielsen, PE. (2006) RNA targeting using peptide nucleic acid. *Handbook of Experimental Pharmacology* Vol. 173, pp.395-403. ISSN: 0171-2004.

Nielsen, P.E. & Egholm M. (1999) An introduction to peptide nucleic acid. *Curent Issues in Molecular Biology* Vol 1, No 2, pp. 89-104. ISSN 1467-3037.

Nielsen, P.E. (2005) Gene targeting using peptide nucleic acid. *Methods in Molecular Biology.* Vol. 288, pp. 343-58. ISSN 1064-3745.

Nielsen, P.E.; Egholm, M.; Berg, R.H. & Buchardt, O. (1991) Sequence-selective recognition of DNA by strand displacement with a thymine-substituted polyamide. *Science* Vol. 254, No. 5037, pp. 1497-500. ISSN 0036-8075.

Oh, S.Y.; Ju, Y.S. & Park, H. (2009) A Highly effective and long-lasting inhibition of miRNA with PNA-based antisense oligonucleotides. *Molecules and Cells* Vol. 28, No. 4, pp 341-345. ISSN 1016-8478.

Orlacchio, A.; Bernardi, G.; Orlacchio, A. & Martino, S. (2007). RNA interference as a tool for Alzheimer's disease therapy. *Mini Reviews in Medicinal Chemistry,* Vol. 7, No. 11, pp. 1166-76. ISSN 1389-5575.

Papagiannakopoulos, T. & Kosik, K.S. (2008 a) MicroRNAs: regulators of oncogenesis and stemness. *BMC Medicine,* Vol. 6, pp. 15. ISSN 1741-7015.

Papagiannakopoulos, T.; Shapiro, A. & Kosik, K.S. (2008 b) MicroRNA-21 Targets a Network of Key Tumor-Suppressive Pathways in Glioblastoma Cells. *Cancer Research* Vol. 68, No 19, pp. 8164-8172. ISSN 0008-5472.

Pedersen, I.M.; Otero, D.; Kao, E.; Miletic, A.V.; Hother, C.; Ralfkiaer, E.; Rickert, R.C.; Gronbaek, K. & David M. (2009) Onco-miR-155 targets SHIP1 to promote TNFalpha-dependent growth of B cell lymphomas. *EMBO Molecular Medicine.* Vol. 1, No.5, pp. 288-95.ISSN. 1757-4676.

Rapireddy, S.; He, G.; Roy, S.; Armitage, B.A. & Ly, D.H. (2007) Strand Invasion of Mixed-Sequence B-DNA by Acridine-Linked, □-Peptide Nucleic Acid (□-PNA) *Journal of the American Chemical Society,* Vol. 129, No. 50 , pp.15596-15600. ISSN 0002-7863.

Rasmussen, F.W.; Bendifallah, N.; Zachar, V.; Shiraishi, T.; Fink, T.; Ebbesen, P.; Nielsen, P.E, & Koppelhus, U. (2006) Evaluation of transfection protocols for unmodified and modified peptide nucleic acid (PNA) oligomers. *Oligonucleotides Vol.* 16, No 1, pp. 43-57. ISSN 1545-4576.

Sahu, B.; Chenna, V.; Lathrop,K.L.; Thomas, S.M.; Zon, G.; Livak, K.J. & Ly, D.H. (2009) Synthesis of conformational preorganized and cell-permeable guanidine-based □-peptide nucleic acid (□GPNAs). *Journal of Organic Chemistry,* Vol. 74, No. 4, pp. 1509-1516. ISSN 0022-3263.

Sahu, N.K.; Shilakari, G.; Nayak, A. & Kohli, D.V. (2007). Antisense technology: a selective tool for gene expression regulation and gene targeting. *Current Pharmaceutical Biotechnology,* Vol. 8, No. 5, pp. 291-304. ISSN 1389-2010.

Sforza, S.; Corradini, R.; Ghirardi, S.; Dossena, A. & Marchelli R. (2000) DNA Binding of a D-Lysine-Based Chiral PNA: Direction Control and Mismatch Recognition. *European Journal of Organic Chemistry.* No.16, pp. 2905-2913. ISSN 1434-193X.

Sforza, S.; Tedeschi, T.; Calabretta, A.; Corradini, R.; Camerin, C.; Tonelli, R.; Pession, A. & Marchelli R. (2010) A Peptide Nucleic Acid Embedding a Pseudopeptide Nuclear Localization Sequence in the Backbone Behaves as a Peptide Mimic. *European Journal of Organic Chemistry* No. 13, pp. 2441-2444. ISSN 1434-193X

Sforza, S.; Tedeschi, T.; Calabretta, A.; Corradini, R.; Camerin, C.; Tonelli, R.; Pession, A. & Marchelli, R.; (2010)A peptide nucleic acid embedding a pseudo peptide nuclear localization sequence in the backbone bahave as a peptide mimic. *European Journal of Organic Chemistry,* No. 13, pp.2441-2444. ISSN 1434-193X.

Sforza, S.; Tedeschi, T.; Corradini, R. & Marchelli R. (2007) Induction of Helical Handedness and DNA Binding Properties of Peptide Nucleic Acids (PNAs) with Two Stereogenic Centres. *European Journal of Organic Chemistry* , No. 35, pp. 5879–5885. ISSN 1434-193X

Shrivastava, N. & Srivastava, A. (2008). RNA interference: an emerging generation of biologicals. *Biotechnology Journal,* Vol. 3, No. 3, pp. 339-53. ISSN. 1860-7314.

Si, M.L.; Zhu, S.; Wu, H.; Lu, Z.; Wu, F. & Mo, Y.Y. (2007) *miR-21* -mediated tumor growth. *Oncogene* Vol. 26, No.19, pp.2799-2803. ISSN 0950-9232.

Sontheimer, E.J. & Carthew, R.W. (2005). Silence from within: endogenous siRNAs and miRNAs. *Cell* , Vol. 122, No. 1, pp. 9–12. ISSN 0092-8674.

Stenvang, J. & Kauppinen, S. (2008) MicroRNAs as targets for antisense-based therapeutics. *Expert Opinions in Biological Therapy,* Vol. 8, No. 1, pp. 59-81. ISSN 1471-2598.

Subramanian, S. & Steer, C.J. (2010) MicroRNAs as gatekeepers of apoptosis. *Journal of Cellular Physiology*, Vol. 223, No. 2, pp. 289-98. ISSN 0021-9541.

Tedeschi, T.; Chiari, M.; Galaverna, G.; Sforza, S.; Cretich, M.; Corradini, R. & Marchelli, R. (2005 b) Detection of the R553X DNA single point mutation related to cystic fibrosis by a "chiral box" D-lysine-peptide nucleic acid probe by capillary Electrophoresis. *Electrophoresis* Vol. 26, No. 22 , pp. 4310–6. ISSN 0173-0835.

Tedeschi, T.; Sforza, S.; Corradini, R. & Marchelli, R. (2005 c) Synthesis of new chiral PNAs bearing a dipeptide-mimic monomer with two lysine-derived stereogenic centres. *Tetrahedron Letters*, Vol. 46, No. 48, pp.8395-9. ISSN 0040-4039.

Tedeschi, T.; Sforza, S.; Dossena, A.; Corradini, R. & Marchelli R. (2005 a) Lysine-based peptide nucleic acids (PNAs) with strong chiral constraint: control of helix handedness and DNA binding by chirality. *Chirality* Vol. 17, No. S196-S204.

Triboulet, R.; Mari, B.; Lin, Y.L.; Chable-Bessia C, Bennasser Y, Lebrigand K, Cardinaud, B.; Maurin, T; Barbry, P.; Baillat, V.; Reynes, J.; Corbeau, P.; Jeang, K.T. & Benkirane, M. (2007) Suppression of microRNA-silencing pathway by HIV-1 during virus replication. *Science*. Vol. 315, No.5818, pp.1579-82. ISSN 0036-8075.

Visone, R.; Russo, L.; Pallante, P.; De Martino, I.; Ferraro, A.; Leone, V.; Borbone, E.; Petrocca, F.; Alder, H.; Croce, C.M. & Fusco, A. (2007) MicroRNAs (miR)-221 and miR-222, both overexpressed in human thyroid papillary carcinomas, regulate p27Kip1 protein levels and cell cycle. *Endocrine-Related Cancer*. Vol. 14, No. 3, pp.791-8.ISSN 1351-0088.

Wang, Y.M. & Blelloch, R. (2009) Cell cycle regulation by MicroRNAs in embryonic stem cells. *Cancer Research* Vol. 69, No. 10, pp.4093-4096. ISSN 0008-5472.

Williams, A.E.; Perry, M.M.; Moschos, S.A. Larner-Svensson, H.M. & Lindsay, M.A. (2008). Role of miRNA-146a in the regulation of the innate immune response and cancer. *Biochemical Society Transactions*, Vol. 36 No. (Pt 6), pp. 1211-5. ISSN. 0300-5127.

Wojciechowski F. & Hudson R.H.E. (2007) Nucleobase modifications in peptide nucleic acids *Current Topics in Medicinal Chemistry*, Vol. 7, No. 7, pp. 667-679. ISSN 1568-0266.

Wojciechowski, F. & Hudson, R.H.E. (2009) Peptide Nucleic Acid Containing a Meta-Substituted Phenylpyrrolocytosine Exhibits a Fluorescence Response and Increased Binding Affinity toward RNA. *Organic Letters* Vol. 11, No. 21,pp. 4878-4881. ISSN 1523-7060.

Woods, K.; Thomson, J.M. & Hammond, S.M. (2007) Direct regulation of an oncogenic micro-RNA cluster by E2F transcription factors. *Journal of Bioogical Chemistry* Vol. 282, No. 4, pp.2130-2134. ISSN 0021-9258.

Yin, H.; Lu, Q. & Wood M. (2008) Effective exon skipping and restoration of dystrophin expression by peptide nucleic acid antisense oligonucleotides in mdx mice. *Molecular Therapy* Vol. 16, No.1, pp. 38-45. ISSN: 1525-0016

Zhang, B.; Pan, X.; Cobb, G.P.; Anderson, T.A. (2007) microRNAs as oncogenes and tumor suppressors. *Developmental Biology* Vol. 302, No. 1 , pp. 1–12. ISSN 0012-1606.

Zhang, C.Z.; Zhang, J.X.; Zhang, A.L.; Shi, Z.D.; Han, L.; Jia, Z.F.; Yang, W.D.; Wang, G.X.; Jiang, T.; You, Y.P.; Pu, P.Y.; Cheng, J.Q. & Kang, C.S. (2010) MiR-221 and miR-222 target PUMA to induce cell survival in glioblastoma. *Molecular Cancer*. Vol. 9, pp. 229. ISSN 1476-4598.

Zhou, P.; Dragulescu-Andrasi, A.; Bhattacharya, B.; O'Keefe, H.; Vatta, P.; Hyldig-Nielsen J. J. & Ly, D.H. (2006) Synthesis of cell-permeable peptide nucleic acids and characterization of their hybridization and uptake properties. *Bioorganic and Medicinal Chemistry Letters*, Vol. 16, No.18, pp. 4931–4935.ISSN 0960-894X.

Zhou, P.; Wang, M.M.; Du, L.; Fisher, G.W.; Waggoner, A. & Ly. D.H. (2003) Novel Binding and efficient Cellular Uptake of Guanidine-Based Peptide Nucleic Acids (GPNA). *Journal of the American Chemical Society*, Vol. 125, No. 23, pp. 6878-6879. ISSN 0002-7863.

Zhu, S.; Si, M.L., Wu, H. & Mo, Y.Y. (2007) *MicroRNA-21* Targets the tumor suppressor gene *Tropomyosin 1 (TPM1)*. *Journal of Biological Chemistry* Vol. 282, No. 19, pp. 14328-14336.ISSN 0021-9258

3

Effective Transgene Constructs to Enhance Gene Therapy with Trichostatin A

Hideki Hayashi et al.*
Nagasaki University
Japan

1. Introduction

Gene therapy has been proposed as a strategy for the treatment of intractable human diseases since the early 1990s. For the expression of a specific transgene in desired cells or tissues with the proper timing, many vectors carrying transgenes have been developed (Mátrai et al., 2010; Nayak & Herzog, 2010; Sliva & Schnierle, 2010). Retroviral, lentiviral, adenoviral, and adeno-associated viral vectors are used in various ways to achieve these goals. However, the introduced transgenes frequently become silenced in the host cells (Harbers et al., 1981; Jähner et al., 1982; Palmer et al., 1991). We searched for bioactive substances from Actinomycetes that enhance transgene expression, and found that trichostatin A (TSA), a histone deacetylase inhibitor (HDACi), enhanced several promoter activities remarkably (Y. Ma et al., 2009).

HDACis have been used as anti-cancer drugs, because they have various effects on tumor cells to arrest cell growth, induce apoptosis, inhibit metastasis, and enhance anti-tumor immunity, by regulating the expression of the relevant genes (Bolden et al., 2006; Haberland et al. 2009; X. Ma et al., 2009; Mai et al., 2005). Here, we developed effective TSA-inducible killer constructs to enhance the anti-cancer effects of TSA, by identifying the TSA-responsive element of the herpes simplex virus thymidine kinase (hsvTK) promoter, and TSA-dependently activating some cell-death-inducing genes. We determined the most relevant regions responsive to TSA, and constructed chimeric promoters with higher fold-increases and greater induced strengths with TSA, by replacing the weak TSA-responsible region (TSA2) of the CMV promoter with two or three copies of the TSA-responsible sites (TSA1) of the hsvTK promoter. In addition, the synthetic intron sequence (0.2kb) from the pRL-TK vector and the long 3'-untranslated region (1.0kb) from the pSV2-neo vector, including the SV40 late polyA site, were important for the basal expression of the transgene and the TSA-induction, respectively.

To create the TSA-inducible killer constructs, we placed the hsvTK gene for combination therapy with the prodrug Ganciclovir, and some strong death-inducing molecules (Bax, caspase8, and TRIF) under the control of the TSA-responsible chimeric promoters. They effectively killed the cells in which they were introduced, in a TSA-dependent manner. To evaluate the utility of the killer constructs for cancer gene therapy, the TSA-dependent death-inducing constructs were transferred to retroviral and adenoviral vectors.

---

*Yuhua Ma[1], Tomoko Kohno[1], Masayuki Igarashi[2], Kiyoshi Yasui[1], Koon Jiew Chua[1],Yoshinao Kubo[1], Motoki Ishibashi[3], Ryuji Urae[3], Shin Irie[3] and Toshifumi Matsuyama[1].
1 Nagasaki University, Nagasaki, Japan,
2 Microbial Chemistry Research Center, Tokyo, Japan
3 MEDICAL CO. LTA, Fukuoka, Japan

2. TSA-induced transgene activation

2.1 Screening of actinomycetes products to enhance the transgene

Actinomycetes are the prime candidates in screens for new natural products as antitumor and antimicrobial bioactive agents, and the achievements have been well reviewed (Jensen et al., 2005; Park et al., 2008; Zheng et al., 2000). We screened the Actinomycetes products for substances that enhance the transgene promoter, using the luciferase reporter, pRL-TK vector (Promega). In the vector, the 0.75kb promoter region of hsvTK was placed upstream of the reporter Renilla luciferase gene. We found that a methanol extract of the MK616-mF5 strain increased the luciferase activity significantly, by about 41-fold, as compared to the control among 2,448 Actinomycetes products. The methanol extract from the Actinomycetes MK616-mF5 strain was purified by chromatography on a silica column and a C18 reverse-phase HPLC column, by monitoring the effects on the hsvTK-driven luciferase activities. Based on NMR and mass spectrometry analyses, we concluded that the natural product is TSA. TSA is a histone deacetylase inhibitor (HDACi), and some HDACis have recently been used in clinical trials for cancer treatment (Hoshino & Matsubara, 2010; X. Ma et al, 2009; Wagner et al., 2010). HDACi is thought to work by changing the acetylation status of core histones and thus modulating the gene expression patterns, including the genes associated with cell cycle arrest, apoptosis, and differentiation. Modifications of the N-terminal tails of core histones (the core histone is an octamer, consisting of an H3-H4 tetramer and two H2A-H2B dimers) play a crucial role in chromatin packing and gene expression. The acetylation of the core histone is illustrated in Fig. 1, although other modifications, including methylation, phosphorylation, and ubiquitination, also affect the chromatin remodeling (Gasper-Maia, et al., 2011; Mai et al., 2005). Generally, the positively-charged lysine residues in the N-terminal core histone tails, which protrude from the surface of the nucleosome, are tightly bound to the phosphate backbone of the DNA, thus maintaining the chromatin in a transcriptionally silent state (closed chromatin). The acetylation status of the core histone is controlled by the competitive activities of histone acetyl transferase (HAT) and histone deacetylase (HDAC). Acetylation neutralizes the positive charges on the core histone, and converts the chromatin to a more open state, enhancing the access of the transcriptional machinery, including RNA polymerase II, to the promoter region for gene expression. HDACis have been used as anti-cancer drugs, because they activate the expression of the TRAIL, Fas, Bid, and p53 genes to induce growth arrest and/or apoptosis of cancer cells (Bandyopadhyay et al., 2004; Nakata et al., 2004; Ogawa et al., 2004; Ruefli et al., 2001; Sonnemann et al., 2007) by inhibiting HDAC activities, and they also have anti-angiogenic and anti-metastatic effects (Bolden et al., 2006). In addition, HDACi can enhance anti-tumor immunity, either by directly affecting malignant cells to make them more attractive immune targets, or by altering immune cell activity and/or cytokine production. HDACi reportedly augments the immunogenicity of tumor cells by upregulating the expression of the major histocompatibility complex (MHC) class I and II proteins and co-stimulatory/adhesion molecules, such as CD40, CD80, CD86 and intercellular adhesion molecule-1 (ICAM-1) ((Maeda et al.,2000; Magner et al., 2000).

On the other hand, HDACis have been used to reactivate virally transduced genes and to amplify the expression of transgenes encoded by recombinant adenoviral or retroviral vectors (Chen et al., 1997; Dion et al., 1997; Khalighinejad et al., 2008; Kikuchi et al., 2007). However, the induction levels of the silenced transgenes were not sufficient to achieve satisfactory results.

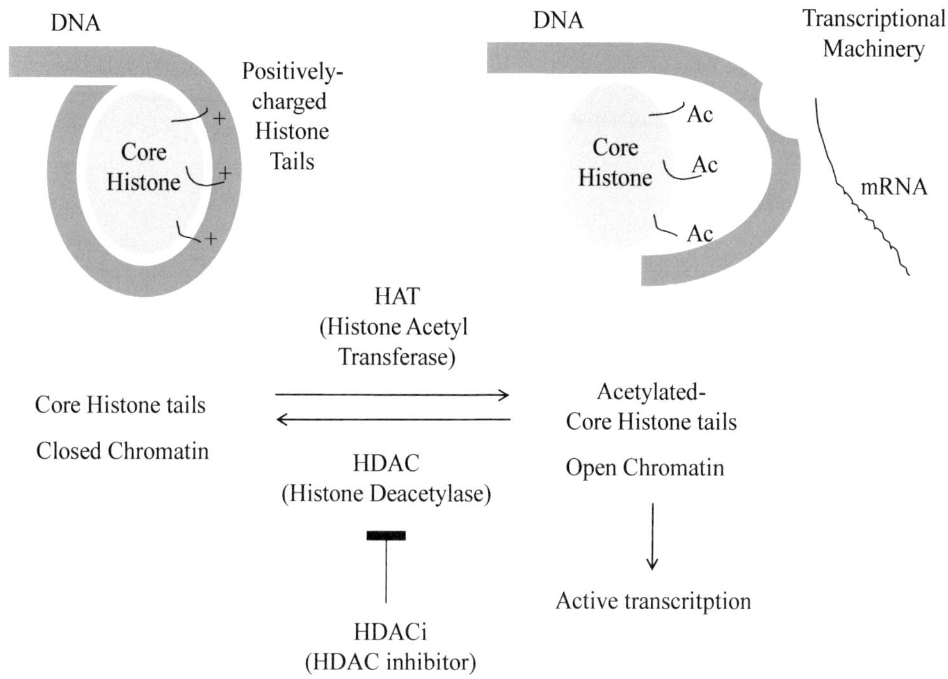

Fig. 1. Effects of HDAC inhibitors on chromatin structure and gene expression. In general, the acetylation of the positively-charged lysine residues within the N-terminal core histone tails, by histone acetyl transferase (HAT), converts the chromatin to a more open form for the access of the transcriptional machinery, including RNA polymerase II, to activate gene expression. In turn, when the acetylation is removed by histone deacetylase (HDAC), the chromatin returns to a closed form (transcriptionally silent). By inhibiting HDAC activities, the HDACi can alter the chromatin structure to an open form, to activate gene expression. —+: positively-charged lysine residues at N-terminal core histone, —Ac: acetylated lysine residues.

To develop effective vectors exhibiting high sensitivities to TSA and sustained strong activities in the presence of TSA, we examined the responsiveness of various promoters to TSA. HeLa cells were treated with 1.0 μg/ml of TSA for 24 hours, after transfections with various Renilla luciferase constructs. The TSA treatment induced remarkable transgene expression with all of the tested promoters, as shown in Fig. 2. The hsvTK promoter exhibited the highest fold-increase, and the RSV and SV40 promoters also showed relatively high fold-increases. The responses of the CMV and β-actin promoters to TSA were poor. In contrast, the CMV promoter showed the greatest strength, but the hsvTK promoter activity was weak, even in the presence of TSA.

2.2 Analyses of the TSA-responsive elements in the hsvTK and CMV promoters

To assess which region of the hsvTK promoter is responsible for the TSA stimulation, we created a series of deletion mutants within the 0.7kb promoter region of the hsvTK gene.

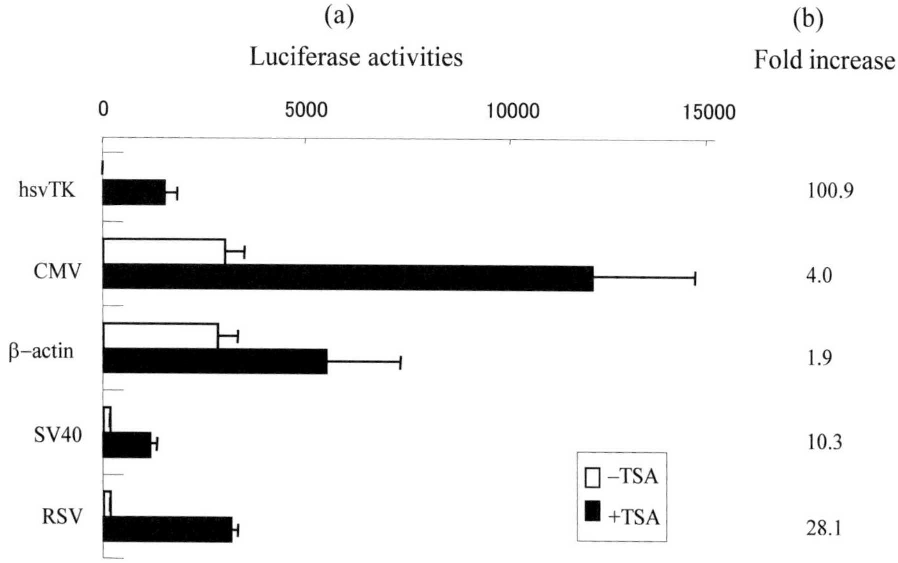

Fig. 2. Treatment with purified TSA leads to the induction of cellular and viral promoters. HeLa cells in a 96-well plate were transfected with 40ng of various constructs in FuGene 6 transfection mixtures. The transfected HeLa cells were treated with/without 1.0 μg/ml of TSA for 24hr, and the reporter assay was performed using a Renilla luciferase assay kit (Promega), according to the manufacturer's instructions. (a) Luciferase activities. (b) Fold increase: the ratio of the luciferase activities in HeLa cells with or without TSA treatment. Promoters: hsvTK, herpes simplex virus thymidine kinase promoter; CMV, cytomegalovirus promoter; SV40, Simian Virus 40 early promoter; and RSV, Rous sarcoma virus LTR promoter. Values are means ± SD. This figure was reproduced from *Int. J. Integ. Biol.*, 5: 108-115, 2009.

They were transfected into HeLa cells, and the Renilla luciferase activities were measured after a 24 hr treatment with 1.0 μg/ml of TSA. The responses to TSA were reduced by the deletion of the region between –231 and –111. Therefore, this region is important for the activation of the HSV-tk promoter by TSA, and we named this region TSA1. The TSA1 region contained an octamer motif (ATTTGCAT), an NF-Y binding site (CCAAT), and a GC box. These elements are also reportedly important for the TSA-activation of other promoters (Hirose et al., 2003), consistent with our results. The TSA treatment also increased the gene expression by the CMV promoter, although the fold-increase was low. The reporter construct deletion mutant -77 almost lost its basal and TSA-induced activities. The region -281 ~ -77 is important for weak activation by TSA, and thus we named it TSA2. The weak TSA-stimulation may be related to the degenerate octamer motif (ATTTGCgT), the partial NF-Y binding site (CCAAg), and the GC box in the TSA2 region.

2.3 Development of chimeric promoters that significantly enhance transgene expression

A strong, drug-inducible promoter is urgently needed for cancer treatments, such as suicide gene therapy. The TSA1 site within the hsvTK promoter was important for the highest fold-increase. On the other hand, the CMV promoter showed the greatest induced strength, and the TSA2 site was relevant to the weak responsiveness to TSA. We succeeded in constructing chimeric promoters with a higher fold-increase and greater induced strength to TSA, by replacing the weak TSA2 site of the CMV promoter with two or three copies of the TSA1 sites of the hsvTK promoter. A schematic representation of the chimeric promoters is shown in Fig. 3a. The reporter assay revealed that the chimeric promoter HC1, containing two copies of TSA1, and the chimeric promoter HC3, containing three copies of TSA1, amplified transgene expression in response to TSA by 220.7-fold and 94.2-fold, respectively (Fig. 3b,c). The two chimeric promoters retained induced strength comparable to that of the CMV promoter.

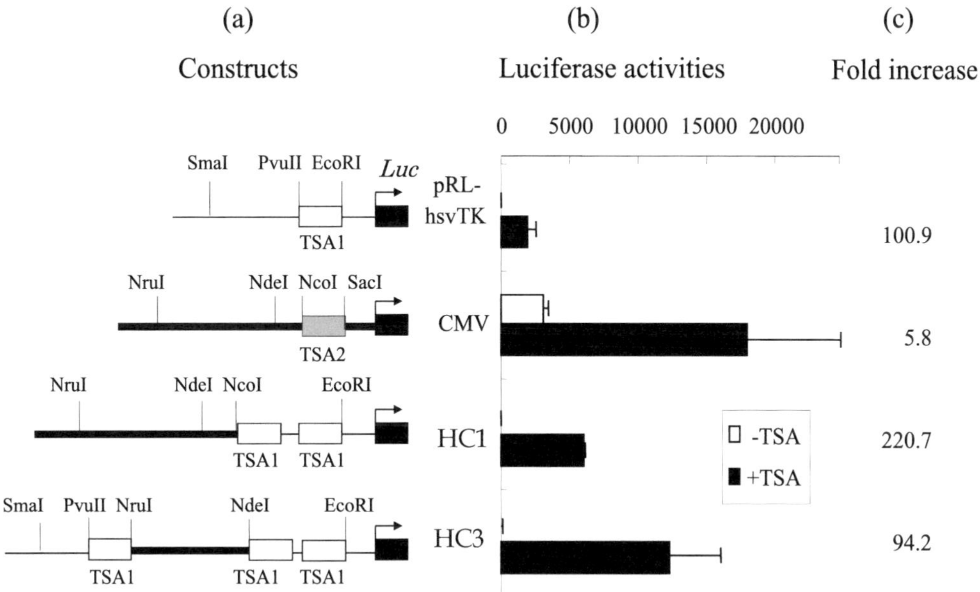

Fig. 3. The chimeric promoter of hsvTK and CMV enhanced transgene expression. (a) Schematic representations of the chimeric promoters. The open horizontal box represents the regulatory region in the hsvTK promoter (shown as a thin line) responsive to TSA (TSA1); the stippled horizontal box represents the regulatory region in the CMV promoter (shown as a thick line) responsive to TSA (TSA2); and the HC1 and HC3 chimeric promoters containing TSA1 and fragments of the CMV promoter are shown as a thick line. The restriction enzyme sites used to make the mutants are indicated. (b) Reporter assay of chimeric promoters. HeLa cells in a 96-well plate were transfected with 40ng of the various constructs in FuGene 6 transfection mixtures. The transfected HeLa cells were treated with/without 1.0 μg/ml of TSA for 24hr, and the Renilla luciferase activities were measured. Experiments were performed in triplicate. Values are means ± SD. (c) Fold increase: the ratio of luciferase activities in HeLa cells with or without TSA treatment. This figure was reproduced from *Int. J. Integ. Biol.*, 5: 108-115, 2009.

As shown in Fig. 4, we also found that a synthetic intron (0.2kb) from the pRL-TK vector and the long 3′-untranslated region (1.0kb) from the pSV2-neo vector are important for the basal expression of the transgene and the TSA-induction, respectively. The long 3′-untranslated region lowered the basal transgene activities in the HC3-L construct, and enhanced the TSA-stimulated transgene activities in all of the constructs (CMV-L, HC1-L, and HC3-L).

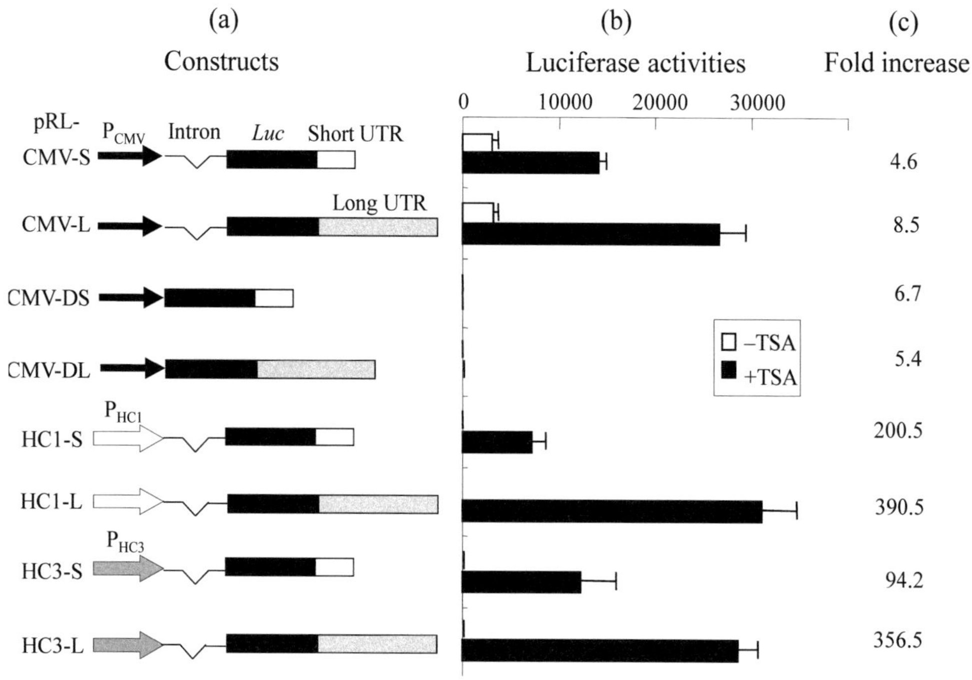

Fig. 4. Development of a modified CMV construct with intron and polyA sequences. (a) Transgene constructs modified with a synthetic intron and short and long 3′-untranslated regions. The closed solid horizontal box (▬) represents Renilla luciferase. The open horizontal box (▭) and the striped horizontal box (▭) represent the short and long 3′-untranslated regions (UTR), respectively. The broken line (¬√¬) represents the synthetic intron. The solid arrow (→), open arrow (⇨), and striped arrow (⇨) represent the CMV, HC1, and HC3 chimeric promoters, respectively. (b) Reporter assay of the constructs. HeLa cells in a 96-well plate were transfected with 40ng of the various constructs in FuGene 6 transfection mixtures. The transfected HeLa cells were treated with/without 1.0 μg/ml of TSA for 24 hr, and the Renilla luciferase activities were measured. Experiments were performed in triplicate. Values are means ± SD. (c) Fold increase: the ratio of luciferase activities in HeLa cells with or without TSA treatment. This figure was reproduced from *Int. J. Integ. Biol.*, 5: 108-115, 2009.

2.4 TSA-dependent induction of the stably integrated transgene under the chimeric promoters to kill target cells by different mechanisms.

Considering the various escape mechanisms employed by cancer cells, we introduced the molecules that can activate different cell death-inducing mechanisms. We placed the hsvTK gene for combination therapy with the prodrug Ganciclovir, and some strong death-inducing molecules (Bax, caspase8, and TRIF) under the TSA-responsible chimeric promoters. Suicide gene therapy has been proposed as a strategy for the treatment of cancer for many years (Culver et al., 1992; Fillat et al., 2003; Mooleten et al., 1990). One of the most widely used prodrug-activating gene therapies is the thymidine kinase gene of the herpes simplex virus (hsvTK), in combination with the non-toxic prodrug Ganciclovir (GCV) (Fig. 5). The principal effect of the hsvTK/GCV system is to generate GCV triphosphate (GCV-PPP) from the non-toxic prodrug GCV, by the introduced hsvTK and several cellular kinases, including guanylate kinase. The produced GCV-PPP inhibits the mammalian DNA polymerase due to its analogy with deoxyguanosine triphosphate, and leads to cell death. The hsvTK is required for the formation of GCV-PPP; however, the GCV treatment eradicated the majority of the population, even though only 10% of the cell population was expressing hsvTK (Freeman et al., 1993). The killing of hsvTK-negative cells by adjacent hsvTK positive cells is called "bystander killing effects", which depend mainly upon gap

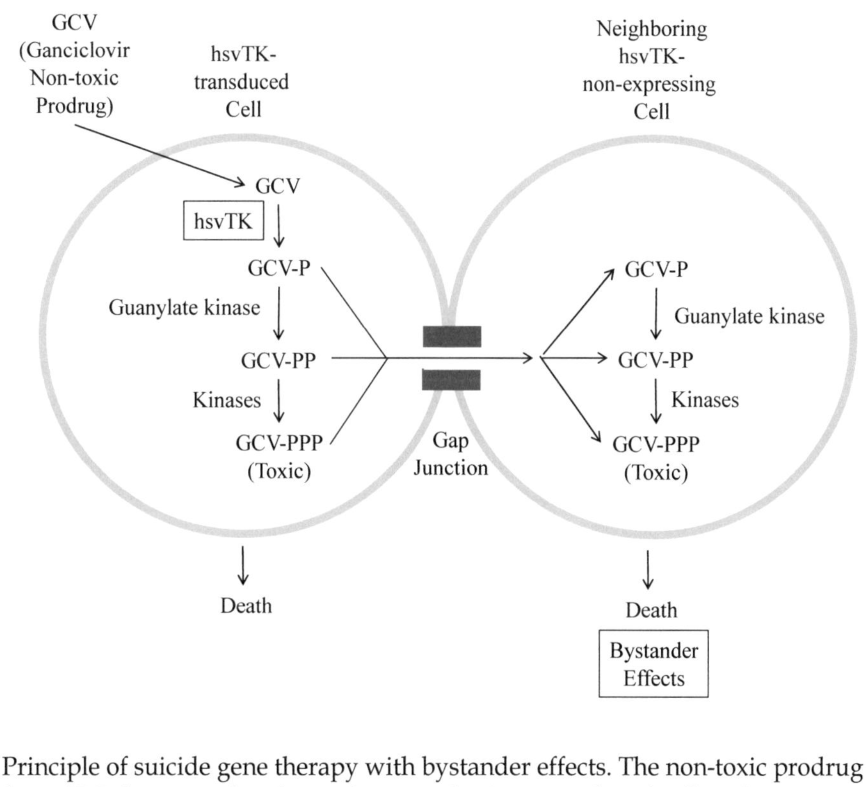

Fig. 5. Principle of suicide gene therapy with bystander effects. The non-toxic prodrug Ganciclovir (GCV) is assimilated into the target hsvTK-transduced cell, and is converted into the toxic triphosphorylated GCV (GCV-PPP) by hsvTK and several cellular kinases. GCV-PPP inhibits the mammalian DNA polymerase due to its analogy with deoxyguanosine triphosphate, and leads to cell death. In addition, GCV-PPP is transferred to the neighboring hsvTK-non-expressing cell via the gap junction, and the neighboring cell is also killed by the toxic GCV-PPP (Bystander killing effects).

junction formation, and has been established as a potentially powerful tool in cancer gene therapy (Fick et al., 1995; Denning & Pitts, 1997; Mesnil et al., 1996). To enhance the killing effects on cancer cells, the hsvTK suicide gene therapy is employed with other anti-cancer treatments, such as chemotherapy, radiotherapy, and immunotherapy. Especially, the combination therapy of hsvTK/GCV and HDAC inhibitors (HDACi) including TSA is promising for cancer therapy (Ammerpohl et al., 2004; Yamamoto et al., 2003), because HDACis have anti-cancer effects by inducing tumor cells to undergo differentiation, growth arrest and/or apoptosis, and by enhancing anti-tumor immunity, by altering gene expression through chromatin structure remodeling.

Other molecules (Bax, Caspase8, and TRIF) that induce apoptosis by activating different pathways should be beneficial for the treatment of various tumors, because each cancer employs various strategies to escape from the host immune surveillance and to gain growth advantages (Liu et al., 2011; Luo et al., 2009; Pavet et al., 2011). As shown in Fig. 6, two core pathways for inducing apoptosis exist: the extrinsic and intrinsic pathways. In the intrinsic pathway, the mitochondrion plays a central role. The mitochondrial membrane integrity is controlled by pro-apoptotic molecules (Bax, Bak, Bid, etc.) and anti-apoptotic molecules (Bcl-2, Bcl-x_L, etc.). The disruption of the membrane integrity by various stimuli, including DNA-damaging agents, increases the permeability and allows the release of cytochrome *c* and second mitochondria-derived activator of caspase (Smac)/direct IAP binding protein with low pH (DIABLO). The cytochrome *c* forms an apoptosome with apoptotic protease-activating factor-1 (Apaf-1) and caspase9 in the cytosol, and the Smac/DIABLO antagonizes the inhibitor of apoptosis proteins (IAPs) to enhance the activation of caspse9 and caspase3. As a result, the executioner caspase3 is effectively activated, to induce cell death. Actually, Bax overexpression has been reported to cause cell death in various cell types (Kitanaka et al., 1997; Tamm et al., 1998; Xiang et al., 1996). Caspase8 is the key enzyme in the extrinsic pathway. When the death receptors (Fas, DR3, DR4, etc.) are activated by their ligands, they recruit caspase8 via an adaptor molecule, Fas-associated death domain (FADD), and form the death-inducing signaling complex (DISC) to activate caspase8. The activated caspase8 not only activates caspase3 directly, but also activates the intrinsic pathway by removing the N-terminal region of Bid, thus producing its active, truncated form (tBid). Both signals work together to induce cell death by activating the executioner caspase3. TIR domain-containing adaptor protein (TRIF) is a key molecule that mediates the signals from pathogens via Toll-like receptor3 (TLR3) and TLR4, to trigger type I interferon production and inflammatory responses via interferon regulatory factor3 (IRF3) and Nuclear factor κB (NFκB), respectively (Kawai & Akira, 2010). Among these molecules related to the innate immune system, TRIF is a strong death-inducing molecule that activates caspse8 via receptor interacting proteins (RIPs) and FADD (Kaiser & Offermann et al., 2005).

To evaluate the utility of these TSA-responsive killer constructs for cancer gene therapy, we introduced the TSA-inducible hsvTK gene constructs to a well-characterized retroviral vector. Retroviral vectors are useful tools for the long-term expression of stably integrated transgenes in target cells, although there are risks due to insertional mutagenesis and the generation of replication competent retroviruses. We used a retroviral vector, pQC (Clontech) that self-inactivates the 5' LTR to avoid promoter interference, and to reduce the risk of transactivation of genome sequences around the integration site. The hsvTK, Bax, Caspase8, and TRIF genes were placed downstream of the chimeric promoters (P_{HC1}, and P_{HC3}), with the P_{PGK}-driven puromycin selection marker (Fig. 7).

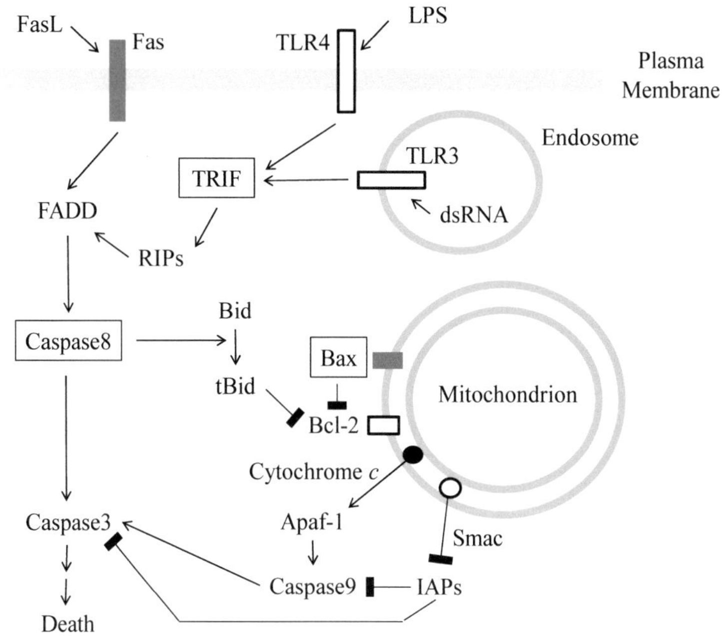

Fig. 6. Apoptosis pathways activated by Bax, Caspase8, and TRIF. Bax activates the intrinsic pathway of apoptosis by antagonizing the anti-apoptotic molecules (Bcl-2, Bcl-x_L, etc.) and increasing the permeability of the mitochondrion. The cytochrome *c* released from the intermembrane space of the mitochondrion forms an apoptosome with Apaf-1 and caspase9 in the cytosol, and leads to cell death by activating the executioner caspase3. Caspase8 is the key enzyme in the extrinsic pathway, where death receptors (Fas, DR4, DR5, etc.) activated by their ligands form the death-inducing signaling complex (DISC) with FADD and caspase8. The activated caspase8 leads to cell death by activating the executioner caspase3. TRIF is not only a key molecule that mediates the signal from pathogens via TLR3 and TLR4 to trigger type I interferon production and an inflammatory response, but also a strong death-inducing molecule by activating caspse8 via RIPs and FADD. Apaf-1, apoptotic protease-activating factor-1; DR4, Death receptor 4; FADD, Fas-associated death domain; TRIF, TIR domain-containing adaptor protein; TLR3, Toll-like receptor 3; RIP, receptor interacting proteins.⟶: stimulatory siganal. ——▮: inhibitory signal.

To verify the activities of the constructs, we examined whether the cells in which these constructs were transiently introduced are killed by TSA treatment. The 293T cells with the P_{HC1}- or P_{HC3}-hsvTK gene showed TSA- and GCV-dependent cell death. The cells with the P_{HC1}- or P_{HC3}-driven Bax, Caspase8, or TRIF genes were also killed with 0.1~0.3 μg/ml TSA treatment. Among them, TRIF triggered the most effective cell death. To examine the effects of TSA on the stably-introduced transgene expression, we obtained stable clones to express the death-inducing molecules under the control of the HC1 and HC3 promoters, by selection with puromycin for several weeks after the retroviral infection. The 293T cells containing the P_{HC1}-TRIF gene showed drastic cell death (apoptosis) upon a treatment with 0.1μg/ml TSA for 24h, as compared to the control 293T cells containing P_{CMV} only (Fig. 8). The chimeric promoter P_{HC1} maintained the TSA-responsiveness after becoming stably-integrated into the genome DNA.

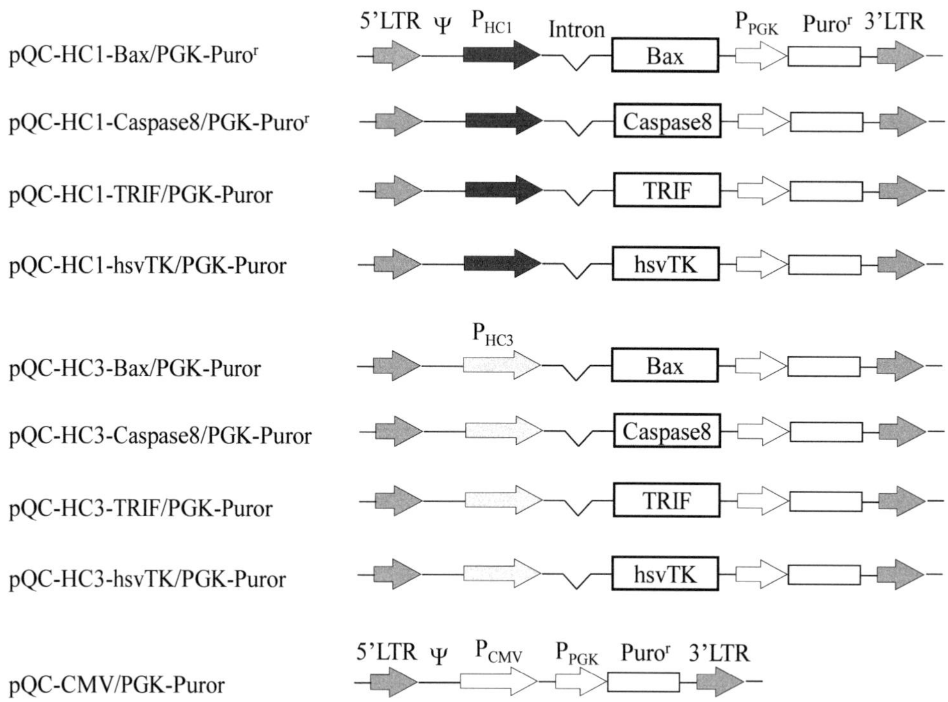

Fig. 7. Retroviral constructs. The retroviral vector, pQC (Clontech), that self-inactivates the 5' LTR to avoid promoter interference, was used to construct the expression plasmids. 5' LTR, the hybrid long terminal repeat, consists of the CMV type I enhancer and the mouse sarcoma virus promoter; Ψ, packaging signal; P_{HC1}, P_{HC3}, and P_{CMV}: the CMV, HC1, and HC3 chimeric promoters, respectively; Intron, the synthetic intron; P_{PGK}-Puro^r, PGK (murine phosphoglycerate kinase) promoter-driven puromycin resistance gene; 3' LTR, the Moloney murine leukemia virus LTR deleted in the U3. The death inducing genes (Bax, Caspase8, TRIF, and hsvTK) are boxed.

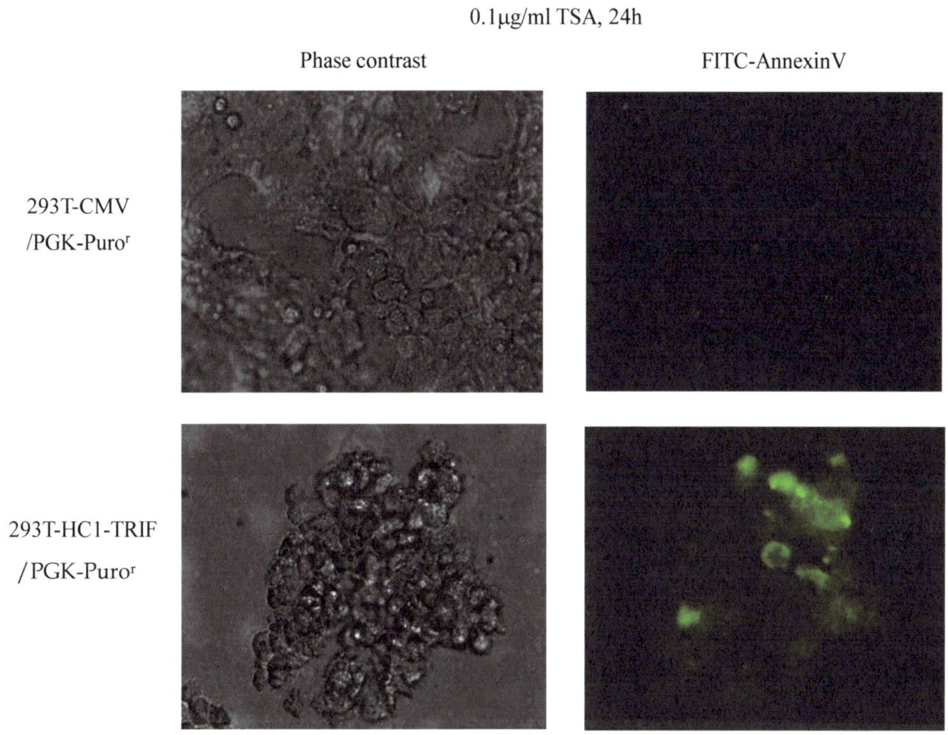

Fig. 8. TSA-induced cell death in the cells stably containing the P_{HC1}-TRIF transgene. The HEK293T cells introduced with the P_{HC1}-TRIF gene, or the control P_{CMV} promoter only, were selected in medium containing 1μg/ml puromycin for more than two weeks to obtain stable clones. The cells were then treated with 0.1μg/ml TSA for 24h to activate the P_{HC1} promoter. To detect the apoptotic cells, FITC-conjugated Annexin V was used according to the manufacturer's instructions. The HEK293T cells containing the P_{HC1}-TRIF gene showed drastic cell death (apoptosis), as compared to the control 293T cells containing P_{CMV} only.

On the other hand, adenoviral or adeno-associated viral vectors are preferable to retroviral or lentiviral vectors, to avoid insertional mutagenesis by the transgene in target cells. In addition, the vectors can be inserted with the long 3'-untranslated region (UTR), to enhance the TSA-responsiveness between the inverted terminal repeats (ITRs). We constructed several adenoviral vectors containing the death-inducing genes (Bax, Caspase8, TRIF, and hsvTK) under the chimeric promoters (P_{HC1} and P_{HC3}) with the long 3' UTR sequence (Fig. 9). To monitor the transfection and infection efficiencies easily, we added the EF1α promoter-driven GFP. The recombinant adenovirus constructs were transferred from a shuttle vector (Clontech) with the specific homing endonucleases I-CeuI and PI-SceI, and showed GFP expression in the HEK293 packaging cells.

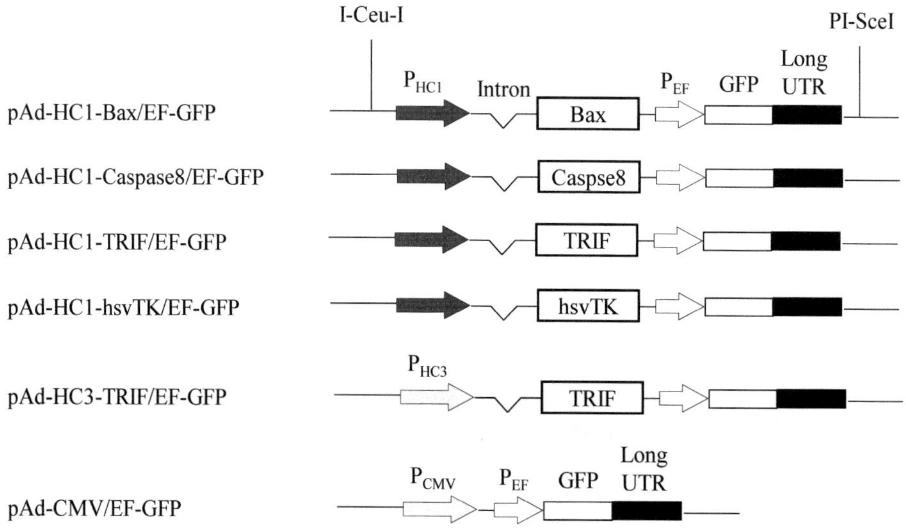

Fig. 9. Adenoviral constructs. The recombinant adenovirus constructs were created by transferring the fragments from a shuttle vector, pTRE-Shuttle2 (Clontech), with the specific homing endonucleases I-CeuI and PI-SceI to an adenoviral vector deleted in the E1 and E3 regions, pAdeno-X (Clontech). P_{HC1}, P_{HC3}, and P_{CMV}: the CMV, HC1, and HC3 chimeric promoters, respectively; Intron, the synthetic intron; P_{PGK}-Puro^r, PGK (murine phosphoglycerate kinase) promoter driving the puromycin resistance gene; Long UTR, long 3′-untranslated region. The death inducing genes (Bax, Caspase8, TRIF, and hsvTK) are boxed.

3. Specific delivery of transgenes to target cells

Another challenge is to deliver the transgene to the desired cells or tissues. Some specific delivery systems have been developed by engineering the viral envelope proteins of Lentivirus or Retrovirus, in a procedure referred to as pseudotyping, and incorporating specific antibodies and ligands (Mátrai et al., 2010). The pseudotyping with vesicular stomatitis virus glycoprotein (VSV-G) as a viral envelope protein has broadened the natural tropism of the virus to infect basically all human and murine cell types (Burns et al., 1993). Using various viral envelopes, the recombinant viruses can be introduced into different target cells, including lymphocytes and nerve cells (Colin et al., 2009; Funke et al., 2009; Miletic et al., 2004). Some viruses have two envelope proteins with distinct functions, to bind to the host receptor and to fuse with the membrane for entry (Buchholz et al., 2009). The E1 and E2 proteins of Sindbis virus (Morizono et al., 2005; Yang et al., 2006), and the H and F proteins of measles virus (Frecha et al. 2008; Funke et al., 2008) have been well characterized for the recombinant virus to infect a desired target cell (retargeting) with high transduction efficiency. The principle of retargeting using the measles H and F proteins is illustrated in Fig. 10. The natural receptor recognition of the measles H protein is ablated, and a ligand is attached that recognizes the cognate receptor on the target cell. Subsequent virus entry is mediated by the F protein pH-independently at the plasma membrane, and the transgene is delivered into the target cell. Using specific markers on target cells (specific epitope and antibody binding, or ligand and receptor binding), the transgene will be retargeted to the desired cell type. By combining this specific delivery system with a suicide gene, selective cell death of the target cells was achieved (Funke et al., 2008). Our TSA-responsible killer gene constructs can be applied to this retargeting system.

Finally, these TSA-responsible killer gene constructs can be used to eliminate the undesirable cells generated by inadvertent insertional mutagenesis in the process of gene therapy, as a biosafety measure.

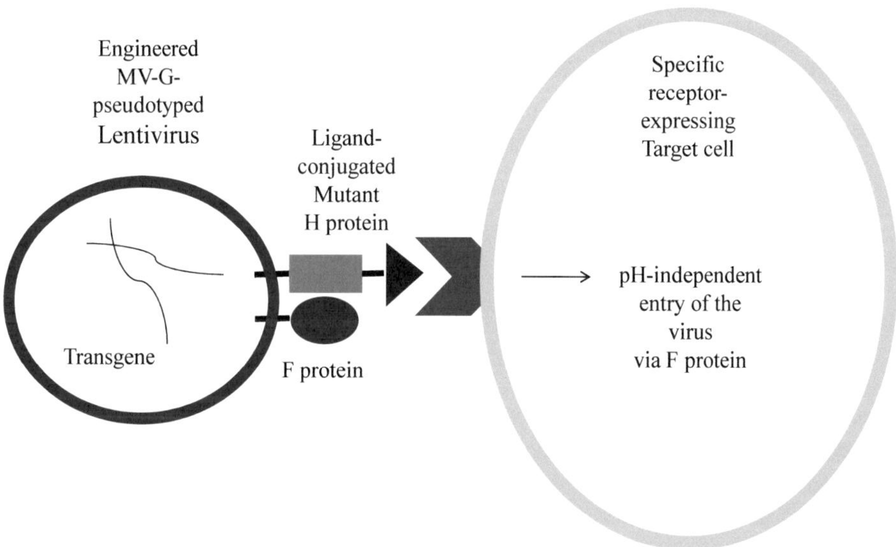

Fig. 10. Specific delivery of a transgene. The natural receptor recognition of the measles H protein is ablated, and a ligand is attached that recognizes the cognate receptor on the target cell. The virus entry is mediated by the F protein pH-independently at the plasma membrane, and the transgene is delivered into the target cell. Using specific epitope and antibody binding, or ligand and receptor binding, the transgene is delivered to the desired target cells.

4. Conclusions

Considering the various anti-cancer effects of TSA, an HDACi with the ability to reactivate silenced transgenes by altering the chromatin structure, we have developed TSA-inducible cell death systems to enhance the anti-cancer effects of TSA. The chimeric promoters P_{HC1} and P_{HC3} showed high TSA-responsiveness to express the death-inducing genes (hsvTK,

Bax, Capase8, and TRIF), and the cells in which the killer constructs were introduced showed TSA-dependent cell death. Combined with specific delivery systems to target cancer cells, these killer constructs will be beneficial for cancer gene therapy. We are planning to investigate the killer efficacies of other HDACis besides TSA, because various HDACis are now available for cancer therapy. The *in vivo* trials of these constructs with HDACis will be the crucial next step.

5. Acknowledgments

This work was supported by Grants-in-Aid from the Ministry of Education, Culture, Sports, Science and Technology of Japan, and by the Global Center of Excellence Program at Nagasaki University.

6. References

Ammerpohl, O.; Thormeyer, D.; Khan, Z.; Appelskog, I.B.; Gojkovic, Z.; Almqvist, P.M. & Ekström, T.J. (2004). HDACi phenylbutyrate increases bystander killing of HSV-tk transfected glioma cells. *Biochem Biophys Res Commun.* Vol.324, No.1 (November 2004), pp.8-14.

Bandyopadhyay, D.; Mishra, A. & Medrano, E.E.(2004). Overexpression of histone deacetylase 1 confers resistance to sodium butyrate-mediated apoptosis in melanoma cells through a p53-mediated pathway. *Cancer Res.* Vol.64, No.21 (November 2004), pp.7706-7710

Bolden, J.E.; Peart, M.J. & Johnstone, R.W. (2006). Anticancer activities of histone deacetylase inhibitors. *Nat Rev Drug Discov.* Vol.5, No.9 (September 2006), pp.769-784

Buchholz, C.J.; Mühlebach, M.D. & Cichutek, K. (2009). Lentiviral vectors with measles virus glycoproteins - dream team for gene transfer? *Trends Biotechnol.* Vol.27, No.5 (May 2009), pp.259-265.

Burns, J.C.; Friedmann, T.; Driever, W.; Burrascano, M. & Yee, J.K. (1993). Vesicular stomatitis virus G glycoprotein pseudotyped retroviral vectors: concentration to very high titer and efficient gene transfer into mammalian and nonmammalian cells. *Proc Natl Acad Sci U S A.* Vol.90, No.17 (September 1993), pp.8033-8037.

Chen, W.Y.; Bailey, E.C.; McCune, S.L.; Dong, J.Y. & Townes, T.M. (1997). Reactivation of silenced, virally transduced genes by inhibitors of histone deacetylase. *Proc Natl Acad Sci U S A.* Vol.94, No. 11 (May 1997), pp.5798-5803.

Colin, A.; Faideau, M.; Dufour, N.; Auregan, G.; Hassig, R.; Andrieu, T.; Brouillet, E.; Hantraye, P.; Bonvento, G. & Déglon, N. (2009). Engineered lentiviral vector targeting astrocytes in vivo. *Glia.* Vol. 57, No. 6 (April 2009), pp.667-679.

Culver, K.W.; Ram, Z.; Wallbridge, S.; Ishii, H.; Oldfield, E.H. & Blaese, R.M. (1992). In vivo gene transfer with retroviral vector-producer cells for treatment of experimental brain tumors. *Science.* Vol.256, No.5063 (June 1992), pp.1550-1552

Denning, C. & Pitts, J.D. (1997). Bystander effects of different enzyme-prodrug systems for cancer gene therapy depend on different pathways for intercellular transfer of toxic metabolites, a factor that will govern clinical choice of appropriate regimes. *Hum Gene Ther.* Vol.8, No.15 (October 1997), pp.1825-1835.

Dion, L.D.; Goldsmith, K.T.; Tang, D.C.; Engler, J.A.; Yoshida, M. & Garver, R.I. Jr. (1997). Amplification of recombinant adenoviral transgene products occurs by inhibition of histone deacetylase. *Virology.* Vol.231, No.2 (May 1997), pp.201-209.

Fick, J.; Barker, F.G. 2nd; Dazin, P.; Westphale, E.M.; Beyer, E.C. & Israel, M.A. (1995). The extent of heterocellular communication mediated by gap junctions is predictive of bystander tumor cytotoxicity in vitro. *Proc Natl Acad Sci U S A.* Vol.92, No.24 (November 1995), pp.11071-11075.

Fillat, C.; Carrió, M.; Cascante, A. & Sangro, B. (2003). Suicide gene therapy mediated by the Herpes Simplex virus thymidine kinase gene/Ganciclovir system: fifteen years of application. *Curr Gene Ther.* Vol.3, No.1 (February 2003), pp.13-26.

Frecha, C., Costa, C., Nègre, D., Gauthier, E., Russell, S.J., Cosset, F.L. & Verhoeyen, E. (2008). Stable transduction of quiescent T cells without induction of cycle progression by a novel lentiviral vector pseudotyped with measles virus glycoproteins. *Blood.* Vol.112, No.13 (December 2008), pp.4843-4852.

Freeman, S.M.; Abboud, C.N.; Whartenby, K.A.; Packman, C.H.; Koeplin, D.S.; Moolten, F.L. & Abraham, G.N. (1993). The "bystander effect": tumor regression when a fraction of the tumor mass is genetically modified. *Cancer Res.* Vol.53, No.21 (November 1993), pp.5274-5283.

Funke, S.; Maisner, A.; Mühlebach; M.D.; Koehl, U.; Grez, M.; Cattaneo, R.; Cichutek, K. & Buchholz, C.J. (2008). Targeted cell entry of lentiviral vectors. *Mol Ther.,* Vol.16, No.8 (August 2008), pp.1427-1436.

Funke, S.; Schneider, I.C.; Glaser, S.; Mühlebach, M.D.; Moritz, T.; Cattaneo, R.; Cichutek, K. & Buchholz, C.J. (2009). Pseudotyping lentiviral vectors with the wild-type measles virus glycoproteins improves titer and selectivity. *Gene Ther.* Vol.16, No.5 (May 2009), pp.700-705.

Gaspar-Maia, A.; Alajem. A.; Meshorer. E. & Ramalho-Santos, M. (2011). Open chromatin in pluripotency and reprogramming. *Nat Rev Mol Cell Biol.* Vol.12, No.1 (January 2011), pp. 36-47.

Haberland M.; Montgomery R.L. & Olson E.N. (2009). The many roles of histone deacetylases in development and physiology: implications for disease and therapy. *Nat Rev Genet.* Vol.10, No.1 (January 2009), pp.32-42

Harbers, K.; Jähner, D. & Jaenisch, R. (1981). Microinjection of cloned retroviral genomes into mouse zygotes: integration and expression in the animal. *Nature.* Vol.293, No.5833 (October 1981), pp.540-542

Hirose, T.; Sowa, Y.; Takahashi, S.; Saito, S.; Yasuda, C.; Shindo, N.; Furuichi K. & Sakai, T. (2003). p53-independent induction of Gadd45 by histone deacetylase inhibitor: coordinate regulation by transcription factors Oct-1 and NF-Y. *Oncogene.* Vol.22, No.49, (October 2003), pp.7762-7773.

Hoshino, I. & Matsubara, H. (2010). Recent advances in histone deacetylase targeted cancer therapy. *Surg Today.* Vol.40, No.9 (September 2010), pp. 809-815.

Jähner, D.; Stuhlmann, H.; Stewart, C.L.; Harbers, K.; Löhler, J.; Simon, I. & Jaenisch, R. (1982). De novo methylation and expression of retroviral genomes during mouse embryogenesis. *Nature.* Vol.298, No.5875 (August 1982), pp.623-628

Jensen, P.R.; Mincer, T.J.; Williams, P.G. & Fenical, W. (2005). Marine actinomycete diversity and natural product discovery. *Antonie Van Leeuwenhoek.* Vol.87, No.1 (January 2005), pp.43-48

Kaiser, W.J. & Offermann, M.K. (2005). Apoptosis induced by the toll-like receptor adaptor TRIF is dependent on its receptor interacting protein homotypic interaction motif. *J Immunol*, Vol.174, No.8 (April 2005), pp. 4942-4952.

Kawai, T. & Akira, S. (2010). The role of pattern-recognition receptors in innate immunity: update on Toll-like receptors. *Nat Immunol.* Vol.11, No.5 (May 2010), pp.373-384.

Khalighinejad, N.; Hariri, H.; Behnamfar, O.; Yousefi, A. & Momeni, A. (2008). Adenoviral gene therapy in gastric cancer: a review. *World J Gastroenterol.* Vol.14, No.2 (January 2008), pp.180-184.

Kikuchi, E.; Menendez, S.; Ozu, C.; Ohori, M.; Cordon-Cardo, C.; Logg, C.R.; Kasahara, N. & Bochner, B.H. (2007). Highly efficient gene delivery for bladder cancers by intravesically administered replication-competent retroviral vectors. *Clin Cancer Res.* Vol.13, No.15 Pt. 1 (August 2007), pp.4511-4518.

Kitanaka, C.; Namiki; T., Noguchi; K., Mochizuki; T., Kagaya, S.; Chi, S.; Hayashi, A.; Asai, A.; Tsujimoto, Y. & Kuchino, Y. (1997). Caspase-dependent apoptosis of COS-7 cells induced by Bax overexpression: differential effects of Bcl-2 and Bcl-xL on Bax-induced caspase activation and apoptosis. *Oncogene.* Vol.15, No.15 (October 1997), pp.1763-1772.

Liu, J.J.; Lin, M.; Yu, J.Y.; Liu, B. & Bao, J.K. (2011). Targeting apoptotic and autophagic pathways for cancer therapeutics. *Cancer Lett.* Vol.300, No.2 (January 2011), pp.105-114.

Luo, J.; Solimini, N.L. & Elledge, S.J. (2009). Principles of cancer therapy: oncogene and non-oncogene addiction. *Cell.* Vol.136, No.5 (March 2009), pp.823-837.

Ma, Y.; Kohno, T.; Igarashi, M.; Yasui, K.; Chua, K.J.; Matsuyama, T. & Hayashi, H. (2009). Effective transgene constructs for combination suicide gene therapy with trichostatin A. I*nt. J. Integ. Biol.* Vol.5, No.2, (February 2009) pp. 108-115, ISSN 0973-8363.

Ma, X.; Ezzeldin, H.H. & Diasio, R.B. (2009). Histone deacetylase inhibitors: current status and overview of recent clinical trials. *Drugs.* Vol.69, No.14, (October 2009), pp.1911-1934

Maeda, T.; Towatari, M.; Kosugi, H. & Saito, H. (2000). Up-regulation of costimulatory/adhesion molecules by histone deacetylase inhibitors in acute myeloid leukemia cells. *Blood.* Vol.96, No.12 (December 2000), pp. 3847-3856

Magner, W.J.; Kazim, A.L.; Stewart, C.; Romano, M.A.; Catalano, G.; Grande, C.; Keiser, N.; Santaniello, F. & Tomasi, T.B. (2000). Activation of MHC class I, II, and CD40 gene expression by histone deacetylase inhibitors. *J Immunol.* Vol.165, No.12 (December 2000), pp.7017-7024.

Mai, A.; Massa, S.; Rotili, D.; Cerbara, I.; Valente, S.; Pezzi, R.; Simeoni, S. & Ragno, R. (2005). Histone deacetylation in epigenetics: an attractive target for anticancer therapy. *Med Res Rev.* Vol.25, No.3 (May 2005), pp.261-309

Mátrai, J.; Chuah, M.K. & VandenDriessche, T. (2010). Recent advances in lentiviral vector development and applications. *Mol Ther.* Vol.8, No.3 (March 2010), pp.477-490.

Mesnil, M.; Piccoli, C.; Tiraby, G.; Willecke, K. & Yamasaki, H. (1996). Bystander killing of cancer cells by herpes simplex virus thymidine kinase gene is mediated by connexins. *Proc Natl Acad Sci U S A.* Vol.93, No.5 (March 1996), pp.1831-1835.

Miletic, H.; Fischer, Y.H.; Neumann, H.; Hans, V.; Stenzel, W.; Giroglou, T.; Hermann, M.; Deckert, M. & Von Laer, D. (2004). Selective transduction of malignant glioma by

Lentiviral vectors pseudotyped with lymphocytic choriomeningitis virus glycoproteins. *Hum Gene Ther.* Vol.15, No.11 (November 2004), pp.1091-1100.

Moolten, F.L.; Wells, J.M.; Heyman, R.A. & Evans, R.M. (1990). Lymphoma regression induced by ganciclovir in mice bearing a herpes thymidine kinase transgene. *Hum Gene Ther.* Vol.1, No.2 (Summer 1990), pp.125-134.

Morizono K.; Xie Y.; Ringpis G.E.; Johnson M.; Nassanian H.; Lee B.; Wu L. & Chen I.S. (2005). Lentiviral vector retargeting to P-glycoprotein on metastatic melanoma through intravenous injection. *Nat Med.* Vol.11, No.3 (March 2005), pp.346-352.

Nakata, S.; Yoshida, T.; Horinaka, M.; Shiraishi, T.; Wakada, M. & Sakai, T. (2004). Histone deacetylase inhibitors upregulate death receptor 5/TRAIL-R2 and sensitize apoptosis induced by TRAIL/APO2-L in human malignant tumor cells. *Oncogene.* Vol.23, No.37 (August 2004), pp.6261-6271.

Nayak, S. & Herzog, R.W. (2010). Progress and prospects: immune responses to viral vectors. *Gene Ther.* Vol.17, No.3 (March, 2010), pp.295-304.

Ogawa, K.; Yasumura, S.; Atarashi, Y.; Minemura, M.; Miyazaki, T.; Iwamoto, M.; Higuchi, K. & Watanabe, A. (2004). Sodium butyrate enhances Fas-mediated apoptosis of human hepatoma cells. *J Hepatol.* Vol.40, No.2 (February 2004), pp.278-284.

Palmer, T.D.; Rosman, G.J.; Osborne, W.R. & Miller, A.D. (1991). Genetically modified skin fibroblasts persist long after transplantation but gradually inactivate introduced genes. *Proc Natl Acad Sci U S A.* Vol.88, No.4 (February 1991), pp.1330-1334.

Park, S.R.; Park, J.W.; Jung, W.S.; Han, A.R.; Ban, Y.H.; Kim, E.J.; Sohng, J.K.; Sim, S.J. & Yoon, Y.J. (2008). Heterologous production of epothilones B and D in Streptomyces venezuelae. *Appl Microbiol Biotechnol.* Vol.81, No.1 (November 2008), pp.109-17.

Pavet V.; Portal M.M. & Moulin J.C., Herbrecht R. & Gronemeyer H. (2011). Towards novel paradigms for cancer therapy. *Oncogene.* Vol.6, No.1 (January 2011), pp.1-20.

Ruefli, A.A.; Ausserlechner, M.J.; Bernhard, D.; Sutton, V.R.; Tainton, K.M.; Kofler, R.; Smyth, M.J. & Johnstone, R.W. (2001). The histone deacetylase inhibitor and chemotherapeutic agent suberoylanilide hydroxamic acid (SAHA) induces a cell-death pathway characterized by cleavage of Bid and production of reactive oxygen species. *Proc Natl Acad Sci U S A.* Vol.98, No.19 (September 2001), pp.10833-10838.

Sliva, K. & Schnierle, B.S. (2010). Selective gene silencing by viral delivery of short hairpin RNA. *Virol J.* Vol.7, No.248 (September 2010).

Sonnemann, J.; Dreyer, L.; Hartwig, M.; Palani, C.D.; Hong, le T.T.; Klier, U.; Bröker, B.; Völker, U. & Beck, J.F. (2007). Histone deacetylase inhibitors induce cell death and enhance the apoptosis-inducing activity of TRAIL in Ewing's sarcoma cells. *J Cancer Res Clin Oncol.* Vol.133, No.11 (November 2007), pp.847-858.

Tamm, I.; Wang, Y.; Sausville, E.; Scudiero, D.A.; Vigna, N.; Oltersdorf, T. & Reed, J.C. (1998). IAP-family protein survivin inhibits caspase activity and apoptosis induced byFas (CD95), Bax, caspases, and anticancer drugs. *Cancer Res.* Vol.58, No.23 (December 1998), pp.5315-5320.

Xiang, J.; Chao, D.T. & Korsmeyer, S.J. (1996). BAX-induced cell death may not require interleukin 1 beta-converting enzyme-like proteases. *Proc Natl Acad Sci U S A.* Vol.93, No.25 (December 1996), pp.14559-14563.

Yamamoto, S.; Yamano, T.; Tanaka, M.; Hoon, D.S.; Takao, S.; Morishita, R.; Aikou, T. & Kaneda, Y. (2003). A novel combination of suicide gene therapy and histone deacetylase inhibitor for treatment of malignant melanoma. *Cancer Gene Ther.* Vol.10, No.3 (March 2003), pp.179-186.

Yang, L.; Bailey, L.; Baltimore, D. & Wang, P. (2006). Targeting lentiviral vectors to specific cell types in vivo. *Proc Natl Acad Sci U S A.* Vol.103, No.31 (August 2006), pp.11479-11484.

Wagner, J.M.; Hackanson, B.; Lübbert, M. & Jung, M. (2010). Histone deacetylase (HDAC) inhibitors in recent clinical trials for cancer therapy. *Clin Epigenetics.* Vol.1, No.3-4 (December 2010), pp. 117-136.

Zheng, Z.; Zeng, W.; Huang, Y.; Yang, Z.; Li, J.; Cai, H. & Su, W. (2000). Detection of antitumor and antimicrobial activities in marine organism associated actinomycetes isolated from the Taiwan Strait, China. *FEMS Microbiol Lett.* Vol.188, No.1 (July 2000), pp.87-91.

4

Suicide Gene Therapy by Herpes Simplex Virus-1 Thymidine Kinase (HSV-TK)

Dilip Dey and Gregory R.D. Evans
Aesthetic and Plastic Surgery Institute, University of California, Irvine, 200 S. Manchester Avenue, Suite 650, Orange, CA 92868 USA

1. Introduction

Suicide gene therapy for cancer treatment proposed by Moolten [1] started more than 25 years ago and has gained momentum with little variations in the original technology. At the current statistics, worldwide 1550 clinical trials of gene therapy have been reported (http://www.wiley.co.uk/genmed/clinical) among them 7% using suicide gene therapy. HSV-TK is the most well characterized suicide gene used for cancer therapy and in other diseases without inducing significant systemic toxicity [2] [3]. Chemotherapeutic drugs used for cancer therapy are problematic because they do not discriminate in their mode of action. Currently available drugs in the market are not cancer specific so functional concentration level in tumors cannot be reached without off-target toxicity level. This is specifically true for solid tumors where vascularization is poor and necrotic at the center of the tumor due to low oxygen and nutrient supply [4][5]. However, when the drug is activated by locally enzymatic reactions in a timely fashion, the metabolite is toxic for the tissue. The most widely used suicide genes are Herpes Simplex Virus-1 Thymidine Kinase (HSV-TK), and Cytosine Deaminase (CD) from the virus Herpes simplex or the bacterium *Escherichia coli* respectively [6][7].

Prior research has focused on the mechanism of initiation and development of tumors. It starts with the mutation of 1 or several genes, then gradually attains more genetic mutation and genomic instability during the evolution of tumor/cancer. Almost all the genes fall in 2 categories - oncogenes (derived from proto-oncogene) and tumor suppressor genes. There are many ways to treat various tumors ranging from benign to metastatic. Among them surgery followed by chemotherapeutic drug treatments is the widely used method of choice that damages the DNA and renders the cells apoptotic. Additionally, tumors can be cured by more subtle ways by restoring the function of tumor suppressor genes or disabling oncogenes, to prime the immune cells to act and down-regulate angiogenesis and metastatic activities. Solid tumors can be treated by intra-tumor delivery of suicide genes. The protein product of these genes catalyzes the formation of highly toxic metabolites following the application of some lesser toxic prodrugs. This leads to apoptosis or programmed cell death of the treated cells [8]. The apoptotic cells invite immune cells that further clear the tumor zone by phagocytosis.

Suicide gene therapy is also known as Gene Directed Enzyme/Prodrug therapy (GDEPT) or as Gene Prodrug Activation Therapy (GPAT). GDEPT can either take the form of CBT (cell based therapy) where nearby cells of the tumor are modified to express suicide gene or the tumor itself expresses the suicide gene therapy. GDEPT can also be used for viral vectors which itself carries the suicide gene. GDEPT (Molecular chemotherapy) has advantages over classical therapy. As only tumor cells posses the enzyme that converts prodrug to active metabolites, it increases the toxicity level several fold inside the tumor whereas the vast majority of the host cells are unaffected. By using tumor specific regulatory elements (promoter) drugs can be activated only in tumor cells [9][10] has used the technique where the drug is only preferentially activated in the hypoxic regions of the tumor. By harnessing the bystander effects, more destruction of tumor cells have been rendered.

2. Properties of suicide gene

To be considered as a suicide gene, the product enzyme should be either absent or present in low concentrations (low expression) in the host. It should have a high catalytic activity, so that tumor cells can convert this prodrug even in low substrate concentration (high K_{CAT}, low K_m). To be considered as an ideal therapeutic agent, it should have/possess the following criteria. 1) The drug should be non-toxic or minimally toxic prior to activation and highly toxic after enzymatic activation. 2) The prodrug should be able to effectively penetrate the tumor, distributed and taken up by individual cells. 3) It should have a high affinity for the transduced suicide gene and low affinity for cellular enzyme. The HSV-TK enzyme has 1000 times more affinity for the substrate GCV than the host cell TK [11]. 4) The metabolite should have a half-life that extends long enough to kill the tumor so that drug is not lost before reaching its concentration.

3. Types of suicide genes for therapy

There are several suicide gene therapies. Among them HSV1-TK and cytodine deaminase are important. Cytidine Deaminase: Cytosine Deaminase (CD) is an enzyme found in some bacteria and fungi that deaminates cytosine to uracil [12]. It can also convert the nontoxic 5-fluorocytosine (5-FC) into the toxic compound 5-fluorouracil (5-FU) [13]. Mammalian cells do not contain CD. This property allows the drug to be used for suicide gene therapy especially for the treatment of cancer. The sensitivity of tumor to CD drug depends on dose, duration etc. This review will mainly focus on HSV-TK gene therapy.

HSV-TK: TK converts GCV into a toxic metabolite that kills cells widely used for cancer therapy. HSV1-TK can also phosphorylate various nucleoside analogs of GCV such as acyclovir, ganciclovir, and penciclovir.

4. Mode of action of HSV-TK

HSV-1 encodes about 70 genes some are immediate early genes. TK is one of the immediate early (IE) genes that give rise to a 376 amino acid long protein. IE genes can be defined as genes that show rapid and transient expression in the absence of *de novo* protein synthesis; some viruses posses IE genes. HSV1 virus is neurotropic (preferentially attacks nerve cells to avoid immune cells) and TK is necessary when the virus goes into the lytic cycle from a dormant stage in the neural cells. During TK suicide gene therapy, GCV is injected systemically way and upon reaching the tumor area, the drug is monophosphorylated by HSV-TK, and further phosphorylation is done by the host cell kinase. This triphosphate form of GCV (deoxythymidine triphosphate) is an analog of purine which inhibits DNA polymerase and is the most toxic. Cancer cells are actively proliferating and synthesizing DNA; the purine analogs GCV triphosphate competes with triphosphate substrate for DNA polymerase and are incorporated in the nascent DNA. This results the DNA polymerase enzyme stall and termination of nuclear and mitochondrial DNA synthesis initiating the cascades of apoptosis paths. [14][1]. The mechanism for cell death with HSV-TK is not completely known. Apoptosis induction or the sensitization of CD95- L, TNF, and TNF-related apoptosis-inducing ligands may contribute to cell death [15]. Yang *et al.* suggested that apoptosis occurred as a result of GCV-induced cell cycle arrests rather than direct chemical effects [16]. Depletion of the T-cells had no effect on the response [17]. The bystander effect causes local inflammation and the apoptotic cells invites dendritic cells and immune effectors (immune response) and further clears the tumor [18][19].

5. Bystander effect mediated by gap junctions

The bystander effect can amplify the effect of toxic drugs several fold. The toxic form of the drug should have diffusible property so that it can kill the non-transduced tumor cells through the bystander effect; in case of absence of diffusion, it should be taken up by surrounding cells by active transport. The action/effect of drug should also be cell cycle independent. Although cancer cells are highly proliferating, at a particular given time only a fraction of cells are dividing. In these cases drug distribution by diffusion is helpful. Moreover, in case of solid tumors only 10% of the cells can be transduced; in that case tumor ablation is mainly dependent on the bystander effect. Phospho-GCV is about a 500 daltons molecule. Such a small molecule should spread to surrounding cells by diffusion. But phospho-GCV is not dissolved in the cell lipid membrane. So, they spread to neighboring cells by gap junction that mainly consists of connexin family of proteins among them connexin-43 is the most studied. Gap junctions are a narrow connecting channel (2-3 nm diameter) between cells that facilitates the exchange of small molecules less than 1.5 kd in size. The gap is bridged by connexins, a family of 21 proteins. Gap junction exchanges small metabolites, second messengers and electric signals through a procedure called Gap Junctional Intercellular Communication (GJIC) [20]. Gap junction allows the ablation of the entire tumor although all cells in the tumor do not contain the suicide gene. This phenomenon is known as bystander effect and has boosted/amplified the toxic effect. Many kinds of cells express gap junction and are connected with neighboring cells. Some of the brain tumors (gliomas) do not express gap junctions or downregulate gap junctions [21]. Several studies have been done to deliver connexin-43 with the suicide gene so that the bystander effect through diffusion of active drug can take place. This was attempted by the pharmacological administration of cAMP analogs, hydroxyurea etc. [22]. Various reports of using connexin-26 and connexin-43 for the augmentation of the bystander effect have been published [23][9]. Solid tumors from both humans and rodents express lower amount of connexin and gap junction [24]. Established cell lines derived from tumors also downregulate expression of connexin and sometimes lack gap junction. Fusion proteins consisting of HSVtk and 11 amino acids from HIV-1 TAT protein have been demonstrated to provide gap-junction independent intercellular trafficking [25].

6. Variations of original HSV-TK approach

HSV1-TK suicide gene therapy is used for glioma [26], prostate cancer [27], leukemia [28] and lymphoma. Potency of original HSV-TK has been improved by the application of various strategies. An approach was made to deliver fusion protein of TK and viral tegument protein VP22 (to increase the bystander effect) [29] and by the use of fusion protein of HIV TAT and TK (that is more stable than wild type TK) [30]. Cerepro (sitimagene ceradenovec) is a recombinant adenoviral vector consisting of HSV-TK and replication deficient (where E1 and part of E3 genes have been deleted). After the brain surgery, this vector was injected immediately. Upon intra-peritoneal administration of GCV, the volume of the tumor was reduced [31]. It is found that GCV is a substrate for ABCG2 (ATP-binding cassette sub-family G member 2, also known as the breast cancer resistance protein) and glioblastoma side population can pump out small molecule drugs like GCV rendering it resistant to therapy whereas non-side populations are susceptible [32]. Due to toxicity of the surrounding healthy tissue especially liver parenchyma cells in liver tumor, the use of TK has limited its clinical usefulness [33]. This problem has been improved by injecting the vector inside the tumor or using engineered HSV-TK under tumor specific promoter like α-fetoprotein. [34]. Ad.TK was injected intratumorally in hepatocellular carcinoma (HCC) and it did not show any toxicity in normal liver tissue and the therapy was well tolerated. Ad.TK can be safely used in HCC patient upto $2X10^{12}$ viral Particles/patient [35]. The HSV-TK gene has been successfully transferred into hepatoma cells (BEL-7402), and the growth potential of these cells was significantly inhibited by the application of GCV [36]. The bystander effect was further boosted by a combination therapy of co-expression of TK and E-cadherin genes in adenoviral vector. E-cadherin expression modulates the gap junction by connexin expression. It is assumed that E-cadherin expression facilitates connexin transport to the plasma membrane thus connexin stabilized and minimize connexin internalization and degradation by lysosomes and proteosome mediated degradation [37]. The role of E-cadherin in suicide gene therapy is established in an in *vivo* model of pancreatic ductal adenocarcinoma. This way it was possible to increase the bystander effect by treating the tumor with HSV-TK+E-cad [38]. Additionally, the increase of E-cad expression. also down regulates bcl-2 (an anti-apoptotic gene) rendering cell death. Non-human primate marmoset is used as a transgenic model for preclinical studies. HSV-TK knock-in marmoset stem cell line (cmES) was established using RMCE (Cre recombinase-mediated cassette exchange). From the cmES cell line-generated tumor cells were effectively destroyed by GCV treatment. Thus, HSV-TK and GCV treatment may ensure safety of stem cell therapy [39]. In NSCLC (non-small cell lung cancer), human telomerase reverse transcriptase hTERT is up-regulated. Thus hTERT promoter controlled E1A (Ad.hTERT-E1A-TK /GCV) gene expression in NSCLC, efficiently killed different types of tumor cells and could be used a safe and potent therapy for NSCLC [40]. One group has used piggyBack vector for HSV-TK delivery and GCV treatment for gene therapy of cervical cancer [41]. Co-transfection of insulin like growth factor-I (IGF-I) and HSVTK by liposome promotes wound healing and minimizes the scar formation [42]. Adenoviral vectors containing HSVTK were transfected into T47D human breast cancer cells [43]. When grown in nude mice, administration of GCV markedly demonstrated regression of tumors over control animals [44]. Fong *et al.* demonstrated that ablation of CT26 tumor cells *in situ* was achieved by directly injecting high-titer HSV-TK retroviral vector preparations into the site of tumor cell inoculation followed by intra-peritoneal delivery of GCV [45]. Chondrosarcoma cells implanted into nude mice were injected with HSV-TK. After 4 weeks, the growth of tumors was significantly prevented [46]. Suicide gene therapy can be used as a tool for molecular biology research. Evans G *et al.* have used HSV-TK suicide gene therapy to shut down Nerve Growth Factor (NGF) when its intended job is done i.e. the bridging of nerve gaps have been achieved [47]. Suicide gene was used as a molecular off switch for growth factor expression in a tissue engineered construct after the successful healing of the defect, both morphologically and functionally. NGF-producing HEK-293 called as hNGF-EcR-293 cells were genetically modified to incorporate HSV-TK gene as a suicide gene for cell kill upon treatment with GCV. The combination of the inducible NGF expression system with the HSV-TK system offers regulation of time and presumed dose-dependent NGF expression at the site of the lesion with a subsequent elimination of genetically engineered cells within the conduit.

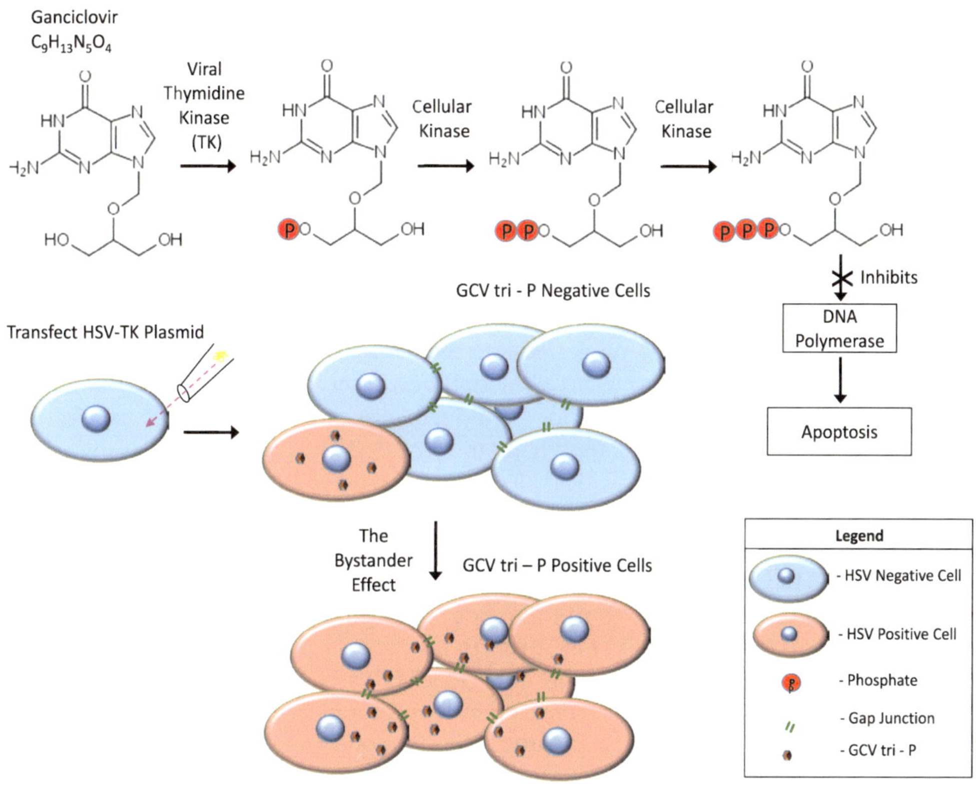

Fig. 1. Conversion of Ganciclovir by HSV-TK and cellular kinase to Ganciclovir triphosphate. The drug GCV is monophosphorylated by HSV-TK, and further phosphorylation is done by the host cell kinase. This triphosphate form of GCV (deoxythymidine triphosphate) is an analog of purine which inhibits DNA polymerase and is the most toxic. The bystander effect is mediated by the intercellular gap junctions present in many kinds of tissues and tumors.

One particular problem with the gene therapy is that retroviral vectors integrate in the genome randomly consequently it may potentially activate a proto-oncogene or silent a tumor suppressor gene rendering the cell to tumorigenesis. Insertion induced mutagenesis is a rare event at a frequency between 10^{-6} and 10^{-8} per insertion event [48]. Adenine

Deaminase (ADA) and Severe Combined Immuno-Deficiency (SCID) are genetic (inherited) disorders where the babies are born with immune deficiency and are vulnerable to common infections that others can resist in their everyday life. Several gene therapy approaches were used to deliver the corrected version of the gene in SCID patients by retroviral delivery. Patients regained immunity within 2-5 months but surprisingly several patients died due to cancer. Upon investigation, it was found that the virus has a preponderance to integrate in the vicinity of the human T-cell oncogene, LMO2 [49]. This probably due to retroviral transgene that has cotransforming role in leukemogenesis by giving advantages of increased cell proliferation or decreased apoptosis. As a cautionary measure, further trial of gene therapy was stopped. Delivery of HSV-TK fused with the therapeutic gene of interest into the therapeutic vector can be used for gene therapy. When the therapeutic gene has done its intended job, the cells harboring the gene and HSV-TK can be selectively eliminated by the administration of GCV. Thus killing the cells after gene therapy can be protective before the oncogene can do any harm. The GCV system has also been utilized in the non-oncologic setting. *In vivo* transduction with HSV-TK adenoviral vector followed by GCV treatment significantly inhibited the development of posterior capsule opacification from hyperplasia of the lens epithelium in the rabbit. Further, HSV-TK plasmid DNA has been injected into the joint space of rabbits with antigen-induced arthritis and when treated with GCV, results demonstrated a reduction in joint swelling in the HSV-TK–transduced knees [50]. Barbier *et al.* in an open and single-arm study on 48 patients, demonstrated that intracerebral injection of HSV-TK carrying cells into glioblastoma multiforme (GBM) did not result in any adverse effects [51]. HSV-TK has also been injected into the white matter of the right frontal lobe in two rhesus monkeys, with no clinical symptoms observed [52]. Murata *et al.* have demonstrated that like the Muristerone A–inducible system, the HSV-TK suicide gene allows for dose- and time-dependent regulation of cell death upon the application of GCV [53].

HSV-TK was modified to be able to migrate to neighboring cells and expand the expression of TK positive cells. A secreting form of HSV-TK was constructed by adding Igkappa leader peptide in the TK gene. An endoplasmic reticulum export signal was added to further increase the secretion. This resulted in the 70% of total protein secreted. However, enzyme activity of the secreted protein was decreased. This may present a hurdle for the development of a transmitted form of TK [54]. Microbubble destruction by ultrasound increases the efficiency of HSV-TK transfection [55]. HCC induces intrahepatic metastatic growth which is difficult to treat and prognosis is poor. A novel approach to introduce chemokine ligand 2/monocyte chemoattractant protein-1 (CCL2/MCP-1) and HSV-TK together increases the efficiency of gene therapy. CCL2/MCP-1 attracts T helper 1-polarized antitumor activity without inducing tumor angiogenesis [56]. By using an IRES sequence, a plasmid was constructed with 2 suicide genes driven by PSMA promoter. The genes are FCY1 and HSV-TK for metabolizing the drug. Introducing the combination of 5-FC and GCV drugs inhibited the growth of prostate tumor compared to each drug individually. In a xenograft mouse model, retarded tumor growth was also observed. This suggests that the combination of multiple suicide genes may be more effective in prostate tumor [57]. Adenovirus mediated HSV-TK is a promising adjuvant therapy for patient's having high grade glioma. This is a choice as surgery for malignant glioma is difficult due to its location and non-metastatic nature of glioma. The HSV-TK attacks the dividing tumor cells without harming healthy neurons which are non-dividing [58]. Pancreatic tumor was treated with mesenchymal stem cells (MSC) containing a CCL5 promoter. Homing of MSC cells into primary pancreatic tumor stroma and activation of the CCL5 promoter takes place. About one week later after stem cell treatment tumor size reduced to 50% and metastasis reduced significantly [59]. Use of undifferentiated embryonic stem (ES) cells may form teratomas thus limiting the use of stem cells in clinical setting. However, HCV-TK with Oct4 promoter construct was injected to ES cells. Upon treatment with GCV, undifferentiated cells die but differentiated cells are free from harm [60]. Combination gene therapy using multidrug resistance (MDR1) shRNA and HPV-TK [61], targeting angiogenesis of hepatocellular carcinoma with GCV treatment has been done [62]. Transfection of wild type p53 makes C6 glioma cells more susceptible to GCV treatment [63]. HIV-1 transactivator protein transduction domain (TAT PTD) can penetrate the cell. Cytotoxicity of GCV was enhanced by the fusion of HSV-TK and TAT PTD [64]. Fusion of mutant HSV-TK (with improved GCV activation) and guanylate kinase enhances prodrug sensitivity [65].

7. Disadvantage or drawback

GCV has toxic side effects especially on bone marrow cells. So, it is administered in lower concentrations [66] and has been used in animal model studies. The disadvantage of using GCV is that although GCV is readily diffusible, its metabolite triphosphate is membrane insoluble and can't diffuse to surrounding cells. However, the bystander effect of the close proximity/neighboring cells happen as triphosphate is transported to nearby cells through the gap junctions.

8. Conclusion

Suicide gene therapy is a method of choice to ablate cells in many diseases including cancer. But like other techniques this method is not fully safe and efficacious. HSV-TK gene therapy is still evolving and the method has been tinkered to be applicable in various cell background and different goal. More works need to be done for future applications.

9. References

[1] F. Moolten. Tumor chemosensitivity conferred by inserted herpes thymidine kinase genes: paradigm for a prospective cancer control strategy. *Cancer Res* 1986; 46: 5276–5281.

[2] C. Fillat, M. Carrio, A. Cascante, B. Sangro. Suicide gene therapy mediated by the Herpes Simplex virus thymidine kinase gene/Ganciclovir system: fifteen years of application. *Curr Gene Ther* 2003; 3: 13–26.

[3] Y. Shen, J. Nemunaitis. Herpes simplex virus 1 (HSV-1) for cancer treatment. *Cancer Gene Ther* 2006; 13: 975–992.

[4] R. Jain, Normalization of tumor vasculature: an emerging concept in antiangiogenic therapy, *Science* 2005; 307; 58–62.

[5] L. Munn. Aberrant vascular architecture in tumors and its importance in drug-based therapies. *Drug Discov. Today* 2003. 8 (9), 396–403.

[6] A. Miller. Human gene therapy comes to age. *Nature* 1992; 357, 455.

[7] M. Black, T. Newcomb, H. Wilson, and L. Loeb. Creation of drug-specific herpes simplex virus type 1 thymidine kinase mutants for gene therapy. *Proc. Natl. Acad. Sci. USA* 1996; 93, 3525.

[8] P. Seth. Vector-mediated cancer gene therapy: an overview. *Cancer Biol. Ther.* 2005; 4 (5), 512–517.

[9] Saukkonen, K., Hemminki, A. Tissue-specific promoters for cancer gene therapy. *Expert Opin. Biol. Ther.* 2004; 4 (5), 683–696.

[10] A. Yakkundi , V. McErlane, M. Murray, H. McCarthy, C. Ward, C. Hughes, L. Patterson, D. Hirst, S. McKeown, T. Robson. Tumor-selective drug activation: a GDEPT approach utilizing cytochrome P450 1A1 and AQ4N. *Cancer Gene Ther.* 2006; 13 (6), 598–605.

[11] G. Elion, P. Furman, J. Fyfe, P. de Miranda, L. Beauchamp, H. Schaeffer. Selectivity of action of an antiherpetic agent, 9-(2-hydroxyethoxymethyl) guanine. *Proc. Natl. Acad. Sci. USA* 1977; 74 (12), 5716–5720.

[12] E. Austin, B. Huber. A first step in the development of gene therapy for colorectal carcinoma: cloning, sequencing, and expression of Escherichia coli cytosine deaminase. *Mol. Pharmacol.* 1993; 43 (3), 380–387.

[13] A. Polak, and H. Scholer. Mode of action of 5-fluorocytosine and mechanisms of resistance. *Chemotherapy* (Basel), 1975; 21: 113-130.

[14] T. Matthews, R. Boehme. Antiviral activity and mechanism of action of ganciclovir. *Rev Infect Dis* 1998; 10(Suppl 3): S490–S494.

[15] C. Beltinger, S. Fulda, T. Kammertoens, E. Meyer, W. Uckert, and K. Debatin. Herpes simplex virus thymidine kinase/ganciclovir induced apoptosis involves ligand inde- pendent death receptor aggregation and activation of cas- pases. *Proc. Natl. Acad. Sci. USA* 1999; 96, 8699.

[16] S. Wei, Y. Chao, Y. Hung, W. Lin, D. Yand, L. Ch'ang, J. Whang-Peng, and W. Yang. S- and G2- phase cell cycle arrest and apoptosis induced by ganciclovir in murine melanoma cells transduced with herpes simplex virus thymidine kinase. *Exp. Cell Res.* 1998; 241, 66.

[17] S. Hall, M. Sanford, G. Atkinson, and S. Chen. Induction of potent antitumor natural killer cell activity by herpes simplex virus thymidine kinase and ganciclovir therapy in an orthotopic mouse model of prostate cancer. *Cancer Res.* 1998; 58, 3221.

[18] A. Kianmanesh, H. Perrin, Y. Panis, M. Fabre, H. Nagy, D. Houssin et al. A "distant" bystander effect of suicide gene therapy: regression of nontransduced tumors together with a distant transduced tumor. *Hum Gene Ther* 1997; 8: 1807–1814.

[19] S. Kuriyama, M. Kikukawa, K. Masui, H. Okuda, T. Nakatani, T. Akahane *et al.* Cancer gene therapy with HSV-tk/GCV system depends on T-cell-mediated immune responses and causes apoptotic death of tumor cells in vivo. *Int J Cancer* 1999; 83: 374–380.

[20] D. Goodenough, & D. Paul. Gap junctions. *Cold Spring Harbor Perspect. Biol.* 1, a 002576 (2009).

[21] T. Jimenez, W. Fox, C. Naus, J. Galipeau, D. Belliveau. Connexin over-expression differentially suppresses glioma growth and contributes to the bystander effect following HSV-thymidine kinase gene therapy. *Cell Commun Adhes* 2006; 13: 79–92.

[22] B. Gentry, P. Boucher, D. Shewach. Hydroxyurea induces bystander cytotoxicity in cocultures of herpes simplex virus thymidine kinase-expressing and nonexpressing HeLa cells incubated with ganciclovir. *Cancer Res.* 2006; 66 (7), 3845–3851.

[23] T. Nicholas, S. Read, F. Burrows, C. Kruse. Suicide gene therapy with Herpes simplex virus thymidine kinase and ganciclovir is enhanced with connexins to improve gap junctions and bystander effects. *Histol. Histopathol.* 2003; 18 (2), 495–507.

[24] D. Laird, P. Fistouris, G. Batist, L. Alpert, T. H. Huynh, G. Carystinos, and M. Alaoui-Jamali. Deficiency of connexin 43 gap junctions is an independent marker for breast tumors. *Cancer Res.* 1999; 59, 4104–4110.

[25] E. Tasciotti, M. Giacca, Fusion of the human immunodeficiency virus type 1 tat protein transduction domain to thymidine kinase increases bystander effect and induces enhanced tumor killing in vivo. *Hum. Gene Ther.* 2005; 16, 1389–1403.

[26] H. Miletic, Y. Fischer, T. Giroglou, et al. Suicide Gene Therapy of Malignant Glioma Normal Brain Cells Contribute to the Bystander Effect in Suicide Gene Therapy of Malignant Glioma. *Clin Cancer Res* 2007;13:6761-6768.

[27] Allan J. Pantuck, Jamie Matherly, Amnon Zisman, David Nguyen, Frank Berger, Sanjiv S. Gambhir, Margaret E. Black, Arie Belldegrun, and Lily Wu. Optimizing Prostate Cancer Suicide Gene Therapy Using Herpes Simplex Virus Thymidine Kinase Active Site Variants. *Human Gene Therapy* 2002; 13:000–000.

[28] M. Blumenthal, D. Skelton, K. Pepper, T. Jahn, E. Methangkool and D. Kohn. Effective Suicide Gene Therapy for Leukemia in a Model of Insertional Oncogenesis in Mice. *Molecular Therapy* 2007; 15, 183–192. doi:10.1038/sj.mt.6300015

[29] M. Dilber, A. Phelan, A. Aints, A. Mohamed, G. Elliott, C. Smith, P. O'Hare. Intercellular delivery of thymidine kinase prodrug activating enzyme by the herpes simplex virus protein, VP22. *Gene Ther.* 1999; 6 (1), 12–21.

[30] L. Cao, J. Si, W. Wang, X. Zhao, X. Yuan, H. Zhu, X. Wu, J. Zhu, G. Shen. Intracellular localization and sustained prodrug cell killing activity of TAT-HSVTK fusion protein in hepatocellular carcinoma cells. *Mol. Cells.* 2006; 21 (1), 104–111.

[31] G. Langford, A. Dayan, S. Yla-Herttuala, D. Eckland. A preclinical assessment of the safety and biodistribution of an adenoviral vector containing the herpes simplex virus thymidine kinase gene (Cerepro) after intracerebral administration. *J Gene Med.* 2009;11(6):468-76.

[32] W. Hu, W. Liu. Side populations of glioblastoma cells are less sensitive to HSV-TK/GCV suicide gene therapy system than the non-side population. In Vitro Cell Dev *Biol Anim.* 2010 Jun;46(6):497-501. Epub 2010 Feb 5.

[33] A. Yakkundi, V. McErlane, M. Murray, H. McCarthy, C. Ward, C. Patterson, M. Herraiz, N. Beraza, A. Solano, B. Sangro, J. Montoya, C. Qian et al. Liver failure caused by herpes simplex virus thymidine kinase plus ganciclovir therapy is associated with mitochondrial dysfunction and mitochondrial DNA depletion. *Hum Gene Ther* 2003; 14: 463–472.

[34] H. Su, R. Lu, J. Chang, Y. Kan. Tissue-specific expression of herpes simplex virus thymidine kinase gene delivered by adeno-associated virus inhibits the growth of human hepatocellular carcinoma in athymic mice. *Proc Natl Acad Sci USA* 1997; 94: 13891–13896.

[35] B. Sangro, G. Mazzolini, M. Ruiz, J. Ruiz, J. Quiroga, I. Herrero, C. Qian, A. Benito, J. Larrache, C. Olagüe, J. Boan, I. Peñuelas, B. Sádaba, J. Prieto. A phase I clinical trial of thymidine kinase-based gene therapy in advanced hepatocellular carcinoma. *Cancer Gene Ther.* 2010 Dec;17(12):837-43.

[36] D. Gao, W. An, and J. Dai. Retrovirus-mediated herpes simplex virus thymidine kinase gene therapy. *Cell Res.* 1999; 9, 225.

[37] H. Qin, Q. Shao, S. Igdoura, M. Alaoui-Jamali, D. Laird. Lysosomal and proteasomal degradation play distinct roles in the life cycle of Cx43 in gap junctional intercellular communication-deficient and -competent breast tumor cells. *J Biol Chem* 2003; 278: 30005–30014.

[38] L Garcia-Rodrı´guez, D Abate-Daga, A Rojas, JR Gonza´lez and C Fillat. E-cadherin contributes to the bystander effect of TK/GCV suicide therapy and enhances its antitumoral activity in pancreatic cancer models. *Gene Therapy* 2011; 18, 73–8.

[39] S. Shiozawa, K. Kawai, Y. Okada, I. Tomioka, T. Maeda, A. Kanda, H. Shinohara, H. Suemizu, HJ. Okano, Y. Sotomaru, E. Sasaki, H. Okano. Gene Targeting and Subsequent Site-Specific Transgenesis at the beta actin locus (ACTB) in common marmoset embryonic Stem Cells. *Stem Cells Dev.* 2011 Jan 16. [Epub ahead of print]

[40] J. Zhang, F. Wei, H. Wang, H. Li, W. Qiu, P. Ren, X. Chen, Q. Huang. Potent anti-tumor activity of telomerase-dependent and HSVTK armed oncolytic adenovirus for non-small cell lung cancer in vitro and in vivo. *J Exp Clin Cancer Res.* 2010 May 20;29:52.

[41] Y. Kang, W. Yu, Q. Sun, X. Zhang, W. Jiang, C. Wu, C. Chen, J. Gu, Y. Zheng, C. Xu. High-level transgene expression mediated by the piggyBack transposon enhances transgenic therapeutic effects in cervical cancer xenografts. *Oncol Rep.* 2010 Oct; 24(4):897-907.

[42] L. Yang, J Wang, J Gao. Study on cotransfection of genes of insulin-like growth factor I and herpes simplex virus thymidine kinase for optimization of wound healing. *Zhonghua Shao Shang Za Zhi.* 2010 Jun;26(3):202-6.

[43] P. Li, D. Ngo, A. Brade, and H. Klamut. Differential chemosensitivity of breast cancer cells to ganciclovir treatment following adenovirus mediated herpes simplex virus thymidine kinase gene transfer. *Cancer Gene Ther.* 1999; 6, 179-90 .

[44] L. Anderson, S. Swaminathan, I. Zackon, A. Tajuddin, B. Thimmapaya, and S. Wetizman. Adenovirus-mediated tissue targeted expression of the HSV-TK gene for the treatment of breast cancer. *Gene Ther.* 1999; 6, 854-64.

[45] B. Howard, H. Kalthoff, and T. Fong. Ablation of tumor cells in vivo by direct injection of HSV-thymidine kinase ret- roviral vector and ganciclovir therapy. *Ann. N. Y. Acad. Sci.* 1999; 880, 352.

[46] M. Seto, H. Wakabayashi, T. Yamazaki, J. Sonoda, Y. Shinto, and A. Uchida. Gene therapy of chondrosarcoma using retrovirus vectors encoding the herpes simplex virus thymi- dine kinase gene. *Int. J. Oncol.* 1999; 14, 1137.

[47] S. Dhar, M. McConnell, N. Gharibjanian, C. Young, J. Rogers, T. Nguyen and G. Evans. Herpes Simplex Virus-Thymidine Kinase–Based Suicide Gene Therapy as a "Molecular Switch Off" for Nerve Growth Factor Production In Vitro. *Tissue Engineering.* Volume 13, Number 9, 2007. 2357-2365.

[48] C. Baum, J. Düllmann, Z. Li, B. Fehse, J. Meyer, D. Williams, and C. von Kalle. Side effects of retroviral gene transfer into hematopoietic stem cells. *Blood* 2003; 101: 2099–2114.

[49] S. Hacein-Bey-Abina. *et al.* LMO2-associated clonal T cell proliferation in two patients after gene therapy for SCID-X1. *Science* 2003; 302: 415–419.

[50] S. Sant, T. Suarez, M. Moalli, B. Wu, M. Blaivas, T. Laing, and B. Roessler. Molecular lysis of synovial lining cells by in vivo herpes simplex virus thymidine kinase gene transfer. *Hum. Gene Ther.* 1998; 9, 2735.

[51] N. Shand, F. Weber, L. Marinai, M. Bernstein, A. Gianella- Borradori, Z. Long, A. Sorensen, and N. Barbier. A phase 1-2 clinical trial of gene therapy for recurrent glio- blastoma multiforme by tumor transduction with the herpes simplex thymidine kinase gene followed by ganciclovir. *Hum. Gene Ther.* 1999; 10, 2325.

[52] M. Driesse, A. Vincent, P. Sillevis-Smith, J. Kros, P. Hoogerbrugge, C. Avezaat, and D. Valerio. Intrace- rebral injection of adenovirus harboring the HSV-TK gene combined with ganciclovir administration: toxicity study in nonhuman primates. *Gene Ther.* 1998; 5, 1122.

[53] I. Kunishige, Y. Samejima, Y. Shiki, A. Moriyama, D. Meruelo, F. Saji, and Y. Murata. Suicide gene therapy for human uterine adenocarcinoma cells using herpes simplex virus thymidine. *Gynecol. Oncol.* 1999; 72, 16.

[54] A. Beerens, M. Rots, B. Bermúdez, E. de Vries, H. Haisma. Secretion of thymidine kinase to increase the effectivity of suicide gene therapy results in the loss of enzymatic activity. *J Drug Target.* 2008 Jan;16(1):26-35.

[55] S. Zhou, S. Li, Z. Liu, Y. Tang, Z. Wang, J. Gong, C. Liu. Ultrasound-targeted microbubble destruction mediated herpes simplex virus-thymidine kinase gene treats hepatoma in mice. *J Exp Clin Cancer Res.* 2010 Dec 23;29:170.

[56] K. Kakinoki, Y. Nakamoto, T. Kagaya, T. Tsuchiyama, Y. Sakai, T. Nakahama, N. Mukaida, S. Kaneko. Prevention of intrahepatic metastasis of liver cancer by suicide gene therapy and chemokine ligand 2/monocyte chemoattractant protein-1 delivery in mice. *J Gene Med.* 2010 Dec;12(12):1002-13.

[57] Q. Yue, X. Hu, Y. Yin, M. Su, X. Cheng, L. Yang, T. Zhou, X. Hao. Inhibition of prostate cancer by suicide gene targeting the FCY1 and HSV-TK genes. *Oncol Rep.* 2009 Dec;22(6):1341-7.

[58] A. Määttä, H. Samaranayake, J. Pikkarainen, T. Wirth, S. Ylä-Herttuala. Adenovirus mediated herpes simplex virus-thymidine kinase/ganciclovir gene therapy for resectable malignant glioma. *Curr Gene Ther.* 2009 Oct;9(5):356-67.

[59] C. Zischek, H. Niess, I. Ischenko, C. Conrad, R. Huss, K. Jauch, P. Nelson, C. Bruns. Targeting tumor stroma using engineered mesenchymal stem cells reduces the growth of pancreatic carcinoma. *Ann Surg.* 2009 Nov;250(5):747-53.

[60] A. Hara, H. Aoki, A. Taguchi, M. Niwa, Y. Yamada, T. Kunisada, H. Mori. Neuron-like differentiation and selective ablation of undifferentiated embryonic stem cells containing suicide gene with Oct-4 promoter. *Stem Cells Dev.* 2008 Aug;17(4):619-27.

[61] S. Park, W. Lee, J. Lee, I. Kim. Combination gene therapy using multidrug resistance (MDR1) gene shRNA and herpes simplex virus-thymidine kinase. *Cancer Lett.* 2008 Mar 18;261(2):205-14. Epub 2007 Dec 21.

[62] B. Li, C. Zhang, Y. Yi, Y. Hao, X. Liu, Q. Ou. Vascular damage and anti-angiogenic effects of tumor vessel-targeted adenovirus-mediated herpes simplex virus thymidine kinase gene. *World J Gastroenterol.* 2007 Aug 7;13(29):4006-10.

[63] Q. Huang, P. Pu P, Z. Xia, Y. You. Exogenous wt-p53 enhances the antitumor effect of HSVTK/GCV on C6 glioma cells. *J Neurooncol.* 2007 May;82(3):239-48. Epub 2006 Nov 11.

[64] O. Rautsi, S. Lehmusvaara, A. Ketola, A. Määttä, J. Wahlfors, R. Pellinen. Characterization of HIV-1 TAT peptide as an enhancer of HSV-TK/GCV cancer gene therapy. *Cancer Gene Ther.* 2008 May;15(5):303-14. Epub 2008 Feb 29.

[65] A. Ardiani, M. Sanchez-Bonilla, M Black. Fusion enzymes containing HSV-1 thymidine kinase mutants and guanylate kinase enhance prodrug sensitivity in vitro and in vivo. *Cancer Gene Ther.* 2010 Feb;17(2):86-96. Epub 2009 Sep 18.

[66] Y. Hasegawa, Y. Nishiyama, K. Imaizumi, N. Ono, T. Kinoshita, S. Hatano, H. Saito, K. Shimokata. Avoidance of bone marrow suppression using A-5021 as a nucleoside analog for retrovirus-mediated herpes simplex virus type I thymidine kinase gene therapy. *Cancer Gene Ther.* 2000 Apr;7(4):557-62.

5

Translational Challenges for Hepatocyte-Directed Gene Transfer

Stephanie C. Gordts, Eline Van Craeyveld, Frank Jacobs and Bart De Geest
Center for Molecular and Vascular Biology, University of Leuven, Leuven, Belgium

1. Introduction

The liver is a central organ in many metabolic processes. Multiple inherited metabolic disorders have their origin in this organ. Therefore, hepatocytes are a key target for gene therapy directed at correction of inborn errors of metabolism and of hemophilia. Inborn errors of metabolism lead to accumulation of toxic products in hepatocytes and extensive hepatotoxicity, as observed in disorders like α_1-antitrypsin deficiency, type I tyrosinemia, or Wilson disease[1]. In other metabolic disorders, such as in Crigler-Najjar syndrome type I, ornithine transcarbamylase deficiency, familial hypercholesterolemia, and hemophilia A and B, manifestations are primarily extrahepatic[1]. In addition, the liver is a target for gene therapy of acquired diseases such as liver cancer and hepatitis[2, 3].

Insights into the determinants of gene transfer efficiency to hepatocytes are therefore required to evaluate the potential of gene therapy for inborn errors of metabolism and for acquired liver diseases. These determinants include innate and adaptive immune responses, cellular and biochemical determinants of hepatocyte transduction such as ligand receptor interactions, and anatomical and histological factors. Here we will first focus on the role of liver sinusoidal cells and sinusoidal fenestrae as determinants of the efficiency in hepatocyte-directed gene transfer. Uptake of gene transfer vectors by Kupffer cells and liver sinusoidal endothelial cells limits hepatocyte transduction[4-11]. However, the presence of fenestrae in liver sinusoidal endothelial cells provides a direct access to the space of Disse and microvillous surface of hepatocytes and may allow transcellular migration of vectors. In the following paragraphs, we provide substantial evidence that the interplay between these opposing forces, i.e. uptake by non-parenchymal liver cells and transcellular migration through fenestrae, is a critical determinant of gene transfer efficiency into hepatocytes.

Before discussing the different parameters that influence the efficiency of hepatocyte-directed gene transfer, it is important to point out that the process of gene transfer to parenchymal liver cells using replication-defective virus-derived vectors or non-viral vectors is fundamentally different from infection of hepatocytes by hepatotropic viruses. After successful infection, viruses replicate, leading to an exponential local increase of viral load. Consequently, a very small inoculum may be sufficient to induce hepatitis. In contrast, the number of transgenes carried by viral gene transfer vectors that pass through fenestrae cannot be amplified in hepatocytes since these vectors are replication defective. The number of vector particles that pass through fenestrae and are subsequently taken up by hepatocytes is therefore a critical determinant of transgene DNA copy number in these cells and of transgene expression levels.

2. Liver anatomy and histology

The liver is the largest internal organ of the human body, weighs about 1.5 kg, and is located in the upper right quadrant of the abdomen. The liver is highly vascularised and the total blood flow through the liver can reach up to 25% of the cardiac output. Approximately 75% of the blood that enters the liver derives from the portal vein that carries oxygen-poor blood. Oxygenated blood entering the liver via the hepatic artery constitutes the remaining 25% of blood supply. The portal vein, the hepatic artery, lymphatic vessels, nerves, and bile ducts enter the liver at the hilus. From the hilus, continuous branching of the hepatic artery and portal vein results in an intricate network of intertwining capillaries, called sinusoids. Histologically, the liver is divided into lobuli, hexagonal functional units formed by hepatocytes and sinusoids surrounding a central vein. Neighbouring lobules are surrounded by portal triads, consisting of branches of the bile duct, the portal vein, and the hepatic artery.

A human liver comprises 4.5×10^{11} cells[12, 13]. A murine liver contains approximately 1.6×10^{8} cells[12] whereas a rabbit liver counts about 1.5×10^{10} cells. These data allow to calculate the ratio of transgene copies contained in a given vector dose versus the number of hepatocytes, which can be calculated as 66% of the total number of liver cells. Empirical determination of the transgene DNA copy number per hepatocyte is hampered by the fact that copy numbers per diploid genome do not accurately reflect transgene DNA copy numbers per hepatocyte. Indeed, hepatocytes are frequently tetraploid or even octoploid and may also have a binuclear nucleus.

3. Liver sinusoidal cells

Sinusoidal cells constitute approximately 33% of the number of resident liver cells whereas parenchymal liver cells or hepatocytes comprise the remaining cells[14-16]. Sinusoidal cells are a compilation of endothelial cells, Kupffer cells (resident liver macrophages), fat-storing cells (also called stellate cells or Ito cells), and pit cells (natural killer cells). Liver sinusoidal endothelial cells comprise 70%, Kupffer cells 20%, stellate cells 10%, and pit cells less than 1% of the number of sinusoidal cells[14, 16, 17]. In the context of hepatocyte-directed gene transfer, we focus here on the role of Kupffer cells and liver sinusoidal endothelial cells that constitute together the reticulo-endothelial cells of the liver. Kupffer cells account for 80% to 90% of resident macrophages in the entire body[18]. They have a diameter of 10-15 µm whereas liver sinusoidal endothelial cells are smaller with a diameter of 7-9 µm[14]. Sinusoidal endothelial cells are scavenger cells that are able to internalize particles up to 0.23 µm under physiologic conditions *in vivo*[19]. Larger particles are taken up by Kupffer cells[19]. Since most gene transfer vectors have a diameter below 0.23 µm, uptake of vectors by both Kupffer cells and liver sinusoidal endothelial cells may attenuate the efficiency of hepatocyte-directed gene transfer.

Most experimental work on the role of liver reticulo-endothelial cells in relation to hepatocyte transduction has been performed with adenoviral vectors. These studies support the dual role of liver reticulo-endothelial cells in hepatocyte-directed gene transfer. On the one hand, the high endocytotic capacity of these cells limits hepatocyte transduction, on the other hand, the presence of fenestrae facilitates hepatocyte transduction[20]. The relevance of these observations for other types of vectors and other modes of gene transfer will subsequently be discussed.

4. *In vitro* and *in vivo* transduction by adenoviral vectors

Efficient hepatocyte transduction by adenoviral vectors requires that two clearly distinct conditions are met. First, adenoviral vectors should have a facilitated access to the space of Disse via sufficiently large sinusoidal fenestrae. Second, vectors in the space of Disse must be able to bind to cellular receptors on hepatocytes for internalisation and transduction. Thus, both the anatomical access of vectors to the space of Disse and the potential for interaction with hepatocyte receptors *in vivo* are necessary but not always sufficient for hepatocyte transduction *in vivo*. Before going into the anatomical access of vectors to the space of Disse, we will first discuss differences between adenoviral transduction *in vitro* and transduction of hepatocytes *in vivo*.

For humans, 51 adenovirus serotypes have been identified, and these serotypes are classified into 6 species (A-F). *In vitro*, uptake of most Ad serotypes belonging to species A, C, D, E, and F, is initiated by binding of the adenovirus fiber protein to coxsackie and adenovirus receptor (CAR) on the cell surface[21, 22]. CD46, a complement regulatory protein that is ubiquitously expressed in humans[23], but only in the testis in mice[24], is a cellular receptor for group B adenoviruses[23]. Human species C adenovirus serotype 5 (Ad5) is the most common viral vector used in clinical studies worldwide[25]. *In vitro*, Ad5 infects cells through binding of the fiber to CAR, followed by binding of an arginine-glycine-aspartic acid (RGD)-motif on the Ad5 penton base with cellular integrins (mainly $\alpha_v\beta_3$ and $\alpha_v\beta_5$) which initiates receptor-mediated endocytosis via clathrin coated pits[26, 27]. However, CAR binding ablation[28, 29] and α_v integrin binding ablation[29, 30] do not significantly reduce liver transduction by adenoviral vectors *in vivo*. The direct Ad binding to hepatic heparan sulfate proteoglycans via the KKTK motif within the fiber shaft domain has been suggested to be the major mechanism of hepatocyte transduction *in vivo*[31, 32]. However, mutation of the KKTK motif in the Ad5 fiber shaft renders the fiber inflexible and prevents internalisation of Ad5 though steric hindrance[33, 34]. *In vitro* and *in vivo* infectivity studies of Ad5-based vectors possessing long Ad31- (species A) or Ad41- (species F) derived fiber shaft domains that lack the KKTK motif, have shown that these vectors transduce hepatocytes with similar efficiency compared to Ad5 vectors[35], consistent with the absence of a critical role of the KKTK motif in hepatocyte transduction.

An important difference between *in vitro* transduction and *in vivo* transduction of liver cells after intravenous injection is that adenoviral vectors are in contact with blood proteins. Treatment of mice with the vitamin K antagonist warfarin, which inactivates several proteins of the coagulation cascade (factor II, factor VII, factor IX, factor X) as well as the anticoagulant protein C, abrogates transduction of hepatocytes by adenoviral serotype 5 vectors[8, 36-38]. These studies suggested that a coagulation protein or coagulation proteins have a bridging function in the entry of liver cells by adenoviral vectors. Only factor X could rescue liver transduction in warfarin anticoagulated mice[39]. Recently, it has been shown that the γ-carboxyglutamic acid domain of factor X binds in a calcium-dependent manner to hexon protein in adenovirus serotype 5[25, 39, 40]. Factor X binds at the cup formed by the center of each hexon trimer. Serotypes with a high affinity for factor X, such as the species C serotypes Ad2 and Ad5, have been shown to efficiently transduce hepatocytes following intravenous administration[41, 42]. In contrast, species B Ad35 and species D Ad26 bind to factor X weakly or not at all, and fail to transduce hepatocytes[39, 43, 44]. More specifically, factor X binds to the adenovirus hexon hypervariable regions (HVRs). Liver infection by the factor X-Ad5 complex is mediated through a heparin-binding exosite in the factor X serine protease domain. Substitution of HVR5 or HVR7 from Ad5 with sequences from the non-factor X binding serotype Ad26 substantially lowered factor X binding and liver transduction *in vivo*[45]. An Ad5 mutant containing an insertion in HVR5 was shown to bind factor X *in vitro* with 10 000-fold reduced affinity compared with unmodified vector and failed to deliver the red fluorescent protein transgene *in vivo*[25]. Taken together, factor X binding to hexon trimer is a necessary prerequisite for hepatocyte transduction *in vivo*[39].

5. Liver trapping of adenoviral vectors

Previous studies have shown that different adenoviral serotypes are rapidly sequestered in the liver after intravenous delivery, independent of their potential to effectively transduce hepatocytes[43, 46, 47]. Trapping of adenoviral vectors in the liver is comparable between wild-type mice and mice treated with warfarin, which shows that factor X-facilitated adenoviral vector entry into hepatocytes is not required for trapping of vectors in the liver[8]. Demonstration of liver sequestration using whole livers does not make a distinction between the presence of vectors extracellularly (in the vascular lumen of the sinusoids or in the space of Disse) or intracellularly (in the non-parenchymal liver cells of the parenchymal liver cells). Cellular uptake of adenoviral vectors after systemic gene transfer occurs predominantly in non-parenchymal liver cells (i.e. mainly liver sinusoidal endothelial cells and Kupffer cells)[4-7]. Kupffer cells may bind adenoviral vectors via multiple mechanisms including scavenger receptor-A, complement, and natural antibodies[9-11] and this uptake is independent of factor X[10, 11]. Interactions of adenoviral vectors with platelets in blood may contribute significantly to sequestration in the reticuloendothelial system of the liver[9]. Nevertheless, the exact mechanisms of adenoviral vector uptake in Kupffer cells have not been elucidated. The amount of Ad vector DNA after intravenous administration was nearly identical in wild-type mice and scavenger receptor-A deficient mice[11] consistent with the presence of multiple pathways leading to Kupffer cell sequestration[10].
Recently, Di Paolo *et al.*[11] showed that simultaneous treatment of mice with warfarin and clodronate liposomes, that deplete Kupffer cells, results in only a minor reduction of sequestration of adenoviral vectors in the liver 1 hour after gene transfer. Transmission electron microsopy showed the presence of vectors in the space of Disse, consistent with anatomical sequestration of vectors. We suggest that the presence of fenestrae is crucial in the liver targeting of adenoviral vectors. In other words, the targeting of adenoviral vectors to the liver reflects predominantly or exclusively anatomical targeting. This also implies that molecular strategies directed at liver detargeting of adenoviral vectors should take into account the existence of anatomical targeting to the liver.

6. Uptake of gene transfer vectors by reticulo-endothelial cells of the liver reduces hepatocyte transduction

Both Kupffer cells and liver sinusoidal endothelial cells take up the large majority of adenoviral vectors after systemic gene transfer[7]. Uptake of vectors by non-parenchymal liver cells (i.e. mainly liver sinusoidal endothelial cells and Kupffer cells) inversely correlates with transduction of parenchymal liver cells[7]. The transgene DNA copy number in the non-parenchymal liver cells at one hour after transfer in Balb/c mice was nearly 6-fold higher than in C57BL/6 mice[7]. This difference in scavenging of vectors between both strains is a major determinant of the approximately 3-fold higher transgene DNA levels in hepatocytes and higher transgene expression levels in C57BL/6 mice compared to Balb/c mice[7]. Based on more refined experiments with isolation of Kupffer cells and liver sinusoidal endothelial cells, we showed that the transgene DNA copy number per diploid genome at 1 hour after transfer in C57BL/6 mice was 2.9-fold higher in liver sinusoidal endothelial cells than in Kupffer cells[7]. In contrast, the copy number in Kupffer cells was 2.6-fold higher than in liver sinusoidal endothelial cells in Balb/c mice. These data indicate that the relative contribution of liver sinusoidal endothelial cells and Kupffer cells to adenoviral vector clearance may be highly dependent on the specific genetic context. One explanation for this difference of uptake of adenoviral vectors by the liver reticulo-endothelial cells of C57BL/6 and Balb/c mice may be the differential modulation of the function of these cells by humoral factors produced by spleen cells. Indeed, a significantly reduced transgene DNA copy number was observed in the liver reticulo-endothelial cells one hour after adenoviral transfer in splenectomized Balb/c mice and in Balb/c rag-2$^{-/-}$ mice compared to control Balb/c mice[7]. This was accompanied by a significantly higher transgene DNA copy number in hepatocytes of splenectomized Balb/c mice and of Balb/c rag-2$^{-/-}$ mice than in hepatocytes of wild-type Balb/c mice[7]. Splenectomy in Balb/c rag-2$^{-/-}$ mice did not result in an incremental effect[7]. This suggests that humoral factors produced by spleen lymphocytes may affect the clearance of adenoviral vectors by liver reticulo-endothelial cells in Balb/c mice. In contrast, no such effects on intrahepatic transgene DNA distribution were observed in splenectomized C57BL/6 mice and in C57BL/6 rag-1$^{-/-}$ mice, suggesting highly heterogeneous effects of humoral factors produced by spleen lymphocytes on liver reticulo-endothelial cells.

Further evidence for a major role of liver reticulo-endothelial cells as a determinant of hepatocyte transduction comes from experiments with clodronate liposomes. Depletion of Kupffer cells and macrophages in the spleen by intravenous administration of clodronate liposomes results in significantly increased transgene DNA levels in parenchymal liver cells[7] and in increased transgene expression[6, 7, 48, 49]. Since liver sinusoidal endothelial cell function may be modified by Kupffer cells[50, 51], it cannot be excluded that part of the effect of clodronate liposomes is due to reduced activation of liver sinusoidal endothelial cells by Kupffer cells. Besides clodronate liposomes, pre-administration of polyinosinic acid, a scavenger receptor A ligand, before gene transfer has been shown to prevent sequestration of adenoviral vectors in Kupffer cells and to enhance parenchymal liver cell transduction[52]. Transient saturation of the reticulo-endothelial system with phosphatidylcholine liposomes or with Intralipid® also reduces uptake of vectors in the non-parenchymal liver cells and augments hepatocyte transduction[7]. Taken together, various interventions that result in reduced uptake of adenoviral vectors in liver reticulo-endothelial cells consistently enhance hepatocyte transduction.

7. Liver sinusoidal endothelial fenestrae

Liver sinusoids are highly specialized capillaries with two critical features: the thin endothelium contains open fenestrae, whereas a basal lamina is lacking[53]. Fenestrae are clustered in sieve plates and provide an open pathway between the sinusoidal lumen and the space of Disse, in which numerous microvilli from parenchymal liver cells protrude[53, 54]. Sinusoidal fenestrae have no diaphragm and visualisation requires perfusion fixation with glutaraldehyde. Scanning electron microscopy analysis has shown that sinusoidal fenestrae

comprise 6–8% of the sinusoidal surface[55]. Compared to the centrilobular area, the diameter of fenestrae is larger but the frequency of fenestrae is lower in the periportal area[55, 56].
The open communication between the sinusoidal lumen and the space of Disse through fenestrae represents a unique route that provides direct access for gene transfer vectors to the surface of hepatocytes. However, fenestrae act as a sieve and will mechanically restrict the transport of gene transfer vectors according to their size. Thus, two parameters must be taken into account when considering the access of gene transfer vectors to hepatocytes namely the diameter of both fenestrae and gene transfer vectors.

8. Species variation of the average diameter of fenestrae

Fenestrae generally measure between 100 nm and 200 nm and significant species differences in their size exist[53-55]. However, the interpretation of the existing literature on species variations of the size of sinusoidal fenestrae is hampered by differences in preparatory methods applied by different investigators. Standardised protocols within one group of investigators are therefore *a conditio sine qua non* for reliable species and strain comparisons. A direct comparative study of the diameter of sinusoidal fenestrae in five species using scanning electron microscopy was performed by Higashi *et al.*[57]. The average diameter of sinusoidal endothelial fenestrae in this study was 45 nm in cows, 52 nm in sheep, 66 nm in guinea pigs, 82 nm in pigs, and 131 nm in dogs[57]. However, these results are based on scanning electron microscopy preparations and are therefore subject to a shrinkage effect in the order of 30% caused by dehydration and drying of the tissue[58]. Accurate measurements of fenestrae can only be obtained by gradually replacing cellular water by plastic during preparation for transmission electron microscopy[59]. Previous studies have shown that this method of preparation leads to accurate measurements of cellular details, such as fenestrae. Visualisation of fenestrae in transmission electron microscopy sections requires that endothelial cells and their sieve plates are cut tangentially so that fenestrae become visible as holes. Using this technology and standardized protocols, it has previously been shown that the average diameter of fenestrae is significantly larger in Sprague Dawley rats (150 nm in the pericentral area and 175 nm in the periportal area)[55] and C57BL/6 mice (141 nm)[60] than in New Zealand White rabbits (103 nm)[60], Fauve de Bourgogne rabbits (105 nm)[61], and humans with a healthy liver (107 nm)[62]. The diameter in Dutch Belt rabbits was intermediate (124 nm)[61]. Taken together, this species comparison demonstrates that the diameter of fenestrae in humans is similar to New Zealand White rabbits and significantly smaller compared to mice and rats, two species that are most frequently used in gene transfer studies. The occurrence of major shrinkage effects in scanning electron microscopy samples is indicated by the significantly lower diameters reported for New Zealand White rabbits (49 nm)[63] and Sprague Dawley rats (89 nm)[63] as compared to diameters obtained in transmission electron microscopy studies[55, 60]. Transmission electron microscopy studies consistently show that the interindividual variation of the average diameter of fenestrae within the same species or strain is low, as indicated by coefficients of variation between 3-8%. In contrast, as will be discussed in the next paragraph, the intraindividual variation of diameters of fenestrae is high.

9. Intraindividual variation of the diameter of fenestrae

The intraindividual variation of the diameter of fenestrae is an important parameter that may complicate investigations on the relation between the diameter of fenestrae and gene transfer efficiency to hepatocytes. The distribution of the diameters of fenestrae within one individual or within one animal follows a Gaussian function with some skewing to the right[20].

Two opposing processes will determine the entrance of vectors into the space of Disse: on the one hand passage through sinusoidal fenestrae and on the other hand endocytosis by Kupffer cells and endothelial cells. Species and strain differences in transendothelial passage will be determined by intrinsic differences of the function of liver reticulo-endothelial cells (e.g. C57BL/6 versus Balb/c mice) as well as the rate passage of vectors through fenestrae. Based on these considerations, one can predict that the ratio of transgene DNA copy number in parenchymal liver cells versus the copy number in sinusoidal liver cells will correlate positively with the diameter of fenestrae. After reviewing data on the diameters of different gene transfer vectors, we will present several lines of experimental evidence that support the critical role of the diameter of fenestrae in hepatocyte transduction.

10. Diameters of gene transfer vectors

To put the importance of the size of fenestrae for hepatocyte-directed gene transfer into perspective, accurate knowledge of the diameter of gene transfer vectors is required. To avoid bias in the measurement of the diameter of adenoviral vectors, we previously vitrified a sample of adenoviral vectors using Vitrobot™ technology and determined the diameter by cryo-electron microscopy[60]. Adenoviral serotype 5 virions were shown to have a diameter of 93 nm with protruding fibers of 30 nm[60]. Using the same imaging techniques, the diameter of a vesicular stomatitis virus-G pseudotyped human immunodeficiency virus-1 derived lentiviral vector was found to be 150 nm[60]. Adeno-associated viral serotype 2 vectors have an average diameter of 22 nm[64]. Herpes simplex virions have been reported to be as large as 180 nm[65]. The diameter of liposomes used for non-viral gene transfer varies between 50 nm and 1000 nm and is highly dependent on production parameters[66, 67].

11. Experimental evidence for a critical role of sinusoidal fenestrae in hepatocyte transduction following adenoviral gene transfer

Based on our prior studies in different strains of rabbits and in different species[60-62], the correlation coefficient between the average diameter of sinusoidal fenestrae in these different strains and species and human apo A-I expression at day 7 after transfer with an adenoviral vector containing a hepatocyte-specific expression cassette was found to be 0.94 ($p<0.01$). This strongly suggests that the diameter of sinusoidal fenestrae is an important determinant of gene transfer efficiency to hepatocytes.

To demonstrate that the difference of human apo A-I plasma levels reflects differences of transgene DNA levels in parenchymal liver cells, we isolated parenchymal and non-parenchymal liver cells at day 3 after transfer in C57BL/6 mice and New Zealand White rabbits. Transgene DNA levels in parenchymal liver cells were much higher in C57BL/6 mice than in New Zealand White rabbits whereas the reverse pattern was observed in non-parenchymal liver cells[60]. Considering the small average diameter of fenestrae in New Zealand White rabbits (103 nm), it appears that the sinusoidal wall constitutes a histological barrier for adenoviral vectors in this species leading to increased uptake by liver reticulo-endothelial cells. In contrast, the larger fenestrae in C57BL/6 mice (141 nm) facilitate access to hepatocytes, leading to increased uptake into hepatocytes and to reduced scavenging by

Kupffer cell and liver sinusoidal endothelial cells. In other words, the size of fenestrae determines the distribution of vectors between sinusoidal and parenchymal liver cells.
Although the relation between the diameter of sinusoidal fenestrae and transgene expression after adenoviral gene transfer may be confounded by substantial differences in genetic background, we showed that interventions that increase the diameter of fenestrae result in New Zealand White rabbits significantly increased transgene expression[60, 61]. These two intervention studies support the view that the correlation between the diameter of fenestrae and transgene expression after adenoviral transfer reflects a causal relationship.
Based on the high degree of similarity of the distribution of the diameter of fenestrae between humans and New Zealand White rabbits[20, 68], one would predict a low efficiency of gene transfer into hepatocytes after adenoviral transfer in humans. In the ornithine transcarbamylase deficiency trial, low levels of gene transfer in hepatocytes were indeed observed[69]. The authors concluded that the level of transgene expression was lower than what would have been predicted based on preclinical animal models[69]. Although histological alterations of the livers in patients with partial ornithine transcarbamylase deficiency may have contributed to low hepatocyte transduction, we speculate that a much smaller size of fenestrae in humans compared to mice and rats is likely the most critical factor in the observed species difference of hepatocyte transduction. On the other hand, the small diameter of fenestrae in humans may be beneficial for the efficacy of molecular strategies directed at liver detargeting of adenoviral vectors since anatomical targeting to the liver will be limited.
Recently, Brunetti-Pierri *et al.*[70] developed a minimally invasive procedure that significantly improves the efficiency of hepatocyte-directed transfer in nonhuman primates. A balloon occlusion catheter was percutaneously positioned in the inferior *vena cava* to occlude hepatic venous outflow[70]. Gene transfer of gutted vectors was performed via a percutaneously placed hepatic artery catheter with an infusion time of 7.5 minutes or 15 minutes. This procedure resulted in approximately 10-fold higher transgene expression levels compared to systemic gene transfer. Increased intrahepatic pressure following occlusion of hepatic outflow of the liver may increase the diameter of fenestrae, similar as observed following hydrodynamic injections in mice[71], and this may contribute to the beneficial effects of this procedure in monkeys.

12. Potential relevance of sinusoidal fenestrae for other modes of hepatocyte-directed gene transfer

Based on the data obtained with adenoviral vectors, it is likely that the large diameter of lentiviral vectors is an important limitation for hepatocyte-directed gene transfer and may restrict passage of vectors even in mice and rats. Indeed, gene transfer efficiency in mice and rats is low after *in vivo* lentiviral gene transfer[72-75]. Although other factors like technological challenges to obtain high titer vector stocks may play a role, it is likely that the large diameter of lentiviral vectors is a limitation for hepatocyte-directed gene transfer. Since this anatomical limitation does not exist for adeno-associated viral vectors, gene transfer efficiency into hepatocytes with this type of vectors will be solely dependent on cellular and molecular determinants of hepatocyte transduction.
Fenestrae may also play a role in naked DNA transfer. Liu *et al.*[76] showed that the murine liver can rapidly extract up to 25 µg of plasmid DNA from the blood during a single pass after simple intravenous injection. Moreover, this study showed that naked DNA is

primarily taken up by the liver endothelial cells, but not by Kupffer cells, and that transfection of hepatocytes can be improved by mechanical massage of the liver, which increases the size of liver sinusoidal fenestrae[76]. Substantial amounts of plasmid DNA are degraded by nucleases in the blood following simple intravenous injection, which can be overcome by hydrodynamic gene transfer. It has also been proposed that fenestrae play a role in the transport of naked DNA into hepatocytes during hydrodynamic gene transfer[71]. Although the exact mechanism of hepatocyte transfection following hydrodynamic gene transfer remains to be elucidated, a general consensus is that the injected volume induces right heart volume overload. This results in a retrograde flow through the *vena cava* and in particular in a retrograde flow into the hepatic veins. As a result, intrahepatic pressure increases and the DNA containing solution is forced out of the hepatic sinusoids into the parenchymal liver cells. Following systemic hydrodynamic gene transfer in mice and rats, the majority of the injected DNA (i.e. >90%) can be retrieved in the liver[77]. In addition, microscopic analysis has indicated that transfected hepatocytes are predominantly located in the pericentral region[78]. This predilection may be explained by the fact that sinusoids are wider and straighter and contain more fenestrae per unit of surface in the pericentral area than in the periportal area[56, 77].

13. Sinusoidal fenestrae and hepatocyte transduction in diseased livers

The unique morphological features of liver sinusoidal endothelial cells may change in pathological conditions. Liver fibrosis and cirrhosis lead to a decreased number of fenestrae[79] and capillarization and perisinusoidal fibrosis leads to the development of a basal lamina, found to be absent in normal sinusoids. A significant reduction in the number of fenestrae and porosity of the sinusoidal endothelial cells was observed in alcoholic liver disease without cirrhosis[80]. In a comparative study, decreased transduction by adenoviral vectors has been observed in cirrhotic rat livers compared to normal livers[81]. Furthermore, hydrodynamic gene transfer was significantly less efficient in rats with a fibrotic liver compared to rats with a healthy liver[82]. Sinusoidal capillarization also occurs in hepatocellular carcinoma[83, 84]. This may constitute a major obstacle for efficient gene therapy for liver cancers.

14. General perspective

Preclinical viral and non-viral gene transfer studies should consider scavenging of vectors by liver reticulo-endothelial cells and as well as the diameter of sinusoidal fenestrae as important determinants of gene transfer efficiency into hepatocytes. Although the diameter of fenestrae may be modulated to some extent, there is currently no safe pharmacological intervention that results in a significant enlargement of fenestrae. The small diameter of fenestrae in humans and alterations of liver sinusoidal endothelial cells in liver disease may constitute a significant and potentially insurmountable obstacle for efficient gene transfer into hepatocytes with several vectors. Both anatomical access of vectors to the space of Disse on the one hand and the potential of vectors for interaction with hepatocyte receptors *in vivo* on the other hand are necessary for efficient hepatocyte transduction *in vivo*. A model on hepatocyte transduction should therefore take into account that both an anatomical prerequisite and a molecular prerequisite have to be met.

15. Innate and adaptive immune responses: an introductory perspective

The use of non-viral gene therapy vectors, including naked DNA and liposomes, results in very low to suboptimal expression levels with the possible exception of hydrodynamic gene transfer[85-87]. However, this latter method is only successful in mice and rats and attempts for implementation of this methodology in larger species have resulted in very low gene transfer efficiencies[88-90]. Therefore, our strategic point of view is that only viral vectors constitute sufficiently potent gene delivery platforms to treat genetic and acquired diseases. Although viral vectors are non-replicative in contrast to wild-type viruses, the immune system is efficient to fight off what it perceives as invading pathogens. Innate immune responses are initiated by recognition of pathogen-associated molecular patters by pattern recognition receptors like Toll-like receptors on the surface of professional antigen presenting cells. Subsequent production of inflammatory cytokines stimulates maturation of antigen presenting cells, enhances their endocytic activity, and upregulates expression of molecules required for antigen processing and presentation and for costimulation. Viral capsid proteins not only elicit innate immunity but are also viable targets for host adaptive immune responses that do not necessarily require *de novo* viral gene expression. Adaptive immune responses against vector-derived antigens may reduce the efficacy of *in vivo* gene transfer and may prevent readministration. Furthermore, many vectors are derived from parent viruses that humans have encountered through natural infection, resulting in pre-existing antibodies and possibly in memory responses against vector antigens. Taken together, adaptive immune responses represent one the most challenging remaining hurdles for the development of viral hepatocyte-directed gene transfer strategies with a sufficient therapeutic index. Besides the issue of adaptive immune responses against the vector and the potential problem of pre-existing immunity, immune responses against the transgene product also constitute a hurdle.

16. Innate immune responses after viral gene transfer

Adenoviral vectors efficiently transduce liver cells after systemic gene transfer and expression levels are generally significantly higher as compared to non-viral, adeno-associated viral, and lentiviral transfer. However, recognition of molecular patterns on adenoviral capsids by pattern recognition receptors on macrophages and dendritic cells triggers innate immune responses and induces the production of several cytokines and chemokines[6, 91-96]. Severe activation of the innate immune system, as observed in patients with systemic microbial infections, severe trauma, or after major surgery, may lead to a systemic inflammatory response syndrome, or even to multiple system organ failure and shock. The development of systemic inflammatory response syndrome and multiple system organ failure after adenoviral transfer is dose and species dependent[69, 94, 97]. Schnell *et al.*[94] demonstrated significant species variation in innate immune responses after adenoviral gene transfer. Mice did not develop clinical symptoms of systemic inflammatory response syndrome at any dose of vector whereas rhesus monkeys developed liver necrosis and coagulopathy at a dose of 10^{13} particles/kg of an E1-deleted vector[94]. The sensitivity of humans to adverse effects of innate immune responses after adenoviral transfer is significantly higher than in rhesus monkeys as significant side-effects have been observed at doses of 6×10^{11} particles/kg or even lower[69].

Interleukin (IL)-6 is not only produced by macrophages and T cells but also by liver sinusoidal endothelial cells[98] and possibly by spleen sinusoidal endothelial cells.

Notwithstanding the fact that Kupffer cells are by large the most numerous population of resident macrophages in the body, we have shown that the predominant source of IL-6 after adenoviral transfer in C57BL/6 mice is the spleen and not the liver or lungs[99]. This finding is based both on gene transfer experiments in splenectomized mice as well as on quantification of IL-6 mRNA levels in different organs following adenoviral transfer[99].

Innate immune responses following adenoviral transfer are dependent on both Toll like receptor (TLR) 2 and TLR9[100]. TLR2 and TLR9 are expressed in Kupffer cells but also in the spleen[101-103] as well as in liver sinusoidal endothelial cells[102].

Depletion of tissue macrophages and dendritic cell subpopulations in liver and spleen by the administration of liposomes encapsulating dichloromethylene-biphosphonate results in reduced plasma levels of IL-6, IL-12, and tumor necrosis factor (TNF)-α[93]. However, this cytotoxic strategy is unlikely to be applicable in humans. Conjugation of adenoviral vectors with activated monomethoxypolyethylene glycols (MPEG) has been shown to reduce IL-6 plasma levels after adenoviral transfer[99, 104]. In addition, we have shown that the combination of PEGylation of adenoviral vectors and administration of methylprednisolone completely suppresses elevations of IL-6 levels after transfer with E1E3E4-deleted adenoviral vectors at a dose of 4×10^{12} particles/kg[99]. This combined strategy also inhibits chemokine expression in the liver, abrogates neutrophil infiltration and T-lymphocyte infiltration in the liver, and reduces elevations of serum transaminases in the early phase after adenoviral transfer[99].

Since dose reduction represents an additional means to attenuate innate immune responses against adenoviral vectors, strategies to enhance the efficiency of hepatocyte transduction are required to obtain therapeutic expression levels at lower doses. Brunetti-Pierri *et al.*[70] developed a minimally invasive procedure that significantly improves the therapeutic index of hepatocyte-directed transfer in nonhuman primates. A balloon occlusion catheter was percutaneously positioned in the inferior *vena cava* to occlude hepatic venous outflow[70]. Gene transfer of gutted vectors was performed via a percutaneously placed hepatic artery catheter with an infusion time of 7.5 minutes or 15 minutes. This procedure resulted in approximately 10-fold higher transgene expression levels compared to systemic gene transfer. At vector doses of 1×10^{10} or 3×10^{10} particles/kg, IL-6 levels were consistently below 100 pg/ml[70].

In contrast to adenoviral gene transfer, adeno-associated viral gene transfer induces very weak or absent innate immune responses to viral capsids both in mice[95] and monkeys[105]. Serum levels of five major inflammatory cytokines (TNF-α, interferon-γ, IL-6, IL-10, and IL-12) were not elevated in macaques after gene transfer with vectors based on adeno-associated virus serotypes 2, 7, and 8[105]. These data suggest that very weak or absent innate immune responses to adeno-associated viral capsids may be a general observation in different species. Nevertheless, some level of innate immune activation occurs even with adeno-associated viral vectors[106].

17. Adaptive immune responses after hepatocyte-directed gene transfer

T helper cell activation is complex. Besides signalling via pattern recognition receptors (signal 0), T cell activation requires interaction of the T cell receptor CD3 complex with antigen presented in Major Histocompatibility Complex II (MHCII) (signal 1), engagement of costimulatory molecules such as CD80/86 on antigen presenting cells with CD28 on T cells or CD40 on antigen presenting cells with CD40 ligand on T cells (signal 2), and a specific cytokine milieu (signal 3) that primes a T helper 1 (Th1) or a T helper 2 (Th2) response. Immunological tolerance is a state in which the immune system is not capable to activate the appropriate cellular or humoral immune responses following antigen exposure. In absence of signal 1, naive T cells are never primed, resulting in immunological ignorance. In the absence of adequate costimulation (signal 2), immunological tolerance is based on anergy/deletion: antigen-specific T cells are primed but are functionally deficient with regard to proliferation and cytokine production. In the absence of signal 3, regulatory T cells (Tregs) may develop. Tregs actively suppress adaptive immune effectors. Taken together, there are multiple requirements for adequate priming of T cells, which offers perspectives for induction of antigen specific tolerance.

Immune responses in mice are highly strain dependent. C57BL/6 mice preferentially develop a predominantly Th1-type immune response whereas Balb/c mice develop a Th2-type immune response[107]. Nevertheless, we have shown that cellular immune responses against adenoviral epitopes do not play a role in transgene DNA kinetics in C57BL/6 mice[108]. This implies that, in the absence of an adaptive immune response against the transgene product, non-immune mechanisms are responsible for the decrease of transgene DNA over time. Whether this is also the case in Balb/c mice, is unknown. Taken together, episomal stability of non-integrated transgenes is an important issue. This is further highlighted by our observations that the persistence of transgene DNA is dependent on the expression cassette design[109-111].

Treatment of genetic diseases by gene replacement therapy is hampered by adaptive immune responses against the transgene product. The risk of antibody formation against the transgene product may be limited in the specific setting of hepatocyte-directed gene transfer[112-114] and specifically by restricting transgene expression to hepatocytes by use of hepatocyte-specific expression cassettes[115, 116].

We consistently observed the absence of antibodies against human apolipoprotein (apo) A-I in all investigated murine strains after gene transfer with vectors containing a hepatocyte-specific expression cassette[110, 115]. This absence of a humoral immune response has also been observed after gene transfer with the same vector in rats[117]. However, this observation cannot be robustly extrapolated to other species. In contrast to findings in mice and rats, we have previously observed a vigorous humoral immune response against human apo A-I in three different rabbit strains following transfer with AdA-I leading to the disappearance of detectable human apo A-I levels within 14 days[61].

18. Development of expression cassettes for hepatocyte-directed gene transfer

The development of potent hepatocyte-specific expression cassettes for gene transfer offers several advantages. First, a therapeutic effect may be obtained at a lower vector dose, thus providing a means to improve the therapeutic index of vectors. Second, hepatocyte-specific expression cassettes represent a very efficient way to restrict transgene expression to hepatocytes, i.e. transcriptional targeting[108, 111, 115]. In contrast, targeting vectors to hepatocytes is significantly more difficult to realise. Third, hepatocyte-specific expression cassettes may lead to immunological unresponsiveness to an immunogenic transgene product via immunological ignorance or immunological tolerance[110, 114, 115, 118, 119].

Optimalisation of transgene expression may be achieved by modulating all levels of expression including transcription, post-transcriptional modification of RNA, RNA export,

RNA stability, and translation. Expression cassettes for hepatocyte-directed transfer have been improved by using new promoter-enhancer combinations[109, 111, 119-123], inclusion of introns[109, 124-127], and inclusion of additional transcriptional sequences like scaffold matrix attachment regions (SMAR) and hepatic control regions (HCR)[126, 128-132]. In a series of studies[87, 108-111, 115, 133], we have performed a direct *in vivo* comparison of nearly 50 different expression cassettes in the context of gene transfer with E1-deleted or E1E3E4-deleted adenoviral vectors using human apo A-I plasma levels in C57BL/6 mice as end-point. These studies represent a continuous improvement of expression cassettes. The conclusion of these investigations is that the *DC172* promoter, consisting of an 890 bp human α_1*-antitrypsin* promoter and two copies of the 160 bp α_1-*microglobulin* enhancer, upstream of the genomic human *apo A-I* sequence and 2 copies of the *HCR-1*, represents at present the most potent expression cassette. After gene transfer with a moderate dose (5×10^{10} particles) of an E1E3E4-deleted vector containing this expression cassette, human apo A-I levels in C57BL/6 mice were more than 3-fold higher than physiological plasma levels in humans[87]. In addition, hydrodynamic gene transfer of minicircles containing this expression cassette resulted in sustained plasma levels in C57BL/6 mice that were equivalent to physiological levels in humans[87].

19. General conclusion

The limited external validity of experimental gene transfer studies with regard to several of the parameters discussed in this review provides a framework to understand why clinical translation of hepatocyte-directed gene transfer is such a major challenge. It is inherent to gene transfer technologies that a wide variety of biological processes affect the ultimate outcome of these interventions. This number of biological determinants is significantly higher compared to classical pharmaceutical therapies or to protein infusion therapies.

Species or strain variation of any of these multiple determinants of the outcome of hepatocyte-directed gene transfer hinders the process of clinical translation. Considering the relative small size of fenestrae in humans, one important parameter that should be considered is the diameter of gene transfer vectors. A progressive increase of fundamental insights into species variations of determinants of the success of hepatocyte-directed gene transfer may provide a solid base for technological advances that may result in more robust technologies and finally in clinical translation. At the present time, it is our view that hepatocyte-directed adeno-associated viral gene transfer has the greatest potential for clinical translation. This view is based on two fundamental properties of these vectors: (1) their size is small enough to pass through human fenestrae that are characterised by a much smaller diameter than those of rodents and (2) innate immune responses are very weak after adeno-associated viral gene transfer. Taken together, the current review contains multiple elements that are a foundation to make stable progress in this field and that provide a realistic perspective on the future of hepatocyte-directed gene transfer.

20. References

[1] Nguyen TH, Ferry N. Liver gene therapy: Advances and hurdles. *Gene Ther*. 2004;11 Suppl 1:S76-84

[2] Hernandez-Alcoceba R, Sangro B, Prieto J. Gene therapy of liver cancer. *Ann Hepatol*. 2007;6:5-14

[3] Grimm D, Kay MA. Therapeutic short hairpin rna expression in the liver: Viral targets and vectors. *Gene Ther.* 2006;13:563-575
[4] Alemany R, Suzuki K, Curiel DT. Blood clearance rates of adenovirus type 5 in mice. *The Journal of general virology.* 2000;81:2605-2609
[5] Tao N, Gao GP, Parr M, Johnston J, Baradet T, Wilson JM, Barsoum J, Fawell SE. Sequestration of adenoviral vector by kupffer cells leads to a nonlinear dose response of transduction in liver. *Mol Ther.* 2001;3:28-35
[6] Wolff G, Worgall S, van Rooijen N, Song WR, Harvey BG, Crystal RG. Enhancement of in vivo adenovirus-mediated gene transfer and expression by prior depletion of tissue macrophages in the target organ. *J Virol.* 1997;71:624-629.
[7] Snoeys J, Mertens G, Lievens J, van Berkel T, Collen D, Biessen EA, De Geest B. Lipid emulsions potently increase transgene expression in hepatocytes after adenoviral transfer. *Mol Ther.* 2006;13:98-107
[8] Waddington SN, Parker AL, Havenga M, Nicklin SA, Buckley SM, McVey JH, Baker AH. Targeting of adenovirus serotype 5 (ad5) and 5/47 pseudotyped vectors in vivo: Fundamental involvement of coagulation factors and redundancy of car binding by ad5. *J Virol.* 2007;81:9568-9571
[9] Stone D, Liu Y, Shayakhmetov D, Li ZY, Ni S, Lieber A. Adenovirus-platelet interaction in blood causes virus sequestration to the reticuloendothelial system of the liver. *J Virol.* 2007;81:4866-4871
[10] Xu Z, Tian J, Smith JS, Byrnes AP. Clearance of adenovirus by kupffer cells is mediated by scavenger receptors, natural antibodies, and complement. *J Virol.* 2008;82:11705-11713
[11] Di Paolo NC, van Rooijen N, Shayakhmetov DM. Redundant and synergistic mechanisms control the sequestration of blood-born adenovirus in the liver. *Mol Ther.* 2009;17:675-684
[12] Knook DL, Blansjaar N, Sleyster EC. Isolation and characterization of kupffer and endothelial cells from the rat liver. *Exp Cell Res.* 1977;109:317-329
[13] Seymour LW, Ferry DR, Anderson D, Hesslewood S, Julyan PJ, Poyner R, Doran J, Young AM, Burtles S, Kerr DJ. Hepatic drug targeting: Phase i evaluation of polymer-bound doxorubicin. *J Clin Oncol.* 2002;20:1668-1676
[14] Do H, Healey JF, Waller EK, Lollar P. Expression of factor viii by murine liver sinusoidal endothelial cells. *J Biol Chem.* 1999;274:19587-19592
[15] Sasse D, Spornitz UM, Maly IP. Liver architecture. *Enzyme.* 1992;46:8-32
[16] Blouin A, Bolender RP, Weibel ER. Distribution of organelles and membranes between hepatocytes and nonhepatocytes in the rat liver parenchyma. A stereological study. *J Cell Biol.* 1977;72:441-455
[17] Knook DL, Sleyster EC. Isolated parenchymal, kupffer and endothelial rat liver cells characterized by their lysosomal enzyme content. *Biochem Biophys Res Commun.* 1980;96:250-257
[18] Arii S, Imamura M. Physiological role of sinusoidal endothelial cells and kupffer cells and their implication in the pathogenesis of liver injury. *J Hepatobiliary Pancreat Surg.* 2000;7:40-48
[19] Shiratori Y, Tananka M, Kawase T, Shiina S, Komatsu Y, Omata M. Quantification of sinusoidal cell function in vivo. *Semin Liver Dis.* 1993;13:39-49

[20] Jacobs F, Wisse E, De Geest B. The role of liver sinusoidal cells in hepatocyte-directed gene transfer. *Am J Pathol*. 2010;176:14-21

[21] Bergelson JM, Cunningham JA, Droguett G, Kurt-Jones EA, Krithivas A, Hong JS, Horwitz MS, Crowell RL, Finberg RW. Isolation of a common receptor for coxsackie b viruses and adenoviruses 2 and 5. *Science*. 1997;275:1320-1323.

[22] Tomko RP, Xu R, Philipson L. Hcar and mcar: The human and mouse cellular receptors for subgroup c adenoviruses and group b coxsackieviruses. *Proc Natl Acad Sci U S A*. 1997;94:3352-3356

[23] Gaggar A, Shayakhmetov DM, Lieber A. Cd46 is a cellular receptor for group b adenoviruses. *Nat Med*. 2003;9:1408-1412

[24] Tsujimura A, Shida K, Kitamura M, Nomura M, Takeda J, Tanaka H, Matsumoto M, Matsumiya K, Okuyama A, Nishimune Y, Okabe M, Seya T. Molecular cloning of a murine homologue of membrane cofactor protein (cd46): Preferential expression in testicular germ cells. *The Biochemical journal*. 1998;330 (Pt 1):163-168

[25] Kalyuzhniy O, Di Paolo NC, Silvestry M, Hofherr SE, Barry MA, Stewart PL, Shayakhmetov DM. Adenovirus serotype 5 hexon is critical for virus infection of hepatocytes in vivo. *Proc Natl Acad Sci U S A*. 2008;105:5483-5488

[26] Wickham TJ, Mathias P, Cheresh DA, Nemerow GR. Integrins alpha v beta 3 and alpha v beta 5 promote adenovirus internalization but not virus attachment. *Cell*. 1993;73:309-319.

[27] Lowenstein PR. With a little help from my f(x)riends!: The basis of ad5-mediated transduction of the liver revealed. *Mol Ther*. 2008;16:1004-1006

[28] Alemany R, Curiel DT. Car-binding ablation does not change biodistribution and toxicity of adenoviral vectors. *Gene Ther*. 2001;8:1347-1353

[29] Mizuguchi H, Koizumi N, Hosono T, Ishii-Watabe A, Uchida E, Utoguchi N, Watanabe Y, Hayakawa T. Car- or alphav integrin-binding ablated adenovirus vectors, but not fiber-modified vectors containing rgd peptide, do not change the systemic gene transfer properties in mice. *Gene Ther*. 2002;9:769-776

[30] Hautala T, Grunst T, Fabrega A, Freimuth P, Welsh MJ. An interaction between penton base and alpha v integrins plays a minimal role in adenovirus-mediated gene transfer to hepatocytes in vitro and in vivo. *Gene Ther*. 1998;5:1259-1264

[31] Smith TA, Idamakanti N, Rollence ML, Marshall-Neff J, Kim J, Mulgrew K, Nemerow GR, Kaleko M, Stevenson SC. Adenovirus serotype 5 fiber shaft influences in vivo gene transfer in mice. *Hum Gene Ther*. 2003;14:777-787

[32] Smith TA, Idamakanti N, Marshall-Neff J, Rollence ML, Wright P, Kaloss M, King L, Mech C, Dinges L, Iverson WO, Sherer AD, Markovits JE, Lyons RM, Kaleko M, Stevenson SC. Receptor interactions involved in adenoviral-mediated gene delivery after systemic administration in non-human primates. *Hum Gene Ther*. 2003;14:1595-1604

[33] Kritz AB, Nicol CG, Dishart KL, Nelson R, Holbeck S, Von Seggern DJ, Work LM, McVey JH, Nicklin SA, Baker AH. Adenovirus 5 fibers mutated at the putative hspg-binding site show restricted retargeting with targeting peptides in the hi loop. *Mol Ther*. 2007;15:741-749

[34] Bayo-Puxan N, Cascallo M, Gros A, Huch M, Fillat C, Alemany R. Role of the putative heparan sulfate glycosaminoglycan-binding site of the adenovirus type 5 fiber shaft on liver detargeting and knob-mediated retargeting. *J Gen Virol*. 2006;87:2487-2495

[35] Di Paolo NC, Kalyuzhniy O, Shayakhmetov DM. Fiber shaft-chimeric adenovirus vectors lacking the kktk motif efficiently infect liver cells in vivo. *J Virol.* 2007;81:12249-12259

[36] Parker AL, Waddington SN, Nicol CG, Shayakhmetov DM, Buckley SM, Denby L, Kemball-Cook G, Ni S, Lieber A, McVey JH, Nicklin SA, Baker AH. Multiple vitamin k-dependent coagulation zymogens promote adenovirus-mediated gene delivery to hepatocytes. *Blood.* 2006;108:2554-2561

[37] Parker AL, McVey JH, Doctor JH, Lopez-Franco O, Waddington SN, Havenga MJ, Nicklin SA, Baker AH. Influence of coagulation factor zymogens on the infectivity of adenoviruses pseudotyped with fibers from subgroup d. *J Virol.* 2007;81:3627-3631

[38] Shayakhmetov DM, Gaggar A, Ni S, Li ZY, Lieber A. Adenovirus binding to blood factors results in liver cell infection and hepatotoxicity. *J Virol.* 2005;79:7478-7491

[39] Waddington SN, McVey JH, Bhella D, Parker AL, Barker K, Atoda H, Pink R, Buckley SM, Greig JA, Denby L, Custers J, Morita T, Francischetti IM, Monteiro RQ, Barouch DH, van Rooijen N, Napoli C, Havenga MJ, Nicklin SA, Baker AH. Adenovirus serotype 5 hexon mediates liver gene transfer. *Cell.* 2008;132:397-409

[40] Vigant F, Descamps D, Jullienne B, Esselin S, Connault E, Opolon P, Tordjmann T, Vigne E, Perricaudet M, Benihoud K. Substitution of hexon hypervariable region 5 of adenovirus serotype 5 abrogates blood factor binding and limits gene transfer to liver. *Mol Ther.* 2008;16:1474-1480

[41] Morral N, O'Neal W, Rice K, Leland M, Kaplan J, Piedra PA, Zhou H, Parks RJ, Velji R, Aguilar-Cordova E, Wadsworth S, Graham FL, Kochanek S, Carey KD, Beaudet AL. Administration of helper-dependent adenoviral vectors and sequential delivery of different vector serotype for long-term liver-directed gene transfer in baboons. *Proc Natl Acad Sci U S A.* 1999;96:12816-12821.

[42] Parks R, Evelegh C, Graham F. Use of helper-dependent adenoviral vectors of alternative serotypes permits repeat vector administration. *Gene therapy.* 1999;6:1565-1573

[43] Sakurai F, Mizuguchi H, Yamaguchi T, Hayakawa T. Characterization of in vitro and in vivo gene transfer properties of adenovirus serotype 35 vector. *Mol Ther.* 2003;8:813-821

[44] Seshidhar Reddy P, Ganesh S, Limbach MP, Brann T, Pinkstaff A, Kaloss M, Kaleko M, Connelly S. Development of adenovirus serotype 35 as a gene transfer vector. *Virology.* 2003;311:384-393

[45] Alba R, Bradshaw AC, Parker AL, Bhella D, Waddington SN, Nicklin SA, van Rooijen N, Custers J, Goudsmit J, Barouch DH, McVey JH, Baker AH. Identification of coagulation factor (f)x binding sites on the adenovirus serotype 5 hexon: Effect of mutagenesis on fx interactions and gene transfer. *Blood.* 2009

[46] Stone D, Ni S, Li ZY, Gaggar A, DiPaolo N, Feng Q, Sandig V, Lieber A. Development and assessment of human adenovirus type 11 as a gene transfer vector. *J Virol.* 2005;79:5090-5104

[47] Stone D, Liu Y, Li ZY, Tuve S, Strauss R, Lieber A. Comparison of adenoviruses from species b, c, e, and f after intravenous delivery. *Mol Ther.* 2007;15:2146-2153

[48] Kuzmin AI, Finegold MJ, Eisensmith RC. Macrophage depletion increases the safety, efficacy and persistence of adenovirus-mediated gene transfer in vivo. *Gene Ther.* 1997;4:309-316.
[49] Schiedner G, Hertel S, Johnston M, Dries V, van Rooijen N, Kochanek S. Selective depletion or blockade of kupffer cells leads to enhanced and prolonged hepatic transgene expression using high-capacity adenoviral vectors. *Mol Ther.* 2003;7:35-43
[50] Niwano M, Arii S, Monden K, Ishiguro S, Nakamura T, Mizumoto M, Takeda Y, Fujioka M, Imamura M. Amelioration of sinusoidal endothelial cell damage by kupffer cell blockade during cold preservation of rat liver. *J Surg Res.* 1997;72:36-48
[51] Deaciuc IV, Bagby GJ, Niesman MR, Skrepnik N, Spitzer JJ. Modulation of hepatic sinusoidal endothelial cell function by kupffer cells: An example of intercellular communication in the liver. *Hepatology.* 1994;19:464-470
[52] Haisma HJ, Kamps JA, Kamps GK, Plantinga JA, Rots MG, Bellu AR. Polyinosinic acid enhances delivery of adenovirus vectors in vivo by preventing sequestration in liver macrophages. *J Gen Virol.* 2008;89:1097-1105
[53] Wisse E. An electron microscopic study of the fenestrated endothelial lining of rat liver sinusoids. *J Ultrastruct Res.* 1970;31:125-150
[54] Braet F, Wisse E. Structural and functional aspects of liver sinusoidal endothelial cell fenestrae: A review. *Comp Hepatol.* 2002;1:1
[55] Wisse E, De Zanger RB, Charels K, Van Der Smissen P, McCuskey RS. The liver sieve: Considerations concerning the structure and function of endothelial fenestrae, the sinusoidal wall and the space of disse. *Hepatology.* 1985;5:683-692
[56] Wisse E, De Zanger RB, Jacobs R, McCuskey RS. Scanning electron microscope observations on the structure of portal veins, sinusoids and central veins in rat liver. *Scan Electron Microsc.* 1983:1441-1452
[57] Higashi N, Ueda H, Yamada O, Oikawa S, Koiwa M, Tangkawattana P, Takehana K. Micromorphological characteristics of hepatic sinusoidal endothelial cells and their basal laminae in five different animal species. *Okajimas Folia Anat Jpn.* 2002;79:135-142
[58] Gatmaitan Z, Varticovski L, Ling L, Mikkelsen R, Steffan AM, Arias IM. Studies on fenestral contraction in rat liver endothelial cells in culture. *Am J Pathol.* 1996;148:2027-2041
[59] Wisse E, Braet F, Duimel H, Vreuls C, Koek G, Olde Damink SW, van den Broek MA, De Geest B, Dejong CH, Tateno C, Frederik P. Fixation methods for electron microscopy of human and other liver. *World J Gastroenterol.* 2010;16:2851-2866
[60] Snoeys J, Lievens J, Wisse E, Jacobs F, Duimel H, Collen D, Frederik P, De Geest B. Species differences in transgene DNA uptake in hepatocytes after adenoviral transfer correlate with the size of endothelial fenestrae. *Gene Ther.* 2007;14:604-612
[61] Lievens J, Snoeys J, Vekemans K, Van Linthout S, de Zanger R, Collen D, Wisse E, De Geest B. The size of sinusoidal fenestrae is a critical determinant of hepatocyte transduction after adenoviral gene transfer. *Gene Ther.* 2004;11:1523-1531
[62] Wisse E, Jacobs F, Topal B, Frederik P, De Geest B. The size of endothelial fenestrae in human liver sinusoids: Implications for hepatocyte-directed gene transfer. *Gene Ther.* 2008;15:1193-1199
[63] Wright PL, Smith KF, Day WA, Fraser R. Small liver fenestrae may explain the susceptibility of rabbits to atherosclerosis. *Arteriosclerosis.* 1983;3:344-348

[64] Chen H. Comparative observation of the recombinant adeno-associated virus 2 using transmission electron microscopy and atomic force microscopy. *Microsc Microanal.* 2007;13:384-389

[65] Szilagyi JF, Berriman J. Herpes simplex virus 1 particles contain spherical membrane-enclosed inclusion vesicles. *J Gen Virol.* 1994;75 (Pt 7):1749-1753

[66] Li S, Rizzo MA, Bhattacharya S, Huang L. Characterization of cationic lipid-protamine-DNA (lpd) complexes for intravenous gene delivery. *Gene Ther.* 1998;5:930-937

[67] Banerjee R. Liposomes: Applications in medicine. *J Biomater Appl.* 2001;16:3-21

[68] Jacobs F, Feng Y, Van Craeyveld E, Lievens J, Snoeys J, De Geest B. Species differences in hepatocyte-directed gene transfer: Implications for clinical translation. *Curr Gene Ther.* 2009;9:83-90

[69] Raper SE, Yudkoff M, Chirmule N, Gao GP, Nunes F, Haskal ZJ, Furth EE, Propert KJ, Robinson MB, Magosin S, Simoes H, Speicher L, Hughes J, Tazelaar J, Wivel NA, Wilson JM, Batshaw ML. A pilot study of in vivo liver-directed gene transfer with an adenoviral vector in partial ornithine transcarbamylase deficiency. *Hum Gene Ther.* 2002;13:163-175

[70] Brunetti-Pierri N, Stapleton GE, Law M, Breinholt J, Palmer DJ, Zuo Y, Grove NC, Finegold MJ, Rice K, Beaudet AL, Mullins CE, Ng P. Efficient, long-term hepatic gene transfer using clinically relevant hdad doses by balloon occlusion catheter delivery in nonhuman primates. *Mol Ther.* 2009;17:327-333

[71] Zhang G, Gao X, Song YK, Vollmer R, Stolz DB, Gasiorowski JZ, Dean DA, Liu D. Hydroporation as the mechanism of hydrodynamic delivery. *Gene Ther.* 2004;11:675-682

[72] VandenDriessche T, Thorrez L, Naldini L, Follenzi A, Moons L, Berneman Z, Collen D, Chuah MK. Lentiviral vectors containing the human immunodeficiency virus type-1 central polypurine tract can efficiently transduce nondividing hepatocytes and antigen-presenting cells in vivo. *Blood.* 2002;100:813-822.

[73] Follenzi A, Sabatino G, Lombardo A, Boccaccio C, Naldini L. Efficient gene delivery and targeted expression to hepatocytes in vivo by improved lentiviral vectors. *Hum Gene Ther.* 2002;13:243-260

[74] Kang Y, Xie L, Tran DT, Stein CS, Hickey M, Davidson BL, McCray PB, Jr. Persistent expression of factor viii in vivo following nonprimate lentiviral gene transfer. *Blood.* 2005;106:1552-1558

[75] Nguyen TH, Aubert D, Bellodi-Privato M, Flageul M, Pichard V, Jaidane-Abdelghani Z, Myara A, Ferry N. Critical assessment of lifelong phenotype correction in hyperbilirubinemic gunn rats after retroviral mediated gene transfer. *Gene Ther.* 2007;14:1270-1277

[76] Liu F, Shollenberger LM, Conwell CC, Yuan X, Huang L. Mechanism of naked DNA clearance after intravenous injection. *J Gene Med.* 2007;9:613-619

[77] Herweijer H, Wolff JA. Gene therapy progress and prospects: Hydrodynamic gene delivery. *Gene Ther.* 2007;14:99-107

[78] Suda T, Gao X, Stolz DB, Liu D. Structural impact of hydrodynamic injection on mouse liver. *Gene Ther.* 2007;14:129-137

[79] Neubauer K, Saile B, Ramadori G. Liver fibrosis and altered matrix synthesis. *Can J Gastroenterol.* 2001;15:187-193

[80] Horn T, Christoffersen P, Henriksen JH. Alcoholic liver injury: Defenestration in noncirrhotic livers--a scanning electron microscopic study. *Hepatology*. 1987;7:77-82
[81] Garcia-Banuelos J, Siller-Lopez F, Miranda A, Aguilar LK, Aguilar-Cordova E, Armendariz-Borunda J. Cirrhotic rat livers with extensive fibrosis can be safely transduced with clinical-grade adenoviral vectors. Evidence of cirrhosis reversion. *Gene Ther*. 2002;9:127-134
[82] Yeikilis R, Gal S, Kopeiko N, Paizi M, Pines M, Braet F, Spira G. Hydrodynamics based transfection in normal and fibrotic rats. *World J Gastroenterol*. 2006;12:6149-6155
[83] Ichida T, Hata K, Yamada S, Hatano T, Miyagiwa M, Miyabayashi C, Matsui S, Wisse E. Subcellular abnormalities of liver sinusoidal lesions in human hepatocellular carcinoma. *J Submicrosc Cytol Pathol*. 1990;22:221-229
[84] Kin M, Torimura T, Ueno T, Inuzuka S, Tanikawa K. Sinusoidal capillarization in small hepatocellular carcinoma. *Pathol Int*. 1994;44:771-778
[85] Liu F, Song Y, Liu D. Hydrodynamics-based transfection in animals by systemic administration of plasmid DNA. *Gene Ther*. 1999;6:1258-1266
[86] Zhang G, Budker V, Wolff JA. High levels of foreign gene expression in hepatocytes after tail vein injections of naked plasmid DNA. *Hum Gene Ther*. 1999;10:1735-1737
[87] Jacobs F, Snoeys J, Feng Y, Van Craeyveld E, Lievens J, Armentano D, Cheng SH, De Geest B. Direct comparison of hepatocyte-specific expression cassettes following adenoviral and nonviral hydrodynamic gene transfer. *Gene therapy*. 2008;15:594-603
[88] Eastman SJ, Baskin KM, Hodges BL, Chu Q, Gates A, Dreusicke R, Anderson S, Scheule RK. Development of catheter-based procedures for transducing the isolated rabbit liver with plasmid DNA. *Hum Gene Ther*. 2002;13:2065-2077
[89] Yoshino H, Hashizume K, Kobayashi E. Naked plasmid DNA transfer to the porcine liver using rapid injection with large volume. *Gene Ther*. 2006;13:1696-1702
[90] Fabre JW, Grehan A, Whitehorne M, Sawyer GJ, Dong X, Salehi S, Eckley L, Zhang X, Seddon M, Shah AM, Davenport M, Rela M. Hydrodynamic gene delivery to the pig liver via an isolated segment of the inferior vena cava. *Gene therapy*. 2008;15:452-462
[91] Lieber A, He CY, Meuse L, Schowalter D, Kirillova I, Winther B, Kay MA. The role of kupffer cell activation and viral gene expression in early liver toxicity after infusion of recombinant adenovirus vectors. *J Virol*. 1997;71:8798-8807.
[92] Muruve DA, Barnes MJ, Stillman IE, Libermann TA. Adenoviral gene therapy leads to rapid induction of multiple chemokines and acute neutrophil-dependent hepatic injury in vivo. *Hum Gene Ther*. 1999;10:965-976.
[93] Zhang Y, Chirmule N, Gao GP, Qian R, Croyle M, Joshi B, Tazelaar J, Wilson JM. Acute cytokine response to systemic adenoviral vectors in mice is mediated by dendritic cells and macrophages. *Mol Ther*. 2001;3:697-707.
[94] Schnell MA, Zhang Y, Tazelaar J, Gao GP, Yu QC, Qian R, Chen SJ, Varnavski AN, LeClair C, Raper SE, Wilson JM. Activation of innate immunity in nonhuman primates following intraportal administration of adenoviral vectors. *Mol Ther*. 2001;3:708-722.
[95] Zaiss AK, Liu Q, Bowen GP, Wong NC, Bartlett JS, Muruve DA. Differential activation of innate immune responses by adenovirus and adeno-associated virus vectors. *J Virol*. 2002;76:4580-4590.

[96] Liu Q, Zaiss AK, Colarusso P, Patel K, Haljan G, Wickham TJ, Muruve DA. The role of capsid-endothelial interactions in the innate immune response to adenovirus vectors. *Hum Gene Ther*. 2003;14:627-643

[97] Nunes FA, Furth EE, Wilson JM, Raper SE. Gene transfer into the liver of nonhuman primates with e1-deleted recombinant adenoviral vectors: Safety of readministration. *Hum Gene Ther*. 1999;10:2515-2526

[98] Kobayashi S, Nagino M, Yokoyama Y, Nimura Y, Sokabe M. Evaluation of hepatic interleukin-6 secretion following portal vein ligation using a minimal surgical stress model. *J Surg Res*. 2006;135:27-33

[99] De Geest B, Snoeys J, Van Linthout S, Lievens J, Collen D. Elimination of innate immune responses and liver inflammation by pegylation of adenoviral vectors and methylprednisolone. *Hum Gene Ther*. 2005;16:1439-1451

[100] Appledorn DM, Patial S, McBride A, Godbehere S, Van Rooijen N, Parameswaran N, Amalfitano A. Adenovirus vector-induced innate inflammatory mediators, mapk signaling, as well as adaptive immune responses are dependent upon both tlr2 and tlr9 in vivo. *J Immunol*. 2008;181:2134-2144

[101] Zhong B, Ma HY, Yang Q, Gu FR, Yin GQ, Xia CM. Decrease in toll-like receptors 2 and 4 in the spleen of mouse with endotoxic tolerance. *Inflamm Res*. 2008;57:252-259

[102] Martin-Armas M, Simon-Santamaria J, Pettersen I, Moens U, Smedsrod B, Sveinbjornsson B. Toll-like receptor 9 (tlr9) is present in murine liver sinusoidal endothelial cells (lsecs) and mediates the effect of cpg-oligonucleotides. *J Hepatol*. 2006;44:939-946

[103] Equils O, Schito ML, Karahashi H, Madak Z, Yarali A, Michelsen KS, Sher A, Arditi M. Toll-like receptor 2 (tlr2) and tlr9 signaling results in hiv-long terminal repeat trans-activation and hiv replication in hiv-1 transgenic mouse spleen cells: Implications of simultaneous activation of tlrs on hiv replication. *J Immunol*. 2003;170:5159-5164

[104] Croyle MA, Le HT, Linse KD, Cerullo V, Toietta G, Beaudet A, Pastore L. Pegylated helper-dependent adenoviral vectors: Highly efficient vectors with an enhanced safety profile. *Gene Ther*. 2005;12:579-587

[105] Gao G, Lu Y, Calcedo R, Grant RL, Bell P, Wang L, Figueredo J, Lock M, Wilson JM. Biology of aav serotype vectors in liver-directed gene transfer to nonhuman primates. *Mol Ther*. 2006;13:77-87

[106] Zhu J, Huang X, Yang Y. The tlr9-myd88 pathway is critical for adaptive immune responses to adeno-associated virus gene therapy vectors in mice. *J Clin Invest*. 2009;119:2388-2398

[107] Muller A, Schott-Ohly P, Dohle C, Gleichmann H. Differential regulation of th1-type and th2-type cytokine profiles in pancreatic islets of c57bl/6 and balb/c mice by multiple low doses of streptozotocin. *Immunobiology*. 2002;205:35-50

[108] Van Linthout S, Lusky M, Collen D, De Geest B. Persistent hepatic expression of human apo A-I after transfer with a helper-virus independent adenoviral vector. *Gene Ther*. 2002;9:1520-1528.

[109] De Geest B, Van Linthout S, Lox M, Collen D, Holvoet P. Sustained expression of human apolipoprotein A-I after adenoviral gene transfer in c57bl/6 mice: Role of apolipoprotein A-I promoter, apolipoprotein A-I introns, and human apolipoprotein e enhancer. *Hum Gene Ther*. 2000;11:101-112.

[110] De Geest B, Van Linthout S, Collen D. Sustained expression of human apo A-I following adenoviral gene transfer in mice. *Gene Ther.* 2001;8:121-127.

[111] Van Linthout S, Collen D, De Geest B. Effect of promoters and enhancers on expression, transgene DNA persistence, and hepatotoxicity after adenoviral gene transfer of human apolipoprotein A-I. *Hum Gene Ther.* 2002;13:829-840.

[112] Nathwani AC, Davidoff A, Hanawa H, Zhou JF, Vanin EF, Nienhuis AW. Factors influencing in vivo transduction by recombinant adeno-associated viral vectors expressing the human factor ix cdna. *Blood.* 2001;97:1258-1265

[113] Mount JD, Herzog RW, Tillson DM, Goodman SA, Robinson N, McCleland ML, Bellinger D, Nichols TC, Arruda VR, Lothrop CD, Jr., High KA. Sustained phenotypic correction of hemophilia b dogs with a factor ix null mutation by liver-directed gene therapy. *Blood.* 2002;99:2670-2676

[114] Mingozzi F, Liu YL, Dobrzynski E, Kaufhold A, Liu JH, Wang Y, Arruda VR, High KA, Herzog RW. Induction of immune tolerance to coagulation factor ix antigen by in vivo hepatic gene transfer. *J Clin Invest.* 2003;111:1347-1356

[115] De Geest BR, Van Linthout SA, Collen D. Humoral immune response in mice against a circulating antigen induced by adenoviral transfer is strictly dependent on expression in antigen-presenting cells. *Blood.* 2003;101:2551-2556

[116] Follenzi A, Battaglia M, Lombardo A, Annoni A, Roncarolo MG, Naldini L. Targeting lentiviral vector expression to hepatocytes limits transgene-specific immune response and establishes long-term expression of human antihemophilic factor ix in mice. *Blood.* 2004;103:3700-3709

[117] Van Linthout S, Spillmann F, Riad A, Trimpert C, Lievens J, Meloni M, Escher F, Filenberg E, Demir O, Li J, Shakibaei M, Schimke I, Staudt A, Felix SB, Schultheiss HP, De Geest B, Tschope C. Human apolipoprotein A-I gene transfer reduces the development of experimental diabetic cardiomyopathy. *Circulation.* 2008;117:1563-1573

[118] Pastore L, Morral N, Zhou H, Garcia R, Parks RJ, Kochanek S, Graham FL, Lee B, Beaudet AL. Use of a liver-specific promoter reduces immune response to the transgene in adenoviral vectors. *Hum Gene Ther.* 1999;10:1773-1781.

[119] Franco LM, Sun B, Yang X, Bird A, Zhang H, Schneider A, Brown T, Young SP, Clay TM, Amalfitano A, Chen YT, Koeberl DD. Evasion of immune responses to introduced human acid alpha-glucosidase by liver-restricted expression in glycogen storage disease type ii. *Mol Ther.* 2005;12:876-884

[120] Al-Dosari M, Zhang G, Knapp JE, Liu D. Evaluation of viral and mammalian promoters for driving transgene expression in mouse liver. *Biochem Biophys Res Commun.* 2006;339:673-678

[121] Guo ZS, Wang LH, Eisensmith RC, Woo SL. Evaluation of promoter strength for hepatic gene expression in vivo following adenovirus-mediated gene transfer. *Gene Ther.* 1996;3:802-810

[122] Kankkonen HM, Vahakangas E, Marr RA, Pakkanen T, Laurema A, Leppanen P, Jalkanen J, Verma IM, Yla-Herttuala S. Long-term lowering of plasma cholesterol levels in ldl-receptor-deficient whhl rabbits by gene therapy. *Mol Ther.* 2004;9:548-556

[123] Wang L, Calcedo R, Nichols TC, Bellinger DA, Dillow A, Verma IM, Wilson JM. Sustained correction of disease in naive and aav2-pretreated hemophilia b dogs: Aav2/8-mediated, liver-directed gene therapy. *Blood.* 2005;105:3079-3086
[124] Brinster RL, Allen JM, Behringer RR, Gelinas RE, Palmiter RD. Introns increase transcriptional efficiency in transgenic mice. *Proc Natl Acad Sci U S A.* 1988;85:836-840
[125] Liu K, Sandgren EP, Palmiter RD, Stein A. Rat growth hormone gene introns stimulate nucleosome alignment in vitro and in transgenic mice. *Proc Natl Acad Sci U S A.* 1995;92:7724-7728
[126] Miao CH, Ohashi K, Patijn GA, Meuse L, Ye X, Thompson AR, Kay MA. Inclusion of the hepatic locus control region, an intron, and untranslated region increases and stabilizes hepatic factor ix gene expression in vivo but not in vitro. *Mol Ther.* 2000;1:522-532.
[127] Palmiter RD, Sandgren EP, Avarbock MR, Allen DD, Brinster RL. Heterologous introns can enhance expression of transgenes in mice. *Proc Natl Acad Sci U S A.* 1991;88:478-482
[128] Agarwal M, Austin TW, Morel F, Chen J, Bohnlein E, Plavec I. Scaffold attachment region-mediated enhancement of retroviral vector expression in primary t cells. *J Virol.* 1998;72:3720-3728
[129] Auten J, Agarwal M, Chen J, Sutton R, Plavec I. Effect of scaffold attachment region on transgene expression in retrovirus vector-transduced primary t cells and macrophages. *Hum Gene Ther.* 1999;10:1389-1399
[130]Dang Q, Auten J, Plavec I. Human beta interferon scaffold attachment region inhibits de novo methylation and confers long-term, copy number-dependent expression to a retroviral vector. *J Virol.* 2000;74:2671-2678
[131] Miao CH, Thompson AR, Loeb K, Ye X. Long-term and therapeutic-level hepatic gene expression of human factor ix after naked plasmid transfer in vivo. *Mol Ther.* 2001;3:947-957
[132] Schiedner G, Hertel S, Johnston M, Biermann V, Dries V, Kochanek S. Variables affecting in vivo performance of high-capacity adenovirus vectors. *J Virol.* 2002;76:1600-1609
[133] De Geest B, Zhao Z, Collen D, Holvoet P. Effects of adenovirus-mediated human apo A-I gene transfer on neointima formation after endothelial denudation in apo E-deficient mice. *Circulation.* 1997;96:4349-4356.

6

Physiologically-Regulated Expression Vectors for Gene Therapy

Olivia Hibbitt and Richard Wade-Martins
University of Oxford, Department of Physiology Anatomy and Genetics
United Kingdom

1. Introduction

Gene-replacement gene therapy has been under development for a number of years. In spite of the large amount of research invested into developing gene therapy for the treatment of recessive genetic disorders only a limited number of patients world-wide have received the benefits. In addition, several high profile adverse events in gene therapy trials have lead to an increasing awareness of the challenges facing gene therapy treatments before they become established in the clinic. This has necessitated the development of novel advances in gene therapy vector design and delivery. This chapter will focus on the development of gene expression vectors incorporating native genomic regulatory elements that ensure transgene expression is physiologically relevant. Three main advances will be discussed here in detail; the use of whole genomic DNA loci to ensure physiologically-regulated transgene expression; development of viral vectors based on the herpes simplex virus type 1 for delivery of whole genomic DNA loci; and the development of genomic mini-gene vectors that contain native regulatory regions for the physiologically-regulated expression of cDNA mini-genes.

The principal aim of gene-replacement gene therapy is to complement the loss of function of an endogenous gene by supplying an exogenous 'working' copy in *trans*. The conventional approach to this is to supply a wild-type cDNA copy of the gene in a small vector in which transgene expression is controlled by a strong heterologous promoter, such as the immediate early promoter of cytomegalovirus (pCMV). The advantage of this approach is that the vectors are easy to use, have high levels of transgene expression, and fit easily into most viral delivery systems such as lentivirus and adenovirus. However, expression from these vectors is characteristically short-term and wide-spread with no tissue specificity or temporal regulation. One alternative to heterologous expression vectors for gene therapy is to utilise native genomic DNA regulatory elements to ensure gene expression that is both spatially and temporally regulated. A highly effective means of achieving gene expression that is physiologically-regulated is through the use of whole genomic loci which contain all introns, exons and regulatory regions in the correct genomic context. Expression from whole genomic loci has been proven to recapitulate endogenous expression. In the context of gene therapy, delivery of whole genomic loci using bacterial artificial chromosomes (BAC) has been shown to be an effective means of complementing gene deficiencies. Delivery of BAC vectors carrying complete loci encoding, for example, the genes for the human low density lipoprotein receptor (*LDLR*), the Friedreich's ataxia (FRDA) frataxin protein (FXN), microtubule associated protein tau (*MAPT*) and hypoxanthine phosphoribosyltransferase (*HPRT*) effectively rescue gene deficiencies *in vitro*. It has also been shown that the complementation of gene deficiency is responsive to changes in the cellular milieu, an important point for conditions where gene expression is controlled by cellular signalling pathways and where over-expression of the gene is toxic.

Historically, BAC vectors have been discounted for gene therapy purposes as there was no viral delivery system with the transgene capacity for a whole genomic locus which may be ≥100 kb. Recently, viral vectors based on the herpes simplex virus type (HSV-1) amplicons have been developed and shown to have a transgene capacity of over 100 kb and a broad cell tropism making them an attractive means of delivering large transgenes for the purposes of gene therapy. Currently HSV-1 amplicons have been used in a number of gene complementation studies which will be reviewed in detail here.

Recent work in our laboratory has adapted the genomic locus approach for the treatment of familial hypercholesterolaemia (FH). FH is a condition caused by mutations in the *LDLR* gene and represents a unique challenge in gene therapy. Over-expression of the LDL receptor leads to a toxic accumulation of intracellular cholesterol. It is therefore essential that *LDLR* transgene expression is appropriately regulated. We have generated gene expression vectors in which expression of the *LDLR* cDNA was controlled by 10 kb of genomic DNA encompassing key regulatory regions in the *LDLR* genomic DNA promoter. These regulatory regions sense the levels of intracellular cholesterol. When cholesterol levels in the cell are high, LDLR expression is low; when the cholesterol stores become depleted, expression of the LDL receptor is high. Delivery of the *LDLR* mini-gene expression vectors in vitro and in vivo lead to efficient and prolonged *LDLR* gene expression in vivo that is sensitive to changes in cellular cholesterol and resulted in a decrease in circulating cholesterol in receptor deficient mice.

2. Physiologically-relevant gene expression vectors: use of a complete genomic locus

The central aim of gene-replacement gene therapy is to complement the loss of function of an endogenous gene by supplying a working copy of that gene *in trans*. Classically this was achieved using cDNA coding for the endogenous gene under the expression control of constitutively active exogenous promoters such as the immediate early promoter from the cytomegalovirus (pCMV). In general transgene expression levels from these vectors are characteristically high and therefore therapeutic effect is seen in some conditions. Clinical trials have demonstrated that these vectors are effective in ameliorating the symptoms of conditions such as haemophilia (Manno et al. 2006) and several severe combined immunodeficiencies (SCID) such as X-linked SCID (Cavazzana-Calvo et al. 2000), adenosine deaminase deficiency (Aiuti et al. 2009) and chronic granulomatous disease (Ott et al. 2006). The SCID trials also demonstrated that delivery of transgenes in the context of small cDNA vectors with no native expression control did have a number of issues including cell transformation.

2.1 Complete genomic locus ensures gene expression in the correct genomic context

There are several issues which may confound the use of cDNA expression cassettes to complement the loss of function of an endogenous gene: aberrant spatial expression dynamics resulting in gene expression in 'off-target' cells; aberrant temporal dynamics resulting in continuous expression of a transgene with possible cytotoxic consequences; transgene over-expression at supra-physiological levels; and, the inability to produce multiple splice variants.

Transgenic mice offer an interesting insight into the benefits of using native genomic loci over cDNA expression systems to investigate the function of genes. For some genes it is essential that they are expressed in the correct spatial, developmental and temporal context to ensure functionality. The β-globin gene cluster is an excellent example of this. This genomic locus consists of five separate genes (5′-ε-^{G}γ-^{A}γ-δ-β-3′) that are expressed at different developmental stages (Huang et al. 2000). The γ genes are expressed in foetal erythroid tissues while the δ and β are expressed in adult haematopoietic cells of the erythroid lineage. The expression of these genes in under the control of a region called the locus control region (Huang, Liu et al. 2000). In mice expressing the β-globin from a cDNA expression plasmid without the locus control region, low levels of protein are detected with no tissue-specificity (Magram et al. 1985; May et al. 2000; Vadolas et al. 2005). The use of the entire genomic locus of the β-globin gene cluster which included the locus control regions resulted in spatial and temporal expression profiles that mimicked the native profile (Porcu et al. 1997; Vadolas, Wardan et al. 2005).

Further examples of the advantages of using the complete genomic locus comes from mice lacking either the frataxin (*Fxn*) gene (Cossee et al. 2000; Miranda et al. 2002) or the cystic fibrosis transmembrane conductance regulator (*Cftr*) gene (Zhou et al. 1994; Manson et al. 1997), mouse models of Friedrich's ataxia and cystic fibrosis, respectively. Mice lacking frataxin die at embryonic day six and crossing heterozygous knock-out mice with mice expressing the full genomic locus of the human *FXN* gene from a bacterial artificial chromosome (BAC) rescues the phenotype and expression patterns of mRNA and protein was physiological (Sarsero et al. 2004). Transgenic mice lacking the endogenous *Cftr* gene but expressing the full 200 kb of the human *CFTR* gene in a yeast artificial chromosome (YAC) show correct expression of CFTR protein in the appropriate spatial and temporal context (Manson, Trezise et al. 1997).

Other examples include comparisons between mice expressing the amyloid precursor protein (APP) as either a cDNA construct or as a complete locus within a YAC. The APP gene is involved with the development of Alzheimer's disease. It is a complex genomic locus comprising 18 exons that are alternatively spliced to give rise to four distinct transcripts (Hsiao et al. 1996). Mice expressing the APP cDNA vector do not express APP protein in the correct genomic context limiting the relevance of biological information obtained from these animals (Lamb 1995; Lamb et al. 1997). Mice expressing APP from the YAC construct displayed physiologically-relevant APP protein expression making them a far superior tool for the study of how APP might contribute to the development of Alzheimer's disease (Lamb, Call et al. 1997).

The advantages of using BAC plasmids to generate transgenic mice is now widely accepted. BAC transgenics have been shown, for example, to rescue knockout phenotypes in mice lacking the Pkd1 gene involved in polycystic kidney disease (Pritchard et al. 2000) and mice lacking β-globin genes (Vadolas et al. 2002; Jamsai et al. 2005; Vadolas, Wardan et al. 2005; Jamsai et al. 2006). BACs have also been useful in investigating novel genomic expression control regions. A negative regulatory region in the Wilson's disease gene was characterised using BAC plasmids (Bochukova et al. 2003). BACs were also used to characterise the locus control regions responsible for the differential expression of Myf5 in skeletal muscle (Carvajal et al. 2001; Zammit et al. 2004). In addition to this, insertion of reporter genes into

BAC plasmids has enabled the understanding of spatial and temporal expression dynamics of many genes such as Nkx2-5 (Chi et al. 2003). Recently BAC transgenesis has been used in studies of immunomodulation (Kulik et al. 2011), blood vessel development (Ishitobi et al. 2010) and in generating mouse models of Parkinson's disease that more closely recapitulate deficits in the human disease (Li et al. 2009). These studies represent a small sub-section of the work being performed using whole genomic loci to better understand gene function. They demonstrate that the use of native regulatory regions can yield more biologically-relevant data than over-expression studies. This is important in the generation of mouse models of disease and also in the development of therapeutic protocols to treat genetic disease.

2.2 Complete genomic locus for therapy

Transgenic animals offer extensive evidence that the use of cDNA expression vectors often does not result in physiologically-relevant expression patterns. In terms of gene therapy the use of these cDNA vectors may not be appropriate for diseases where the correct physiological expression of the transgene is vital for therapeutic effect and to protect cells from ectopic or cytotoxic over-expression, where proteins expressed with no control result in pathological changes in the transduced cell.

The use of a complete genomic DNA region in the design of gene therapy vectors is still a relatively new field. Manipulation and use of such large pieces of DNA can be challenging. Success has been seen however with a range of genes using a number of different techniques to isolate and deliver the locus. *In vitro* studies demonstrated that it was possible to achieve gene expression following non-viral BAC plasmid delivery. The gene involved in Lesh-Nyan syndrome, hypoxanthine phosphoriribosyltransferase (*HPRT*) was delivered to *HPRT* deficient fibroblasts and resulted in sustained physiological levels of *HPRT* (Wade-Martins et al. 2000). Lipofection and an integrin targeting peptide were used to deliver a 143 kb BAC encompassing the locus of Nijmegen breakage syndrome gene (*NBS1*) resulting in expression of the *NBS1* gene product, nibrin (White et al. 2003). BACs have also been generated that contain the *CFTR* locus (Kotzamanis et al. 2009) delivery of which to CMT-93 cells resulted in mRNA expression that was correctly spliced (Kotzamanis, Abdulrazzak et al. 2009).

In vivo non-viral delivery of plasmids containing large genomic DNA inserts has been achieved in two studies. In the first study hydrodynamic tail vein injection or lipofection was used to successfully deliver plasmids containing 150 kb of non-gene specific DNA (Magin-Lachmann et al. 2004). We have also demonstrated efficient delivery of a 135 kb genomic insert containing the full human low density lipoprotein receptor (*LDLR*) genomic locus for the treatment of Familial Hypercholesterolaemia (FH). We showed that up to 4 months following hydrodynamic tail vein injection, human LDLR protein was detectible in the livers of recipient mice (Hibbitt et al. 2007).

Alternatives to BAC plasmids for delivery of large genomic inserts are also being investigated. Human artificial chromosomes (HACs) for example offer advantages over the bacterial counterparts. HAC vectors are able to replicate and segregate without integration into the host-cell chromosomes and are capable of carrying very large amounts of DNA. HACs have been shown to be an effective means of generating transgenic mice (Suzuki 2006). They have also been used to express *HPRT* (Moralli et al. 2006) and *CFTR* complete genes (Rocchi et al. 2010). In addition a HAC containing the entire 2.4 Mb genomic locus of the human dytrophin gene was used to stably maintain expression of human dystrophin in mouse embryonic stem cells (Hoyshiya 2009) without any integration into the host cell chromosomes. These cells were used to generate chimeric mice analysis of which showed correct tissue-specific dystrophin expression. As the HACs are stable they could be useful in cell therapies in the future.

Viral vectors have also been developed to achieve infectious delivery of large genomic sequences. A gutless adenovirus with a transgene capacity of 36 kb was used to deliver the whole locus of the human α1 antitrypsin gene (*SERPINA1*) to mice (Schiedner et al. 1998). Vectors based on the Epstein Barr virus have also been used to deliver 120 kb of genomic DNA to cells of lymphoblast and B-cell lineage (White et al. 2002). Other viral systems have been under investigation, such as CMV which has a very large transgene capacity of around 210 kb and a strong haematopoietic cell tropism (Borst and Messerle 2000; Borst and Messerle 2003). However, the best characterised is amplicon vectors based on Herpes Simplex 1 (HSV-1).

2.3 Infectious delivery of a complete genomic locus – HSV-1 amplicons

The large size of a compete genomic locus precludes their use with most viral vector systems which typically have a transgene capacity of less than 20 kb. Vectors based on the herpes virus family however have a much larger transgene capacity. HSV-1 in particular is well described and widely used. Wild-type HSV-1 infects mucosa and establishes a latent phase in sensory neurons. HSV-1 infection produces cold sores in symptomatic infected individuals and 90% of the population has circulating antibodies (Corey and Spear 1986; Bowers et al. 2003). The HSV-1 genome consists of 152 kb of double stranded DNA. Of this only two non-coding regions are required for the packaging of DNA plasmids into HSV-1 virions (Spaete and Frenkel 1982; Spaete and Frenkel 1985). Inclusion of these two packaging signals, the *OriS* and *pac*, into DNA plasmids will promote their packaging into HSV-1 virions in the presence of the HSV-1 genome in *trans*. Plasmids are packaged head to tail in concatemers up to 150 kb. The average size of a human genomic locus is around 40 kb and the 150 kb capacity of HSV-1 amplicons potentially allows delivery of up to 90% of genomic loci as infectious particles, making the vector a highly versatile viral packaging system (Senior and Wade-Martins 2005; Hibbitt and Wade-Martins 2006).

HSV-1 amplicons are capable of infecting dividing and non-dividing cells including, but not limited to; neurons, such as those of the dorsal root ganglion (Marsh et al. 2000), thalamus (Costantini et al. 1999), cortex (Agudo et al. 2002), hippocampus (Adrover et al. 2003), glial cells (Marsh, Dekaban et al. 2000), gliomas (Shah et al. 2004), skeletal muscle (Wang et al. 2000; Wang et al. 2002) and osteoblasts (Xing et al. 2004). HSV-1 amplicons also retain their ability for retrograde transport in neuronal axons allowing for the possibility of peripheral delivery for centrally located targets. For example inoculation of the foot pad in diabetic rats with HSV-1 amplicons expressing nerve growth factor (NGF) resulted in NGF expression in the dorsal root ganglion and protected against diabetes associated peripheral neuropathy (Goss et al. 2002).

One of the key concerns with any viral vector system is safety. HSV-1 amplicons are non-integrating viruses which thus avoids issues of cell transformation by insertional mutagenesis. The packaging of *OriS* and *pac* containing plasmids into HSV-1 amplicons requires the presence of the HSV-1 genome in *trans*. To improve vector safety helper virus-free HSV-1 amplicon packaging systems have been developed. The supply of the HSV-1 genome in *trans* has been achieved by the use of BAC plasmids encompassing the full genome and lacking the packaging signal (Saeki et al. 1998; Stavropoulos and Strathdee

1998). Further safety mechanisms were then added to the system. One recent packaging BAC now widely used has both the packaging signal (*pac*) and the essential gene, ICP27, deleted, and is also oversized to preclude its inclusion into HSV-1 virions (Saeki et al. 2003). It has also been demonstrated that this packaging system is an efficient means of generating infectious BAC (iBAC) particles that have been successfully used for gene expression in vivo and *in vitro*. Overall, helper virus-free packaging systems for HSV-1 amplicons result in vector stocks with a much reduced immune-response *in vivo* (Olschowka et al. 2003).

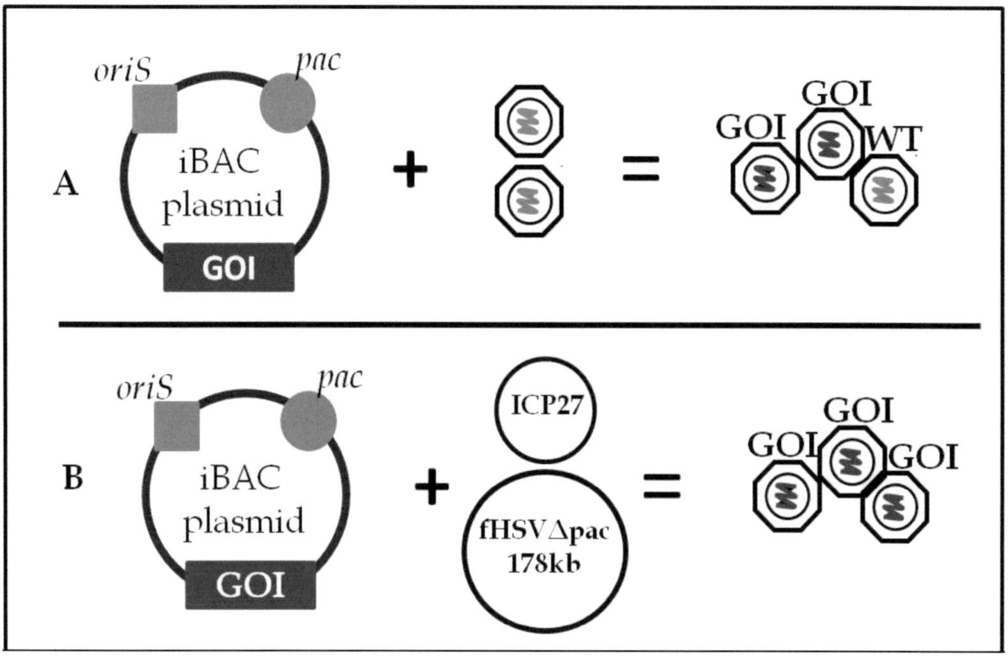

Fig. 1. Packaging of HSV-1 amplicons.

Schematic showing packaging of OriS and pac containing plasmids into HSV-1 virions. A) AniBAC plasmid containing the gene of interst (GOI) is packaged using packaging virus to supply the HSV-1 genome in trans. This results in viral stocks that contain virions only carrying the iBAC GOI plasmid and wild-type-like virus. B) An improved packaging system using two plasmids in place of the wild-type-like virus. An oversized, ICP27 deleted BAC plasmid and a small plasmid that contains ICP27. This results in viral stocks that only contain virions with GOI containing iBAC.

HSV-1 delivers DNA to the cell as an extrachromosomal element and hybrid vectors have been designed to promote persistence of episomal vector DNA (Figure 2). The best described of these is the HSV-1/EBV hybrid vectors. The inclusion of the EBV latent origin of replication *OriP* and the EBV nuclear antigen (EBNA-1) promotes replication and segregation of DNA during cell division (Wang and Vos 1996; Wade-Martins et al. 2001; Wade-Martins et al. 2003; Muller et al. 2005). Mammalian-based systems have also been investigated. The inclusion of scaffold matrix attachment regions (SMARs) to an iBAC containing the human *LDLR* gene resulted in the establishment of stable, episomal *LDLR* expression in cell lines (Lufino et al. 2007). Successful delivery and establishment of HACs has been shown in cells transduced with iBAC vectors carrying alpha satellite DNA inserts (Moralli, Simpson et al. 2006).

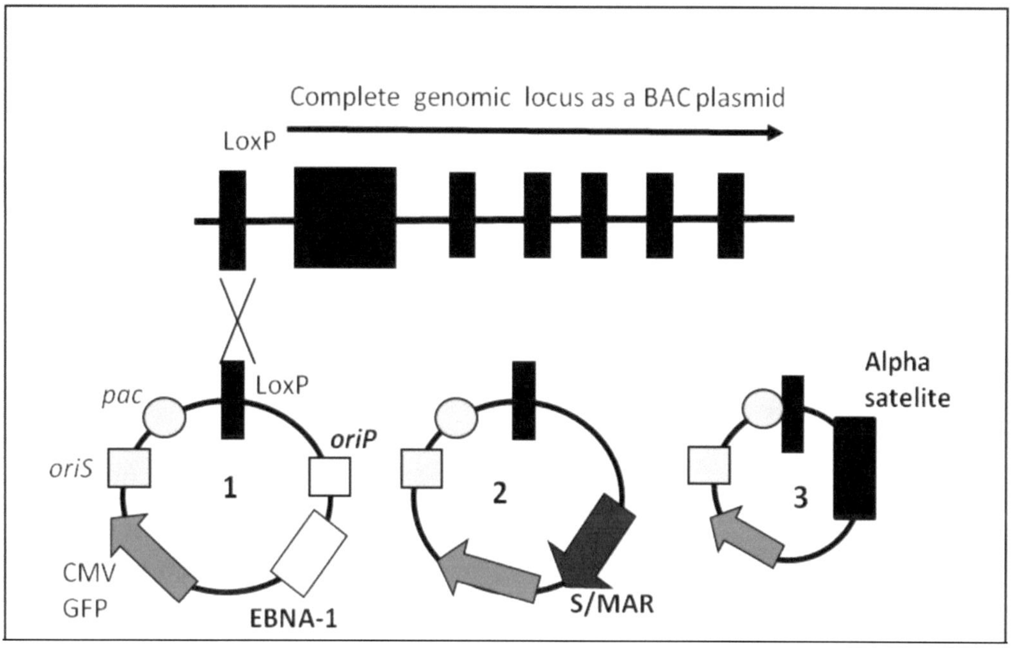

A BAC plasmid containing complete genomic locus can be retrofitted using cre-LoxP recombination with small plasmids containing elements essential for extrachromosomal maintance of delivered plasmids. Suggested in this figure is the incorpation of a CMV-green fluorescence protein (CMVGFP) reporter gene cassette to allow for assessment of delivery. The HSV-1 packaging signals (*pac* and *oriS*) and retention elements. ; 1) Contains the episomal retention elements from the Epstein Barr virus (EBNA-1 and oriP), 2) contains the S/MAR retention elements, 3) Alpha satelite DNA promotes the generation of human artificial chromosomes following delivery.

Fig. 2. Extrachromosomal retention elements.

The use of iBAC vectors in gene therapy is still evolving and a number of studies have demonstrated that these vectors are capable of efficient delivery and genetic complementation. Recent work has used the delivery and expression of the complete genomic of two genes key to the development of Alzheimer's disease and Parkinson's disease, microtubule associated protein tau (*MAPT*) and alpha synuclein (*SNCA*) to study gene function. Amplicon iBAC vectors carrying the 143 kb *MAPT* locus or the 135 kb *SNCA* locus were used to infect cellular models of neurodegeneration (Peruzzi et al. 2009). Expression of *MAPT* and *SNCA* in cells infected with the iBAC vectors was similar to endogenous human levels. It was found by comparing transgene expression in primary neuronal and glial cultures that expression from the *MAPT* locus was strictly regulated by developmental time-point and cell type. Multiple transcripts were observed which mimicked the expression pattern seen in humans. Infection of *MAPT*-deficient neurons in culture with the *MAPT* iBAC vector rescued the cellular phenotype, restoring the normal response to Aβ-peptide (Peruzzi, Lawler et al. 2009). This delivery system provides an effective means of investigating neurodegeneration in cell models.

Success had already been seen previously using iBAC vectors coding for the *HPRT* (Wade-Martins, Smith et al. 2001) as described in Section 2.2 or bone morphogenic protein 2 *(BMP2)* (Xing, Baylink et al. 2004) loci. The role of *BMP2* in osteoblast formation was investigated using iBAC delivery of the complete *BMP2* locus (Xing, Baylink et al. 2004). *BMP2* has been implicated in the differentiation of osteoblasts by altering alkaline phosphatase activity in precursor cells (Thies et al. 1992). When the iBAC-*BMP2* vector was used to infect a preosteoblast cell line differentiation was observed consistent with appropriate BMP2 expression (Xing, Baylink et al. 2004).

Small cDNA-based vectors are not suitable to express loci which undergo complex splicing, such as the *MAPT* locus discussed above. Another example is the human *CDKN2* genomic locus, an especially complex region. Expression from the *CDKN2* locus results in five different genes from only six exons (Sharpless and DePinho 1999). Two of the genes $p16^{INK4a}$ and $p14^{ARF}$ are particularly complex. Two separate promoter regions control expression of each gene. Separate first exons are spliced with second and third exons which are shared between the two transcripts (Sharpless and DePinho 1999). Both of these genes are involved in cell cycle control. They are being investigated as potential targets for cancer gene therapy. The 132 kb *CDKN2* locus was delivered as a iBAC vector to *CDKN2* knockout glioma cells. Cells transduced with the iBAC vector has physiological levels of expression and correct splicing of three gene products of the *CDKN2* locus, *p15*, $p16^{INK4a}$ and $p14^{ARF}$ (Inoue et al. 2004). Cells also displayed a phenotype of reduced growth consistent with expression of cell cycle arrest genes (Inoue, Moghaddam et al. 2004).

HSV-1 amplicons have been used to deliver the complete genomic locus of the *LDLR* gene to cell models of FH (Wade-Martins, Saeki et al. 2003; Lufino et al. 2007; Lufino, Manservigi et al. 2007). It was shown that delivery of the *LDLR* locus as an iBAC to *Ldlr* deficient CHO cells and FH patient fibroblasts lead to attenuation of the cellular phenotype as seen by normalisation of uptake and internalisation of LDL (Wade-Martins, Saeki et al. 2003; Lufino, Manservigi et al. 2007). Long-term expression was achieved by the use of the EBV episomal retention elements (Wade-Martins, Saeki et al. 2003) or scaffold matrix attached regions (Lufino, Manservigi et al. 2007). Both episomal retention systems promoted efficient establishment of the *LDLR* locus as a extrachromosomal element (Wade-Martins, Saeki et al. 2003; Lufino, Manservigi et al. 2007). Expression from this locus was down-regulated by sterol treatment through interaction with response elements in the promoter region (Wade-Martins, Saeki et al. 2003; Lufino, Manservigi et al. 2007).

The first example of *in vivo* infectious delivery of a whole genomic locus using the iBAC delivery system was recently described (Gimenez-Cassina et al. 2011). The entire 135 kb *FXN* gene was delivered as an iBAC directly to mouse cerebellum using intracranial injection. Analysis of expression of the *LacZ* reporter gene expressed from within the *FXN* locus showed large numbers of transduced cells in the cerebellum up to 75 days post-injection. This was also compared to reporter gene expression from the viral HSV-1 IE4/5 promoter which was short-lived *in vivo* from the same vector. This work is an elegant demonstration of the potential of BAC plasmid delivery in vivo to result in high-level sustained transgene expression.

The *LDLR* expression and *FXN* iBAC delivery studies represent an interesting proof of principle in the use of complete genomic regions to treat genetic disease via gene therapy. Delivery of the whole genomic locus is an elegant way to provide the therapeutic gene in its correct genomic context, ensuring that complementation can be physiologically-relevant, cell-specific and temporally-regulated. This has the potential effect of decreasing genotoxicity and improving the safety and efficacy of gene therapy vectors. However, the use of large genomic inserts can be technically challenging. Work is underway to develop gene expression vectors that combine the gene-regulation of a large insert with the convenience of a small mini-gene vector.

4. Physiologically-relevant gene expression vectors: use of native regulatory regions

Whole genomic loci represent an excellent means of ensuring physiologically-relevant expression in target cells. However, the large size of BAC plasmids precludes their use in all but a few viral vector systems. Although, non-viral systems such as hydrodynamic tail vein injection offer excellent means of delivery to target certain tissues, for many applications BAC-sized plasmids may not be practical. Many studies have attempted to combine the advantages of cDNA vectors (small size, high transduction or transfection efficiency, and high levels of protein expression) with an advantage of a whole genomic locus, being regulated physiologically-relevant expression. Depending on the gene of interest it may be necessary only to ensure expression of the transgene is restricted to a particular cell type; alternatively, it may be necessary to ensure transgene expression also tracks changes in cell physiology to ensure therapeutic and not pathologic transgene expression.

There has been extensive research into targeting gene expression to desired tissues using transcriptional restriction. Such work uses well-characterised promoters and enhancer regions that limit transgene expression to certain desired cell types where they are active. Liver-directed gene expression for example has been achieved using the promoter regions from either the albumin (Follenzi et al. 2002) or α1 antitrypsin genes (Le et al. 1997) to target expression of clotting factors to the liver to treat the haemophilia family of diseases. Targeting gene expression to cells in vascular wall is possible using endothelial cell restricted expression through the use of promoter such as VE-cadherin or VEGFR-1 (Quinn et al. 2000; Nicklin et al. 2001). Vascular smooth muscle specific expression has been achieved using promoters like the SM22 promoter (Imai et al. 2001) and was successfully used to target expression of heme oxygenase 1 to the vascular endothelium.

For some diseases it is not enough to limit expression to cell type. The temporal dynamics of gene expression is also important. One novel way of achieving physiological expression using small cDNA vectors is to generate a genomic mini-gene construct that uses native gene expression elements with a cDNA transgene. Wiskott-Aldrich syndrome (WAS) is an excellent example of the need for native regulatory elements to ensure correct expression dynamics. WAS is an X-linked recessive disease caused by mutations in the WAS protein gene (*WAS*) and defined by thrombocytopenia. *WAS* is expressed in haematopoietic cells at different concentrations depending on the cell type (Toscano et al. 2008). Over-expression in non-haematopoietic cells has been shown to be cytotoxic (Toscano, Frecha et al. 2008). Lentiviral delivery of *WAS* cDNA vectors where expression is governed by different fragments of the *WAS* gene promoter ranging from 500 bp to 1600 bp has demonstrated restricted expression of WASP in haematopoietic cells (Dupre et al. 2004; Martin et al. 2005; Leuci et al. 2009). These vectors were also able to correct the genetic defect in *Was* knockout mice and transduce haematopoietic cells from WAS patients. However, these relatively small promoter fragments were unable to achieve complete physiological regulation and some target cell types did not exhibit correct transgene expression profiles (Frecha et al. 2008). This may be because the promoter fragment was too small to contain all necessary machinery for all target cells.

One example in which clinical success has been seen with a vector containing native regulatory elements is in treatment of Leber's congenital amaurosis, a group of recessive congenital rod-cone dystrophies. Mutations in a retinal pigment epithelium specific gene called *RPE65* causes impaired vision from birth that degenerates to complete blindness later in life. An adeno-associated virus was constructed that contained the *RPE65* cDNA under the expression control of 1600 bp human *RPE65* promoter (Le Meur et al. 2007). The use of the native promoter region of the RPE65 gene effectively targeted expression to the retinal epithelium. This was shown to be effective at improving vision in a naturally occurring animal model; the Swedish Briard dog. This vector is now in clinical trials to treat this condition in humans (Bainbridge et al. 2008).

These two examples use only a minimal promoter region, which may be appropriate for those genes where regulatory elements are located in a small region proximal to the start of the coding region. However, as was seen in the WAS example, a larger portion of genomic DNA may be necessary for full physiological regulation. In our laboratory we have investigated the use of a 10 kb piece of genomic DNA to ensure fully physiological expression of the low density lipoprotein receptor gene (*LDLR*) for functional complementation *in vitro* and *in vivo* for the treatment of familial hypercholesterolaemia (FH). FH is caused by mutations in the LDL receptor which binds and internalises LDL cholesterol in response to low intracellular cholesterol levels. Gene therapy for FH been under investigation for a number of years with many published investigations reporting lowering of plasma cholesterol following delivery of cDNA vectors where expression is driven by heterologous promoters and delivery is achieved by virus-mediated liver-directed transduction with retrovirus (Miyanohara et al. 1988; Wilson et al. 1988; Chowdhury et al. 1991; Grossman et al. 1995; Kankkonen et al. 2004), adenovirus (Ishibashi et al. 1993; Kozarsky et al. 1994; Li et al. 1995; Kozarsky et al. 1996; Nomura et al. 2004; Jacobs et al. 2008; Van Craeyveld et al. 2011) and adeno-associated virus (Lebherz et al. 2004; Kassim et al. 2010). These previous studies included a clinical trial (Grossman, Rader et al. 1995) that showed no evidence of long-term therapeutic effect.

FH represents a significant challenge for gene therapy due to the regulation of *LDLR*. There are three issues that need to be overcome by a therapeutic protocol. Firstly, cholesterol biosynthesis in the liver is constitutive. This means any gene therapy protocol needs to supply an agent that is not only capable of clearing cholesterol already present in the serum, it needs to clear all future cholesterol that will be synthesised by the liver. This puts huge demands on the transduced cells. The second issue is that the *LDLR* locus is tightly regulated by a negative feedback system. Expression from the *LDLR* genomic locus is controlled by levels of intracellular cholesterol. When intracellular levels of cholesterol fall *LDLR* expression is triggered by the binding of sterol response element binding proteins (SREBP) to the sterol response elements in the promoter region (Sudhof et al. 1987; Briggs et al. 1993; Horton et al. 2002). This drives expression of the LDL receptor which binds and internalises LDL particles from the circulation. As cellular cholesterol stores become replete the SREBP become less active and expression from the *LDLR* locus is repressed. There is evidence that suggests hepatocytes are only metabolically able to deal with a certain amount of cholesterol influx. Delivery of cDNA vectors with strong viral promoters driving *LDLR* expression into cells, and animals, using adenovirus results in immediate, dramatic lowering of cholesterol. The initial lowering of cholesterol is slowly eroded over time as intracellular cytotoxic accumulation of cholesterol leads to apoptotic cell death and loss of the transduced population of cells. The third confounding factor is the physiological expression itself. It is apparent that physiologically-relevant expression of the LDLR is important for the function of the hepatocytes and the nature of the expression plasmid may limit its ability to clear large amounts of cholesterol from the blood. As the cholesterol stores in transduced cells become replete the expression of the LDLR transgene will be repressed effectively 'switching off' that particular cell's cholesterol processing ability, this could reduce the therapeutic effectiveness of physiological vectors.

We have previously shown that an iBAC vector containing the 135 kb *LDLR* genomic locus encompassing all 18 exons, intervening introns, sterol response elements and other regulatory elements all in the correct genomic context was capable of rescuing the genetic defect in cell models of FH (Wade-Martins, Saeki et al. 2003; Lufino, Manservigi et al. 2007). When we moved the focus of the work into animal models of FH we found that non-viral gene transfer via hydrodynamic tail vein injection to be an efficient means of vector delivery. Delivery of the *LDLR* BAC using hydrodynamic tail vein injection resulted in long-term expression of human LDLR in the liver over the full four month course of the experiment (Hibbitt, Harbottle et al. 2007). However, the level of hepatocyte transduction was insufficient to result in therapeutic lowering of cholesterol.

The challenge was to maintain physiologically-regulated expression while improving transfection efficiency using hydrodynamic tail vein injection. We built genomic DNA mini-gene vectors that contained 10 kb of genomic DNA encompassing the full genomic DNA promoter of the human *LDLR* gene (Hibbitt et al. 2010). This consisted of the 5' untranslated region, three sterol response elements, the transcription initiation sequence and eight kb upstream of genomic DNA that may contain as yet undescribed enhancer elements (Figure 3a). This genomic DNA promoter region was used to drive the cDNA of either the luciferase or human *LDLR* genes. We have shown *in vitro* that the 10 kb *LDLR* promoter provides stable, long-term, physiological expression and provides functional complementation in cell culture in *Ldlr* deficient CHO cells and FH patient fibroblasts (Figure 3b). Physiological *LDLR* promoter induction was demonstrated using either luciferase expression, or specific LDL binding and internalisation assays in the presence of modifiers of receptor expression, sterols or statins. Statins are specific inhibitors of the de novo cholesterol synthesis pathway. They act on the LDL receptor by decreasing the amount of cholesterol in the cell thereby up-regulating expression from the *LDLR* promoter. Incubation of cells with statins lead to a five-fold up-regulation of expression from the 10 kb promoter element. Sterols down-regulate LDL receptor expression through association with sterol response elements in the *LDLR* promoter region. Incubation with sterols lead to a 50% down-regulation of expression from the 10 kb promoter element.

Liver-directed delivery of LDLR mini-gene vectors in vivo using hydrodynamic tail vein injection resulted in expression from the *LDLR* promoter element that was sensitive to drug administration in vivo. Pravastatin administration resulted in a five-fold increase in luciferase expression five days after delivery (Figure 3c). The inclusion of EBV episomal retention elements ensured long-term expression up to 240 cell cycles *in vitro* and 9 months *in vivo* (Hibbitt, McNeil et al. 2010).

This work describes the successful combination of genomic DNA regulatory elements with a mini-gene cDNA vector. Expression from this vector is physiologically-regulated by intracellular cholesterol levels. Delivery of the smaller-sized mini-gene vector is more efficient than with the full BAC and highlights the possibility of combining gene replacement gene therapy with traditional medical treatments. Combining gene delivery with treatment that will reduce the amount of cholesterol being synthesised by the liver could increase the power of the gene delivery ensuring efficient binding and internalisation of LDL to reduce plasma cholesterol levels. We have demonstrated *in vivo* that treatment with statin drugs increases the activity of the *LDLR* promoter. We have also investigated the feasibility of using a more targeted approach. Statins work by inhibiting the conversion of HMG CoA to mevalonate by 3-hydroxy-3-methylglutaryl Coenzyme A reductase (HMGCR), the rate limiting step in cholesterol synthesis inhibitors. We have investigated whether knock-down of HMGCR might have a more specific effect leading to a greater reduction in cholesterol synthesis and therefore greater induction of LDLR. We have demonstrated that treatment with HMGCR-specific small-interferring RNAs and synthetic microRNAs leads to a ten-fold induction of the LDLR promoter *in vitro* and *in vivo* which resulted in a greater reduction in circulating LDL cholesterol in *Ldlr* knockout mice (Hibbitt et al. Accepted).

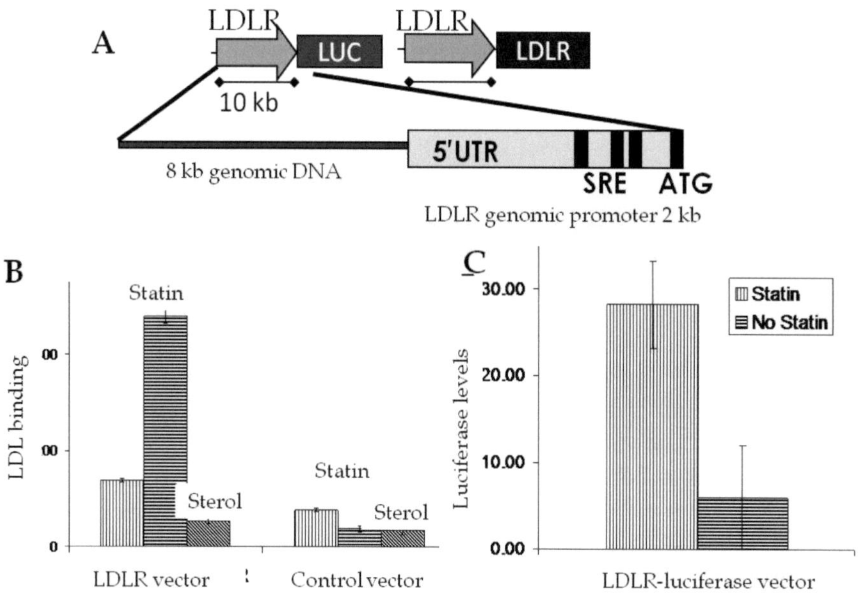

Generation of LDLR genomic mini-gene vectors. A) A 10kb Icece of genomic DNA encompassing the LDLR promoter the promoter region (UTR) and 8kb upstream of genomic DNA was cloned into vectors containing the cDNA of either luciferase or LDLR. B) Following delivery of LDLR cDNA containing vectors to patient fibroblasts binding and internalisation of LDL was observed. Increased binding was seen after cells were treated with statins. Decreased binding was observed with cells treated with sterols. Cells transduced with a control vector that did not contain the LDLR expression cassette showed no binding and internalisation of LDL. C) Animals injected with luciferase expressing vectors and treated with statins show a 5 fold induction of LDLR promoter activity compared to animals no treated with statin. Results were obtained using live animal luciferase imaging. Figure modified from (Hibbitt et. al.,2010).

Fig. 3. Genomic mini-gene vectors

3. Conclusion

Gene replacement gene therapy has been under investigation for a number of years and is emerging as a potentially potent tool to treat genetic disease. Most gene therapy protocols involve the use of small cDNA vectors where expression of the transgene is constitutive and unregulated. While for some conditions this may be adequate, others will require the expression of therapeutic genes to be regulated spatially, temporally and physiologically to circumvent issues with genotoxicity, loss of expression, and lack of therapeutic effect in animal models.

Several advances have been made in recent years to address these issues. The use of transcriptional restriction is now wide-spread with many studies employing cell-specific promoters to ensure gene expression is limited to target cells. There have also been developments in the use of whole genomic DNA loci transgenes. This opens the possibility of using vectors for gene therapy which completely recapitulate endogenous expression. Advances in viral vectors based on helper virus-free HSV-1 amplicons mean that viral delivery of large genomic loci >100 kb is now possible in vivo. Finally, the development of novel vectors which incorporate genomic DNA elements to achieve physiological expression in a mini-gene vector format will push the use of genomic regulatory elements in gene therapy vectors closer to a clinical reality.

A greater body of work *in vivo* is now needed using genomic regulatory vectors. Work is currently underway in our laboratory to assess the feasibility of using genomic mini-gene vectors to correct genetic defects in vivo long-term. We believe that these vectors represent a major addition to the gene therapy field and will be applicable to a wide range of genetic conditions.

4. Acknowledgements

Our work on gene therapy and vector development has been supported by the British Heart Foundation, the Medical Research Council, the Biotechnology and Biological Sciences Research Council, the Friedreich's Ataxia Research Alliance, and the Wellcome Trust.

5. References

Adrover, M. F., V. Guyot-Revol, et al. (2003). "Hippocampal infection with HSV-1-derived vectors expressing an NMDAR1 antisense modifies behavior." *Genes Brain Behav* 2(2): 103-113

Agudo, M., J. L. Trejo, et al. (2002). "Highly efficient and specific gene transfer to Purkinje cells in vivo using a herpes simplex virus I amplicon." *Hum Gene Ther* 13(5): 665-674

Aiuti, A., F. Cattaneo, et al. (2009). "Gene therapy for immunodeficiency due to adenosine deaminase deficiency." *N Engl J Med* 360(5): 447-458.1533-4406 (Electronic) 0028-4793 (Linking)

Bainbridge, J. W., A. J. Smith, et al. (2008). "Effect of gene therapy on visual function in Leber's congenital amaurosis." *N Engl J Med* 358(21): 2231-2239.1533-4406 (Electronic) 0028-4793 (Linking)

Bochukova, E. G., A. Jefferson, et al. (2003). "Genomic studies of gene expression: regulation of the Wilson disease gene." *Genomics* 81(6): 531-542

Borst, E. and M. Messerle (2000). "Development of a cytomegalovirus vector for somatic gene therapy." *Bone Marrow Transplant* 25 Suppl 2: S80-82.0268-3369 (Print) 0268-3369 (Linking)

Borst, E. M. and M. Messerle (2003). "Construction of a cytomegalovirus-based amplicon: a vector with a unique transfer capacity." *Hum Gene Ther* 14(10): 959-970

Bowers, W. J., J. A. Olschowka, et al. (2003). "Immune responses to replication-defective HSV-1 type vectors within the CNS: implications for gene therapy." *Gene Ther* 10(11): 941-945

Briggs, M. R., C. Yokoyama, et al. (1993). "Nuclear protein that binds sterol regulatory element of low density lipoprotein receptor promoter. I. Identification of the protein and delineation of its target nucleotide sequence." *J Biol Chem* 268(19): 14490-14496

Carvajal, J. J., D. Cox, et al. (2001). "A BAC transgenic analysis of the Mrf4/Myf5 locus reveals interdigitated elements that control activation and maintenance of gene expression during muscle development." *Development* 128(10): 1857-1868

Cavazzana-Calvo, M., S. Hacein-Bey, et al. (2000). "Gene therapy of human severe combined immunodeficiency (SCID)-X1 disease." *Science* 288(5466): 669-672.0036-8075 (Print) 0036-8075 (Linking)

Chi, X., S. X. Zhang, et al. (2003). "Expression of Nkx2-5-GFP bacterial artificial chromosome transgenic mice closely resembles endogenous Nkx2-5 gene activity." *Genesis* 35(4): 220-226

Chowdhury, J. R., M. Grossman, et al. (1991). "Long-term improvement of hypercholesterolemia after ex vivo gene therapy in LDLR-deficient rabbits." *Science* 254(5039): 1802-1805

Corey, L. and P. G. Spear (1986). "Infections with herpes simplex viruses (1)." *N Engl J Med* 314(11): 686-691

Cossee, M., H. Puccio, et al. (2000). "Inactivation of the Friedreich ataxia mouse gene leads to early embryonic lethality without iron accumulation." *Hum Mol Genet* 9(8): 1219-1226

Costantini, L. C., D. R. Jacoby, et al. (1999). "Gene transfer to the nigrostriatal system by hybrid herpes simplex virus/adeno-associated virus amplicon vectors." *Hum Gene Ther* 10(15): 2481-2494

Dupre, L., S. Trifari, et al. (2004). "Lentiviral vector-mediated gene transfer in T cells from Wiskott-Aldrich syndrome patients leads to functional correction." *Mol Ther* 10(5): 903-915.1525-0016 (Print) 1525-0016 (Linking)

Follenzi, A., G. Sabatino, et al. (2002). "Efficient gene delivery and targeted expression to hepatocytes in vivo by improved lentiviral vectors." *Hum Gene Ther* 13(2): 243-260.1043-0342 (Print) 1043-0342 (Linking)

Frecha, C., M. G. Toscano, et al. (2008). "Improved lentiviral vectors for Wiskott-Aldrich syndrome gene therapy mimic endogenous expression profiles throughout haematopoiesis." *Gene Ther* 15(12): 930-941.1476-5462 (Electronic) 0969-7128 (Linking)

Gimenez-Cassina, A., R. Wade-Martins, et al. (2011). "Infectious delivery and long-term persistence of transgene expression in the brain by a 135-kb iBAC-FXN genomic DNA expression vector." *Gene Ther*.1476-5462 (Electronic) 0969-7128 (Linking)

Goss, J. R., W. F. Goins, et al. (2002). "Herpes simplex-mediated gene transfer of nerve growth factor protects against peripheral neuropathy in streptozotocin-induced diabetes in the mouse." *Diabetes* 51(7): 2227-2232

Grossman, M., D. J. Rader, et al. (1995). "A pilot study of ex vivo gene therapy for homozygous familial hypercholesterolaemia." *Nat Med* 1(11): 1148-1154
Hibbitt, O., S. Agkatsev, et al. (Accepted). "RNAi-mediated knockdown of HMG CoA reductase enhances gene expression from physiologically-regulated low density lipoprotein receptor (LDLR) therapeutic vectors in vivo." *Gene Ther*
Hibbitt, O. C., R. P. Harbottle, et al. (2007). "Delivery and long-term expression of a 135 kb LDLR genomic DNA locus in vivo by hydrodynamic tail vein injection." *J Gene Med* 9(6): 488-497
Hibbitt, O. C., E. McNeil, et al. (2010). "Long-term physiologically regulated expression of the low-density lipoprotein receptor in vivo using genomic DNA mini-gene constructs." *Mol Ther* 18(2): 317-326.1525-0024 (Electronic) 1525-0016 (Linking)
Hibbitt, O. C. and R. Wade-Martins (2006). "Delivery of large genomic DNA inserts >100 kb using HSV-1 amplicons." *Curr Gene Ther* 6(3): 325-336
Horton, J. D., J. L. Goldstein, et al. (2002). "SREBPs: activators of the complete program of cholesterol and fatty acid synthesis in the liver." *J Clin Invest* 109(9): 1125-1131
Hsiao, K., P. Chapman, et al. (1996). "Correlative memory deficits, Abeta elevation, and amyloid plaques in transgenic mice." *Science* 274(5284): 99-102
Huang, Y., D. P. Liu, et al. (2000). "Proper developmental control of human globin genes reproduced by transgenic mice containing a 160-kb BAC carrying the human beta-globin locus." *Blood Cells Mol Dis* 26(6): 598-610
Imai, T., T. Morita, et al. (2001). "Vascular smooth muscle cell-directed overexpression of heme oxygenase-1 elevates blood pressure through attenuation of nitric oxide-induced vasodilation in mice." *Circ Res* 89(1): 55-62.1524-4571 (Electronic) 0009-7330 (Linking)
Inoue, R., K. A. Moghaddam, et al. (2004). "Infectious delivery of the 132 kb CDKN2A/CDKN2B genomic DNA region results in correctly spliced gene expression and growth suppression in glioma cells." *Gene Ther* 11(15): 1195-1204
Ishibashi, S., M. S. Brown, et al. (1993). "Hypercholesterolemia in low density lipoprotein receptor knockout mice and its reversal by adenovirus-mediated gene delivery." *J Clin Invest* 92(2): 883-893
Ishitobi, H., K. Matsumoto, et al. (2010). "Flk1-GFP BAC Tg mice: an animal model for the study of blood vessel development." *Exp Anim* 59(5): 615-622.1881-7122 (Electronic) 1341-1357 (Linking)
Jacobs, F., E. Van Craeyveld, et al. (2008). "Adenoviral low density lipoprotein receptor attenuates progression of atherosclerosis and decreases tissue cholesterol levels in a murine model of familial hypercholesterolemia." *Atherosclerosis* 201(2): 289-297.1879-1484 (Electronic) 0021-9150 (Linking)
Jamsai, D., F. Zaibak, et al. (2005). "A humanized mouse model for a common beta0-thalassemia mutation." *Genomics* 85(4): 453-461
Jamsai, D., F. Zaibak, et al. (2006). "A humanized BAC transgenic/knockout mouse model for HbE/beta-thalassemia." *Genomics* 88(3): 309-315
Kankkonen, H. M., E. Vahakangas, et al. (2004). "Long-term lowering of plasma cholesterol levels in LDL-receptor-deficient WHHL rabbits by gene therapy." *Mol Ther* 9(4): 548-556

Kassim, S. H., H. Li, et al. (2010). "Gene therapy in a humanized mouse model of familial hypercholesterolemia leads to marked regression of atherosclerosis." *PLoS One* 5(10): e13424.1932-6203 (Electronic) 1932-6203 (Linking)

Kotzamanis, G., H. Abdulrazzak, et al. (2009). "CFTR expression from a BAC carrying the complete human gene and associated regulatory elements." *J Cell Mol Med* 13(9A): 2938-2948.1582-4934 (Electronic) 1582-1838 (Linking)

Kozarsky, K. F., K. Jooss, et al. (1996). "Effective treatment of familial hypercholesterolaemia in the mouse model using adenovirus-mediated transfer of the VLDL receptor gene." *Nat Genet* 13(1): 54-62

Kozarsky, K. F., D. R. McKinley, et al. (1994). "In vivo correction of low density lipoprotein receptor deficiency in the Watanabe heritable hyperlipidemic rabbit with recombinant adenoviruses." *J Biol Chem* 269(18): 13695-13702

Kulik, L., K. Chen, et al. (2011). "Human complement receptor type 2 (CR2/CD21) transgenic mice provide an in vivo model to study immunoregulatory effects of receptor antagonists." *Mol Immunol* 48(6-7): 883-894.1872-9142 (Electronic) 0161-5890 (Linking)

Lamb, B. T. (1995). "Making models for Alzheimer's disease." *Nat Genet* 9(1): 4-6

Lamb, B. T., L. M. Call, et al. (1997). "Altered metabolism of familial Alzheimer's disease-linked amyloid precursor protein variants in yeast artificial chromosome transgenic mice." *Hum Mol Genet* 6(9): 1535-1541

Le, M., T. Okuyama, et al. (1997). "Therapeutic levels of functional human factor X in rats after retroviral-mediated hepatic gene therapy." *Blood* 89(4): 1254-1259.0006-4971 (Print) 0006-4971 (Linking)

Le Meur, G., K. Stieger, et al. (2007). "Restoration of vision in RPE65-deficient Briard dogs using an AAV serotype 4 vector that specifically targets the retinal pigmented epithelium." *Gene Ther* 14(4): 292-303.0969-7128 (Print) 0969-7128 (Linking)

Lebherz, C., G. Gao, et al. (2004). "Gene therapy with novel adeno-associated virus vectors substantially diminishes atherosclerosis in a murine model of familial hypercholesterolemia." *J Gene Med* 6(6): 663-672

Leuci, V., L. Gammaitoni, et al. (2009). "Efficient transcriptional targeting of human hematopoietic stem cells and blood cell lineages by lentiviral vectors containing the regulatory element of the Wiskott-Aldrich syndrome gene." *Stem Cells* 27(11): 2815-2823.1549-4918 (Electronic) 1066-5099 (Linking)

Li, J., B. Fang, et al. (1995). "In vivo gene therapy for hyperlipidemia: phenotypic correction in Watanabe rabbits by hepatic delivery of the rabbit LDL receptor gene." *J Clin Invest* 95(2): 768-773

Li, Y., W. Liu, et al. (2009). "Mutant LRRK2(R1441G) BAC transgenic mice recapitulate cardinal features of Parkinson's disease." *Nat Neurosci* 12(7): 826-828.1546-1726 (Electronic) 1097-6256 (Linking)

Lufino, M., O. Hibbitt, et al. (2007). Long-term regulated functional complementation of LDLR deficiency in cells using iBAC-SMAR-LDLR, a novel infectious genomic DNA episomal vector. American Society for Gene Therapy Annual Main Meeting, Seattle, Washington.

Lufino, M. M., R. Manservigi, et al. (2007). "An S/MAR-based infectious episomal genomic DNA expression vector provides long-term regulated functional complementation of LDLR deficiency." *Nucleic Acids Res* 35(15): e98

Magin-Lachmann, C., G. Kotzamanis, et al. (2004). "In vitro and in vivo delivery of intact BAC DNA -- comparison of different methods." *J Gene Med* 6(2): 195-209

Magram, J., K. Chada, et al. (1985). "Developmental regulation of a cloned adult beta-globin gene in transgenic mice." *Nature* 315(6017): 338-340

Manno, C. S., G. F. Pierce, et al. (2006). "Successful transduction of liver in hemophilia by AAV-Factor IX and limitations imposed by the host immune response." *Nat Med* 12(3): 342-347.1078-8956 (Print) 1078-8956 (Linking)

Manson, A. L., A. E. Trezise, et al. (1997). "Complementation of null CF mice with a human CFTR YAC transgene." *Embo J* 16(14): 4238-4249

Marsh, D. R., G. A. Dekaban, et al. (2000). "Herpes simplex viral and amplicon vector-mediated gene transfer into glia and neurons in organotypic spinal cord and dorsal root ganglion cultures." *Mol Ther* 1(5 Pt 1): 464-478

Martin, F., M. G. Toscano, et al. (2005). "Lentiviral vectors transcriptionally targeted to hematopoietic cells by WASP gene proximal promoter sequences." *Gene Ther* 12(8): 715-723.0969-7128 (Print) 0969-7128 (Linking)

May, C., S. Rivella, et al. (2000). "Therapeutic haemoglobin synthesis in beta-thalassaemic mice expressing lentivirus-encoded human beta-globin." *Nature* 406(6791): 82-86

Miranda, C. J., M. M. Santos, et al. (2002). "Frataxin knockin mouse." *FEBS Lett* 512(1-3): 291-297

Miyanohara, A., M. F. Sharkey, et al. (1988). "Efficient expression of retroviral vector-transduced human low density lipoprotein (LDL) receptor in LDL receptor-deficient rabbit fibroblasts in vitro." *Proc Natl Acad Sci U S A* 85(17): 6538-6542

Moralli, D., K. M. Simpson, et al. (2006). "A novel human artificial chromosome gene expression system using herpes simplex virus type 1 vectors." *EMBO Rep* 7(9): 911-918.1469-221X (Print) 1469-221X (Linking)

Muller, L., O. Saydam, et al. (2005). "Gene transfer into hepatocytes mediated by herpes simplex virus-Epstein-Barr virus hybrid amplicons." *J Virol Methods* 123(1): 65-72

Nicklin, S. A., P. N. Reynolds, et al. (2001). "Analysis of cell-specific promoters for viral gene therapy targeted at the vascular endothelium." *Hypertension* 38(1): 65-70.1524-4563 (Electronic) 0194-911X (Linking)

Nomura, S., A. Merched, et al. (2004). "Low-density lipoprotein receptor gene therapy using helper-dependent adenovirus produces long-term protection against atherosclerosis in a mouse model of familial hypercholesterolemia." *Gene Ther* 11(20): 1540-1548

Olschowka, J. A., W. J. Bowers, et al. (2003). "Helper-free HSV-1 amplicons elicit a markedly less robust innate immune response in the CNS." *Mol Ther* 7(2): 218-227

Ott, M. G., M. Schmidt, et al. (2006). "Correction of X-linked chronic granulomatous disease by gene therapy, augmented by insertional activation of MDS1-EVI1, PRDM16 or SETBP1." *Nat Med* 12(4): 401-409.1078-8956 (Print) 1078-8956 (Linking)

Peruzzi, P. P., S. E. Lawler, et al. (2009). "Physiological transgene regulation and functional complementation of a neurological disease gene deficiency in neurons." *Mol Ther* 17(9): 1517-1526.1525-0024 (Electronic) 1525-0016 (Linking)

Porcu, S., M. Kitamura, et al. (1997). "The human beta globin locus introduced by YAC transfer exhibits a specific and reproducible pattern of developmental regulation in transgenic mice." *Blood* 90(11): 4602-4609

Pritchard, L., J. A. Sloane-Stanley, et al. (2000). "A human PKD1 transgene generates functional polycystin-1 in mice and is associated with a cystic phenotype." *Hum Mol Genet* 9(18): 2617-2627

Quinn, G., T. Ochiya, et al. (2000). "Mouse flt-1 promoter directs endothelial-specific expression in the embyroid body model of embryogenesis." *Biochem Biophys Res Commun* 276(3): 1089-1099.0006-291X (Print) 0006-291X (Linking)

Rocchi, L., C. Braz, et al. (2010). "Escherichia coli-cloned CFTR loci relevant for human artificial chromosome therapy." *Hum Gene Ther* 21(9): 1077-1092.1557-7422 (Electronic) 1043-0342 (Linking)

Saeki, Y., X. O. Breakefield, et al. (2003). "Improved HSV-1 amplicon packaging system using ICP27-deleted, oversized HSV-1 BAC DNA." *Methods Mol Med* 76: 51-60

Saeki, Y., T. Ichikawa, et al. (1998). "Herpes simplex virus type 1 DNA amplified as bacterial artificial chromosome in Escherichia coli: rescue of replication-competent virus progeny and packaging of amplicon vectors." *Hum Gene Ther* 9(18): 2787-2794

Sarsero, J. P., L. Li, et al. (2004). "Human BAC-mediated rescue of the Friedreich ataxia knockout mutation in transgenic mice." *Mamm Genome* 15(5): 370-382

Schiedner, G., N. Morral, et al. (1998). "Genomic DNA transfer with a high-capacity adenovirus vector results in improved in vivo gene expression and decreased toxicity." *Nat Genet* 18(2): 180-183

Senior, S. L. and R. Wade-Martins (2005). "Herpes simplex virus type 1 amplicon vectors for the infectious delivery and expression of genomic DNA loci." *Curr Opin Mol Ther* 7(4): 337-345

Shah, K., C. H. Tung, et al. (2004). "In vivo imaging of HIV protease activity in amplicon vector-transduced gliomas." *Cancer Res* 64(1): 273-278

Sharpless, N. E. and R. A. DePinho (1999). "The INK4A/ARF locus and its two gene products." *Curr Opin Genet Dev* 9(1): 22-30

Spaete, R. R. and N. Frenkel (1982). "The herpes simplex virus amplicon: a new eucaryotic defective-virus cloning-amplifying vector." *Cell* 30(1): 295-304

Spaete, R. R. and N. Frenkel (1985). "The herpes simplex virus amplicon: analyses of cis-acting replication functions." *Proc Natl Acad Sci U S A* 82(3): 694-698

Stavropoulos, T. A. and C. A. Strathdee (1998). "An enhanced packaging system for helper-dependent herpes simplex virus vectors." *J Virol* 72(9): 7137-7143

Sudhof, T. C., D. W. Russell, et al. (1987). "42 bp element from LDL receptor gene confers end-product repression by sterols when inserted into viral TK promoter." *Cell* 48(6): 1061-1069

Thies, R. S., M. Bauduy, et al. (1992). "Recombinant human bone morphogenetic protein-2 induces osteoblastic differentiation in W-20-17 stromal cells." *Endocrinology* 130(3): 1318-1324

Toscano, M. G., C. Frecha, et al. (2008). "Hematopoietic-specific lentiviral vectors circumvent cellular toxicity due to ectopic expression of Wiskott-Aldrich syndrome protein." *Hum Gene Ther* 19(2): 179-197.1043-0342 (Print) 1043-0342 (Linking)

Vadolas, J., H. Wardan, et al. (2005). "Transgene copy number-dependent rescue of murine beta-globin knockout mice carrying a 183 kb human beta-globin BAC genomic fragment." *Biochim Biophys Acta* 1728(3): 150-162

Vadolas, J., H. Wardan, et al. (2002). "Development of sensitive fluorescent assays for embryonic and fetal hemoglobin inducers using the human beta -globin locus in erythropoietic cells." *Blood* 100(12): 4209-4216

Van Craeyveld, E., S. C. Gordts, et al. (2011). "Regression and stabilization of advanced murine atherosclerotic lesions: a comparison of LDL lowering and HDL raising gene transfer strategies." *J Mol Med*.1432-1440 (Electronic) 0946-2716 (Linking)

Wade-Martins, R., Y. Saeki, et al. (2003). "Infectious delivery of a 135-kb LDLR genomic locus leads to regulated complementation of low-density lipoprotein receptor deficiency in human cells." *Mol Ther* 7(5 Pt 1): 604-612

Wade-Martins, R., E. R. Smith, et al. (2001). "An infectious transfer and expression system for genomic DNA loci in human and mouse cells." *Nat Biotechnol* 19(11): 1067-1070

Wade-Martins, R., R. E. White, et al. (2000). "Stable correction of a genetic deficiency in human cells by an episome carrying a 115 kb genomic transgene." *Nat Biotechnol* 18(12): 1311-1314.1087-0156 (Print) 1087-0156 (Linking)

Wang, S. and J. M. Vos (1996). "A hybrid herpesvirus infectious vector based on Epstein-Barr virus and herpes simplex virus type 1 for gene transfer into human cells in vitro and in vivo." *J Virol* 70(12): 8422-8430

Wang, Y., S. M. Camp, et al. (2002). "Herpes simplex virus type 1/adeno-associated virus rep(+) hybrid amplicon vector improves the stability of transgene expression in human cells by site-specific integration." *J Virol* 76(14): 7150-7162

Wang, Y., C. Fraefel, et al. (2000). "HSV-1 amplicon vectors are a highly efficient gene delivery system for skeletal muscle myoblasts and myotubes." *Am J Physiol Cell Physiol* 278(3): C619-626

White, R. E., R. Wade-Martins, et al. (2003). "Functional delivery of large genomic DNA to human cells with a peptide-lipid vector." *J Gene Med* 5(10): 883-892

White, R. E., R. Wade-Martins, et al. (2002). "Infectious delivery of 120-kilobase genomic DNA by an epstein-barr virus amplicon vector." *Mol Ther* 5(4): 427-435

Wilson, J. M., D. E. Johnston, et al. (1988). "Correction of the genetic defect in hepatocytes from the Watanabe heritable hyperlipidemic rabbit." *Proc Natl Acad Sci U S A* 85(12): 4421-4425

Xing, W., D. Baylink, et al. (2004). "HSV-1 amplicon-mediated transfer of 128-kb BMP-2 genomic locus stimulates osteoblast differentiation in vitro." *Biochem Biophys Res Commun* 319(3): 781-786

Zammit, P. S., J. J. Carvajal, et al. (2004). "Myf5 expression in satellite cells and spindles in adult muscle is controlled by separate genetic elements." *Dev Biol* 273(2): 454-465

Zhou, L., C. R. Dey, et al. (1994). "Correction of lethal intestinal defect in a mouse model of cystic fibrosis by human CFTR." *Science* 266(5191): 1705-1708

7

PLP-Dependent Enzymes: a Potent Therapeutic Approach for Cancer and Cardiovascular Diseases

Ashraf S. El-Sayed and Ahmed A. Shindia
Microbiology Department, Faculty of Science, Zagazig University, Zagazig, Egypt

1. Introduction

The evolution on the field of biotechnology and proteomics create a novel therapeutic field (Enzymo-therapy) for treatment of various types of disease, particularly in the last fifty years. Exploitation of enzymes as anticancer, anti-cardiovascular, anticoagulants, antimicrobials and antioxidants (Vellard, 2003) was absolutely approved by Food and Drug Administration (FDA). Practically, almost of tumor cells were reported to be auxotrophs for L-methionine, glutamine, asparagine and arginine, due to the absence of intrinsic enzymatic systems synthesizing these amino acids, thus it depends for their growth and proliferation on the exogenous supply of these amino acids, that usually from diets (Hoffman and Erbe, 1976, Mecham et al., 1983, Pasut et al., 2007, El-Sayed, 2010). Consequently, L-methioninase, L-glutaminase, L-asparaginase and arginine deiminase were frequently used as common anticancer agents by sequestering their corresponding amino acids from the blood plasma (Hoffman, 1985, Klimberg and McClellan, 1996, Agrawal et al., 2003, Cheng et al., 2005).

Additionally, hyperaccumulation of certain metabolic intermediates as homocysteine and cystathionine usually associated with various cardiovascular diseases and complex disorders (Zou and Banerjee, 2005, Wang and Hegele, 2003). Cystathionine β-synthase and cystathionine γ-lyase are potential for sequestering homocysteine and cystathionine via transsulfuration metabolic pathways for production of glutathione and other antioxidants, so, these enzymes were described as anti-cardiovascular agents (Stipanuk, 2004, Zhu et al., 2008).

Unlike traditional approaches, Enzymo-therapy seems to be the promising therapeutic technology for their great specificity and affinity towards a clue substrate on specific metabolic pathway. However, the structural and conformational complexity of these enzymes makes it more vulnerable to extrinsic parameters, modulators, immunogenicity and proteolysis (Tan et al., 1996, Sun et al., 2003, Pasut et al., 2007). In addition, purification and formulation of these therapeutic enzymes, due to the economic expenses may add further complications.

Therefore, the various approaches for stabilization of these enzymes in situ and decreasing their immunogenicity were the objective of this context. The structural and catalytic identity of pyridoxal phosphate enzymes, molecular aspects to enhance their therapeutic potentiality, in addition to our prospectives will be exploited.

2. Pyridoxal 5'-phosphate dependent enzymes: classification and catalytic identities

Pyridoxal 5'-Phosphate (PLP) dependent enzymes, a group of versatile enzymes including about 145 distinct enzyme, 4% of the total cellular enzymatic activities (www.brenda.com) (Thornton et al., 2000, Percudani and Peracchi, 2003) which mainly uses PLP as covalent co-enzyme. PLP is an active phosphorylated derivative of vitamin B6 (pyridoxine) (Heyl et al., 1951). According to the international biochemical, molecular classification of enzymes (Enzyme Commission) (www.chem.qmul.ac.uk/iubmb), PLP-dependent enzymes were distributed in to five groups; 1- Oxido-reductase (EC 1; one enzyme), 2-Transferase (EC 2; eighty enzymes), 3- Hydrolase (EC 3; two enzymes), 4-Lyase (EC 4; Forty nine enzyme), and 5-Isomerase (EC 5; Thirteen enzyme) as totally 145 enzyme (Grishin et al., 1995, Percudani and Peracchi, 2003) as shown in Fig.1.

Practically, all the PLP-dependent-enzymes are mainly involved in amino acids transformation as decarboxylation, transamination, racemization, β, γ-elimination and β, γ-substitution (Percudani and Peracchi, 2003). The multiple functional catalytic modes of PLP-enzymes according to the position of net reaction were summarized in Table 1. PLP coenzyme has a pivotal role in catalysis of various enzymatic reactions. Pyridoxal phosphate can be synthesized de novo from preexisting precursor in bacteria (Brewke and Leistner, 2001), fungi (Bean et al., 2001, Ehrenshaft and Daub, 2001) and plants (Galperin and Koonin, 1997) from erythrose 4-phosphate, pyruvate and D-glyceraldhyde 3-phosphate. However, in human PLP cannot be synthesized de novo, it must be supplemented from the diet as pyridoxine, pyridoxamine and/or pyridoxal. PLP can be formed from pyridoxal via phosphorylation by action of kinase (PdxK; EC. 2.7.1.35), from oxidation of pyridoxamine/ pyridoxine by oxidase (EC. 1.4.3.5) (Choi et al., 1983, Bahn et al., 2002). Structurally, aldehyde group of PLP are bound covalently as internal aldimine (Schiff base)/ imine linkage to the Ɛ-amino group of lysine residues, close to *N*-terminus (Lopez et al., 2010) as in Fig. (2).

The role of PLP, during catalysis, is to reduce the energy for conversion of amino acids substrates to a zwitterionic carbonion (Richard and Amyes, 2004), substantially the apoenzyme catalyze the cleavage of substrate target bond yielding the product as reviewed by Richard et al. (2011). Regarding to the native internal aldimine of PLP-enzyme, the catalytic process started with formation of external aldimine linkage of amino group of substrate and pyridoxal phosphate coenzyme forming coenzyme-substrate Schiff base, replacing the Ɛ-amino group of lysine-enzyme (Schirch et al., 1993).This external aldimine of Co-enzyme-substrate Schiff base is the common intermediate for all PLP-dependent enzymes. Interestingly, pyridoxal phosphate without apo-enzyme, can slowly mediate many of reactions while the enzyme can ensure the substrate specificity and catalysis (Toney, 2005, Lopez et al., 2010), that justifies the lack of apoenzyme activity, with potentiality to recover its catalytic state upon supplementation by external PLP (El-Sayed, 2011). Since the formation of external aldimine, the pyridoxal phosphate is bounded tightly to the apoenzyme via nine hydrogen bonds (Johnson et al., 1990, Palm et al., 1990). The PLP extremely withdraw electrons, stabilizing the negative charge at α-carbon (carbanion) of the substrate as transition state that commonly referred as Quinonoid intermediates (Metha and Christen, 2000, Hult and Berglund, 2007). The catalytic promiscuity of PLP-dependent enzymes mainly depends on the mechanistic consequence of quinonoid intermediates (Alexander et al., 1994, Toney, 2005) as shown in Fig. (3).

Depending of crystallographic structures and topological studies, PLP-dependent enzymes were categorized in to five distinct folds (I-V) (Alexander et al., 1994, John, 1995, Jansonius, 1998) as illustrated in Table 2. The five independent fold types of PLP-enzymes were: Fold type I; Aspartate Aminotransferase (AAT) family; the most functionally diverse type containing α and γ-families of PLP-enzymes in which the internal aldimine was formed at lysine of *N*-terminus of the short helix at β-strand (Percudani and Peracchi, 2003). On AAT family, pyridine nitrogen is protonated and stabilized by interaction with enzyme aspartic and glutamic acid (Casanovas et al., 2009). Methionine γ-lyase, cystathionine β-synthase, cystathionine γ-lyase were belongs to this family. Fold type II; Tryptophan Synthase β-family, this family represented tryptophan synthase (Hyde et al., 1988), threonine deaminase (Gallagher et al., 1998) and *O*-acetylserine sulfhydrylase (Burkhard et al., 1998). The internal aldimine was at lysine residues of α-helix on the *N*-terminal domain. The apoenzyme was stabilized by interaction of its serine and threonine residues with pyridine ring of PLP (Percudani and peracchi, 2003). Fold type III; Alanine Racemase family; that represented by alanine racemase (Shaw et al., 2000), ornithine decarboxylase (Kern et al., 1999). Physically, the pyridine ring PLP, coenzyme, was interacted with NH moiety of arginine residues of apo-enzyme (Le-Magueres et al., 2005). Fold type IV; D-Amino Acid Aminotransferase family, that involve D-amino acid aminotransferase (Sugio, 1995), branched chain amino acid amino transferase (Okada et al., 1997) and 4-amino-4-deoxychorismate lyase (Nakai et al., 2000) as reviewed by Denesyuk et al. (2002). Like Type I, pyridine of PLP was interacted with glutamic acid of apoenzyme by hydrogen bonds (Sugio, 1995). Fold type V; Glycogen Phosphorylase Family; that contains glycogen phosphorylase (Sprang and Fletterick, 1979, Palm et al., 1990) and maltodextrin phosphorylase (Watson et al., 1999).

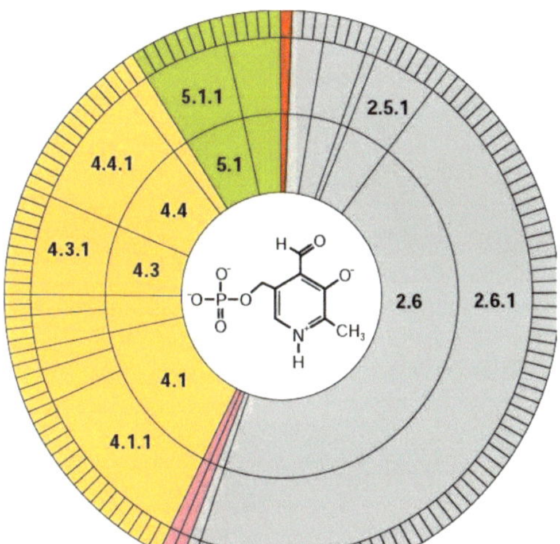

PLP-dependent enzymes were within five classes according to enzyme classification system (Enzyme Commission (EC) 1-Oxidoreductases, one enzyme (Red), 2-Transferase, 80 enzyme (faint blue), 3-Hydrolase, two enzymes (faint red), 4-Lyase, 49 enzyme (yellow) and 5-Isomearse, 13 enzyme (green). The catalytic diversity of PLP-dependent enzymes was described by Thornton et al. (2000) and Percudani and Peracchi (2003).

Fig. 1. Pyridoxal Phosphate Dependent Enzymes.

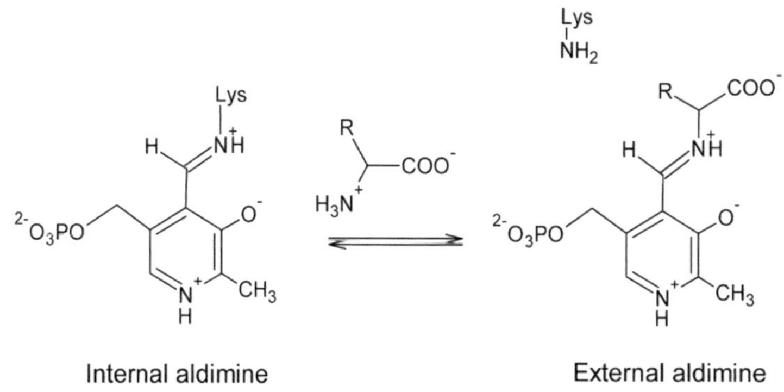

Fig. 2. Internal and External aldimine linkage of Pyridoxal Phosphate with enzyme and substrate, respectively

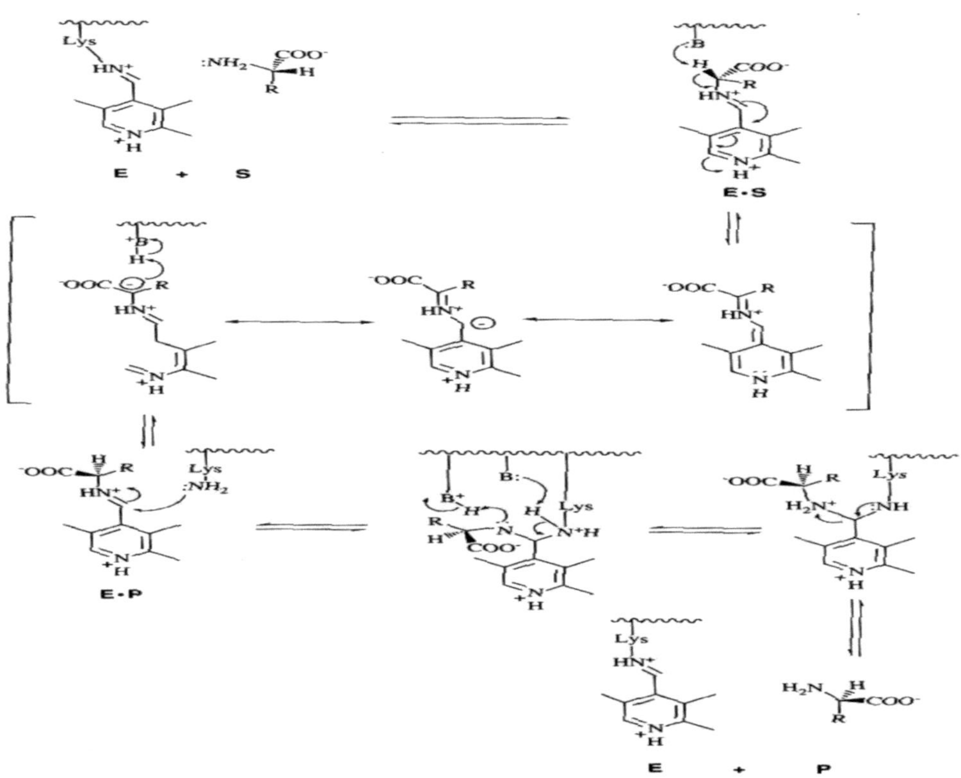

Fig. 3. Mechanism of PLP-enzyme catalysis via Quinonoid intermediates.

Reaction site	Reaction type	Mechanism of Reaction	Example of PLP-Enzyme
α-Position	Racemization	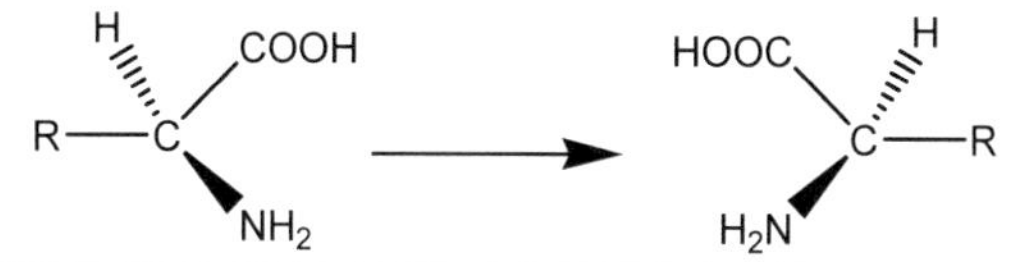	Alanine racemase
	Decarboxylation	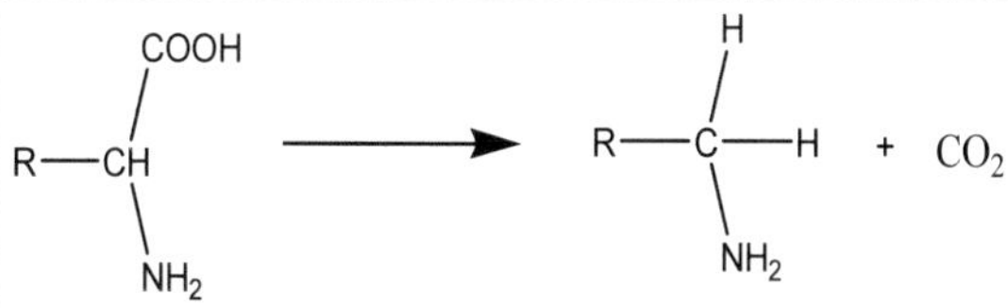	Ornithine decarboxylase
	Transamination	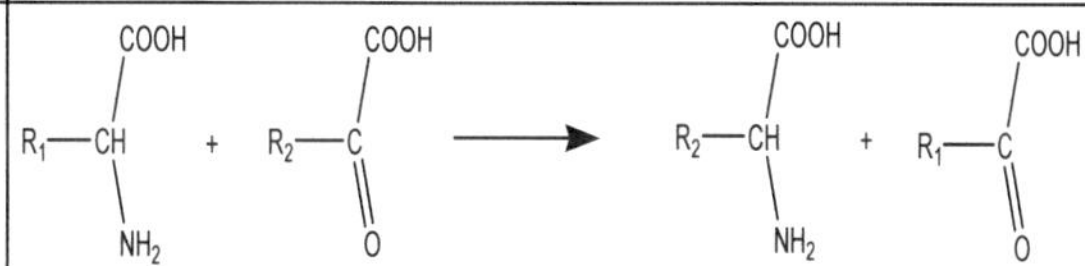	Tyrosine aminotransferase
	Elimination	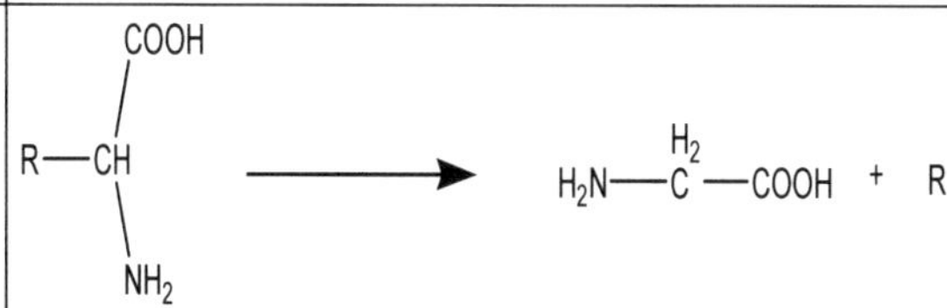	Serine hydroxylmethyltransferase
β-Position	Replacement	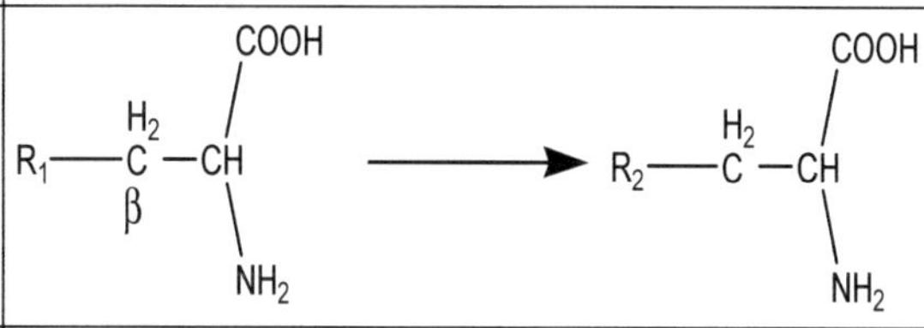	Tryptophan synthase
	Elimination	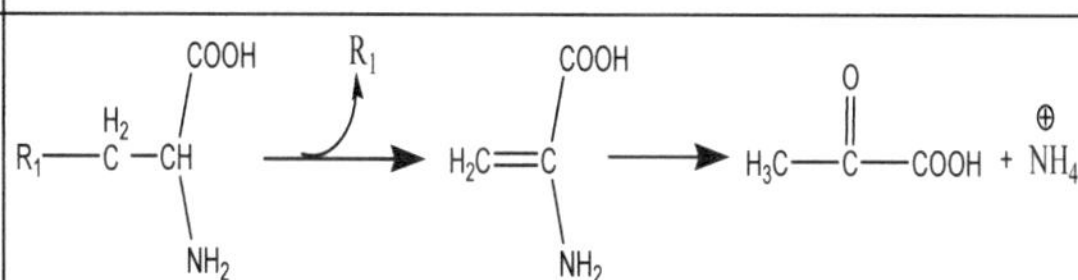	Serine dehydratase
γ-Position	Replacement	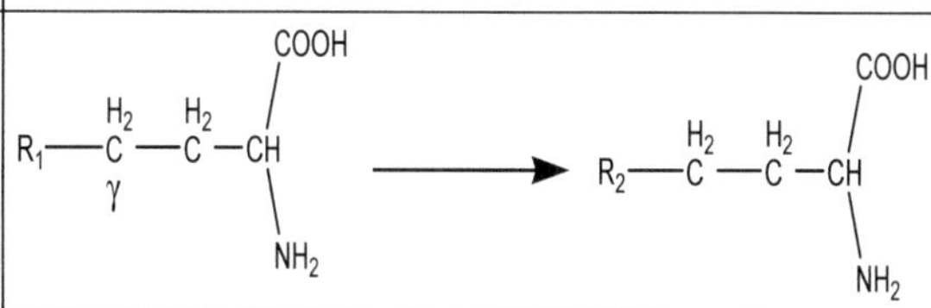	Cystathionine γ-synthase
	Elimination	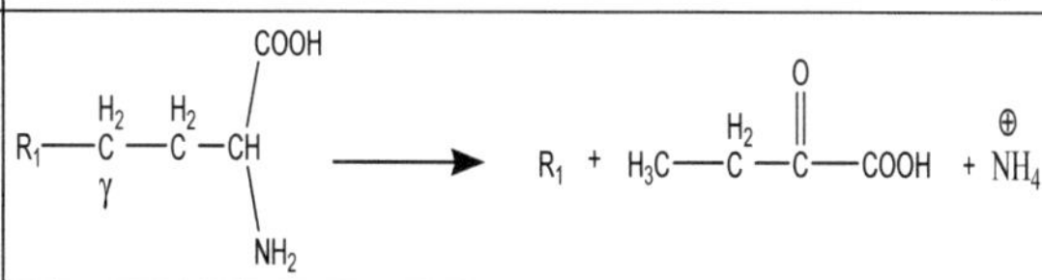	Methionine γ-lyase

Table 1. Functional catalytic modes of PLP-enzymes according to the position of net reaction

No.	Fold Type I	No.	
1	Glycine dehydrogenase	50	Tyrosine decarboxylase
2	Glycine hydroxymethyltransferase	51	Glutamate decarboxylase b
3	Threonine aldolase	52	Histidine decarboxylase b
4	Trptophanase	53	Ornithine decarboxylase 1
5	Tyrosine phenol lyase	54	Arginine decarboxylase 1
6	Selenocysteine lyase	55	Lysine decarboxylase
7	Glyoxylate aminotransferase	56	Allinase
8	Serine aminotransferase		
9	Phosphoserine aminotransferase		
10	Amino ketobutyrate CoA ligase		Fold Type II
11	Aminolevulinate Synthase	1	Aminocyclopropane-carboxyl deaminase
12	Amino oxononanoate synthase	2	Tryptophan synthase β
13	Serine palmitoyltransferase	3	Cystathionine β-synthase
14	Kvnureninase	4	O-Acetylserine sulfhydrylase
15	Isopenicillin *N*-epimerase	5	D-Serine dehydratase
16	Cysteine desulfurase	6	L-serine dehydratase
17	Splicing protein SPL1	7	Threonine dehydratase
18	Cystathionine γ-Synthase	8	Threonine synthase 1
19	*O*-Succinylhomoserine sulhydrase	9	Diaminopropionate lyase
20	Methionine γ-Lyase	10	Threonine synthase 2
21	Cystathionine γ-Lyase	11	D-Alanine aminotransferase
22	Cystathionine β-Lyase	12	Amino deoxychorismate lyase
23	Aspartate aminotransferase a	13	Branched amino acid aminotransferase
24	Aromatic amino acid aminotransferase		
25	Tyrosine aminotransferase		
26	Alanine aminotransferase		Fold Type III
27	*malY* gene product	1	Ornithine decarboxylase 2
28	Phenylpuruvate aminotransferase	2	Diaminopimelate decarboxylase
29	Aminocyclopropane carboxylate synthase	3	Arginine decarboxylase
30	Rhizopine regulatory protein		alanine racemase
31	Aspartate aminotransferase b		
32	Aspartate aminotransferase c		
33	Histidinol phosphate aminotransferase		Fold Type IV
34	cobC gene product	1	D-amino acid aminotransferase
35	Valine-Pyruvate aminotransferase	2	branched chain amino acid amino transferase
36	Acetylornithine aminotransferase	3	4-amino-4-deoxychorismate lyase
37	Succinylornithine aminotransferase		
38	Ornithine aminotransferase		
39	Alanine glyoxylate aminotransferase		
40	Dialkylglycine decarboxylase		Fold type V

41	Alanine pyruvate aminotransferase	1	Glycogen phosphorylase
42	Aminooxononanoate aminotransferase	2	Maltodextrin phosphorylase
43	DNTP hexose aminotransferase		
44	Glutamate semialdehyde aminomutase		
45	Aminobutyrate aminotransferase		
46	Lysine Ɛ-aminotransferase		
47	Diaminobutanoate aminotransferase		
48	Glutamate decarboxylase a		
49	Histidine decarboxylase a		

Table 2. Families of Pyridoxal Phosphate dependent enzymes

No hydrogen bonds between pyridine nitrogen and apoenzyme (Percudani and Percacchi, 2003). The systematic and catalytic promiscuity of the five fold types PLP-dependent enzymes as adopted by Metha and Christen (2000) and Percudani and Peracchi (2003), were illustrated in Table 2.

Regarding to our previous work (Khalaf and El-Sayed, 2009, El-Sayed, 2009, 2010, 2011a, b), the subsequent section was focused on the metabolic interactions of sulfur containing amino acid by PLP-dependent enzymes of Aspartate Aminotransferase Family.

3. Metabolic interactions of sulfur-containing amino acids by PLP-dependent enzymes: Biochemical identity of normal and tumor cells

Sulfur-containing amino acids are pivotal compounds for almost of metabolic cellular process. In contrary to humans, plants and microorganisms can synthesize their sulfur containing amino acids from the inorganic precursor as sulfate, sulfite and sulfide via reduction or activation (Beinert, 2000, Kessler, 2006). In humans, methionine and cysteine were described as conditional essential amino acids for normal various biological aspects (Baylin et al., 1998, Davis and Uthus, 2004). The prominent sulfur containing amino acids on living cell are cysteine and methionine, that crucially incorporated on the synthesis of Co-enzyme, vitamins, epigenetic DNA modulators, DNA stabilizers and antioxidants (El-Sayed, 2010 and Cellarier et al., 2003). Additionally, cysteine is the essential source for H_2S biogenesis that critically acts as neuro-modulators, cardio-protector, relaxing muscle regulators, and vasodiolator for vascular system (Wang, 2002, Kimura, 2010, Predmore and Lefer, 2010 and Gadalla and Snyder, 2010). The general metabolic interactions of sulfur containing amino acids and their derivative by PLP-enzymes were illustrated in Fig. (3). Methionine can be metabolized via different ways that collectively regulated by PLP-dependent enzymes as methionine γ-lyase, cystathionine β, γ-synthases and cystathionine β, γ-lyases. In plants and microbes, methionine can be undergoes oxidative deamination/ demethiolation forming methanethiol, α-ketobutyrate and ammonia (Tanaka et al., 1977) via the action of L-methioninase. L-Methioninase was frequently reported as a substrate induced extracellular enzyme for various microbial cultures (Tanaka et al., 1977, Soda et al., 1983; Nikulin et al., 2008, Khalaf and El-Sayed, 2009), while it is absent in mammalian cells (Cooper, 1983). Biochemically, methionine was activated by methionine adenosyltransferase forming *S*-adenosylmethionine as a key intermediate for the following metabolic pathways;

4. Transmethylation pathway and methionine synthesis

S-Adenosylmethionine undergoes de-methylation by glycine-*N*-methyltransferase forming *S*-adenosyl homocysteine (Luka et al., 2006). This reaction is the source for more than 100 biological methylation reactions including epigenetic DNA regulation and protein posttranslational modifications, in living cell (Choi and Mason, 2002) Moreover, in microbial cells, the methyl group from adenosylmethionine can switch the formation of Siroheme via methylation followed by oxidation of Uroporphyrinogen II (Thomas et al., 1997, Hansen et

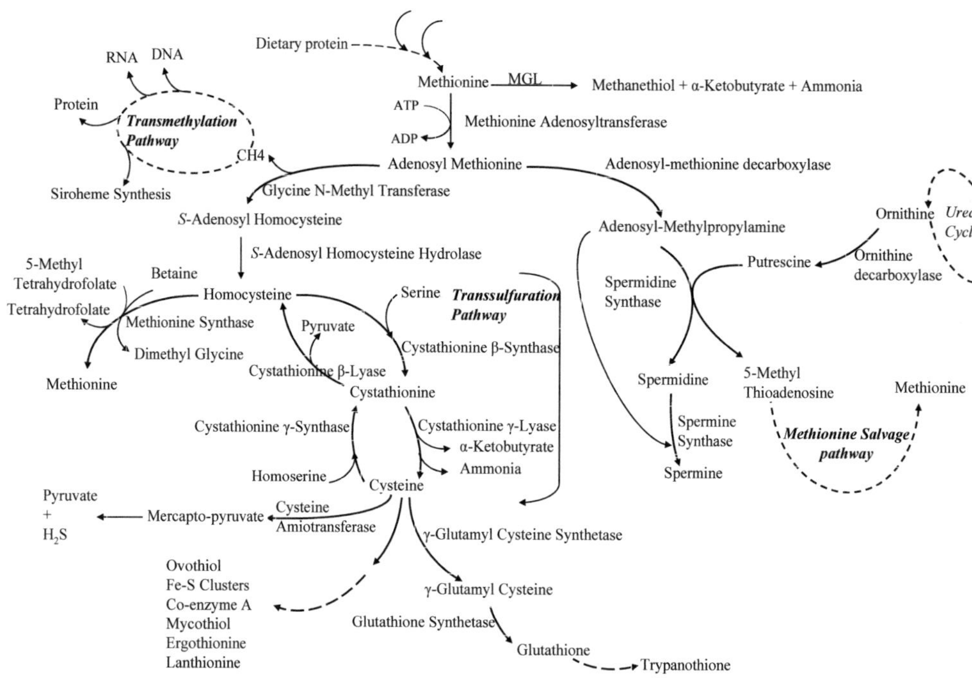

Fig. 3. Metabolic Interactions of sulfur-containing amino acids, as supplied from the diet or intracellular, via different cellular pathways. Except human, L-methionine was undergoes oxidative deamination and demethiolation by L-methioninase (EC 4.4.1.11) in various microorganisms and plants. In all living cells, adenosyl methionine, activated form of L-methionine, was implicated in various pathways: 1- Transmethylation, adenosylmethionine by glycine *N*-methyltransferase is demethylated to adenosyl-homocysteine that involved in methylation of DNA, RNA, and protein. 2- Transsulfuration pathway, forming glutathione and trypanothione as cellular antioxidants, cysteine was involved on formation of several S-containing compounds. 3- Polyamine synthesis, S-adenosylmethionine was decarboxylated by decarboxylase forming adenosyl methylpropylamine that condensate with putrescine forming spermidine by spermidine synthase, then forming spermine by spermine synthase.

al., 1997). Physiologically, tumors are genetically abnormal cells with uncontrolled rapidly growth and proliferation, for mutation on some genes encoding amino acids metabolizing enzymes, comparing to the corresponding normal cells (Hoffman, 1985). Elevated requirements of methionine are the common biochemical criteria by tumor cells comparing to corresponding normal ones, to fulfill their high protein synthesis and regulation of DNA expression (Stern et al., 1984, Swisher et al., 2009). Practically, hypermethylation of DNA is usually correlates with transcriptional silencing of many of tumor suppressor genes, P_{53} genes, thus disrupting DNA repairing systems and cell signaling modulators (Jones and Baylin, 2002, Santini et al., 2001) as reviewed by El-Sayed (2010). Also, methylation of tumor DNA change the identity of CpG islands, thus altering the expression of DNA repairing and apoptosis controlling genes (Sun et al., 1997, Matsukura et al, 2003) and changing of CpG islands (Swisher et al., 2009). On other hand, suppression of methionine synthase genes are a reliable cellular criteria in various cells as bladder, breast, kidney, lung and hematological tumors (Mecham et al., 1983, Hoffman, 1985, Kreis and Goodenow, 1978), thus it described as methionine dependent cells. In contrast, the normal cells have an active methionine synthase with the ability to form methionine from homocysteine in the presence of methyl tetrahydro folate and betaine as methyl group donors (Kenyon et al., 2002). Consequently, the tumor cells have no ability to grow on homocysteine, comparing to the normal growth of healthy cells. The different argumentations for methionine dependency of tumor cells and biochemical identity of L-methioninase as therapeutic agent were comprehensively interpreted by our previous studies (El-Sayed, 2010).

5. Polyamines synthesis

S-Adenosylmethionine was decarboxylated by adenosylmethionine decarboxylase forming *S*-adenosyl-methylpropylamine (Gilmour, 2007) that subsequently reacts with putrescine forming spermidine by spermidine synthase (Fig. 3). Subsequently, S-adenosyl-methyl propylamine react with spermidine forming spermine by action of spermine synthase (Martinez-Lopez et al., 2008). Putrescine residues are catabolically products of ornithine/ arginine as intermediates of urea cycle by action of decarboxylases. Polyamines are biogenic molecules that tightly bound to the poly-anionic macromolecules as DNA, RNA and phospholipids (Igarashi et al., 1982), regulating the gene expression and protein processing. Biochemically, it crucially involved in stabilization of DNA: Chromatin conformational structures (Davidson et al., 1999), reprogramming of some genes by translational frame-shifting mechanism and expression of the targeted overlapped open reading frames (such as nuclear phospholipids P_{53}) (Coffino, 2000). Also, it essentially interact with membrane phospholipids regulating the membrane linked enzyme transporters (Moruzzi et al., 1993), maintaining the proper membrane potentials. In contrast, high levels of polyamines usually associated with high carcinogenesis of skin, breast, liver, kidney (O'Brien, 1976, Pegg, 1988) and over apoptosis (Hoet and Nemery, 2000). Practically, elevated levels of ornithine decarboxylase a pyridoxal phosphate-dependent enzyme, is significantly correlates with high ratio of polyamines that usually used as relevant carcinogenesis marker (Persson et al., 1998).

6. Transsulfuration pathway

Transsulfuration is the main metabolic pathway for transformation of homocysteine to glutathione, and trypanothione (Cellarier et al., 2003), involving two pyridoxal phosphate dependent enzymes, cystathionine β-synthase and γ-lyase (Fig. 3). By cystathionine β-synthase, homocysteine condensates with serine moiety forming cystathionine, that subsequently oxidized to cysteine, α-ketobutyrate and ammonia by cystathionine γ-lyase (Zou and Baerjee, 2005). Biochemically, transsulfuration pathway contributes in maintaining the cellular balance of cysteine-homocysteine pool that participates in about 50% of total antioxidant formation (Zhu et al., 2008). Practically, inactivation of cystathionine β-synthase causes hyperaccumulation of homocysteine that is a visual risk of cardiovascular diseases, damage to vascular endothelia (De Bree et al., 2002, Wald et al., 2002) and Alzheimer's disease (Morris, 2003). Moreover, the deficiency of cystathionine γ-lyase results in accumulation of cystathionine, known as Cystathioninuria that usually accompanied with diabetes, Down's syndrome, neuroblastoma (Wang and Hegele, 2003, Zhu et al., 2008). Glutathione was synthesized by γ-glutamylation (El-Sayed et al., 2010) of cysteine by γ-glutamyl cysteine synthetase, then complexation with glycine forming glutathione by glutathione synthetase (Cellarier et al., 2003) as reviewed by El-Sayed (2010). Trypanothione as dimmer of glutathione molecules joined by sperimidine linker, as powerful antioxidants against stress (Tover et al., 2003).

7. Rationality of PLP dependent enzymes as antitumor and anti-cardiovascular agents

The absolute dependence of tumor cells on the exogenous supply of plasma L-methionine, not homocysteine, due to their lacks to active methionine synthase is the biochemical target for many therapeutic strategies (Cellarier et al., 2003). Unlike the inactivity of methionine synthase in tumor cells, this enzyme was very active in normal cells ensuring their ability for synthesizing required methionine from homocysteine (Anderson, 1998). The argumentation of biochemical dependence of tumors on methionine synthase or their coenzymes for various cell lines corresponding to the normal cells was comprehensively documented (Liteplo et al., 1991; Fiskerstrand et al., 1994, El-Sayed, 2010). Several approaches were designed for triggering the methionine dependency of tumor cells, for example, starvation of the tumor cells from methionine using methionine-free diets that displays a reliable efficacy against various types of tumor cells (Goseki et al. 1992). However, this strategy is practically inefficient for many technical, therapeutical and economical considerations (Hoffman, 1985, Tan et al., 1996, Hoshiya et al., 1997). Consequently, application of L-methioninase for removal of plasma L-methionine is the potent justifiable strategy towards various methionine dependent tumor cells (Anderson, 1998 and Kokkinakis, 2006). Methionine depletions cause arresting of tumor cell growth on the late of S-G2 phase undergoing eventually apoptosis (Guo et al., 1993, Nagahama et al., 1998). Biochemically, nutrients with depleted or enriched specific amino acid affect on the growth of normal/tumor cells, according to Harper's concept of amino acid balance. Malnutrition of patient is closely associated with severe amino acid metabolic disorders, uncorrectable nitrogen balance with low activity of immune system (Nitenberg and Raynard, 2000). Interestingly, methionine/ valine depleted, tyrosine lowered and arginine enriched was the most rationalized form for inhibition of tumor growth (Chen et al., 2001, He et al., 2003). L-Methioninase was extensively tested a potent anti-proliferative enzyme towards Lewis lung (Yoshioka et al., 1998), human colon (Tan et al., 1998), glioblastoma (Kokkinakis et al., 2001), neuroblastoma (Hu and Cheung, 2009) as reviewed by Sato and Nozaki (2009) and El-Sayed (2010). Recently, Parenteral nutrition is a common co-supportive strategy for various aspects of tumor therapy (Buchman et al., 2006).

L-Methioninase was purified and characterized from different bacterial isolates (Hoffman and Erbe, 1976; Tanaka et al., 1977, Soda et al., 1983, Nikulin et al., 2008), particularly, *Pseudomonas putida* enzyme that extensively structurally studied via crystallographic studies (Ito et al., 1976, Tanaka et al., 1977, Nakayama et al., 1984, Lishko et al., 1993, Motoshima et al., 2000, Kudou et al., 2007). However, the therapeutic response of bacterial enzymes usually associated with high immunogenic reactions, rapid plasma clearance and proteolysis especially with multiple dosing (Tan et al., 1996; Sun et al., 2003), making the patient is more vulnerable to secondary immunogenic disorders by opportunistic pathogens. Also, as result of deaminating activity of this enzyme, extra amounts of ammonia (hyper-ammoniemia) was released during the course of tumor therapy, causing additional hazardous effects to the kidney and liver, as observed for many of anticancer deaminating enzymes (Balcao et al., 2001). Biochemically, hyperaccumulation of ammonia anticipates on formation of extra amounts of arginine and ornithine, via urea cycle, promoting the polyamines synthesis that indirectly induces tumorgenesis (Pegg, 1988, Gerner and Meyskens, 2004). The immunogenic reactions of bacterial enzyme could be attributed to their structural stereo-conformation during the enzyme posttranslational modifications, prokaryotic nature, making distinct epitopes immunogenic sites on the surface of the enzyme as assumed from the phylogenetic analysis of their amino acids (El-Sayed, 2010). Depending on database, the structural amino acid identity of *Arabidopsis thaliana* L-methioninase was similar to that of *Pseudomonas putida* by less than 25 %, suggesting the differences on the surface amino acid constitution (El-Sayed, 2010). Accordingly, L-methioninase was classified structurally in two forms; First, *Pseudomonas-Trichomonas* group that contain six subgroups namely; *Pseudomonas, Bacillus, Brevibacterium, Trichomonas, Rhizobium* and *Aeromonas*. Second; *Arabidopsis* group which represented by *A. thaliana*. Interestingly, the similarity of amino acid composition of L-methioninase is closely related to the systematic morphological and physiological position of the organism. Actually, the amino acid composition of the fungal L-methioninase open reading frame, nor crystallographic studies was not studied. Therefore, regarding to the therapeutic implications of currently applied L-methioninase, the searching for a novel enzyme with less immunogenic activity and high therapeutic potentiality or modifications of the currently used enzymes is a challenge for many biotechnologists.

8. Different approaches to increase the therapeutic potentiality of l-methioninase

8.1 PEGylation of L-methioninase

Immobilization of the therapeutic enzymes on polyethylene glycol (PEG), PEGylation, is one of the most successful strategies that originated in 1970 (Abuchowski et al., 1977). PEGylation of albumin and catalase was the milestone for the development and globalization of this technique, as efficient method for modification of the structural and immunogenic identities of proteins (Abuchowski et al., 1977). Polyethylene glycol is a neutral, water soluble, hydrophilic polyether with less immunogenicity that ensure various pharmacological properties as increasing half-life time, reducing the kidney clearance, protecting protein from proteolysis by via steric hindrance, reduce the immunogenicity of protein, increasing the solubility of target therapeutic agent (Reddy, 2000, Veronese and Pasut, 2005, Fee and Van Alsteine, 2004, Pasut and Veronese, 2009). The therapeutic behavior of PEGylated-enzyme was illustrated (Fig. 4). PEGylated-enzyme have a reduced kidney excretion, with more plasma half-life time for the increasing of its molecular size (hydrodynamic radii), masking the sensitive amino to chemical modification, shielding the critical surface active sites from proteolysis, antibodies recognition and/or interaction with inhibitors (Harris, 1991; Zalipsky, 1995; Harris et al., 2001; Veronese and Harris, 2002), comparing to free enzyme. Also, PEGylation reduce the protein opsonization and adhesion to liposomes, microparticles (Fee and Van Alstine, 2004). Currently, PEGylation become a well developed technique for formulations of biopharmaceuticals for improving their solubility, bioavailability and decreasing their immunogenic properties as approved by FDA organization (Pasut et al., 2007). PEGylated forms of therapeutic enzymes as *Escherichia coli* asparaginase (Abuchowski et al., 1979), arginine deiminase (Izzo et al., 2007), *Bacillus subtilis* arginase (Cheng et al., 2005), *Aspergillus flavus* uricase (Bayol et al., 2002) displays affordable therapeutic potentialities comparing to corresponding free enzymes, as declared by FDA.

PEGylation of *Pseudomonas putida* L-methioninase was extensively studied (Tan et al., 1998 and Sun et al., 2003). The half-life time of PEG-L-methioninase was increased to 160 min, comparing to 80 min to the unmodified enzyme. However, the activity of L-methioninase was relatively not inhibited by PEGylation as appeared from the IC_{50} values against human lung and kidney tumors (Tan et al., 1998). In addition, PEGylation enhance the half-life times of the recombinant L-methioninase by about 20 fold and rate of serum methionine depletion by about 12 fold (Sun et al., 2003). Apparently, the degree of enzyme PEGylation usually correlate with the decreasing on enzyme immunogenicity and prolonged half-life time, in vivo. For example, the in vivo half-life times was increased from 12, 18 to 38 h upon degree of PEGylation of L-methioninase by 30/1, 60/1 and 120/1 molar ratios, respectively, comparing to the 2 h for the naked L-methioninase. PEGylation decreases the titer of IgG by about 10 and 10000 fold for PEG-rMETase 30/1 and 120/1 molar ratios, degree of PEGylation comparing to free enzyme (Sun et al., 2003). Also, administration of external pyridoxal phosphate remarkably confers the half-life times and activity of PEG-rMETase. The significant decrease on the enzyme immunogenicity was appeared from the titer of anti-PEG-METase as significantly reduced comparing to the native enzyme. As could be deduced, the more degree of PEGylation, the more masking of the superficial antigenic, epitopes, sites of the enzyme (Sun et al., 2003, Yang et al., 2004). The decrease on the activities of native of PEG-L-methioninase *in vivo* may attributed to dissociation of PLP Co-enzyme (Yang et al., 2004), that being confirmed by our results *in vitro* (El-Sayed, 2011). However, L-methioninase and co-enzyme being easily re-associate upon external supplementation of pyridoxal phosphate as appeared by A420/280 ratio parallel to spectroscopic analysis for determination of the enzyme activity (El-Sayed, 2011). Thus, the combination of PEG-L-methioninase and pyridoxal phosphate infusion, or periodical supplementation of PLP by external osmotic pump, may exhibit a new strategy for prolonging the half-life time, for maximum enzyme therapeutic exploitation. L-Methioninase displays two absorption maxima at 280 nm, as aromatic amino acids containing protein, and at 420 nm due to the internal aldimine linkage of the aldhyde group of pyridoxal phosphate and ε-amino group of lysine N-terminal domain of PLP-enzyme. The absorption spectra of bacterial and fungal L-methioninase (Tanaka et al., 1977, Johnston et al., 1979, El-Sayed, 2011) are typically to other pyridoxal-dependent enzymes (Bertoldi et al., 2002; Saha et al., 2009). The pyridoxal phosphate co-enzyme was dissociate from the apo-enzyme by incubation with 10 mM hydroxylamine, giving one peak at 280nm, with disappearance of the 420 nm peak due to the dissociation of the PLP and hydrolysis of the internal aldimine bond. To evaluate the structural reconstitution potentiality of fungal L-methioninase, different doses of PLP was supplemented to the apo-enzyme, the structural and catalytical efficiency was monitored. The ratio of A280/420 was decreased from 4.01 to 1.7, upon addition of pyridoxal phosphate (0.2 mM) to the apo-enzyme, indicating the full reconstitution of the active holo-enzyme (El-Sayed, 2011) (Fig.5). Johnston et al. (1979) reported that upon freezing and thawing the ratio of A280/420 of *Pseudomonas ovalis* L-methioninase was increased from 3.90 to 4.7, due to the dissociation of pyridoxal phosphate. *P. ovalis* L-methioninase lacks the ability to restore its original activity by dialysis against pyridoxal phosphate (Johnston et al., 1979), while that of *Trichomonas vaginalis* enzyme restore more than 90 % of its activity by 0.1mM PLP (Lockwood and Coombs, 1991). However, *A. flavipes* L-methioninase has the ability to reconstitute its fully structural catalytic state upon addition of pyridoxal phosphate (0.2mM), similarly to cystathionine γ-lyase (Zhu et al., 2008).

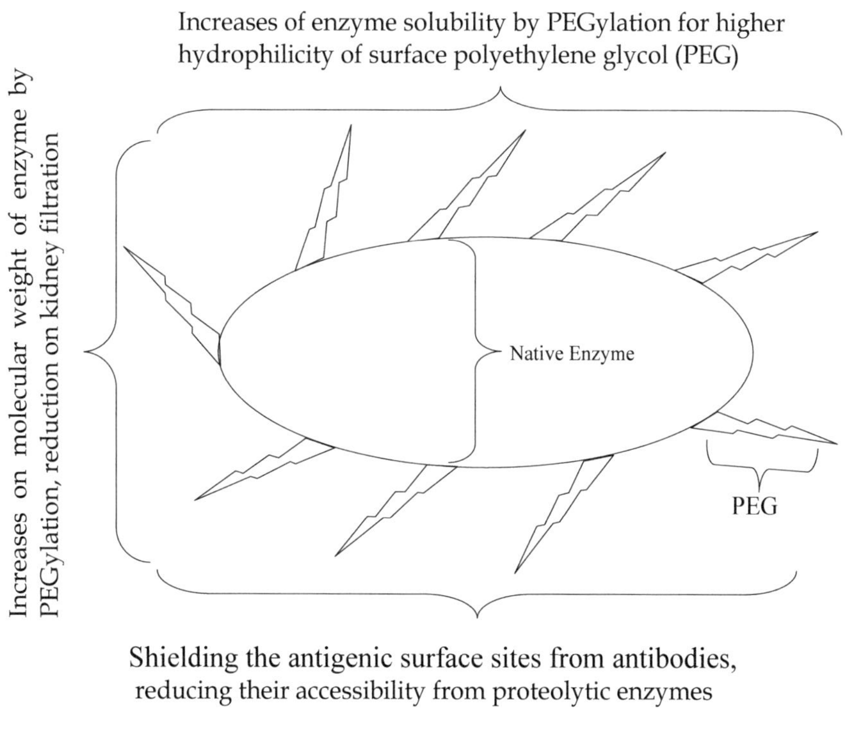

Fig. 4. Prospective of enzyme PEGylation

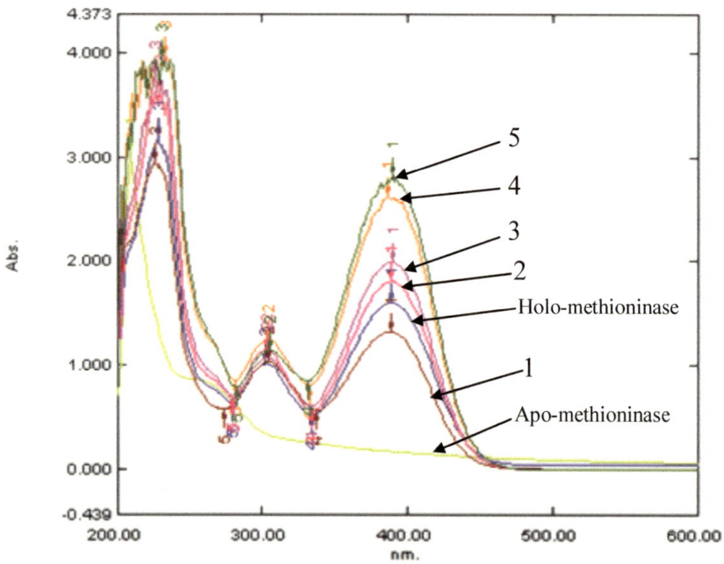

Fig. 5. Absorption spectra of holo and apo-methioninase from *A. flavipes* (El-Sayed, 2011). Apo-methioninase obtained by preincubation of the holo-enzyme (2.2 mg/ml) in potassium phosphate buffer (pH 7.8) with 10 mM hydroxylamine. Reconstruction of the holo-enzyme by incubation of the apo-methioninase with 0.04 mM PLP (1), 0.08 mM PLP (2), 0.1 mM PLP (3), 0.15 mM PLP (4) and 0.2 mM PLP (5).

9. Combination between L-methioninase and chemotherapeutic agents

Synergism between L-methioninase and chemotherapeutic agents present a new strategy against various types of tumors (Yoshioka et al., 1998). Biochemically, starvation of the tumor cells to L-methionine, by action of L-methioninase or L-methionine depleted diets usually make the tumor cells more vulnerable to any biochemical modulator as reviewed by El-Sayed (2010). Methionine starvation and simultaneous phase-specific chemotherapeutic agent is an overall concept for all therapeutic strategies. 5-Fluorouracil, common biochemical modulator, an analogue to thiamine, that competitively bind to thymidylate synthetase, causing prompted suppression to DNA synthesis of tumor cells (Poirson-Bichat et al., 1997). The sensitivity of Lewis lung carcinoma to L-methioninase was increased by about 4.5 fold by addition of 5-fluorouracil (Hoshiya et al., 1997, Tan et al., 1998, Yoshioka et al., 1998). Similarly, doxorubicin as intercalating agent blocks the cell cycle, greatly improves the activity of L-methioninase against human lung carcinoma H460 (Gupta et al., 2003). Ethionine, as methionine analogue, in combination with methionine starved diets display a potent activity against human colon and lung tumors, that attributed to inhibition of methyltransferase leading to DNA, RNA, protein hypomethylation (Razin and Riggs, 1980 and Poirson-Bichat et al., 2000). Also, methionine free diets potentiality against human prostate and glioma was strongly augmented by supplementation of ethionine that attributed to reduction of ATP pool and glutathione synthesis (Guo et al., 1996, Poirson-Bichat et al., 1997). Also, methionine deprivation induce the hypomethylation reactions that lowers the glutathione and alters folate metabolism causing selective arresting to the cell cycle in the late of S/G2 phase, strongly modulate the efficiency of Cisplatin against human breast carcinoma (Hoshiya et al., 1996). However, continuous starvation of human serum to methionine may exert hazardous implications to liver (Kokkinakis, 2006). Biochemically, combination of methioninase with various therapeutic agents, for methionine starvation, as doxorubicin (Stern et al., 1984), 5-fluoruracil, mitomycin C (Goseki et al., 1992), nitrosoureas (Kokkinakis et al., 2001) and BCNU (Kokkinakis et al. 1997), display a new approach for treatment of methionine dependent tumor cells.

10. L-Methioninase gene therapy and selenomethionine as prodrugs

Introduction of the L-methioninase encoding genes to tumor cells with regulating their expression one of the recent challenges for treating of tumor cells as reviewed by El-Sayed (2010). Transduction of bacterial L-methioninase gene via developed adenoviral vector, with exogenous L-methioninase, display a powerful activity towards human ovarian cancer cells (Miki et al., 2000a). The potentiality of gene therapy for methionine dependent tumors based on deprivation of the tumor cells from the intrinsic L-methionine, so this technique significantly intensified by combination with external L-methioninase, to remove the serum L-methionine. A plausible anti-proliferative activity towards human lung cancer by transduction of *P. putida* L-methioninase gene via retroviral vectors, in combination with methioninase treatment, was observed (Miki et al., 2000b). Transduction of *P. putida* L-methioninase gene to human lung carcinoma using retroviral victors and their therapeutic implications were extensively studied by Tan et al., 1997, Miki et al., 2000a,b, 2001). In contrary to hypomethylation by extrinsic starvation of L-methionine, introduction of p53 genes using retroviral, adenoviral, lipid based delivery, displays an efficient strategy against various types of p53 regulated tumors (Miki et al., 2001). Unfortunately, different genetic therapeutical trials is rarely occurred without signs of biochemical implications as low clinical efficiency and lethal toxicity (Fox, 1999), due to the production of some anti-apoptic mitochondrial proteins that counteract the introduced methioninase gene (Yamamoto et al., 2003). Mitochondrial protein (Bc1-2) is the common released anti-apoptotic proteins that hinder the release of mitochondrial cytochrome *c* to cytosol thus counteracting different gene therapeutic approaches (Hamel et al., 1996, Carsten et al., 2000). Additionally, the low transduction efficiency by retroviral L-methioninase gene hinders their therapeutic potentiality. Recently, a novel strategy for reduction the clinical hazardous and augmentation of the pharmacokinetic impact of this enzyme via combination of gene therapy and selenomethionine as prodrugs as reported by Miki et al. (2001) and Yamamoto et al. (2003). In addition to intracellular and extracellular depletion of L-methionine, introduction of selenomethionine, as non-toxic prodrug, plausibly maximize the therapeutic potentiality of this approach, against tumor cells. Selenomethionine, methionine analogue, is a prodrug that under γ-elimination forming a powerful toxic methylselenol, α-ketobutyrate and ammonia (El-Sayed, 2010). Subsequently methylselenol catalyzes thiols oxidation generating reactive oxygen species as superoxide causing mitochondrial swelling, releasing cytochrome *c*, activation of *caspase* inducing prompt cell apoptosis (Green and Reed, 1998, Miki et al., 2001, Yamamoto et al., 2003). Methylselenol released from L-methioninase gene transduced tumor cell can easily adsorbed by surrounding cells, bystander effect, generating the same toxicity on mitochondrial system (Miki et al., 2001) as reviewed by El-Sayed (2010). Unlike the sensitivity of tumor cells to methylselenol, the normal human cells were not being affected for their lack to L-methioninase (Hoffman, 1984). The sensitivity of tumor cells to transduction by adenovirus methioninase gene and selenomethionine as prodrug was increased by 1000 fold (Miki et al., 2000a) comparing to only gene transduced cells.

Currently, in a revolution of biotechnology in the fight against cancer, directing of the enzyme via antibodies to the target tumor cells for removal of extracellular methionine in addition to transduced enzyme gene and selenomethionine as prodrug is the promising strategy against various types of tumors (Napier et al., 2000, Zhao et al., 2006). This novel approach referred as Antibody Directed Enzyme Prodrug Therapy (ADEPT) that is reliable strategy to avoid the systemic clinical and therapeutical limitations of the traditional approaches (Sharma et al., 2005). However, several trials for construction of enzyme antibodies models (Bagshawe, 1987, Stener and Springer, 2001, Bagshawe et al., 2004) were experimented. However, the design of enzyme-antibody without interactions on the enzyme catalytic sites and specific to receptors on the surface of tumor cells is main challenge by biotechnologists, for approving this strategy. After transduction of L-methioninase gene to the target tumor cells, the enzyme-antibody was introduced to the human plasma followed by injection of selenomethionine as planned by several trials as reviewed by El-Sayed (2010).

11. Exploitation of L-methioninase as a target for antimicrobial drugs

Uniqueness distribution of L-methioninase as intracellular enzyme among all microbial pathogens, but not humans makes this enzyme is a novel target for antibacterial, antifungal and anti-protozoal therapies (Ali and Nozaki, 2007, Sato and Nozaki, 2009). Trifluoromethionine (TFM), a fluorinated methionine that undergoes β, γ-elimination forming trifluoro-methanethiol (CF_3SH) that converted to carbonothionic difluoride which subsequently interacted with primary amino groups of the enzymes lysine moieties, causing cellular toxicities (Alston and Bright, 1983, Sato et al., 2008). TFM was reported as a potent antibacterial agent towards the growth of *Mycobacterium smegmatis*, *M. phlei* and *Candida lipolytica* (Zygmunt and Tavormina, 1966, Sato and Nozaki, 2009), *P. gingivalis, F. nucleatum* (Yoshimura et al., 2002) and antiprotozoal agent *Entaemoba histolytica* (Coombs and Mottram, 2001). Also, TFM is highly effective against many anaerobic bacteria as *Clostridium botulinum* (botulism), *C. difficile* (colitis), *Porphyromonas* sp (tooth decay) and *Bacteroides* sp (intra-abdominal infections) (Finegold and Wexler, 1996). Methionine and TFM was activated by methionine adenosyltransferase for further metabolic biochemical pathways. Mammalian cystathionine γ-lyase doesn't affected by the presence of TFM (Alston and Bright, 1983). Myrsinoic acid B and terpeno-benzoic acid extracted from *Myrisine seguinii,* were reported as potent anti-methioninase, anti-inflammatory and anti-edema agents (Hirota et al., 2002, Ito et al., 2008). Myrsinoic acid exhibits a significant activities against *F. nucleatum* (IC_{50} 0.39 μm), *T. denticoal* (IC_{50} 30.3 μM) and *P. gingivalis* (IC_{50} 82.4 μM), it used as powerful anti-malodor and periodontal disease (Sato and Nozaki, 2009). Propargylglycine as cysteine analogues, was widely reported as suicide L-methioninase catalytic inhibitor, *in vitro* (El-Sayed, 2011), with relatively low deleterious effect on whole growth of amoebic trophozites, *E. histolytica* (Ali and Nozaki, 2007), suggesting alternative shunt for sulfur amino acid metabolism other than L-methioninase (Coombs and Mottram, 2001). Thus, for unique distribution of L-methioninase as intracellular enzyme among pathogenic microbes, the searching for various inhibitors with reliable specificity to this enzyme will be a justifiable new trend of antimicrobials agents.

12. Pyridoxal phosphate-dependent enzymes deficiency and cardiovascular diseases

Biochemically, transsulfuration and reverse-transsulfuration pathways are the pivotal mechanisms for proper accumulation of homocysteine and cystathionine. As shown in Fig.

(3), these pathways are controlled by four PLP-dependent enzymes namely; cystathionine β, γ-synthases and cystathionine γ, β-lyases. Inactivation of transsulfuration enzymes as cystathionine β-synthase causes hyperaccumulation of homocysteine (homocysteinuria) that is a visual risk of cardiovascular diseases, damage to vascular endothelia, increases to the risk of abnormal blood clots and skeletal abnormalities (De Bree et al., 2002; Wald et al., 2002) and Alzheimer's disease (Morris, 2003). Also, homocysteinuria usually associated with intellectual disability, seizures and megaloblastic anemia (Mudd et al., 1985). Practically, it commonly reported as genetic or metabolic disorders that affect on the metabolism of protein, generally one to 200,000 babies are born with genetic disorders. Homocysteinuria is a biochemically disorder due to the deficiency of cystathionine β-synthase, owing to the genetically inborn error of the transsulfuration pathway that increases the homocysteine and methionine, with crucial decreasing to the cysteine pool (Mudd et al., 1985). The major clinical implication of homocysteinuria includes mental retardation, dislocation of the optic lenses, skeletal abnormalities (Schuh et al., 1984). Dietary therapy relying of deprivation of methionine and supplementation of cysteine display a reliable positive result in delaying the clinical manifestations (Pullon, 1980). However, supplementation of cystathionine β-synthase was the potent relevant therapy for dramatically conversion of homocysteine to cystathionine (Zhu et al., 2008). Since cystathionine β-synthase is a PLP-dependent enzyme and the rapid dissociation of PLP as coenzyme from the apoenzyme is a common structural and catalytic criteria (El-Sayed, 2010, 2011), external supplementation of pyridoxal phosphate, vitamin B6 gave a plausible results for decreasing the amount of homocysteine, assuming the reassociation of apo-cystathionine β-synthase forming the holo-enzyme (Barber and Spaeth, 1967). Moreover, the deficiency of cystathionine γ-lyase results in accumulation of cystathionine (Cystathioninuria) that usually accompanied with diabetes, Down's syndrome, neuroblastoma (Wang and Hegele, 2003) as reviewed by Zhu et al. (2008).

13. Industrial application of l-methioninase: methanethiol production

Methanethiol has enormous biotechnological applications such as key gradient in gas odorants, jet fuel additives and coke formation in steel mill furnaces (Welirnan 1966). Recently, it is used for preparation of modified gold biosensors, manufacturing of plastics and pesticides (Jin et al. 2005, Nakamura et al. 2006). Also, it is the precursor for dimethyltrisulfide, *S*-methylthio-esters and 2,4-dithiapentane production (Chin and Lindsay 1994, Amarita *et al.* 2004), as presulfiding, hydrocracking catalysts, extracting solvents, manufacturing of ion-exchange resins and as modifier of Nylon fibers (Herschler 1962; Stewart and Lasis 1965) (www.gaylardchemical.com).

Chemically, methanethiol can be synthesized by reaction of methanol with hydrogen sulfide (Scott et al., 1955). The reaction was preceded at 380°C (716°F) in the presence of K_2MoSO_4/SiO_2 as catalyst and 2MPa. By chemical methods usually methanethiol accompanied with formaldehyde, requiring more steps for purification, especially with higher solubility of methanethiol in water (Yang et al., 1998). Commercially, the price of methanethiol salt is about eighteen fold higher than L-methionine, also one gram of sodium methanethiolate is 3.6 folds more than one liter of methanol (Sigma-Aldrich Co 2010).

Consequently, the enzymatic method, using L-methioninase seems to be a plausible process for large scale production of methanethiol from the technical and economical point of views. For the high expense of enzyme purification from the microbial cultures, immobilization is a promising technique for enzyme stabilization and continuous production of methanethiol (El-Sayed and Shindia, 2011). Among the tested methods, polyacrylamide (42.2%), Ca-alginate (40.9%) and chitin (40.8%) displaying the highest *A. flavipes* L-methioninase immobilization efficiency. Chitin-enzyme gave a plausible stability till 4th cycle for production of methanethiol under controlled system. Applying GC and HNMR analysis, methanethiol has identical chemical structure to the standard compound. A new method for continuous production of pure methanethiol using a simple low expense enzymatic method was developed (El-Sayed and Shindia, 2011).

14. Prospectives for improving the therapeutic potentiality of PLP-dependent enzymes

Regarding to publications describing the structural and catalytic identities of PLP-dependent enzymes and their wide therapeutic and pharmaceutical applications, the immunogenicity and relative instability were the common limitations from pharmacokinetic point of view. Actually, all of these enzymes that receive considerable attention as therapeutic agent were of bacterial sources as reviewed by El-Sayed (2010). However, the crystallographic and biochemical studies for various therapeutic enzymes reveal a reliable distinction on the enzyme conformational structural of surface amino acids and immunogenic sites, from prokaryotes to eukaryotes (Kusakabe et al., 1979). Unlike the extensive studies of bacterial PLP-dependent enzymes, no more publications for biochemical characterization and crystal structures of these enzymes from eukaryotes, in spite of their distinct structural identity from eukaryotes as revealed from amino acid constitution (El-Sayed, 2010). Thus, further biochemical and crystallographic studies to elucidate the catalytic identity and tertiary structure of eukaryotic PLP-enzymes for the maximum therapeutic exploitation of these enzymes need to be resolved. The plausible re-association of PLP coenzyme with the apo-L-methioninase with full activity, comparing to lower to inability to re-association of the corresponding enzymes from prokaryotes, is an obscure, and their authorization with greatly participates in explanation of their catalytic and immunogenic identities. In addition, immobilization and co-immobilization studies of these enzymes will significantly maximize their biotechnological and therapeutical applications. Regarding to gene therapy, PEGylation and directing of these enzymes to specific tumors via targeting by modified antibodies or nao-particles is the main challenge for our ongoing research.

15. References

Abuchowski A., Van ES, T., Palczuk,N.C. and Davis F.F. (1977): Alteration of immunological properties of bovine serum albumin by covalent attachment of polyethylene glycol. J. Biol. Chem. 252: 3578-3581.

Abuchowski A., Van ES T., Palczuk N.R., McCoy J.R. and Davis F.F. (1979): Treatment of L5178Y tumor-bearing BDF1 mice with a non-immunogenic L-glutaminase-L-asparaginase. Cancer Treat. Rep. 63: 1127-1132.

Agrawal N.R., Bukowski R.M., Rybicki L.A, Kurtzberg J., Cohen L.J. and Hussein M.A. (2003): A phase I-II trial of polyethylene glycol-conjugated L-asparaginase in patients with multiple myloma. Cancer 98:94-99

Alexander F.W., Sandmeier E., Mehta P.K. and Christen P. (1994): Evolutionary relationships among pyridoxal-5-phosphate-dependent enzymes. Regio-specific alpha, beta and gamma families. Eur. J. Biochem. 219: 953-960.

Ali V. and Nozaki T. (2007): Current Therapeutics, Their problems, and sulfur-containing amino acid metabolism as a novel target against infections by Amitochondriate Protozoan parasites. Clinical Microbiology Rev. 20: 164-187.

Alston T.A. and Bright H.J. (1983): Conversion of trifluoromethionine to a cross-linking agent by gamma-cystathionine. Biochem. Pharmacol., 32: 947-950.

Amarita F., Yvon M., Nardi M., Chambellon E., Delettre J. and Bonnarme P. (2004): Identification and functional analysis of the gene encoding methionine-γ-lyase in *Brevibacterium linens.* Appl. Environ. Microbiol. 70: 7348-7354.

Anderson ME (1998): Glutathione: an overview of biosynthesis and modulation. Chem. Biol. Interact 112: 1-14.

Bagshawe K.D. (1987): Antibody directed enzyme revive anticancer prodrug concept. Br. J. cancer, 56: 531-532.

Bagshawe K.D., Sharma S.K., Begent R.H.J. (2004): Antibody-directed enzyme prodrug therapy (ADEPT) for cancer. Expert. Opinion Biol. Ther. 4: 1777-1789.

Bahn J.H., Kwon O.S., Joo H.M., Jang S.H., Park J., Hwang I.K., Kang T.C., Won M.H., Kwon H.Y., Kwok F., Kim H.B., Cho S.W. and Choi S.Y. (2002): Production of monoclonal antibodies and immuno histochemical studies of brain pyridoxine-5-phosphate oxidase. Brain Res. 925: 159-168.

Balcao V.M., Mateo C., Fernandez-Lafuente R., Malcata F.X. and Guisan J.M. (2001): Co-immobilization of L-asparaginase and glutamate dehydrogenase onto highly activated supports. Enz. Microbial. Technol. 28: 696-704.

Barber G.W. and Spaeth G.L. (1967): Pyridoxine therapy in homocysteinuria. Lancet 1: 337

Baylin S.B., Herman J.G., Graff J.R., Vertino P.M., Issa J.P. (1998): Alteration in DA methylation: a fundamental aspect of neoplasia. Adv. Cancer Res. 72: 141-196.

Bayol A., Capdevielle J., Malazzi P., Buzy A., Bonnet M.C., Colloc'h N., Mornon J.P., Layaux D. and Ferrara P. (2002): Modification of a reactive cysteine explains differences between rasburicase and uricozyme, a natural *Aspergillus flavus* uricase. Biotechnol. Appl. Biochem. 36: 21-31.

Bean L.E., Dvorachek W.H., Braun E.L., Erret A., Saenz G.S., Giles M.D., Erner-Washburne M., Nelson M.A. and Nativg D.O. (2001): Analysis of the *pdx-1 (snz-1/sno-1)* region of the *Neurospora crassa* genome: correlation of pyridoxine-requiring phenotypes with mutations in two structural genes. Genetics 157: 1067-1075.

Beinert H. (2000): Iron-sulfur proteins: ancient structures, still full of surprises. J. Biol. Inorg. Chem. 5: 2-15.

Bertoldi M., Cellini B., Clausen T. and Voltattorni C.B. (2002): Spectroscopic and kinetic analyses reveal the pyridoxal 5-phosphate binding mode and the catalytic features of *Treponema denticola.* Biochem. 41: 9153-9164

Brewke C. and Leistner E. (2001): Biosynthesis of vitamin B6 and structurally related derivatives. Vitam. Horm. 61: 121-155.

Buchman A.L., Lyaer K., Fryer, J. (2006): Parenteral nutrition-associated liver disease and the role for isolated intestine and intestine/liver transplantation. Hepatology 43: 9-19.

Burkhard P., Rao G.S., Hohenester E., Schnackerz K., Cook P.F. and Jansonius J.N. (1998): Three-dimensional structure of O-acetylserine sulfhydrolase from *Salmonella typhimurium.* J. Mol. Biol. 283: 121-133.

Carsten F., Christph S., Barbara H. et al., (2000): Bcl-2 expression in high-grade human glioma: Clinical and exprimental study. J. Neurooncol. 48: 207-216.

Casasnovas R., Salva A., Frau J., Donoso J. and Munoz F. (2009): Therotical study on the distribution of atomic charges in the Schiff base of 3-hydroxypyridine-4-aldehyde and alanine. The effect of the protonation state of the pyridine and imine nitrogen atoms. Chemical Physics. 355: 149-156.

Cellarier E., Durando X., Vasson M.P., Farges M.C., Demiden A., Maurizis J.C., Madelmont J.C., Chollet P. (2003): Methionine dependency and cancer treatment. Cancer Treat Rev 29: 489-499

Cheng P.N., Leung Y.C., Lo W.H., Tsui S.M. and Lam K.C. (2005): Remission of hepatocellular carcinoma with arginine depletion induced by systemic release of endogenous hepatic arginase due to trans-heptic arterial embolisation, augmented by high-dose insulin: arginase as a potential drug candidate for hepatocellular carcinoma. Cancer Lett. 224: 67-80.

Chin H.W. and Lindsay R.C. (1994): Ascorbate and transition-metal mediation of methanethiol oxidation to dimethyldisulfide and dimethyltrisulfide. Food Chem. 49: 387-392..

Choi S.W. and Mason J.B. (2002): Folate status: effects on pathways of colorectal carcinogenesis: J. Nut. 132: 2413-2418

Choi J.D., Bowers-Komoro M., Davis D.M., Edmondson D.E., McCormick D.B. (1983): Kinetic properties of pyridoxamine (pyridoxine)-5-phosphate oxidase from rabbit liver. J. Biol. Chem. 258: 840-845.

Coffino P. (2000): Polyamines in spermigenesis: Not now, darling. Proc. Natl. Acad Sci. USA. 97: 4421-4423.

Coombs G.H. and Mottram J.C. (2001): Trifluoromethionine, a prodrug designed against methionine gamma-lyase-containing pathogens, has efficacy *in vitro* and *in vivo* against *Trichomonas vaginalis*. Antimicrobial Agents Chemotherapy 45: 1743-1745.

Cooper A.J.L. (1983): Biochemistry of sulfur-containing amino acids. Annual Rev. Biochem 52: 187-222

Davidson N.E., Hahm H.A., McCloskey D.E., Woster P.M., Casero Jr R.A. (1999): Clinical aspects of cell death in breast cancer: the polyamine pathway as a new target for treatment. Endocr. Relat. Cancer 6: 69-73.

Davis C.D. and Uthus E.O. (2004): DNA methylation, cancer susceptibility and nutrient interactions. Exp. Biol. Med. 229: 988-995.

De Bree A., Verscuren W.M., Kromhout D., Kluijtmans L.A. and Blom H.J. (2002): Homocysteine determinates and the evidence to what extent homocysteine determines the risk of coronary heart disease. Pharmacol. Rev. 54: 599-618.

Denesyuk A.I., Denessiouk K.A., Korpela T. and Johnson M.S. (2002): Functional attributes of the phosphate group binding cup of pyridoxal phosphate-dependent enzymes. J. Mol. Biol. 316: 155-172.

Denesyuk A.I., Denessiouk K.A., Korpela T., and Johnson M.S. (2003): Phosphate group binding cup of PLP-dependent and non-PLP-dependent enzymes: Leitmotif and variations. Biochimica et Biophysica Acta, 1647: 234-238.

Dominy J.E. and Stipanuk M.H. (2004): New roles for cysteine and transsulfuration enzymes: production of H2S, a neuromodulator and smooth muscle relaxant. Nutr. Rev., 62: 348-53.

Ehrenshaft M. and Daub M.E. (2001): Isolation of PDX2, a second novel gene in the pyridoxine biosynthesis pathway of eukaryotes, archaebacteria, and a subset of eubacteria. J. Bacterial. 183: 3383-3390.

El-Sayed A.S.A. (2009): L-Methioninase production by *Aspergillus flavipes*: under solid state fermentation. J. Basic Microbiol. 49: 331-341.

El-Sayed A.S.A. (2010): Microbial L-Methioninase, molecular characterization, and therapeutic applications. Appl. Microbiol. Biotechnol. 86: 445-467.

El-Sayed A.S.A. (2011): Purification and characterization of new L-methioninase from solid cultures of *Aspergillus flavipes*. J. Microbiol. 49: 130-40.

El-Sayed A.S.A. and Shindia A.A. (2011): Characterization and immobilization of purified *Aspergillus flavipes* l-methioninase: continuous production of methanethiol. J. Appl. Microbiol. DOI: 10.1111/j.1365-2672.2011.05027.x.

El-Sayed A.S.A., Fujimoto S., Yamada C. and Suzuki H. (2010): Enzymatic synthesis of γ-glutamylglutamine, a stable glutamine analogue, by γ-glutamyl-traspeptidase from *Escherichia coli* K-12. Biotechnol. Letter 32: 1877-1881.

Fee C.J. and Van Alsteine J.M. (2004): Prediction of the viscosity radius and the size exclusion chromatography behavior of PEGylated proteins. Bioconjug. Chem. 15: 1304-1313.

Finegold S.M. and Wexler H.M. (1996): Present studies of therapy for anaerobic infections. Clinic. Infect. Dis. 23: S9-S14.

Fiskerstrand T., Christensen B., Tysnes O.B., Ueland P.M. and Refusm H. (1994): Development and reversion of methionine dependence in a human glioma cell line: relation to homocysteine remethylation and cobalamin status. Cancer Res. 54: 4899-4906.

Fox J.L. (1999): Gene Therapy safety issues come to fore. Nature Biotechnology 17: 1153

Gadalla M.M. and Snyder S.H. (2010): Hydrogen sulfide as a gasotransmitter. J. Neurochem. 113: 14-26.

Gallagher D.T. Gilliland G.L., Xiao G., Zondlo J., Fisher K., Chinchilla D. and Eisenstein E. (1998): Structure and control of pyridoxal phosphate dependent allosteric threonine deaminase. Structure 6: 465-475.

Galperin M.Y. and Koonin E.V. (1997): Sequence analysis of an exceptionally conserved operon suggests enzymes for a new link between Histidine and purine biosynthesis. Mol. Micrbiol. 24: 443-445.

Gerner E.W. and Meyskens Jr., F.L. (2004): Polyamines and cancer: Old molecules, new understanding. Nature Rev. Cancer 4: 781-792.

Gilmour S.K. (2007): Polyamines and nonmelanoma skin cancer. Toxicol. Appl. Pharmacol. 224: 249-256.

Goseki N., Yamazaki S., Endo M., Onodera T., Kosaki G., Hibino Y., Kuwahata T. (1992): Antitumor effect of methionine-depleting total parenteral nutrition with doxorubicin administration on Yoshida sarcoma-bearing rats. Cancer 69: 1865-1872.

Green D.R., and Reed J.C. (1998): Mitochondria and apoptosis. Science 281: 1309-1312.

Grishin N.V., Phillips M.A. and Goldsmith E.J. (1995): Modeling of the spatial structure of eukaryotic ornithine decarboxylase. Protein Sci. 4: 1291-1304.

Guo H., Lishko V.K., Herrera H., Groce A., Kubota T. and Hoffman R.M. (1993): Therapeutic tumor-specific cell cycle block induced by methionine starvation in vivo. Cancer Res. 53: 5676-5679.

Guo H., Tan Y., Kubota T., Moossa, A.R. and Hoffman, R.M. (1996): Methionine depletion modulates the antitumor and antimetastatic efficiency of ethionine. Anticancer Res., 16: 2719-2723.

Gupta A., Miki K., Xu M., Yamamoto N., Mossa A.R., Hoffman R.M. (2003): Combination efficiency of doxorubicin and adenoviral methioninase gene therapy with prodrug selenomethionine. Anticancer Res. 23: 1181-1188

Hamel W., Magnelli L., Chiarugi V.P. and Israel M.A. (1996): Herpes simplex virus thymidine kinase/ ganciclovir-mediated apoptosis death of bystander cells. Cancer Res. 56: 2697-2702.

Hansen J., Muldbjerg M., Cherest H. and Surdin-Kerjan Y. (1997): Siroheme biosynthesis in *Saccharomyces cerevisiae* requires the products of both MET1 and MET8 gene. FEBS Lett. 401: 20-24.

Harris J.M., Martin N.E. and Modi M. (2001): PEGylation: a novel process for modifying pharmacokinetics. Clin. Pharmacokinetic. 40: 539-551.

Harris M.J. (1991): Poly (Ethylene glycol) Chemistry: Biotechnical and biomedical Applications. Plenum Press, New York.

Herschler R.J.U.S. (1962) Patent 3,023, 074, Feb. 27.

Heyl D.L., Harris E. and Folkers K. (1951): Phosphates of vitamin B6 group I. The structure of Co-decarboxylase. J. American Chemical Society. 73: 3430-3433.

Hirota M., Miyazaki S., Minakuchi T., Takagi T. and Shibata H. (2002): Myrsinoic acids B, C and F, anti-inflammatory compounds from *Myrsine seguinii*. Biosci. Biotechnol. Biochem. 66: 655-659.

Hoet P.H. and Nemery B. (2000): Polyamines in the lung: polyamine uptake and polyamine-linked pathological or toxicological conditions. Cell Mol. Physiol. 278: 417-433.

Hoffman R.M. (1985): Altered methionine metabolism and transmethylatin in cancer. Anticancer Res. 5: 1-30

Hoffman R.M. (1984): Altered methionine metabolism, DNA methylation, and oncogene expression in carcinogenesis: A review and synthesis. Biochem. Biophys Acta 738: 49-87.

Hoffman R.M. and Erbe R.W. (1976): High in vivo rate of methionine biosynthesis in transformed human and malignant rat cells auxotrophic for methionine. Proc. Natl. Acad .Sci. USA 73: 1523-1527.

Hoshiya Y., Kubota T., Inada T., Kitajima M. and Hoffman R.M. (1997): Methionine-depletion modulates the efficiency of 5-fluorouracil in human gastric cancer in nude mice. Anticancer Res. 17: 4371-4375.

Hu J. and Cheung N.K. (2009): Methionine depletion with recombinant methioninase: in vitro and in vivo efficacy against neuroblastoma and its synergism with chemotherapeutic drugs. Int. J. Cancer. 124: 1700-1706.

Hult K. and Berglund P. (2007): Enzyme Promiscuity: Mechanism and applications. TRENDS in Biotechnol. 25: 231-238.

Hyde C.C., Ahmed S.A., Padlan E.A., Miles E.W. and davis D.R. (1988): Three-dimensional structure of the tryptophan synthase alpha 2 bet 2 multi-enzyme complex from *Salmonella typhimurium*. J. Biol. Chem. 263: 17857-17871.

Igarashi K., Sakamoto I., Goto N., Kashiwangi K., Honma R. and Hirose S. (1982): Interaction between polyamines and nucleic acids or phospholipids. Arch. Biochem. Biophys. 219: 438-443.

Ito S., Narise A. and Shimura S. (2008): Identification of a methioninase inhibitor, myrsinoic acid B, from *Myrsine seguinii* Lev., and its inhibitor activities. Biosci. Biotechnol. Biochem. 72: 2411-2414.

Izzo F., Montella A.P., Orlando A.P. Nasti G. Beneduca G. and Castello G. (2007): PEGylated arginine deiminase lowers hepatitis C viral titers and inhibits nitric oxide synthesis. J. Gastroenterol. Hepatol. 22: 86-91.

Jansonius J.N. (1998): Structure, evolution and action of vitamin B6-dependent enzymes. Current Opinion Structure Biol. 8: 759-769.

Jin B., Ding S., Kametani K. and Nakamura T. (2005): The preparation and electrochemical behavior of density-controlled gold nano-particles self assembled interface. Chem Lett 34: 302-303.

John R.A.(1995): Pyridoxal phosphate-dependent enzymes. Biochim. Biophys Acta. 1248: 81-96.

Johnson L.N., Acharya K.R., Jorrdan M. D. and McLaughlin P.J. (1990): Refined Crystals structure of the phosphorylase-heptulose 2-phosphate oligosaccharide-AMP complex. J. Mol. Biol. 211: 645-661.

Johnston M., Jankowski D., Marcotte P., Tanaka H., Esaki N., Soda K. and Walsh C. (1979): Suicide inactivation of bacterial cystathionine γ-synthetase and methionine γ-lyase during processing of L-propargylglycine. Biochemistry 18: 4690-4701.

Jones P.A. and Baylin S.B. (2002): The fundamental role of epigenetic events in cancer. Nat Rev Genetic 3: 415-428.

Kenyon S.H., Waterfield C.J., Timbrell J.A. and Nicolaou A. (2002): Methionine synthase activity and sulphur amino acid levels in the rat liver tumor cells HTC and Phi-1. Biochem Pharmacol. 63: 381-391.

Kern A.D., Oliveira M.A. Coffino P. and Hackert M.L. (1999): Structure of mammalian ornithine deacrboxylase at 1.6°A resolution: Sterochemical implications of PLP-dependent amino acid decarboxylase. Structure 7: 567-581.

Kessler D. (2006): Enzymatic activation of sulfur for incorporation into biomolecules in prokaryotes. FEMS Microbiol. Rev. 30: 825-840.

Kimura H. (2010): Hydrogen sulfide: from brain to gut. Antioxid. Redox Sigal. 12: 1111-1123.

Klimberg V.S. and McClellan J.L. (1996): Glutamine, Cancer and its therapy. Am. J. Surg. 172: 418-424.

Khalaf S.A. and El-Sayed A.S.A. (2009): L-Methioninase production by filamentous fungi: I-Screening and optimization under submerged conditions. Curr. Microbiol. 58: 219-226.

Kokkinakis D.M. (2006): Methionine-stress: a pleiotropic approach in enhancing the efficacy of chemotherapy. Cancer Lett. 233: 195-207.

Kokkinakis, D.M., Hoffman, R.M., Frenkel, E.P., Wick, J.B., Han, Q., Xu, M., Tan, Y. and Schold, S.C. (2001): Synergy between xenografts in athymic mice. Cancer Res. 61: 4017-4023.

Kreis W. and Goodenow M. (1978): Methionine requirement ad replacement by homocysteine in tissue cultures of selected rodent and human malignant and normal cells. Cancer Res 38: 2259-2260.

Kudou D., Misaki S., Yamashita M., Tamura T., Takakura T., Yoshioka T., Yagi S., Hoffman R.M., Takimoto A., Esaki N. and Inagaki K. (2007): Structure of the antitumor enzyme L-methionine γ-lyase from *Pseudomonas putida* at 1.8 °A resolution. J. Biochem. 141:535-544

Kusakabe H., Kodama K., Machida H., Midorikawa Y., Kuninaka A., Misono H. and Soda K. (1979): Occurrence of a novel enzyme, L-lysine oxidase with antitumor activity in culture extract of *Trichoderma viride*. Agric. Biol. Chem. 43: 337-343.

Le Magueres, P., Im, H., Ebalunode, J., Strych, U., Benedik, M.J., Briggs, J.M., Hohn, H. and Krause K.L. (2005): The 1.9 Å crystal structure of alanine racemase from *Mycobacterium tuberculosis* contains a conserved entryway into the active site. Biochemistry 44: 1471-1481.

Lishko V.K., Lishko O.V. and Hoffman R.M. (1993): The preparation of endotoxin-free L-methionine-α-deamino-γ-mercaptomethane-lyase (L-Methioninase) from *Pseudomonas putida*. Protein Expr. Purif. 4: 529-533.

Liteplo R.G., Hipwell S.E., Rosenblatt D.S., Sillaots S. and Lue-Shing H. (1991): Changes in cobalamine metabolism are associated with the altered methionine auxotrophy of highly growth autonomous human melanoma cells. J. Cell Physiol. 149: 332-338.

Lockwood B. and Coombs G. (1991): Purification and Characterization of methionine γ-lyase from *Trichomonas vaginalis*. Biochem. J. 279: 675-682.

Lopez C., Rios S.D., Lopez-Santin J., Caminal G. and Alvaro G. (2010): Immobilization of PLP-dependent enzymes with cofactor retention and enhanced stability. Biochem. Engin. J. 49: 414-421.

Luka Z., Capdevila A., Mato J.M. and Wagner C. (2006): A glycine N-methyltransferase knockout mouse model for humans with deficiency of this enzyme. Transgenic Res. 15: 393-397.

Martinez-Lopez N., Varela-Rey M., Ariz U., Embade N., Vazquez-Chantada M., Fernandez-Ramos D., Gomez-Santos L., Lut S.C., Mato J.M. and Martinez-Chantar M.L. (2008): *S*-adenosylmethionine and proliferation: new pathways, new targets. Biochem. Soci. Trans. 63: 848-852.

Matsukura S., Soejima H., Nakagawachi T., Yakushiji H., Ogawa A., Fukuhara M., Miyazaki K., Nakabeppu Y., Sekiguchi M. and Mukai T. (2003): CpG methylation of MGMT and hMLH1 promotor in hepatocellular carcinoma associated with hepatitis viral infection. British J. Cancer 88: 521-529.

Mecham J.O., Rowitch D., Wallace C.D., Stern P.H. and Hoffman R.M. (1983): The metabolic defect of methionine dependence occurs frequently in human tumor cell lines. Biochem. Biophys Res. Comm. 117: 429-434.

Metha P.K. and Christen P. (2000): The molecular evolution of pyridoxal 5'-phosphate-dependent enzymes. Adv. Enzymol. 74: 129-184.

Miki K., Al-Refaie W., Xu M, Jiang P., Tan Y., Bouvet M., Zhao M., Gupta A., Chishima T., Shimada H., Makuuchi M., Mossa A.R. and Hoffman R.M. (2000a): Methioninase gene therapy of human cancer cells is synergistic with recombinant methioninase treatment. Cancer Res. 60: 2696-2702.

Miki K., Xu M., An Z., Wang X., Yang M., Al-Refaie W., Sun X., Baranov E., Tan Y., Chishima T., Shimada H., Mossa A.R. and Hoffman R.M. (2000b): Survival efficacy of the combination of the methioninase gene and methioninase in a lung cancer orthotopic model. Cancer Gene Therp. 2: 332-338.

Miki K., Xu M., Gupta A., Ba Y., Tan Y., Al-Refaie W., Bouvet M., Makuuchi M., Mossa A.R. and Hoffman R.M. (2001): Methioninase cancer gene therapy with selenomethionine as suicide prodrug substrate. Cancer Res. 61: 6805-6810.

Morris M.S. (2003): Homocysteine and Alzheimer's disease. Lancet. Neurol. 2: 425-428.

Moruzzi M.S., Marverti G., Piccini G., Frassineti C. and Monti M.G. (1993): Effect of spermine on membrane-associated and membrane-inserted forms of protein kinase C. Mol. Cell Biochem. 124: 1-9.

Motoshima H., Inagaki K., kumasaka T., Furuichi M., Inoue H., Tamura T., Esaki N., Soda K., Tanaka N., Yamamoto M. and Tanaka H. (2000): Crystal structure of the pyridoxal 5'-phosphate dependent L-methioninase γ-lyase from *Pseudomonas putida*. J. Biochem. 128: 349-354.

Mudd S.H., Skovby F., Levy H.L., Pettigerw K.D., Wilcken B., Pyeritz R.E., Andria G., Boers G.H.J., Bromberg I.L., Cerone R., Fowler B., grobe H., Schimidt H. and Schweitzer L. (1985): The natural history of homocysteinuria due to cystathionine β-synthase deficiency. Am. J. Hum. Genet. 37: 1-31.

Nagahama T., goeski N. and Endo M. (1998): Doxorubicin and vincristine with methionine depletion contributed to survival in the Yoshida sarcoma bearing rats. Anticancer Res. 18: 25-31.

Nakai T., Mizutani H., Miyahara I., Hirotsu K., Takeda S. and Jhee K.H. (2000): Three-dimensional structure of 4-amino-4-deoxychorismate lyase from *Escherichia coli*. J. Biochem. 128: 29-38.

Nakamura T., Ren J., Zhu K-M., Kawara S. and Jin B. (2006): Application of the nanogold-4, 4'-bis (methanethiol) biphenyl modified gold electrode to the determina-tion of tyrosinase-catechol reaction kinetics in acetonitrile. Anal. Sci. 22: 1261-1264.

Nakayama T., Esaki N., Lee W-J., Tanaka I., Tanaka H. and Soda K. (1984): Purification and properties of L-Methioninase γ-lyase from *Aeromonas* sp. Agric. Biol. Chem. 48:2367-2369.

Napier M.P., Sharma S.K., Springer C.J., Bagshawe K.D., Green A.J., Martin J., Stribbling S.M., Cushen N., OMalley D. and Begent R.H.J. (2000): Antibody-directed enzyme prodrug therapy: Efficacy and mechanism of action in colorectal carcinoma. Clinical Cancer Res. 6: 765-772.

Nikulin A., Revtovich S., Morozova E., Neveskaya N., Nikonov S., Garber M. and Demidkina T. (2008): High resolution structure of methionine γ-lyase from *Citrobacter freundii*. Acta Crystallogr. 64: 211-218.

Nitenberg G. and Raynard B. (2000): Nutritional support of the cancer patient: issues and dilemmas. Critical Rev. Oncology Hematology, 34: 137-168.

O'Brien T.G. (1976): The induction of ornithine decarboxylase over expression is a sufficient condition for tumor promotion in mouse skin. Cancer Res. 57: 2630-2637.

Okada K., Hirotsu K., Sato M., Hayashi H. and Kagamiyama H. (1997): Three-dimensional structure of *Escherichia coli* branched-chain amino acid aminotransferase at 2.5°A resolution. J. Biochem. 121: 637-641.

Palm D., Klein H.W., Schinzel R., Buehner M. and Helmreich E.J.M. (1990): The role of pyridoxal-5-phosphate in glycogene phosphorylase catalysis. Biochemistry 29: 1099-1107.

Pasut G. and Veronese F.M. (2009): PEG-Conjugates in clinical development or use as anticancer agents: An overview. Advan Drug Delivery Reviews 61: 1177-1188.

Pasut G., Sergi M. and Veronese F.M. (2007): Anti-cancer PEG-enzymes: 30 years old, but still a current approach. Advanced Drug Delivery Reviews

Pegg A.E. (1988): Polyamine metabolism and its importance in neoplastic growth as a target for chemotherapy. Cancer Res. 48: 759-774.

Percudani R. and Peracchi A. (2003): Agenomic overview of pyridoxal-phosphate dependent enzymes. EMBO Reports 4: 850-854.

Persson L., Wallstrom E.L. and Nasizadeh S. (1998): Regulation of mammalian ornithine decarboxylase. Biochem. Soc. Tran. 26: 575-579.

Poirson-Bichat F., Lopez R., Bras Goncalves R.A., Miccoli L., Bourgeois Y., Demerseman P., Poisson M., Dutrillaux B. and Poupon M.F. (1997): Methionine deprivation and methionine analogs inhibit cell proliferation and growth of human xenografted gliomas. Life Sci. 60: 919-931.

Poirson-Bichat F., Bras Goncalves R.A., Miccoli L., Dutrillaux B. and Poupon M.F. (2000): Methionine Depletion Enhances the Antitumoral Efficacy of cytotoxic agents in Drug-resistant Human Tumor Xenografts. Clinical Cancer Research 6: 643-653.

Predmore B.L. and Lefer D.J. (2010): Development of hydrogen sulfide-based therapeutics for cardiovascular disease. J. Cardiovascular Transl. Res. 3: 487-498.

Pullon D.H.H. (1980): Homocystinuria and other methioninemias, in neonatal screening for inborn errors of metabolism, edited by Bickel H, Guthrie R, hammersen G, New York, Springer-Verlag, pp: 29-44.

Razin A. and Riggs A.D. (1980): DNA methylation and gene function. Science (Washington DC), 210: 604-610.

Reddy K.R. (2000): Controlled-release, pegylation, liposomal formulations: new mechanisms in the delivery of injectable drugs. Ann. Pharmacother. 34 915-923.

Richard J.P. and Amyes T.L. (2004): On the importance of being zwitterionic: enzymic catalysis of decarboxylation and deprotonation of cationic carbon. Bioorg. Chem. 32: 354-366.

Saha B., Mukherjee S. and Das A.K. (2009): Molecular characterization of *Mycobacterium tuberculosis* cystathionine gamma synthase-Apo-and holoforms. Internat. J. Biological Macromol. 44: 385-392.

Santini V., Kantarjian H. and Issa J.P. (2001): Changes in DNA methylation in neoplasia: Patho-physiology and therapeutic implications. Annual Intern. Med. 134: 573-586.

Sato D., Yamagata W., Harada S. and Nozaki T. (2008): Kinetic characterization of methionine γ-lyase from the enteric protozoan parasite *Entamoeba histolytica* against physiological substrates and trifluoromethionine, a promising lead compound against amoebiasis. FEBS J. 275: 548-560.

Sato D. and Nozaki T. (2009): Methionine gamma-lyase: the unique reaction mechanism, physiological roles, and therapeutic applications against infectious disease and cancers. IUBMB Life 61: 1019-1028.

Schirch D., Fratte D. Lurescia S., Iurescia S., Angelaccia S. Contestabile R. Bossa F. and Schirch V. (1993): Function of the active site lysine in *Escherichia coli* serine hydrox-methyltransferase. J. Biological Chem. 268: 23132-23138.

Schuh S., Rosenblatt D.S. and Cooper B.A. (1984): Homocysteinuria and megaloblastic anemia responsive to vitamin B12 therapy. N. Eng. J. Med. 310: 686-690.

Scott C.B., Dorsey W.S. and Huffman H.C. (1955): Methyl mercaptan from methyl chloride. Industr. Engin. Chem. 47: 876-877.

Sharma S.K., Begshawe K.D. and Begent R.H.J. (2005): Advances in antibody-directed enzyme prodrug therapy. Current Opin. Investig. Drugs 6: 611-615.

Shaw J.P. Petsko G.H. et al., (2000): Determination of the structure of alanine racemase from *Bacillus stearothermophilus* at 1.9 °A resolution. Biochemistry 36: 1329-1342.

Soda A., Tanaka, H. and Esaki N. (1983): Multifunctional biocatalysis: methionine-γ-lyase. Trends Biochem. Sci. 8: 214-217.

Sprang S. and Fletterick R.J. (1979): The structure of glycogen phosphorylase alpha at 2.5°A resolution. J. Mol. Bio. 131: 523-551

Stener P.D. and Springer C.J. (2001): Selective activation of anticancer prodrugs by monoclonal antibody-enzyme conjugates. Adv. Drug. Deliv. 53: 247-264.

Stern P.H., Wallace C.D. and Hoffman R.M. (1984): Altered methionine metabolism occurs in all members of a set of diverse human tumor cell lines. J. Cell Phys. 119: 29-34.

Stewart RA, Lasis E (1965) US. Patent 3,196,143, July 20, 1965

Stipanuk M.H. (2004): Sulfur amino acid metabolism: pathways for production and removal of homocysteine and cysteine. Ann. Rev. Nutr. 24: 539-577.

Sugio S., Petsko G.A., Manning J.M. and Soda D. (1995): Crystal structure of a D-amino acid aminotransferase: How the protein controls stereoselectivity. Biochemistry, 34: 9661-9669.

Sun X., Yang Z., Li S., Tan Y., Zhang N., Wang X., Yagi S., Yoshioka T., Takimoto A., Mitsushima K., Suginaka A., Frankel E.P. and Hoffman R.M. (2003): In vivo efficiency of recombinant methioninase is enhanced by the combination of polyethylene glycol conjugation and pyridoxal 5-phosphate supplementation. Cancer Res. 63: 8377-8383.

Sun L., Hui A.M., Kanai Y., Sakamoto M. and Hirohashi S. (1997): Increased DNA methyltransferase expression is associated with an early stage of human hepato-carcinogenesis. Jpn. J. Cancer Res. 88: 1165-1170.

Swisher E.M., Gonzalez R.M., Taniguchi T., Garcia R.L., Wash T., Goff B.A. and Welcsh P. (2009): Methylation and protein expression of DNA repair genes: association with chemotherapy exposure and survival in sporadic ovarian and peritoneal carcinomas. Mol Cancer 8: 1-11

Tan Y., Sun X., Xu M., An Z., Tan X., Tan X., Han Q., Miljkovic D.A., Yang M. and Hoffaman R.M. (1998) : Polyethylene glycol conjugation of Recombinant methioninase for cancer therapy. Protein Expr. Purif. 12: 45-52.

Tan Y., Xu M., Guo H., Sun X., Kubota T. and Hoffman R.M. (1996): Anticancer efficiency of methioninase in vivo. Anticancer Res. 16: 3931-3936

Tanaka H., Esaki N. and Soda K. (1977): Properties of L-methionine γ-lyase from *Pseudomonas ovalis*. Biochem. 16: 100-106.

Thomas D., Barbey R. and Surdin-Kerjan Y. (1997): Gene enzyme relationship in the sulfate assimilation pathway of *Saccharomyces cerevisiae*. Study of the 3-phosphoadenosylsulfate reductase structural gene. J. Biol. Chem. 265: 15518-15524.

Thornton J.M., Todd A.E., Milburn D., Borkakoti N. and Orengo C.A. (2000): From structure to function: approaches and limitations. Nature Struct. Biol. 7: 991-994.

Toney M.D. (2005): reaction specificity in pyridoxal phosphate enzymes. Arch. Biochem. Biophys 433: 279-287.

Tover J., Leon-Avila G., Sachez L.B., Sutak R., Tachezy J., Van der Giezen M., Hernadez M., Muller, M. and Lucocq J.M. (2003): Mitochondrial remnant organelles of Giardia function in iron-sulphur protein maturation. Nature 426: 172-176.

Vellard M. (2003): The enzyme as drug: application of enzymes as pharmaceuticals. Curr. Opin Biotechnol. 14: 444-450.

Veronese F.M. and Harris J.M. (2002): Theme issue on peptide and protein PEGylation I. Adv. Drug Deliv. Rev. 54: 453-609.

Veronese F.M. and Pasut G. (2005): PEGylation, successful approach to drug delivery. Drug Discovery Today 21: 1451-1458.

Wald D.S., Law M. and Morris J.K. (2002): Homocysteine and cardiovascular disease: evidence on causality from a meta-analysis. BMJ 325: 1202-1206.

Wang J. and Hegele R.A. (2003): Genomic basis of cystahioninuria (MIM 219500) revealed by multiple mutations in cystathionine gamma lyase (CTH). Human Genetic 112: 404-408.

Wang R. (2002): Two's Company, three's a crowd: can H_2S be the third endogenous gaseous transmitter? FASEB J. 16: 1792-1798.

Watson K.A., McCleverty C., Germia S., Cottaz S., Driguez H. and Johnson L.N. (1999): Phosphorylase recognition and phosphorolysis of its oligosaccharide substrate: Answers to a long outstanding question. EMBO J. 18: 4619-4632.

Welirnan H.B. (1966) U. S. Patent 3, 236, 046, Feb. 22.

Yamamoto N., Gupta A., Xu M., Miki K., Tsugimoto Y., Tsuchiya H., Tomita K., Mossa A.R. and Hoffman A.R. (2003): Methioninase gene therapy with selenomethionine induces apoptosis in bcl-2-overproducing lung cancer cells. Cancer Gene Therp. 10: 445-450.

Yang Z., Wang J., Yoshioka T., Li B., Lu Q., Li S., Sun X., Tan Y., Yagi S., Frankel E.P. and Hoffman R.M. (2004): Pharmacokinetics, methionine depletion, and antigenicity of recombinant methioninase in primates. Clinical Cancer Res. 10: 2131-2138.

Yang Y-Q., Yuan Y-Z., Dai S-J., Wang B. and Zhang H-B. (1998): The catalytic properties of supported K2MoS4/SiO2 catalyst for methanethiol synthesis from high H_2S-content syngas. Catalysis Lett. 54: 65-68.

Yoshimura M., Nakano Y. and Koga T. (2002): L-Methionine-gamma-lyase, as a target to inhibit malodorous bacterial growth by trifluoromethionine. Biochem. Biophys. Res. Commun. 292: 964-968.

Yoshioka T., Wada T., Uchida N., Maki H., Yoshida H., Ide N., Kasai H., Hojo K., Shono K., Maekawa R., Yagi S., Hoffman R.M. and Sugita K. (1998): Anticancer efficiency in vivo and in vitro, synergy with 5-fluorouracil, and safety of recombinant methioninase. Cancer Res. 58: 2583-2587.

Zalipsky S. (1995): Functionalized poly(ethylene glycol) for preparation of biologically relevant conjugates. Bioconjug. Chem. 6: 150-165.

Zhao R., Domann F.E., Zhong W. (2006): Apoptosis induced by selenomethionine and methioninase is superoxide-mediated and p53-dependent in human prostate cancer cells. Mol. Cancer Therp. 5: 3275-3284.

Zhu W., Lin A. and Banerjee R. (2008): Kinetic properties of polymorphic variants and pathogenic mutants in human cystathionine γ-lyase. Biochemistry 47: 6226-6232.

Zou C. G. and Banerjee R. (2005): Homocysteine and redox signaling. Antioxidant Redox Sig. 7: 547-559.

Zygmunt W.A. and Tavormina P.A. (1966): Dl-S-Trifluoromethyl-homocysteine, a novel inhibitor of microbial growth. Can. J. Microbiol. 12: 143-148.

8

Improvement of FasL Gene Therapy *In Vitro* by Fusing the FasL to Del1 Protein Domains

Hisataka Kitano, Atsushi Mamiya and Chiaki Hidai
Nihon University
Japan

1. Introduction

Gene delivery, transfection, cytotoxicity, and many other factors influence the ability of gene therapy to treat cancer. In addition, as with pharmacologic agents, longer exposure to higher concentrations of gene products should intensify their effects (Wada et al., 2007). Cytotoxic gene products, such as FasL and TRAIL, may remain in tissues after the death of the transfected cells, and they are known to induce apoptosis in both transfected cells and neighbouring cells (Hyer et al., 2003; Kagawa et al., 2001). They have been examined for use in cancer gene therapy and its effects have been examined *in vitro* and *in vivo* (Elojeimy et al., 2006; Griffith et al., 2009). FasL delivered via a viral vector can reduce tumour size and improve prognosis in an explanted tumour model.

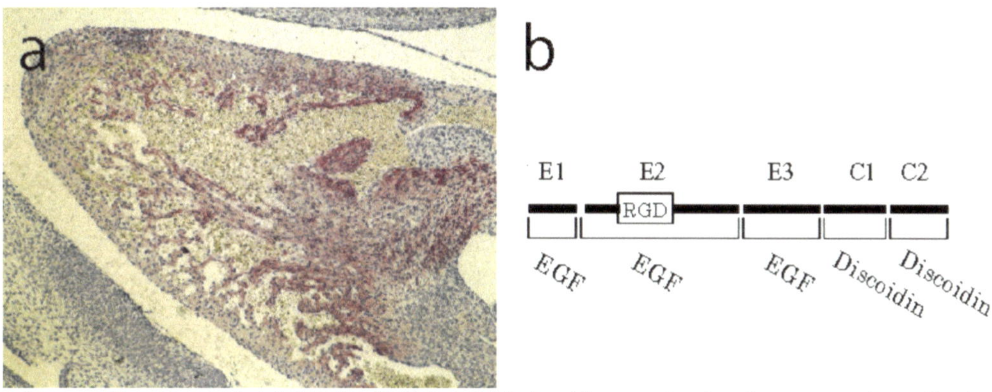

a. Immunohistochemical staining for Del1 in a 14.5 dpc (days post coitum) mouse embryo. Sections were stained with anti-Del1 antibody, followed by an alkaline phosphatase-conjugated secondary antibody and naphthol red as a colorimetric substrate. Immunoreactive protein appears red. Staining for Del1 appeared in the subendocardial region. b. The domain structure of Del1 protein. The RGD sequence in the second EGF motif is indicated.

Fig. 1. Expression and structure of Del1 protein

Currently, multiple injections with a gene therapeutic agent are needed because it is unlikely for a single injection to eliminate a cancer. Therefore, gene therapeutic agents need to be not only safe but inexpensive. Non-viral vectors represent a possible safe and inexpensive way of delivering genes for gene therapy (Lungwitz et al., 2005). However, the

gene transfer efficiency of non-viral vectors remains low. New non-viral vectors that are non-carcinogenic, non-immunogenic, and highly efficient are currently being developed.
Here, we discuss the use of non-viral vectors encoding Del1 in cancer gene therapy. Del1 is an extracellular matrix (ECM) protein expressed by embryonic endothelial cells and hypertrophic chondrocytes (Fig. 1a) (Hidai et al., 1998). We examined the biological functions of Del1 domains by generating non-viral vectors encoding fragments of the Del1 gene.

2. Del1 and its application in cancer gene therapy

Del1 is a 480-amino acid protein made up of five regions, including three epidermal growth factor (EGF) repeats (E1-3) at its N-terminus and two discoidin domains (C1 and C2) at its C-terminus (Fig. 1b). The C1 domain is essential for the deposition of Del1 in the ECM, and E3 enhances the ECM deposition mediated by C1 (Hidai et al., 2007). Proteins fused to the E3 and C1 domains are deposited in the ECM, where they accumulate. The E3 domain can also increase the endocytosis of transfected genes, and at high concentrations, E3 induces apoptosis (Kitano et al., 2008, 2010). We therefore examined the possible application of Del1 in cancer gene therapy by transfecting a squamous cell carcinoma line with cDNA encoding a FasL-E3C1 fusion protein. This protein was deposited in ECM, increased apoptosis, and enhanced the efficiency of a following second transfection *in vitro*.

2.1 E3 enhances the efficiency of gene transfection

Although viral vectors are highly efficient for gene transfer, they can be carcinogenic and immunogenic (Check, 2002). They also require more time and are more expensive than non-viral vectors. However, non-viral vectors are less efficient for gene transfer. Various methods have been made to improve the efficiency of non-viral vectors. For example, novel chemical transfection reagents have been developed to improve extracellular binding. Also, vectors have been modified with chemicals, growth factor peptides, extracellular matrix proteins, and viral proteins to improve uptake via receptor-mediated endocytosis (Al-Taei et al., 2006; Kikuchi et al., 1996; Nam et al., 2009; Oba et al., 2007).
Although the characteristics of the transfection reagents are important, differences between cell types are a more important determinant of transfection efficiency; some cells are always more easily transfected than others (Von Gersdorff et al., 2006). In this regard, the biological state of a given cell type, such as which endocytic pathways are functional in the cell prior to treatment, may be an important factor in endocytosis-mediated gene transfer. Molecules that initiate and enhance endocytosis are needed to improve endocytosis as a method for delivering exogenous molecules.
Del1 protein is one such a factor that increases the efficiency of transfection *in vitro* and *in vivo* (Kitano et al., 2008). We have found that conditioned medium containing Del1 increases *LacZ* gene transfection using several non-viral gene transfer systems, including lipoplex and polyplex systems. Experiments using deletion mutants and fragments of Del1 have shown that domain E3 of Del1 mediates the enhancement of gene transfer. Incubation of culture cells with as low as 16 pM of recombinant E3 is sufficient to enhance transfection, and 1 nM recombinant E3 enhances the transfection 12-fold. This effect of E3 was observed in every cell type tested. E3 enhanced transfection even when it was administrated to the cell culture medium before transfection. The effects of Del1 on gene transfer are inhibited by both of nystatin, an inhibitor of caveolin-dependent endocytosis, and chlorpromazine, an inhibitor

of clathrin-dependent endocytosis. Furthermore, the addition of E3 to cell culture medium increases phagocytosis *in vitro* (Fig. 2). These results indicate that E3 activates several kinds of endocytosis.

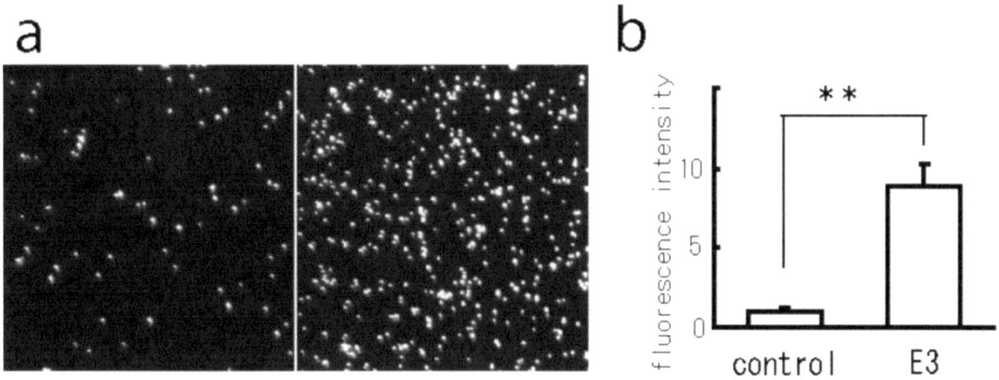

a. Confluent COS-7 cells were cultured with 1-µm diameter fluorescent beads (Invitrogen, Carlsbad, CA) and 1 nM of an alkaline phosphatase (AP)-E3 fusion protein (left side of panel a) for 1 h, washed with PBS, and visualized by fluorescence microscopy. AP protein was used as a negative control (right side of panel a). b. Fluorescence intensity evaluated using image analysis software (AquaCosmos, Hamamatsu photonics, Hamamatsu, Japan). Fluorescence was normalized by the control samples. Results represent means ± SEM (n=6). The results show that recombinant E3 increases phagocytosis.

Fig. 2. Effect of recombinant E3 on phagocytosis

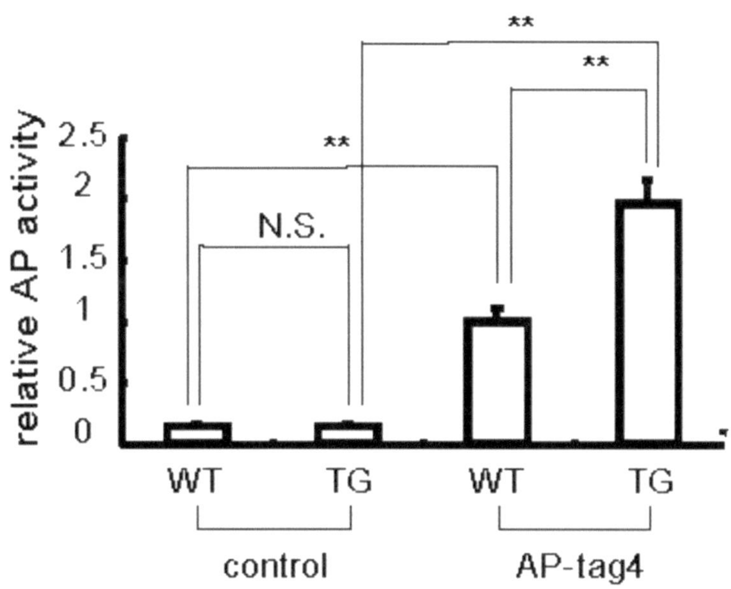

Fig. 3. Effect of recombinant E3 on gene transfer *in vivo*

The effects of Del1 on gene transfer were observed *in vivo*. We found two-fold higher serum alkaline phosphatase activity following transfection with a heat-stable alkaline phosphatase (AP) cDNA in mice over-expressing Del1 compared wild-type littermates (Fig. 3). These

results suggest that the E3 fragment of Del1 in ECM can be used as a general enhancer of non-viral gene transfer.
Del1 over-expressing mice (TG) and wild-type mice (WT) were intravenously injected with a cDNA encoding AP using jet-PEI (Polyplus-transfection, San Marco, CA, USA). Mice injected with an empty vector were used as negative controls. After 24 h, serum AP activity was measured. AP activities were normalized by the AP activity of wild-type mice. Results represent means ± SEM (n=6). N.S., not significant. These results revealed that Del1 increased the susceptibility to gene transfer *in vivo.*

2.2 E3 induces apoptosis

Del1 is present in branchless cavities, such as the heart and umbilical veins, as well as in avascular tissue with hypertrophic chondrocytes in developing embryos (Hidai et al., 1998). In transgenic mice, constitutive expression of Del1 decreases the total volume of the vascular bed (Hidai et al., 2005). These findings suggest that Del1 is inhibits angiogenesis activity. However, some evidence suggests that Del1 promotes angiogenesis. Zhong et al. reported that Del1 can stimulate angiogenesis in animal models of ischemia (Zhong et al., 2003). Additionally, Del1 can accelerate tumor growth by enhancing vascular formation (Aoka et al., 2002). Del1 has seemed to have ambiguous characteristics.
We have found that Del1 induces cell death *in vitro* (Fig. 4) (Kitano et al., 2010). Treatment of cells with Del1 results in chromatin condensation and DNA laddering, suggesting apoptosis. Experiments using TUNEL and annexin V staining also suggest that Del1 induces apoptosis. The apoptosis-inducing activity of Del1 is localized in E3. As little as 25 pM recombinant E3 is sufficient to induce apoptosis, and we have found that E3 induces apoptosis in all adhesive cell types examined. Because of this ability to induce cell death, the E3 domain of Del1 might be useful for cancer gene therapy.

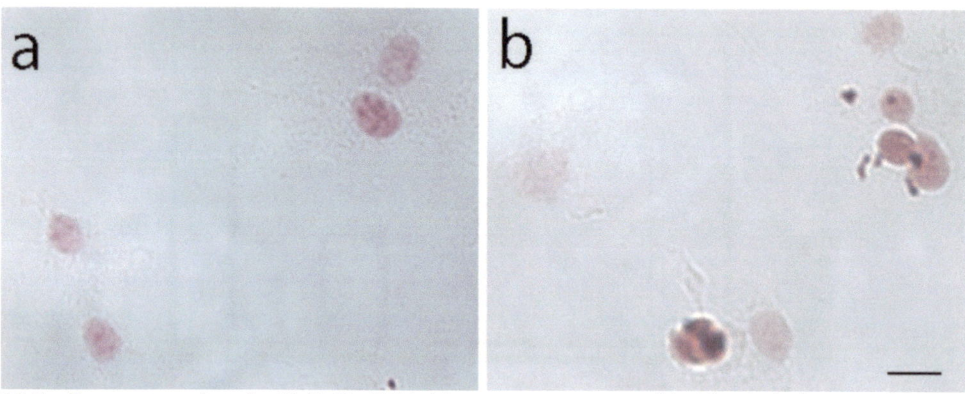

COS-7 cells were transfected with Del1 cDNA (a) or an empty vector. (b). After 24 h, fragmented DNA was detected with a TACS2 TdT-blue label *in situ* apoptosis detection kit (Trevigen, Gaithersburg, MD, USA). Cells were counterstained with Nuclear Fast Red. Bar , 20 μm.

Fig. 4. *In situ* detection of DNA fragmentation induced by a recombinant E3

The C1 domain of Del1 also mediates apoptosis. Hanayama et al. reported that the C1 domain binds to phosphatidylserine (PS), a component of the plasma membrane (Hanayama et al., 2004). In healthy cells, PS is maintained on the inner leaflet of the plasma membrane lipid bilayer. However, in apoptotic cells, PS is present in the outer leaflet. Del1 may link phagocytes with apoptotic cells via the integrin-binding RGD sequence in the E2 domain and the PS-binding C1 domain, which can bind to apoptotic cells. Thus, Del1 can both initiate apoptosis and enhance the elimination of apoptotic cells.

2.3 C1 as a deposition domain

The ECM is a critical factor in morphogenesis (Fujiwara et al., 2011; Sakai et al., 2003). Because the organization of the ECM directly influences the structure of tissues and organs, determining how ECM organization is regulated can help clarify the process of morphogenesis. We therefore investigated how Del1 is assembled in the ECM using an AP-Del1 fusion protein. We found that the fusion protein is secreted from cells and deposited in the ECM (Fig. 5).

Fig. 5. Del1 deposition domain can immobilize AP protein

CHO cells were cultured and transfected with cDNA of an AP-Del1 fusion protein. Cells were removed from tissue culture plates with EDTA and the ECM remaining was collected with a cell scraper, followed by centrifugation. Collected ECM pellets were incubated with p-nitrophenyl phosphate in microcentrifuge tubes. The ECM pellet on the left was collected from wild-type cells, the pellet in the middle from cells transfected with a cDNA encoding AP, and the pellet on the right from cells transfected with cDNA encoding the AP-Del1 fusion protein. The pellet on the right was stained purple indicating that the AP-Del1 fusion protein was present in the ECM.

Using various Del1 deletion mutants, we have found that the C-terminus of the C1 domain, which contains a lectin-like structure, mediates ECM deposition (Hidai et al., 2007). The efficiency of deposition is influences by the presence of other domains in Del1. A fragment containing E3 and C1 (E3C1) had the highest level of ECM deposition, with approximately 70% of the secreted AP fusion protein deposited in the ECM. In contrast, fragments containing C2, which is highly homologous to C1, were present at much lower levels in the ECM. The E3C1 fragment was deposited in the ECM by all cell types examined, although the efficiency varied. Digestion of the ECM with bovine testis hyaluronidase released Del1 from ECM, suggesting that glycosaminoglycans are involved in the deposition of Del1.

In vivo gene transfer experiments in mice showed that the deposition domain of Del1 dramatically alters the distribution of exogenous proteins. The AP activity in liver was 8 times

higher and the serum activity 30 times lower in mice injected intravenously with a cDNA encoding an AP-E3C1 fusion protein than in mice injected with a cDNA encoding AP alone.
In addition to AP protein, the E3C1 sequence of Del1 can immobilize several proteins, including yellow fluorescent protein (YFP) (Fig. 6). Therefore, the E3C1 sequence should be a powerful tool for targeting therapeutic proteins to target tissues and thereby increasing the efficacy and decreasing side-effects.

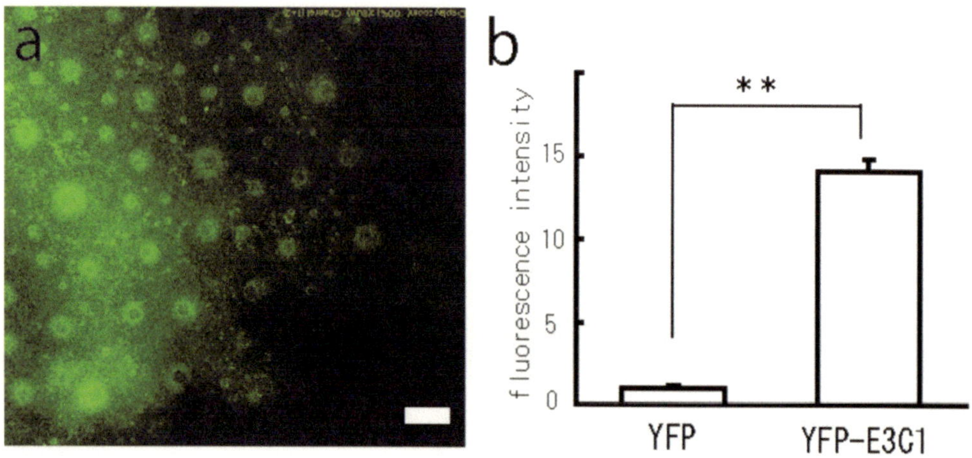

a COS-7 cells were transfected with cDNA encoding YFP fused with E3C1. After 48 h, cells were removed with EDTA and observed by fluorescence microscope. Bar, 10 μm. Specific staining of the ECM was observed. b. Fluorescence intensity in the ECM. Values were corrected by the fluorescence from unconditioned ECM. Values were normalized to the fluorescence from cells expressing cDNA encoding YFP alone. Results represent mean ± SEM (n=6). The data indicate that E3C1 can immobilize YFP protein in ECM.

Fig. 6. YFP-E3C1 fusion stains the ECM

To examine whether the E3C1 domain interferes with the function of fused enzymes, we fused it to 3α-hydorxysteroid dehydrogenase and expressed it in the prostatic cancer-derived, androgen-dependent cell line LNCap (Hidai et al., 2009). The 3α-hydorxysteroid dehydrogenase-E3C1 fusion protein was localized in the ECM and metabolized dihydrotestosterone in the medium, inhibiting cell growth. Thus, the E3C1 domain can target proteins to the ECM without interfering with their function.

2.4 Potential of a FasL-E3C1 fusion protein in cancer gene therapy

We next considered fusing the E3C1 domain to FasL, a cytotoxic protein that has been studied for cancer gene therapy. A FasL-E3C1 fusion protein was deposited and concentrated in the ECM and enhanced the efficiency of subsequent transfections with the same plasmid (Fig. 7).
SCCKN oral squamous cell carcinoma cells (Urade et al., 1992) were transfected with a non-viral vector encoding a FasL-E3C1 fusion protein or encoding FasL alone (control). Three days later, the cells were transfected with a cDNA encoding AP. E3C1 was expected to target FasL to the ECM, increase cytotoxicity, and increase the efficiency of the secondary transfection with AP.

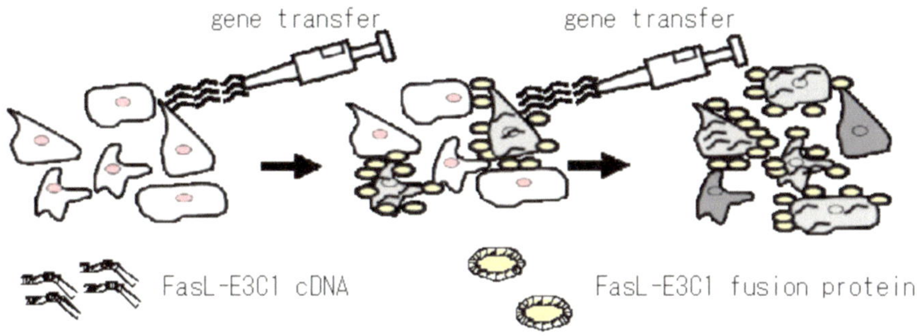

Fig. 7. Scheme describing repetitive gene therapy using a FasL-E3C1 fusion protein.

2.4.1 The E3C1 sequence of Del1 targets FasL to the ECM

2.4.1.1 Materials and methods

Cell culture

CHO cells were purchased from ATCC and grown in α-minimum essential medium (Invitrogen, Carlsbad, CA) supplemented with 10% fetal bovine serum (Invitrogen). The human oral squamous cell carcinoma cell line, SCCKN, a gift from Dr. Hayashido, Hiroshima university, was grown in RD medium (45% Dulbecco's modified Eagle's medium [Invitrogen], 45% RPMI 1640 medium (Invitrogen), and 10% fetal bovine serum. Cells were cultured in 5% CO_2 at 37°C.

DNA constructs

Mouse FasL cDNA was a gift of Dr. Tagawa, Chiba cancer center. Mouse Del1 cDNA in pcDNA3 (Invitrogen, Carlsbad, CA) was a gift from Dr. Quertermous, Stanford university. First, a cDNA fragment encoding the mouse FasL gene was amplified by reverse transcriptase-PCR using the forward primer 5′-TACCGAGCTCGGATCCATGCAGCAGCCCATGAATTAC and the reverse primer 5′-GGCACTGTGCTGGATATCAAGCTTATACAAGCCGAA and then cloned into pcDNA3D (Invitrogen), resulting in pFasL. Next, a fragment encoding the E3 and D1 sequence (E3D1, amino acids 122–316 of mouse Del1) was amplified with the forward primer 5′-TGTGAAGCTGAGCCTTGCAGAATGGCCGGA and the reverse primer 5′-ACAGCCTGAGAGCTCACAGCCAAGAAGTT and cloned into the 3′-end of the FasL gene in pFasL, resulting in pFasL-E3D1. The recombinant proteins expressed by these constructs also had a V5 epitope tag at their C-terminal ends.

Immunoblotting

Immunoblotting was used to determine whether E3C1 can target FasL protein to the ECM. CHO cells were used for the experiment because they are more efficiently transfected than SCCKN cells. CHO cells was cultured in 60-mm tissue culture plates and transfected with pFasL-E3D1, pFasL, or a empty vector using jet-PEI (PolyPlus-transfection; San Marcos, CA). Six hours later, the medium was replaced with 3 ml of fresh medium. After 72 h, cells were harvested by incubation with 10 mM EDTA and then solubilized with SDS-sample buffer. Next, the remaining ECM was fixed with 1 ml of 10% trichloroacetic acid in PBS (Wako, Osaka, Japan) and harvested with a cell scraper. One-fourth of the protein from the samples was analyzed by SDS-polyacrylamide gel electrophoresis, after which protein was transferred to a poluvinylidene difluoride membrane (ATTO, Tokyo, Japan). After blocking and incubation with anti-V5 antibody (Invitrogen), anti-laminin antibody (Sigma, Saint Louis, MO), or anti-tubulin antibody (Oncogene, San Diego, CA), and HRP conjugated secondary antibody (Cell signaling technology, Denvers, MA). an ECL advance western blotting detection kit (Amersham, Piscataway, NJ) was used to detect immunoreactive protein.

2.4.1.2 Results

Immunoblotting of cell lysate showed that the recombinant FasL and FasL-E3C1 fusion proteins had the expected sizes (Fig. 8a). Immunoblotting of conditioned ECM remaining after cell removal showed that FasL-E3C1 fusion protein but not FasL was present in the ECM (Fig. 8b).

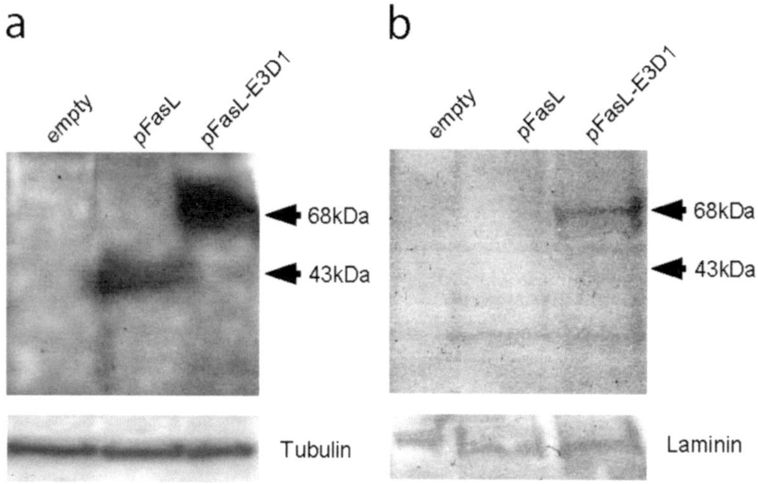

Fig. 8. Immunoblotting

Immunoblotting of cell lysate (a) and ECM (b) from CHO cells transfected with empty vector, pFasL, or pFasL-E3C1. Immunoblotting for tubulin and laminin was used to confirm equal loading.

2.4.2 The E3C1 fragment of Del1 improved the effects of FasL

2.4.2.1 Materials and methods

Induction of apoptosis by FasL fusion proteins

SCCKN cells were plated on a 24-weel plate at 30% confluency. After 1 or 4 days, cells were transfected with an empty vector, pFasL, or pFasL-E3C1. Cells were co-transfected with pAP-tag4 (GenHunter, Nashville, TN) as a control for transfection efficiency. After 48 h, cell death was analyzed by measuring lactate dehydrogenase (LDH) in the cell medium using a LDH cytotoxicity detection kit (Takara) according to the manufacturer's protocol (Decker and Lohmann-Matthes, 1988; Legrand et al., 1992). Percent cell death was calculated as 100% x [(LDH activity for the test condition – LDH activity for the negative control)/LDH activity in cells treated with 1% Triton X-100 (positive control)]. LDH activity was normalized to the heat stable AP activity, which was measured as follows. Conditioned medium (20 µl/well) was added to a 96-well plate, heated at 65ºC for 30 min to inactivate endogenous AP activity, and mixed with 200 µl/well of 1 mg/ml p-nitrophenyl phosphate (Sigma, St Louis, MO) in 1 mM $MgCl_2$ and 1 M diethanolamine, pH 9.8. The absorbance at 405 nm was measured after 30 to 60 min.

2.4.2.2 Results

In a first set of experiments, cells were transfected with plasmids 1 day after plating (Fig. 9a). In this experiment, expression of the FasL-E3C1 fusion protein was as cytotoxic as FasL. Because the deposition activity of Del1 varies between cells, possibly because of the composition and amount of ECM, we repeated the experiment with transfection 4 days after plating to allow them to produce sufficient ECM (Fig. 9b). Under these conditions, transfection with pFasL-E3C1 was twice as effective as transfection with pFasL at inducing cell death.

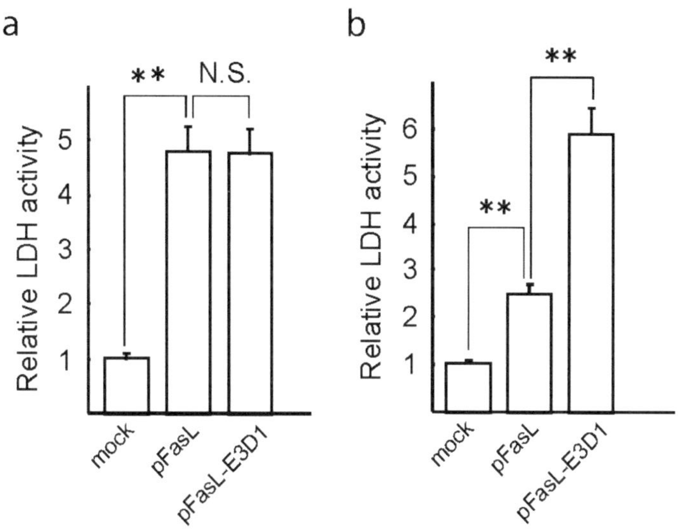

Fig. 9. Effect of E3C1 on the cytotoxicity of FasL

KN cells were transfected 1 (a) or 4 (b) days after plating with an empty vector, pFasL, or pFasL-E3C1. Results represent means ± SEM (n=8). N.S., not significant. Asterisk, $P<0.01$.

2.4.3 The E3C1 fragment of Del1 enhances the efficiency of a following transfection

2.4.3.1 Materials and methods

Evaluation of the effects of FasL-E3C1 on the efficiency of a second gene transfer

SCCKN cells were cultured at 30% confluency in 96-well plates for 4 days. The cells were transfected with 1 µg of pFasL, pFasL-E3C1, or empty vector (negative control) using jet-PEI. After the cells were cultured for 72 h, the cells that survived the first transfection were transfected with pAPtag-4. Next, the cells were cultured for 24 h before analysis. The AP activity in medium was measured as described above. To count the number of cells, cells were harvested with trypsin EDTA, stained with Trypan blue, and counted using a counting chamber. The AP activity was calculated as the total AP activity in medium/cell numbers.

2.4.3.2 Results

The efficiency of the second transfection was evaluated by measuring the secreted AP activity per cells (Fig. 10). Efficiency increased in the following order: empty vector < pFasL

< pFasL-E3C1. Because cells transfected with empty vector during the first transfection were cultured for 8 days without significant cell death, they may have been too dense to allow for an efficient second transfection, which could explain the higher efficiency of secondary transfection in the pFasL-transfected cells than in the control cells.

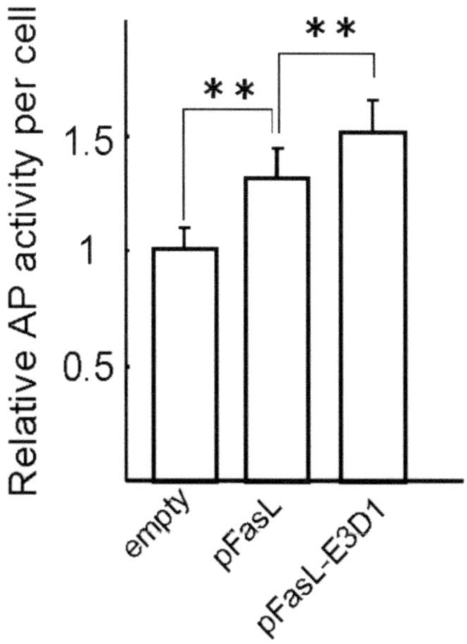

Fig. 10. Effect of E3C1 on secondary transfection with AP

Results represent mean ± SEM (n=8). N.S., not significant. Asterisk, P<0.01.

2.5 Discussion

Expression of Del1 is cell- and tissue-specific. As some reports suggest that Del1 promotes angiogenesis, whereas other reports suggest that it inhibits it, Del1 may be bifunctional. Furthermore, the E3 and C1 domains of Del1 have distinct functions and can act on a variety of cells, and they might be useful as fusion partners to enhance gene therapy using FasL or other proteins.

Neck and esophageal cancer can cause obstruction. Although they can be treated using radiation therapy, its use is limited by the total dosage. As an alternative treatment, we designed a fusion protein of FasL and E3C1 to allow multiple rounds of cancer gene therapy with non-viral vectors. Further study of this fusion protein in the treatment of cancer needs is warranted and should be explored *in vivo* using an explanted tumor model.

3. Conclusion

The E3C1 fragment of Del1 can substantially improve the efficiency of cancer gene therapy using FasL.

4. Acknowledgment

This work was supported by Grant 04-162 from the Japan Science and Technology Agency.

5. References

Al-Taei, S., Penning, N. A., Simpson, J. C., Futaki, S., Takeuchi, T., Nakase, I.& Jones, A. T. (2006). Intracellular Traffic and Fate of Protein Transduction Domains Hiv-1 Tat Peptide and Octaarginine. Implications for Their Utilization as Drug Delivery Vectors. *Bioconjug Chem*, Vol.17, No.1, (February 2006), pp.(90-100), ISSN 1043-1802

Aoka, Y., Johnson, F. L., Penta, K., Hirata Ki, K., Hidai, C., Schatzman, R., Varner, J. A.& Quertermous, T. (2002). The Embryonic Angiogenic Factor Del1 Accelerates Tumor Growth by Enhancing Vascular Formation. *Microvasc Res*, Vol.64, No.1, (July 2002), pp.(148-161), ISSN 0026-2862

Check, E. (2002). Gene Therapy: Shining Hopes Dented - but Not Dashed. *Nature*, Vol.420, No.6917, (December 2002), pp.(735), ISSN 0028-0836

Decker, T.& Lohmann-Matthes, M. L. (1988). A Quick and Simple Method for the Quantitation of Lactate Dehydrogenase Release in Measurements of Cellular Cytotoxicity and Tumor Necrosis Factor (Tnf) Activity. *J Immunol Methods*, Vol.115, No.1, (November 1988), pp.(61-69), ISSN 0022-1759

Elojeimy, S., Mckillop, J. C., El-Zawahry, A. M., Holman, D. H., Liu, X., Schwartz, D. A., Day, T. A., Dong, J. Y.& Norris, J. S. (2006). Fasl Gene Therapy: A New Therapeutic Modality for Head and Neck Cancer. *Cancer Gene Ther*, Vol.13, No.8, (August 2006), pp.(739-745), ISSN 0929-1903

Fujiwara, H., Ferreira, M., Donati, G., Marciano, D. K., Linton, J. M., Sato, Y., Hartner, A., Sekiguchi, K., Reichardt, L. F.& Watt, F. M. (2011). The Basement Membrane of Hair Follicle Stem Cells Is a Muscle Cell Niche. *Cell*, Vol.144, No.4, (February 2011), pp.(577-589), ISSN 1097-4172

Griffith, T. S., Stokes, B., Kucaba, T. A., Earel, J. K., Jr., Vanoosten, R. L., Brincks, E. L.& Norian, L. A. (2009). Trail Gene Therapy: From Preclinical Development to Clinical Application. *Curr Gene Ther*, Vol.9, No.1, (February 2009), pp.(9-19), ISSN 1566-5232

Hanayama, R., Tanaka, M., Miwa, K.& Nagata, S. (2004). Expression of Developmental Endothelial Locus-1 in a Subset of Macrophages for Engulfment of Apoptotic Cells. *J Immunol*, Vol.172, No.6, (March 2004), pp.(3876-3882), ISSN 0022-1767

Hidai, C., Kawana, M., Habu, K., Kazama, H., Kawase, Y., Iwata, T., Suzuki, H., Quertermous, T.& Kokubun, S. (2005). Overexpression of the Del1 Gene Causes Dendritic Branching in the Mouse Mesentery. *Anat Rec A Discov Mol Cell Evol Biol*, Vol.287, No.2, (December 2005), pp.(1165-1175), ISSN 1552-4884

Hidai, C., Kawana, M., Kitano, H.& Kokubun, S. (2007). Discoidin Domain of Del1 Protein Contributes to Its Deposition in the Extracellular Matrix. *Cell Tissue Res*, Vol.330, No.1, (Octtober 2007), pp.(83-95), ISSN 0302-766X

Hidai, C., Kitano, H.& Kokubun, S. (2009). The Del1 Deposition Domain Can Immobilize 3alpha-Hydroxysteroid Dehydrogenase in the Extracellular Matrix without Interfering with Enzymatic Activity. *Bioprocess Biosyst Eng*, Vol.32, No.5, (August 2009), pp.(569-573), ISSN 1615-7605

Hidai, C., Zupancic, T., Penta, K., Mikhail, A., Kawana, M., Quertermous, E. E., Aoka, Y., Fukagawa, M., Matsui, Y., Platika, D., Auerbach, R., Hogan, B. L., Snodgrass, R.& Quertermous, T. (1998). Cloning and Characterization of Developmental Endothelial Locus-1: An Embryonic Endothelial Cell Protein That Binds the Alphavbeta3 Integrin Receptor. *Genes Dev*, Vol.12, No.1, (January 1998), pp.(21-33), ISSN 0890-9369

Hyer, M. L., Sudarshan, S., Schwartz, D. A., Hannun, Y., Dong, J. Y.& Norris, J. S. (2003). Quantification and Characterization of the Bystander Effect in Prostate Cancer

Cells Following Adenovirus-Mediated Fasl Expression. *Cancer Gene Ther*, Vol.10, No.4, (April 2003), pp.(330-339), ISSN 0929-1903

Kagawa, S., He, C., Gu, J., Koch, P., Rha, S. J., Roth, J. A., Curley, S. A., Stephens, L. C.& Fang, B. (2001). Antitumor Activity and Bystander Effects of the Tumor Necrosis Factor-Related Apoptosis-Inducing Ligand (Trail) Gene. *Cancer Res*, Vol.61, No.8, (April 2001), pp.(3330-3338), ISSN 0008-5472

Kikuchi, A., Sugaya, S., Ueda, H., Tanaka, K., Aramaki, Y., Hara, T., Arima, H., Tsuchiya, S.& Fuwa, T. (1996). Efficient Gene Transfer to Egf Receptor Overexpressing Cancer Cells by Means of Egf-Labeled Cationic Liposomes. *Biochem Biophys Res Commun*, Vol.227, No.3, (October 1996), pp.(666-671), ISSN 0006-291X

Kitano, H., Hidai, C., Kawana, M.& Kokubun, S. (2008). An Epidermal Growth Factor-Like Repeat of Del1 Protein Increases the Efficiency of Gene Transfer in Vitro. *Mol Biotechnol*, Vol.39, No.3, (July 2008), pp.(179-185), ISSN 1073-6085

Kitano, H., Kokubun, S.& Hidai, C. (2010). The Extracellular Matrix Protein Del1 Induces Apoptosis Via Its Epidermal Growth Factor Motif. *Biochem Biophys Res Commun*, Vol.393, No.4, (March 2010), pp.(757-761), ISSN 1090-2104

Legrand, C., Bour, J. M., Jacob, C., Capiaumont, J., Martial, A., Marc, A., Wudtke, M., Kretzmer, G., Demangel, C., Duval, D.& Et Al. (1992). Lactate Dehydrogenase (Ldh) Activity of the Cultured Eukaryotic Cells as Marker of the Number of Dead Cells in the Medium [Corrected]. *J Biotechnol*, Vol.25, No.3, (September 1992), pp.(231-243), ISSN 0168-1656

Lungwitz, U., Breunig, M., Blunk, T.& Gopferich, A. (2005). Polyethylenimine-Based Non-Viral Gene Delivery Systems. *Eur J Pharm Biopharm*, Vol.60, No.2, (July 2005), pp.(247-266), ISSN 0939-6411

Nam, H. Y., Park, J. H., Kim, K., Kwon, I. C.& Jeong, S. Y. (2009). Lipid-Based Emulsion System as Non-Viral Gene Carriers. *Arch Pharm Res*, Vol.32, No.5, (May 2009), pp.(639-646), ISSN 0253-6269

Oba, M., Fukushima, S., Kanayama, N., Aoyagi, K., Nishiyama, N., Koyama, H.& Kataoka, K. (2007). Cyclic Rgd Peptide-Conjugated Polyplex Micelles as a Targetable Gene Delivery System Directed to Cells Possessing Alphavbeta3 and Alphavbeta5 Integrins. *Bioconjug Chem*, Vol.18, No.5, (September 2007), pp.(1415-1423), ISSN 1043-1802

Sakai, T., Larsen, M.& Yamada, K. M. (2003). Fibronectin Requirement in Branching Morphogenesis. *Nature*, Vol.423, No.6942, (June 2003), pp.(876-881), ISSN 0028-0836

Urade, M., Ogura, T., Mima, T.& Matsuya, T. (1992). Establishment of Human Squamous Carcinoma Cell Lines Highly and Minimally Sensitive to Bleomycin and Analysis of Factors Involved in the Sensitivity. *Cancer*, Vol.69, No.10, (May 1992), pp.(2589-2597), ISSN 0008-543X

Von Gersdorff, K., Sanders, N. N., Vandenbroucke, R., De Smedt, S. C., Wagner, E.& Ogris, M. (2006). The Internalization Route Resulting in Successful Gene Expression Depends on Both Cell Line and Polyethylenimine Polyplex Type. *Mol Ther*, Vol.14, No.5, (November 2006), pp.(745-753), ISSN 1525-0016

Wada, A., Tada, Y., Kawamura, K., Takiguchi, Y., Tatsumi, K., Kuriyama, T., Takenouchi, T., J, O. W.& Tagawa, M. (2007). The Effects of Fasl on Inflammation and Tumor Survival Are Dependent on Its Expression Levels. *Cancer Gene Ther*, Vol.14, No.3, (March 2007), pp.(262-267), ISSN 0929-1903

Zhong, J., Eliceiri, B., Stupack, D., Penta, K., Sakamoto, G., Quertermous, T., Coleman, M., Boudreau, N.& Varner, J. A. (2003). Neovascularization of Ischemic Tissues by Gene Delivery of the Extracellular Matrix Protein Del-1. *J Clin Invest*, Vol.112, No.1, (July 2003), pp.(30-41), ISSN 0021-9738

9

Feasibility of BMP-2 Gene Therapy Using an Ultra-Fine Needle

Kenji Osawa, Yasunori Okubo, Kazumasa Nakao, Noriaki Koyama and Kazuhisa Bessho
Department of Oral and Maxillofacial Surgery, Graduate School of Medicine, Kyoto University
Japan

1. Introduction

Bone morphogenetic proteins (BMPs) belong to the transforming growth factor β superfamily and have the unique ability to control the differentiation of mesenchymal stem cells into osteoblastic cells [1]. Bone morphogenetic protein-2 (BMP-2), an osteoinductive member of the BMP family, plays an important role in bone growth and regeneration [2], and the clinical applications of recombinant human BMP-2 (rhBMP-2) are being investigated [3,4]. However, a large quantity of the recombinant protein and carrier are necessary, and the carriers often have problems with antigenicity, biocompatibility, biodegradability, and infection. An alternative, more efficient approach, gene transfer, may be able to target specific cells with specific promoters, and appropriate vectors to attain sustained gene expression. BMP-2 gene transfer with adenovirus have been investigated extensively [5-7]. Although the adenovirus vector is very efficient, potential toxicity and immunogenicity may limit its clinical application [8]. Furthermore, its therapeutic application would require efficient and reliable manufacture of viral vectors that are free of helper viruses and a reduction in immunogenicity. On the other hand, nonviral methods are safe and do not require immunosuppression for successful gene delivery, but suffer from lower transfection efficiencies. DNA injection followed by application of electric fields (electroporation) has been more effective for introducing DNA into muscle tissue than the use of simple intramuscler DNA injection [9]. Although this method should have the highest potential for clinical application, there is a concern that the electric pulse causes tissue damage. In addition, this method requires special equipment, and optimization of the parameters is necessary. Recently, ultrasound-enhanced gene transfer (sonoporation) has been investigated [10]. We recently reported osteoinduction by microbubble enhanced transcutaneous sonoporation of BMP-2 plasmid DNA [11]. Although this method seems to be safer than electroporation, it also requires special equipment and it is necessary to optimize the parameter of ultrasound. In this chapter, we report the human BMP-2 gene transfer using an ultra-fine needle and describe the feasibility of BMP-2 gene therapy using this new apparatus.

2. Materials and methods

To obtain human BMP-2 cDNA, a polymerase chain reaction (PCR) was performed using a pUC BMP-2 plasmid [12] and the following primers: 5′-AGA GAG AG *GAATTC* G TCG

ACC ATG GTG GCC GGG ACC CGC T (ATG, initial codon) and human BMP-2 reverse primer, 5'-AGA GAG AG *GAATTC* CTA GCG ACA CCC ACA ACC CTC CAC AA (CTA, stop codon). Both primers had EcoRI recognition sites (italicized). The PCR protocol consisted of 25 cycles of 15 sec at 98°C, 2 sec at 65°C, and 30 sec at 74°C with KOD DNA polymerase (Toyobo, Osaka, Japan). The PCR product was digested using EcoRI and ligated into the EcoRI-digested cloning site of the pCAGGS expression vector, which contains CAG (cytomegalovirus immediate-early enhancer/chicken β-actin hybrid) promoter [13], to yield pCAGGS-BMP-2. The 1197-bp insert sequence was confirmed by DNA sequencing. As a control, pCAGGS-lacZ, which causes the cytoplasmic expression of E.coli β-galactosidase [13], was used. The plasmid vectors were grown in Escherichia coli DH5α and prepared with a Qiagen Plasmid Giga Kit (Qiagen GmbH, Hilden, Germany) according to the manufacturer's protocol. To verify the identity and purity of the plasmid vectors, agarose-gel electrophoresis was performed after restriction endonuclease digestion. The plasmid DNA concentration was determined using a UV/visible spectrophotometer (DU-530, Beckman, Fullerton, CA).

To determine the effect of the ultra-fine needle transfection on mammalian cells, C3H10T1/2 (passage 9-10), a mouse fibroblastic cell line, was obtained from RIKEN Cell Bank (Tsukuba, Japan). The cells were maintained in DMEM supplemented with 10% fetal bovine serum and penicillin, streptomycin and ampicillin (PSA). The cell cultures were grown at 37°C in a humidified atmosphere of 95% air-5% CO2. Once confluent, the cells were reseeded into 35-mm glass bottom dishes and incubated 24 hours. Then the medium is replaced with Hank's balanced salt solution (HBSS) supplemented with the plasmid DNA (0.1, 0.2, and 0.3 mg/ml) to be delivered. The cells cultured on a dish were set on a stage and pierced the plasma membrane with the apparatus.

In the present study, we used the ultra-fine needle transfection apparatus SU100 (Olympus, Tokyo, JAPAN) attached to an inverted confocal microscope (IX81, Olympus, Tokyo, Japan). This apparatus was attached to an inverted microscope. A target cell was placed under the needle by the x-y stage controller. To pierce the cell membrane, the needle was lowered vertically by z-stage controller. The needle tip stayed inside the cell for one second. Then, cells were washed with fresh culture medium a few times, followed by incubation in a CO2.

First, to optimize the amount of the plasmid DNA in the medium, the lacZ gene, which causes the cytoplasmic expression of E.coli β-galactosidase, was transferred using pCAGGS-lacZ. As many as 100 cells were transfected under various concentration of the lacZ-encoding plasmid. On day 2 after transfection, the cells were fixed for 5 min in 2% formaldehyde and 0.2% glutaraldehyde in phosphate-buffered saline (PBS) at room temperature. They were subsequently washed with PBS and stained for 2 hours at 37°C in 5-Bromo-4chloro-3-indolyl-β-D-galactopyranoside (X-gal) staining solution containing 1 mg/ml X-gal, 2 mM MgCl2, 5 mM K3Fe(CN)6 and 5 mM K4Fe(CN)6⊙3H2O in PBS (pH 7.4). Experiments were performed in triplicate. Cells expressing β-galactosidase were counted and the results were presented as the mean and standard deviation Difference in the β-galactosidase activity was assessed by analysis of variance.

Next, BMP-2 gene transfer was performed using pCAGGS-BMP-2 and pCAGGS-LacZ as a control. The cells were harvested one day after transfection. RNA was isolated from the cells using a Qiagen RNeasy Mini Kit (Qiagen GmbH, Hilden, Germany). Human BMP-2 mRNA and glyceraldehydes-3-phosphate dehydrogenase (GAPDH) mRNA were detected by reverse transcription-polimerase chain reaction (RT-PCR) using the following primers: human BMP-2 forward, 5'-TCTGACTGACCGCGTTACTC-3'; human BMP-2 reverse, 5'-

TCTCTGTTTCAGGGCCGAACA-3' ; GAPDH forward, 5'-ACTCCACTCACGGCAAATTC-3'; and GAPDH reverse, 5'-CCTTCCACAATGCCAAAGTT-3'. The human BMP-2 forward primer was designed to hybridize with the sequence immediately downstream of the transcriptional start site of the CAG promoter to ensure that the PCR products were not contaminated by plasmid DNA and genomic DNA. The PCR products were analyzed by 2% agarose gel electrophoresis to detect the 285-bp human BMP-2 mRNA and 682-bp GAPDH mRNA. In addition, to determine early osteoblastic differentiation, alkaline phosphatase (ALP) staining was performed using a Sigma diagnostic ALP kit (Sigma, St.Louis, MO) on 7 days after transfection. Moreover, to confirm the terminal differentiation of osteoblast, von Kossa staining, which stains phosphates and the carbonates deposited in mineralized tissue, was performed on 21 days after transfection. For von Kossa staining, cells in dishes were fixed with 4% paraformaldehyde and were then soaked in 0.1M $AgNO_3$ solution for 15 min. After exposure to ultraviolet light at least 5 min, the dishes were washed with PBS.

3. Results

On day 2 after lacZ gene transfer, we found that X-gal positive cells were present in all of the groups performed transfection (Figure 1). In 0.1 mg/ml group, transfection efficiency reached 40.2±22.4%. In addition, 0.2 mg/ml group, the transfection efficiency significantly enhanced ($p<0.05$ versus 0.1mg/ml group) and reached 71.2±16.8%. In 0.3mg/ml group, moreover, transfection efficiency significantly ($p<0.01$ versus 0.1mg/ml group) and reached 100%. It was suggested that when 0.3 mg/ml of plasmid DNA was used, gene transfer was performed most efficiently.

According to the results of lacZ gene transfer, we performed transfection with BMP-2-encoding plasmid DNA at the concentration of 0.3 mg/ml. We detected human BMP-2 mRNA expression by RT-PCR one day after transfection (Figure 2). On day 7 after transfection, ALP-positive cells were found (Figure 3). Furthermore, on day 21 after gene transfer, von Kossa positive areas were also found (Figure 4).

4. Discussion

We have demonstrated the transfer of the human BMP-2 gene to mouse fibroblastic cells by cell membrane perforation with an ultra-fine needle, and have shown that it caused the expression of human BMP-2 mRNA one day after transfection. On day 7 after transfection, we saw an increase in ALP activity. On day 21 after transfection, moreover, calcification was seen. It is known that rhBMP-2 can induce the differentiation of non-osteogenic cell lines into osteoblastic cells, indicating that the BMP-2 gene could be transfected into C3H10T1/2 cells with an ultra-fine needle to induce the differentiation of fibroblast into osteoblast.

Our previous studies demonstrated that implantation of rhBMP-2 with a carrier matrix [14], *in vivo* adenovirus-mediated gene transfer [15], and *in vivo* plasmid DNA-mediated gene transfer, such as electroporation [16], sonoporation [11], or repeat plasmid injection [17], could cause osteoinduction. However, the above techniques showed some limitations in practical usage. The purification of rhBMP-2 was laborious and expensive, and carrier matrices created problems with antigenicity, biocompatibility, biodegradability, and infection. In addition, surgical procedures were required in order to implant a carrier matrix. The direct delivery of human BMP-2 genes using adenoviral vectors caused an immune response that needed to be systemically or locally suppressed. Non-viral gene transfer using naked plasmid DNA is a useful technique to reduce the side effect of gene therapy. However, the low transfection efficiency is a major obstacle to the clinical application. Numerous attempts have been made to overcome the relatively low transfection efficiency, including the application of electric pulses and / or ultrasonic devices. Although these techniques are efficient to some degree, using a large amount of plasmid DNA is needed to enhanced the effect [11, 17]. In addition, direct injection of naked plasmid DNA into the animal or human body is associated with toxicity and immunogenicity [18]. However, this technique is also limited due to the low transfection efficiency. It is necessary to repeat the transfection procedure to raise the efficiency [11, 17].

There are two general strategies in BMP-2 gene therapy: BMP-2-encoding vector is directly delivered to the body (*in vivo*) or genetically transduced cells by BMP-2-encoding vector are transplanted (*ex vivo*). In the case of the *in vivo* approach, it is difficult to control the specific cell population transduced genetically [19] and significant antibody response to the vector can be caused [20]. Concerning this issue, an *ex vivo* approach has the ability to overcome these problems. Previous studies showed that transfer of BMP-2-encoding vector into a mesenchymal cell line stimulated the osteogenic pathway via autocrine and paracrine mechanisms *in vitro* [21] and *in vivo* [22], and that cell mediated BMP-2 gene transfer using the stably transfected mesenchymal progenitor cell line C3H10T1/2 resulted in enhanced bone defect repair in a mice nonunion fracture model [23]. Another previous *ex vivo* gene transfer experiment suggested that neighbouring cells including periosteal cells and non-transfected mesenchymal stem cells were affected by paracrine mechanisms, and BMP-2-producing cells may themselves differentiate into osteoprogenitor cells in an autocrine activity [24]. In this study, we demonstrated efficient gene transfer without using chemical reagent and / or physical energy. This technique was simple to pierce the plasma membrane and resulted in extremely high efficiency, with the efficiency reaching to 100%. Thus, human BMP-2 gene transfer using an ultra-fine needle may be a feasible method for the *ex vivo* gene therapy of musculoskeletal disorders. However this technique is low-throughput. Future improvement of this apparatus in order to raise the throughput is indicated. In addition, injection of transfected cells is necessary and can cause damage to the target tissue. Injection of transfected cells with naked plasmid DNA into target tissue causes various degrees of damage and inflammatory reaction, depending on factors such as the needle size, the nature of solutions. One of the purposes for local growth factor application by gene delivery is production of growth factor at a defined site, thereby avoiding potentially negative effects on other organs and immune reactions. However, after direct injection, extensive spread of the vector DNA was observed. In the liver and in the spleen, reporter gene expression could be detected histochemically in several cells. In both of these organs as well as the lung, vector DNA was detected by nested PCR in all animals examined at 3 days and at 14 days after direct intraarticular injection. This indicated a broad systemic distribution of viral particles. Nevertheless, it was reported that no external DNA could be detected in the lung, the liver, or the spleen of most animals that have received cells infected *ex vivo* [20].

Our results suggest that BMP-2 gene transfer using an ultra-fine needle may allow gene delivery to be used for bone regeneration. The response to the procedure could be monitored with clinical examinations (e.g., X-ray). These findings showed that transfection using an ultra-fine needle with BMP-2-encoding plasmid caused the expression of the human BMP-2 gene in transfected cells, which demonstrated a feasibility of initiating the cascade of events to enhance bone induction. This study has suggested the possibility of the clinical application of gene therapy using an ultra-fine needle. Furthermore, the clinical application of BMP-2 gene therapy is consequently facilitated.

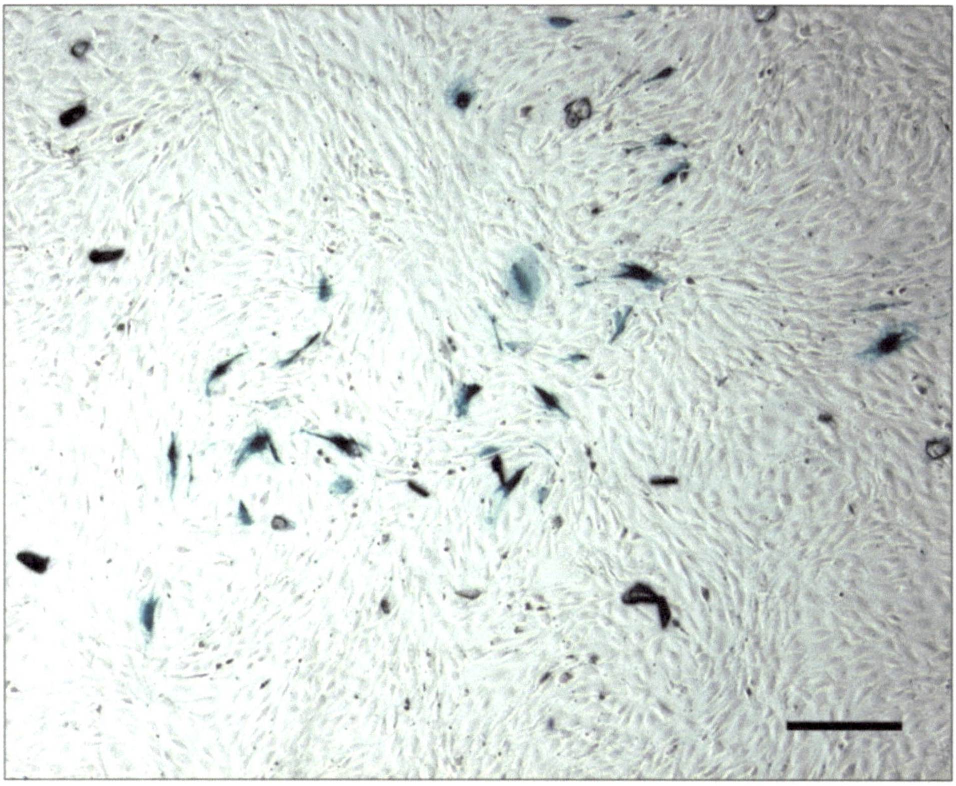

Fig. 1. Beta-galactosidase expression in C3H10T1/2 cells using an ultra-fine needle apparatus. X-gal staining was performed two days after transfection. Blue-stained cells were counted to examine the transfection efficiency and the maximum efficiency reached to 100%. Scale bar: 250 µm.

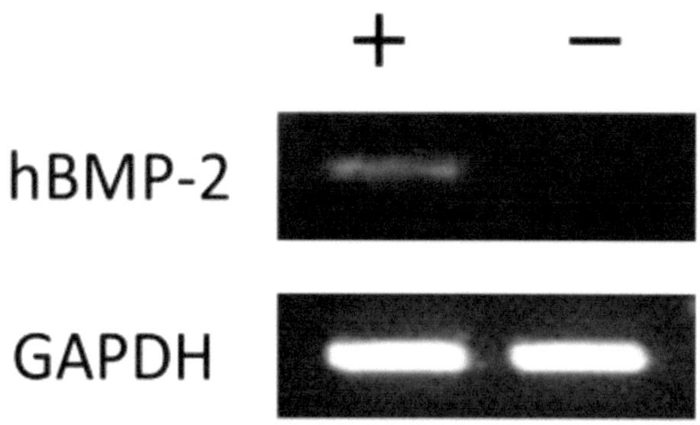

Fig. 2. Expression of the human BMP-2 transgene following the ultra-fine needle transfection was detected. RT-PCR was performed a day after transfection.

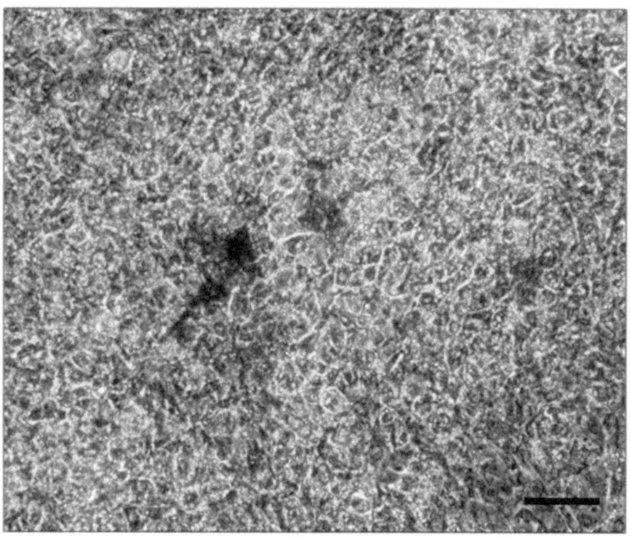

Fig. 3. ALP activity was observed in the region of the transfected cells. ALP staining was performed 7days after transfection. Skale bar: 100 μm

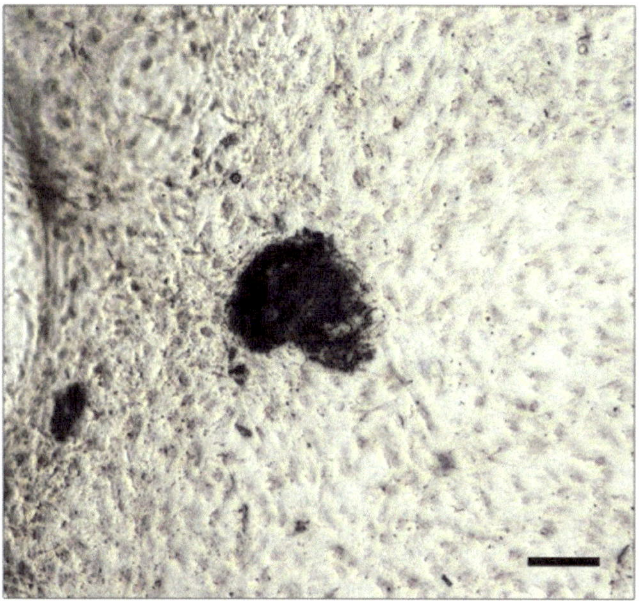

Fig. 4. Von Kossa staining was performed 21 days after transfection. Calcium deposition was confirmed in the region of the transfected cells. Skale ber: 100μm

5. References

[1] Katagiri T,Yamaguchi A, Komaki M, *et al. J Cell Biol* 1994; 127: 1755-1766.
[2] Wang EA, Rosen V, D'Alessandro JS, *et al. Proc Natl Acad Sci USA* 1990; 87: 2220-2224.
[3] Bessho K, Carnes DL, Cavin R, *et al. J Biomed Mater Res A* 2002; 61:61-65.
[4] Govender S, Csimma C, Genant HK, *et al. J Bone Joint Surg Am* 2002; 84: 2123-2134.
[5] Riew KD, Wright NM, Cheng S, *et al. Calcif Tissue Int* 1998; 63: 357-360.
[6] Baltzer AW, Lattermann C, Whalen JD, *et al. Gene Ther* 2000; 7: 734-739
[7] Engstrand T, Daluiski A, Bahamonde ME, *et al. Hum Gene Ther* 2000; 11: 205-211.
[8] Marshall E. *Science* 1999; 286: 2244-2245.
[9] Aihara H and Miyazaki J. *Nat Biotechnol* 1998; 16: 867-870.
[10] Kim HJ, Greenleaf JF, Kinnick RR, *et al. Hum Gene Ther* 1996; 7: 1339-1346.
[11] Osawa K, Okubo Y, Nakao K, *et al. J Gene Med* 2009; 11: 633-641.
[12] Okubo Y, Bessho K, Fujimura K, *et al. Biochem Biophys Res Commu*n 1999; 262: 739-743.
[13] Niwa H, Yamamura K, and Miyazaki J. *Gene* 1991; 108:193-199.
[14] Fujimura K, Bessho K, Kusumoto K, *et al. Biochem Biophys Res Commun* 1995; 208: 316-322.
[15] Okubo Y, Bessho K, Fujimura K, *et al. Biochem Biophys Res Commu*n 1995; 208: 316-322.
[16] Kawai M, Bessho K, Kaihara S, *et al. Hum Gene Ther* 2003; 14: 1547-1556.
[17] Osawa K, Okubo Y, Nakao K, *et al. J Gene Med* 2010; 12: 937-944.
[18] Wolff JA, Ludtke JJ, Acsadi G, *et al. Hum Mol Genet* 1992; 1: 363-369.
[19] Franceschi RT, Wang D, Krebsbach PH, et al. J Cell Biochem 2000; 78: 276-286.
[20] Gelse K, Jiang QJ, Aigner T, *et al. Arthritis and Rheum* 2001; 44: 1943-1953.
[21] Wang EA, Israel DI, Kelly S, *et al. Growth Factors* 1993; 9: 57-71.
[22] Gazit D, Turgeman G, Kelley P, *et al. J Gene Med* 1999; 2: 121-133.

[23] Moutsatsos IK, Turgeman G, Zhou S, *et al. Mol Ther* 2001; 3: 449-461.
[24] Park J, Ries J, Gelse K, *et al. Gene Ther* 2003; 10: 1089-1098.

Part 2

Gene Therapy of Cancer

10

Current Strategies for Cancer Gene Therapy

Yufang Zuo, Xiaofang Ying, Hui Wang, Wen Ye,
Xiangqi Meng, Hongyan Yu, Yi Zhou,
Wuguo Deng and Wenlin Huang
*State Key Laboratory of Oncology in South China, Cancer Center,
Sun Yat-sen University, Guangzhou,
PR China*

1. Introduction

Cancer is one of the most lethal diseases in the world. Traditional methods for cancer treatment are surgery, chemotherapy and radiotherapy. Early stage cancer patients may be cured by radical surgery and (or) chem(radio-)therapy. However, advanced cancer patients usually suffer from chem(radio-)resistance or metastasis, most of which can not be controlled by current therapy. Furthermore, traditional chem(radio-)therapy will bring patients with severe side effects as they not only kill cancer cells, but also normal cells.

Many investigators believe the potential to make great progress in cancer treatment lies in understanding the molecular biology of cancer and exploiting effective agents targeting abnormal molecules which regulate the growth and metastasis of tumor (Ku and Ilson, 2010). This is called targeting therapy, which can selectively kill cancer cells with minor side effects. Effective targeting therapy lies on good targets chosen and the methods used to deliver targets into the tumor mass safely and efficiently. During the past decades, various important tumor targets were exploited.

2. Targeting tumors by dysfunctional pathways

Overexpression of receptors and the abnormal activation of intracellular kinase mutations, resulting downstream of signaling pathways enhanced, leading to cell transformation, proliferation, resistance to apoptosis and eventually promote tumorigenesis. Therefore, signaling pathway has become a potential therapeutic target for cancer.

2.1 Targeting the EGFR signaling pathway

EGFR pathway mediates many important physiological processes in both normal and cancerous cells. Because of the function of the EGFR pathway, a number of therapeutic agents have been developed aiming to target EGFR. To date, five EGFR-targeted agents have been approved by the FDA for treating cancer patients. Erlotinib (OSI-774, Tarceva) was approved to treat metastatic non-small cell lung cancer (NSCLC) as single agent and to be used in combination with gemcitabine for pancreatic cancer. Another small molecule EGFR kinase inhibitor, Gefitinib (ZD1839, Iressa), is being used for locally advanced and metastatic NSCLC (Lo). Lapatinib (GW572016, Tykerb/Tyverb) is an EGFR/HER2-dual targeting small molecule inhibitor, it used in combination with other drugs, for patients with advanced or metastatic breast cancer whose cancer is HER2 positive and has failed to respond to other drugs (Moy et al., 2007).

2.2 Targeting the NF-κB pathway

Many cancer cells show aberrant or constitutive NF-κB activation which mediates resistance to chemo- and radio-therapy. Based on the pivotal role of the NF-κB pathway in the tumor progression, the NF-κB signaling pathway has become a potential target for pharmacological intervention. Strategies for blocking NF-κB include a NF-κB targeting strategy and an upstream strategy. The NF-κB targeting strategy involves blocking the activation of NF-κB signaling pathway, includes: (a) glucocorticoids used to block the transactivation of NF-κB (D'Acquisto et al., 1998). (b) decoy oligodeoxynucleotides (ODNs) used to block the DNA binding of NF-κB (Karin et al., 2004). On the other hand, the upstream strategy includes: (a) IKK inhibitors NSAIDs, sulfasalazine, arsenic trioxide, curcumin, thalidomide; (b) proteasome inhibitors PS-341, MG132; (c) the recombinant adenovirus-mediated overexpression of the IκBα gene. (d) cell-permeable peptides SN-50; (e) antioxidants disulfiram, glutathione (Chen et al., 2002; Tomita et al., 2003).

2.3 Targeting the PTEN/PI3K/AKT signaling pathway

PTEN/PI3K/AKT constitutes an important pathway regulating the signaling of cell proliferation, survival, apoptosis, and metabolism. Many components of this pathway have been described as causal forces in cancer. Once the activity of mTOR induced by disfunction of PTEN/PI3K/AKT pathway, the promotion of tumor proliferation and growth are achieved through its downstream targets. A number of basic research studies and clinical trials have investigated that rapamycin, the potential of the selective mTOR inhibitor could inhibit activity of both mTOR and AKT, suggesting that it may be an effective therapeutic blockade of PI3K signaling (Guertin and Sabatini, 2007). PI3K inhibitors, TGX115, LY294002 derivatives have shown to have greater solubility, lower toxicity, improved pharmacodynamics, and more specific PI3K selectivity than LY294002 (Granville et al., 2006). In addition, PX-866a, wortmannin derivative has more potent and less toxic effects than wortmannin (Jiang and Liu, 2008). SF1126 is a small molecule inhibitor that can inhibit all isoforms of PI3K class. In preclinical studies, it has been identified to be effective for tumor treatment in a variety of mouse tumor models, including prostate, breast, lung, multiple myeloma, and other cancers (Hennessy et al., 2005). Lipid-based inhibitors of Akt were the first group of inhibitors to be developed. Perifosine is the best-characterized Akt inhibitor, which inhibits the translocation of Akt to the cell membrane. It can inhibit the cell growth in different solid tumors (Martelli et al., 2003). Several other Akt inhibitors such as the indazole-pyri-dine A-443654 and 9-methoxy-2-methylellipticinium acetate (API-59-OMe) have been identified. A-443654 was shown to increase the effect of paclitaxel treatment both *in vitro* and *in vivo* (Han et al., 2007). API-59-OMe can inhibit cell growth and induce apoptosis of several different human cancer cells, including prostate, breast, endometrial and ovarian cancers (Jin et al., 2004; Tang et al., 2006).

2.4 Targeting the MAPK signaling pathway

The RAS–mitogen activated protein kinase (MAPK) signaling pathway not only promotes cell proliferation, but also mediates cell survival. The activity of this pathway was reported to be upregulated in a broad spectrum of human tumors. In this signalling pathway, RAS,

RAF and MEK proteins have unique features that make it a good therapeutic target. By inhibiting the post-translational addition of farnesyl group to RAS by farnesyltransferase, it was thought that Farnesyltransferase inhibitors (FTIs)would be able to target human tumors in which RAS was constitutively activated (Sebolt-Leopold and Herrera, 2004). Several FTIs such as BMS-214662, Sarasar and Zarnestra have been studied in patients diagnosed with a range of cancers. FTIs could be specific and effective therapeutic agents, however, clinical data obtained so far leads us to conclude that these agents do not represent a viable approach to blocking signal transduction through the RAS–MAPK pathway. Therefore, several small molecule RAF inhibitors have now been reported. According to published reports, only BAY 43-9006 has reached the clinical testing stage. It has completed Phase I and Phase II trials. It has been reported that this agent is generally well tolerated. However, the toxicities involving the gastrointestinal track and the skin have existed. Phase III trials to be focusing on patients with renal-cell carcinoma indicated that BAY 43-9006 lack of specificity. So, although BAY 43-9006 has promise as an anticancer agent, it is difficult to assess the impact of RAF inhibition on observed clinical outcomes. The first MEK inhibitor reported to inhibit tumor growth *in vivo* was CI-1040 (Sebolt-Leopold et al., 1999). There was evidence of antitumor activity in the Phase I trial, however, similar results were not observed in Phase II trials, so PD0325901, which is structurally highly similar to CI-1040, was subsequently developed. The anticancer activity of PD0325901 was improved compared with CI-1040. The longer duration and greater solubility leading to improved bioavailability, and increased metabolic stability. Therefore, PD0325901 viewed as a significantly more potent MEK inhibitor (Sebolt-Leopold and Herrera, 2004).

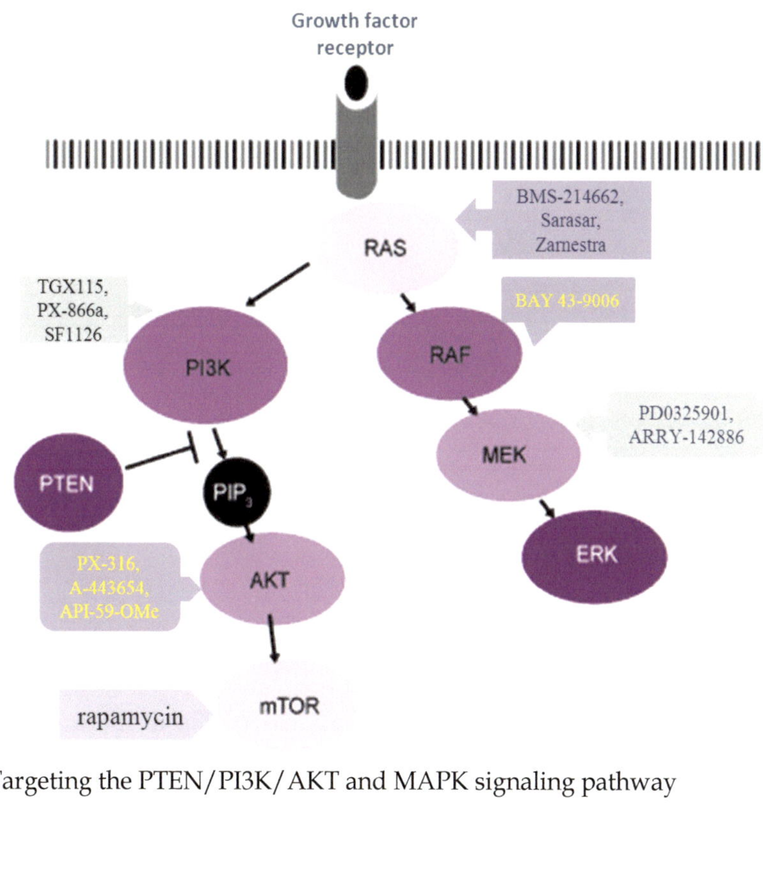

Fig. 1. Targeting the PTEN/PI3K/AKT and MAPK signaling pathway

3. Targeting tumors with tumor suppress gene p53

Clinical studies have shown that p53 is a tumor suppressor which mutates in about 50% of human cancers, and where the gene itself is not mutated, its signal pathway functionally inactivated. Three decades of researches in p53 have reached an understanding of p53 playing a key role in the regulations of many different genes in response to a wide variety of epigenetic stresses.

3.1 Regulation of p53 expression

In normal cells, p53 restrains its expression and function to maintain normal homeostasis. Critical for the control of p53 function are its two main negative regulators: Mdm2 and Mdmx. Duplicated from a single ancestral gene, Mdm2 and Mdmx have similar sequences. They bind to p53 via an N-terminal hydrophobic pocket, thus inhibiting transactivation function of p53 (Kruse and Gu, 2009). The C-terminal of both Mdm2 and Mdmx contain a RING domain which has intrinsic E3 ubiquitin ligase activity and it targets p53 for ubiquitin-dependent degradation by proteasome both in nucleus and cytoplasm (Deshaies and Joazeiro, 2009). Mdm2 and Mdmx also induce the exportation of p53 from the nucleus to the cytoplasm. Thus, these two proteins negatively regulate p53 by both suppression of transactivation and post-translational destabilization.

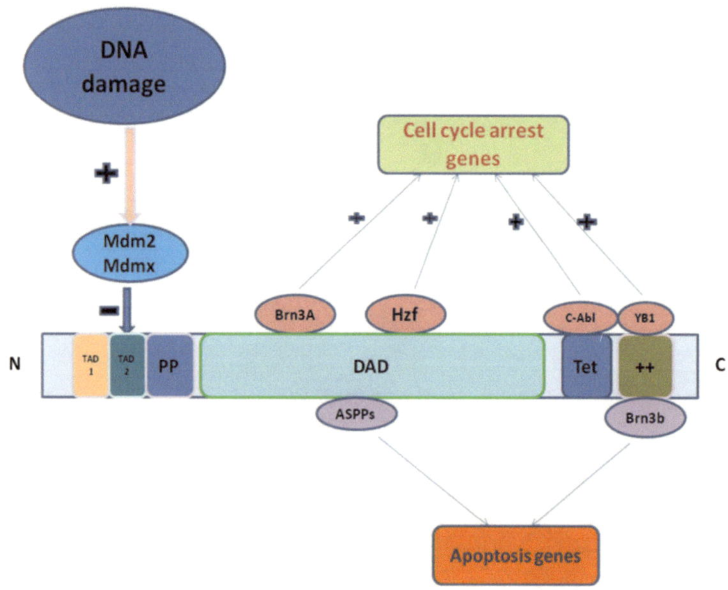

Fig. 2. Targeting tumors with tumor suppress gene p53

3.2 Conformation of p53

The p53 protein contains three main functional domains: N-terminal harbors transcriptional activation domain 1 (TAD1, residues 20-40), TAD2 (residues 40-60) which interacts with Mdm2 and Mdmx, and the proline domain (PP, residues 60-90); in the middle lies the central core sequence-specific DNA-binding domain (DAD, residues 100-300), it interacts with its target genes or proteins; and C-terminal contains the tetramerization domain (Tet, residues 325-356) and lysine-rich basic C-terminal domain (++, residues 363-393) which regulates DNA-binding. Interacts mainly with sequence-specific DNA binding sites of its target agents, p53 starts series of cellular responses: cell-cycle arrest, apoptosis, DNA-repair and so on. For example, Brn3A and Hzf with DAD, C-Abl with Tet, YB1 and p18/Hamlet with ++ selectively induce p53 activation of cell-cycle arrest genes like p21. Conversely, ASPPs with DAD and Brn3b, and so on with the p53 C-terminal selectively induce apoptotic genes like PUMA and Bax (Vousden and Prives, 2009).

3.3 Function of p53

Here comes to questions: When do cells perform cell-cycle arrest, and when do they bring about senescence and apoptosis? Some researches hypothesis that the outcome of p53 activation mostly depends on the type of tissue and stress, how severe the stress is, the microenvironment, and the post-transcriptional modification. With mild impact to DNA, p53 may stabilize the genes, including DNA repair and activating anti-oxidant genes. As a result, p53 acts as a protector by preventing the generation of oncogenic lesions. Conversely, once severe stress happens, like oncogene activation, lethal DNA damage or hypoxia, p53 may start senescence and apoptosis, eliminating badly injured cells which cannot be rescued by cell-cycle arrest (Vousden and Lu, 2002).

3.4 Wild-type p53 in cancers

In tumors which have wild-type p53 reduced, disturbing the interaction between p53 and Mdm2/Mdmx may rationally restore p53 function and may enhance sensitivity of tumors to chemotherapy and radiotherapy.

Nutlins, a well studied inhibitor family of the Mdm2-p53 complex, are highly selective for Mdm2 and they can tightly bind to their receptors (Dickens et al.). In the Nutlin family there is Nutlin-3, it competes for binding to Mdm2, so displaces p53 protein and releases it to function normally in cancer cells derived from hematologic malignancies (Secchiero et al., 2008). The molecular pathways in the Nutlin-3 induced responses still wait to be explored.

A small molecular compound, RITA, induces wild-type p53 activation and accumulation thus programs apoptosis in different tumor cell lines of colon, lung, breast, etc both in vitro and in vivo. It prevents interaction between p53 and Mdm2 through binding to the 1-63 residues of the p53 protein N-terminal (Issaeva et al., 2004).

3.5 Mutant p53 in cancers

A large-scale sequencing of various tumor cells proved that p53 mutations, mostly DNA binding domain mutations are common events.

Small molecular compounds for mutant p53 reactivation via different mechanisms have been identified in recent years. CP-31398, stabilizes the conformation of DNA binding domain to restore the function of several p53 mutants. Foster. et al reported that CP-31398 suppressed the growth of both human tumor cells in vitro and xenograft tumors in mice (Foster et al., 1999).

Similar with CP-31398, PRIMA-1 also serves to suppress tumor cell growth by reactivating the transcriptional function of mutant p53 and inducing cofactors responsible in p53-mediated apoptosis like PUMA, Noxa, and Bax, which induce caspase activation, especially caspase-2 (Bykov et al., 2002). Rescue tumor suppression function of p53 will pave the way for future anti-cancer therapy.

For the purpose of inducing p53 activities in a desirable way, a wide range of unknown fields from the p53 posttranscriptional modifications, cofactors to network of targeted agents wait to be fetched.

4. Targeting tumors by anti-angiogenesis

Cytotoxic approaches to killing tumor cells, based on their increased rate of proliferation relative to normal cells, have been the mainstay of cancer therapy for decades. However, over 30 years ago, as proposed by Folkman in 1971, angiogenesis is required for tumor, so targeting angiogenesis is a significant approach in inhibiting solid tumor growth and hence, limit cancer progression (Folkman, 1971).

Angiogenesis is the formation of new blood vessels from pre-existing ones. The understanding of the angiogenic mechanisms and the successful use of several angiogenesis inhibitors in animal models, have led to clinical applications of anti-angiogenic therapy. This strategy has several advantages over traditional chemotherapy, in principle, including side effects and less toxicity, a reduced risk for development of resistance, and a general broad spectrum of activity. More important, anti-angiogenic approaches can efficiently target both low and high proliferating tumor cells, so unlike conventional cytotoxic chemotherapies that are more effective against fast growing tumors, anti-angiogenic therapy could act against a broader range of cancers. The expected results are different from traditional cancer therapies, the first aim of anti angiogenesis is to stabilize the disease rather than to eradicate the tumor mass, unlike radiotherapy or chemotherapy; however these strategy can be used in concert (Bisacchi et al., 2003).

4.1 Potential anti-angiogenic factors for gene therapy

Induction of the angiogenic switch depends on a local change in the balance between inhibitors and activators of angiogenesis. The switch to an angiogenic phenotype of tumor requires downregulation of angiogenesis inhibitors and upregulation of angiogenic factors (Dell'Eva et al., 2002). Until now, many angiogenic peptides have been identified, including vascular endothelial growth factor (VEGF) and vascular permeability factor (VPF), basic and acidic fibroblast growth factor (FGF), epidermal growth factor (EGF), platelet-derived epidermal cell growth factor (PD-ECGF), platelet-derived growth factor (PDGF), insulin-like growth factors (IGFs), interleukin-8 (IL-8),transforming growth factor-α and β (TGF-α and -β), heparin growth factor, granulocyte colony stimulating factor, E-selectin, angiogenin, tumor necrosis factor-α (TNF-α). Angiogenic factors released by tumor cells stimulate endothelial cells (EC) which become activated, providing growth factors (FGF-1,-2) and matrix metalloproteinases (MMPs). Proteolytic activities of the MMPs degrade the surrounding tissue and vascular membrane, leading to EC proliferation, migration and new capillary formation.

Thus, the goal of anti-angiogenic gene therapy is to switch the local balance between angiogenic factors and angiogenic inhibitors in tumor microenvironment to the anti-angiogenic phenotype, targeting one or more events of angiogenesis cascade. The more attractive angiosuppressive factors for clinical trials are: naturally occurring inhibitors of angiogenesis, agents that interfere with vascular basement membrane and extracellular matrix MMP inhibitors, angiostatic steroids and others, anti-adhesion molecules antibodies and miscelllaneous drugs that modulate angiogenesis by diverse mechanisms of action (O'Reilly et al., 1997).

4.2 Clinical trials targeting tumor angiogenesis

The greatest clinical success with the antiangiogenic strategy to date, has been achieved with bevacizumab, the antibody to VEGF. Bevacizumab blocks the binding of VEGF-A to its receptors, VEGFR-1 and VEGFR-2. In rectal cancer patients, this VEGF signaling inhibitor reduced tumor microvessel density, blood flow and interstitial pressure, and increased the percentage of vessels covered by pericytes (Willett et al., 2004).

Endostatin is a 20-kDa proteolytic COOH-terminal fragment derived from collagen XVIII58. Endostatin reduces endothelial cell proliferation and migration, significantly reduces invasion of endothelial as well as tumor cells into the reconstituted basement membrane and acts as a potent inhibitor of angiogenesis and tumor growth. In preclinical studies, expression of endostatin decreased tumor vascularization 3-fold with a concomitant 3-fold increase in the number of apoptotic cells. Endostatin is the first endogenous angiogenesis inhibitor to enter clinical trials. The earliest phase I trials were published in 2002 and 2003 at The University of Texas M.D. Anderson Cancer Center. The final results show that the anti-angiogenic drug was safe and reduced blood flow in patients. There was some shrinkage of tumors among the participants, and two patients showed encouraging results (Thomas et al., 2003). A Chinese phase III trial using recombinant endostatin in combination with chemotherapy in NSCLC has exhibited a significant increase in response rates and time to progression. Another potent angiogenesis inhibitor is angiostatin (38kDa), which is generated as a result of proteolytic cleavage of plasminogen and comprises the first four triple loop disulphide-linked structures of plasminogen, termed kringle domains (O'Reilly et al., 1994). Currently, phase II/III clinical trials of endostatin and angiostatin are ongoing, and preliminary data analysis show minimal toxicities but anti-tumor results are inconsistent.

Now, more than 300 anti-angiogenic molecules targeting different signalling pathways and over 20 angiogenic growth factors are being tested for their potential anti-cancer efficacies at preclinical and clinical stages. Eight new drugs in which anti-angiogenic activity is considered to be central to their therapeutic effects have been approved by the FDA in the United States for the treatment of cancer (Table 1) (Park and Dilda).

4.3 Perspectives

Antiangiogenic methods have changed the landscape in traditional cancer therapy after the initial clinical success of bevacizumab in 2004. Future development of antiangiogenic drugs targeting various pathways with different principles, particularly in combination therapy settings, is expected to significantly improve therapeutic efficacies. One of the important approaches of increasing therapeutic efficacy is to optimize the drug delivery systems that enable accurate drug release only in malignant tissues, persistent release and tightly controlled release of antiangiogenic agents. Long-term delivery is particularly advantageous for clinical benefits as withdrawal of these drugs might cause a rebound angiogenic activity in tumors. However, persistent release of the same drug in cancer patients might elicit evasive refractoriness to antiangiogenic therapy. This dilemma may be resolved using a smart microchip delivery system that simultaneously or sequentially releases multiple drugs targeting different pathways.

Angiogenic inhibitor	Target	FDA approved for
Avastin/bevacizumab (Genentech)	VEGF	Non-small cell lung carcinoma, metastatic colorectal cancer and breastcancer
Cetuximab/Erbitux (Bristol-Myers Squibb ImClone)	EGFR	Metastatic colorectal carcinoma and head and neck cancer
Panitumumab/Vectibix (Amgen)	EGFR	Metastatic colorectal carcinoma
Erlotinib/Tarceva (Genentech OSI Roche)	EGFR	Non-small cell lung carcinoma and pancreatic cancer
Sunitinib/Sutent (Pfizer)	Multi-kinase inhibitor	Advanced renal cell carcinoma and gastrointestinal tumours
Sorafenib/Nexavar (Bayer Onyx)	Multi-kinase inhibitor	Advanced renal cell carcinoma and advanced hepatocellular carcinoma

Table 1. Anti-angiogenic therapeutics FDA approved for the treatment of cancer.

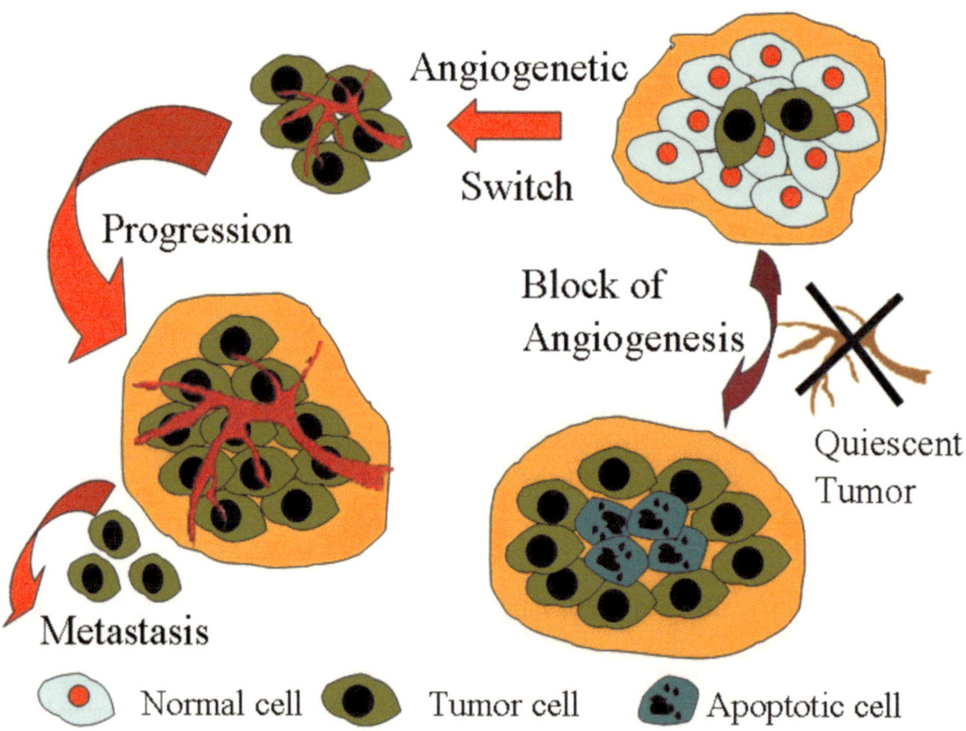

Fig. 3. Targeting tumor by antiangiogenesis

5. Targeting tumors with monocloning antibody

For several decades, antibodies has been hoped to become a 'magic bullets' to cure patients, and this vision came true with the development of hybridoma technology by Kohler and Milstein (Kohler and Milstein, 1975). The antibodies are Y-shaped proteins with two identical light chains and two identical heavy chains. The arms of the Y identify antigens, and the stem of Y alerts and recruits the components to attack the molecular targets once bounded.

Present, more than 400 mAbs entered commercial clinical development and anticancer mAbs comprised almost half of the total mAbs (Reichert et al., 2005). To date, a dozen of anticancer mAbs have been approved for marketing by FDA. There are two modes that mAbs destroy the target tumor cells, one is direct way by conjugating radioactive toxins or triggering apoptosis. Another is the indirect way through activating immune system components or blockade of critical receptors.

The conjugated mAbs can increase the specificity of chemo- or radiation therapy. Drugs composed of the conjugate can be produced by chemical linkers, while the proteins can be produced by either chemosynthesis or genetic engineering. However, some challenges exist in the development of immunotoxins since the protein toxins can lead to immunogenic action in human and the drug toxins which may lack potency for the little doses degrade in the way to the tumor site. Another limitation is that immunotoxins require internalization to gain a cytotoxic effect on tumor cells.

In the recent data, over half of the mAbs are unmodified mAbs. The characteristics like average half-life, vary with the isotype of the unmodified mAbs are determined to be the crystallizablefragment (Fc) region. A common mode of mAbs function is to activate the components of the human immune system attacking the target cancer cells. Once binding to target, mAbs can call up effector cells to activate the complement. These actions are known as antibody-dependent cell cytotoxicity (ADCC) and complement-dependent cytotoxicity (CDC), and they are mediated by the Fc portion of mAbs.

5.1 Targets in solid tumors

EGFR family includes EGFR(c-erbB-1), HER2/*neu* (c-erbB-2), HER3(c-erbB-3), and HER4 (c-erbB-4). EGFR overexpressed in many solid tumors, such as non-small cell lung cancer, colorectal cancer, breast cancer, head and neck cancer, and prostate cancer. Some anti-EGFR mAbs can inhibit tumor cell growth and activate tyrosine kinases. Cetuximab, a chimeric form of anti-EGFR antibody can objective anti-tumor responses alone, or in combination with other treatment strategies for the overexpressing EGFR cancers. A second EGFR-targeted mAbs, Panitumumab, was produced in a muse while the genes of antibody came from human (Mendez et al., 1997).

bold (HER2/neu) is overexpressed in 25% of breast cancer cells, and in other adenocarcinomas of the ovary, lung, prostate and gastrointestinal tract (Baselga et al., 1996). Trastuzumab is a humanized mAb that derived from the murine mAb4D5, which combined with chemotherapy in the randomized phase 3 trial shows a 25% increase in survival after 29 months than chemotherapy alone. It had also been shown activity in Trastuzumab combination with small- molecule drugs such as vinorelbine, docetaxel and paclitaxel.

Ep-CAM (epithelial cell adhesion molecule) is highly expressed in colorectal, non-small cell lung and prostatic cancer and so on. Edrecolomab, came from murine and transformed into human chimeric construct, is a manual antibody for Ep-CAM. The clinical testing showed the chimeric construct increased mononuclear cell-mediated ADCC and prolonged half-life than the murine mAb. In addition, it develops no human anti-mouse antibodies (Hartung et al., 2005).

5.2 Targets in lymphomas

The mAb direct against human B cell lymphoma-associated antigen have shown enormous power on clearance circulating tumor cells with rare objective clinical responses. The mechanisms underlying responses to these mAb are complex and have not been completely elucidated now, while the main mechanisms could include ADCC and disturbance transductional signals. Another target, CD52, a glycopeptides exists on T and B lymphocytes, has been tested as a target for mAb in the treatment of numerous lymphomas which decreased the response from allogeneic transplant grafts.

5.3 Toxicity of mAb

mAb are paid more attention as the clinical tests were shown with less toxicity than the normal cytotoxic chemotherapy and radiotherapy. But cytotoxic always emergence through two ways, one is mechanism-dependent and the other is mechanism-independent. Mechanism-independent occur for the mAb proteins produced by the xenogeneic gene. The primary toxicity of mAbs is mechanism-dependent toxicity that exaggerated pharmacology of blocking or enhancing the activities of the target cells or tissues target molecule. Toxicity is also resulted from binding to the target in normal tissues other than cancer tissues alone. Treatment with cetuximab can cause the skin toxicity (acneiform rash) and the cardiotoxicity observed with trastuzumab due to skin and cardiac muscle respectively expressing the same target antigens.

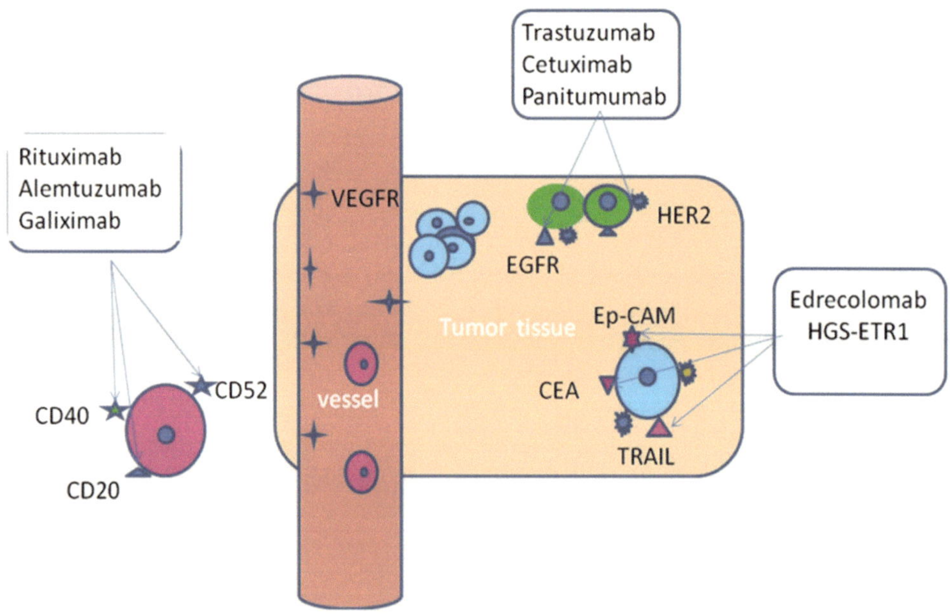

Fig. 4. Targets in solid tumors and lymphomas

5.4 Further exploration

Nowadays mAbs have achieved significantly success compared with the disappointment of failure in decades ago. Despite these accomplishments, the clinical response remains, such as the toxicity on the normal cells. Regardless of these challenges, each new anticancer mAb approved represents more choice and potential benefit to patients. With the development of biotechnology, the efficient and safe mAb for cancer patients may be produced. "We have a long way to go before the story is finished," says Winter (Gura, 2002).

6. Viral vector for gene delivery

Cancer is a multigenic disorder involving activation of oncogenes and inactivation of suppressor genes. Many data has suggested that cancer can be arrested or reversed by treatment with gene transfer vectors that carrying therapeutic genes. The vectors used for gene therapy include viral or non-viral vectors. Viruses have been the most common vectors for gene therapy and about 70% of gene therapy clinical trials use viral vectors. The main viral vectors used in clinic include retroviruses, adenovirus, adeno-associated virus, herpesvirus and poxvirus.

Retrovirus is an enveloped RNA virus. The genome of retrovirus contains two identical single-stranded RNAs about 7-10 kb. There are three open reading frames, gap, pol and env, and two long terminal repeats (LTRs) in retroviral genome (Baum et al., 2006). Replication-defective retroviral vectors (RDR) lack genes required for self-replication and the capability of cell-to-cell spreading. RDR vectors have used to deliver therapeutic genes into immunodeficiency disease. Replication-competent retrovirus (RCR) vectors can duplicate in dividing cells and result cell lysis. Retrovirus may randomly integrate to host genome and results insertional mutagenesis. Many methods has been explored to improve the safety of RCR vectors, such as using tissue-specific regulatory sequences replace the viral promoter elements; using inducible regulatory sequences to control transcription.

Lentivirus is a kind of slow viruses of the Retroviridae family. In contrast with simple retrovirus, lentivirus has evolved the ability to infect nondividing cells (Cockrell and Kafri, 2007). Recently, the inducible tet-on/off lentivirus expression system has been structured by researchers. Using this system, researchers can control gene expression, so this system is a powerful tool to research transgene expression.

Adenovirus is a linear, double-stranded and non-enveloped DNA virus. The genome of adenovirus is about 36 kb. Over 50 serotypes of human Adenovirus have been identified, among which Ad5 is the most commonly used vector. Unlike the retrovirus, adenovirus genomes do not integrate into the host chromosome, so it is a safe vector for transient transgene expression. Replication-defective adenoviruses have been used to transfer tumor-suppressor genes, anti-angiogenesis genes, immunostimulatory genes, prodrug-activating genes. In 2004, replication-deficient recombinant adenovirus (Ad)-p53 was approved to use for head and neck squamous cell carcinoma (HNSCC) by China's State Food and Drug Administration. In china another cancer gene therapy agentia Ad-endostatin (E10A) has been finished the class I clinical trial for solid cancers and no dose-limiting toxicity was developed (Lin et al., 2007).

Adeno-Associated Virus (AAV) is a small, nonenveloped DNA virus. Its genome is a linear single-stranded DNA of 4.7 kb. AAV produces infection only in the presence of adenovirus or herpesvirus. In the absence of helper virus, AAV can set up latency by integrating into chromosome 19q13.4 (Lai et al., 2002). AAV vectors have successfully delivered targeting genes into varieties of dividing and quiescent cells, including in the muscle, liver, lung, brain, eye, retina and heart. The therapeutic genes that AAV vectors contain are no more than 5kb. Researchers invent a new AAV vectors system which uses head-to-tail heterodimers of the two rAAV vectors form via recombination in the ITRs, which can improves the packaging capacity of AAV vectors to 10 kb. This vector has been successfully used for gene expression in the retina, lung and muscle diseases.

Herpes Simplex Virus (HSV) is double-strand DNA virus. HSV-1 is the common vector in gene therapy. The genome of HSV includes long and short unique regions, each flanked by inverted repeats. The neurotropic ability of HSV makes this vector for the design of gene therapies that target cancers of the CNS (Shen and Nemunaitis, 2006). The replication-defective HSV vector lacks one or several essential immediate-early (IE) genes. Some researchers have used replication-defective HSV vector with suicide genes, such as thymidine kinase (TK) gene or cytosine deaminase (CD), treat CNS malignant tumors. Conditionally replicating HSV vector delete some genes for virus replication, but this vector can duplicate in cancer cells where it gains the enzymes of replication. This vector is an oncolytic HSV vector and has widely used to treat the squamous cancers in head and neck, malignant glioma, colorectal cancer, pancreatic cancer and prostate cancer.

Poxvirus is a kind of complex DNA virus. The genome is linear double-stranded DNA and the size of the different poxvirus species is variable from 130kb to 160kb. The dsDNA molecule contains the open reading frame (ORF) and the inverted terminal repeats (ITRs) in the terminal regions of the genome (Lefkowitz et al., 2006). Poxvirus as a transgene vector with tumor-associated antigens or tumor-specific antigens has been used in cancer therapy, which can improve hose anti-cancer ability.

7. Nonviral vector for gene delivery

During the past two decades, gene therapy has gained rapid development as a promising therapeutic modality for the treatment of genetic and acquired disorders (Al-Dosari and Gao, 2009). However, the rate-limiting step is lack of a suitable vector for gene delivery. Although viral vectors are attractive in initial research due to its high efficiency, nonviral gene-delivery carriers have gained increasing attention in recent years because their safety and easy preparation advantages over viral vectors.

Nonviral vectors for gene therapy have been categorized as expression vector and delivery vector. Among the nonviral vectors, the most widely used expression vector is plasmid DNA. Methods of nonviral gene delivery contained direct injection of naked plasmid DNA, physical and chemical approaches (Gao et al., 2007). Physical approaches employing mechanical (particle bombardment or gene gun), electric (electroporation), ultrasonic, or hydrodynamic (hydrodynamic gene transfer) have been explored in recent years. Chemical methods mediate gene uptake by membrane fusion and/or receptor-mediated endocytosis. Chemical vectors such as cationic lipids and cationic polymers form condense complexes with negatively charged DNA through electrostatic interactions (Al-Dosari and Gao, 2009; Ohlfest et al., 2005).

7.1 Nonviral therapeutics in clinical trials

Although adenoviral- and retroviral-mediated transfections are currently the most widely used strategies for gene therapy in clinical trials, there are more than 400 clinical trials using nonviral vectors so far (www.wiley.co.uk/genmed/clinical). Lipid and polymer-mediated gene delivery has been used to successfully target both genetic diseases as well as cancer. With extensive effort being put into designing nonviral vectors with higher gene transfer efficiency, synthetic gene carriers may become superior to viral analogues in clinical trials in the near future.

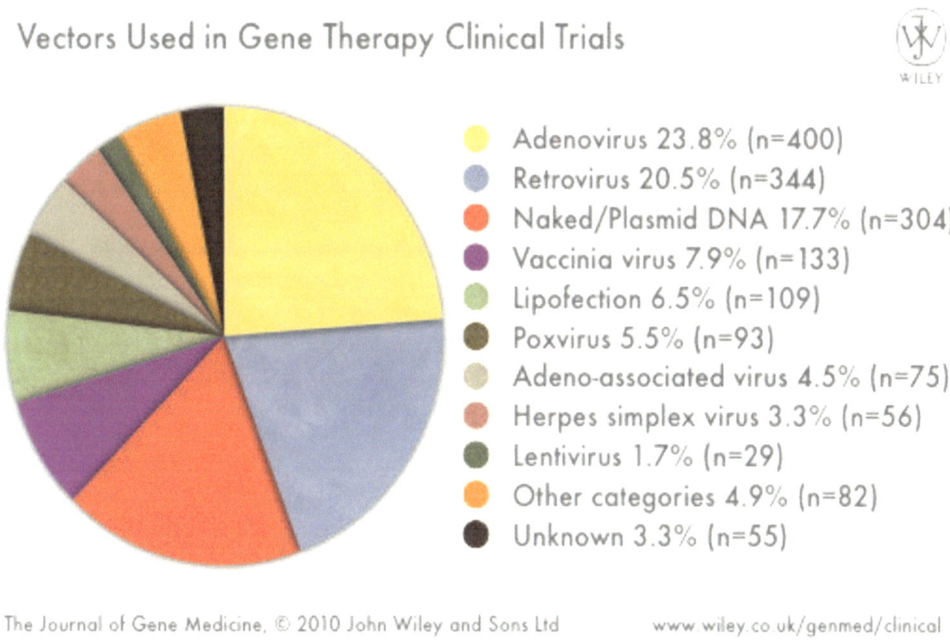

Fig. 5. Vectors used in gene therapy

8. Future direction and challenge

Single targeted cancer therapy can not be expected to yield optimal outcomes as tumorigenesis is a multistep process and its molecular pathogenesis is not linked to the defect of a single target. Therefore, multi-targeted therapy through the combination of agents targeting distinct molecules might be the goals for targeting therapy in the near future. This could overcome the issues of tumour heterogeneity and maintain the selectivity of treatment at the same time. In addition, monotherapy is further evolving to single inhibitor which can target several molecules simultaneously. It seems promising that with our better understanding of tumor biology, more efficacious combinations for targeted therapy will emerge in the immediate future (Imai and Takaoka, 2006).

Another new aspect of cancer-targeted therapy is employing cancer stem cells as the target. It was reported that mTOR inhibition by rapamycin selectively eliminated leukaemic stem cells without affecting normal haematopoietic stem cells (Zhang et al., 2006). Therefore, targeting abnormal signalling pathway in cancer stem cells might offer an effective approach for targeting therapies. Besides, it is of great importance to identify predictive markers for the response to targeted therapy (Swain, 2011). Beyond its obvious clinical benefits for cancer patients, the identification of predictive markers can also reduce the costs of cancer treatments (Warren et al., 2008).

9. References

Al-Dosari, M.S. and Gao, X. (2009) Nonviral gene delivery: principle, limitations, and recent progress. *Aaps J*, 11, 671-681.

Baselga, J., Tripathy, D., Mendelsohn, J., Baughman, S., Benz, C.C., Dantis, L., Sklarin, N.T., Seidman, A.D., Hudis, C.A., Moore, J., Rosen, P.P., Twaddell, T., Henderson, I.C. and Norton, L. (1996) Phase II study of weekly intravenous recombinant humanized anti-p185HER2 monoclonal antibody in patients with HER2/neu-overexpressing metastatic breast cancer. *J Clin Oncol*, 14, 737-744.

Baum, C., Schambach, A., Bohne, J. and Galla, M. (2006) Retrovirus vectors: toward the plentivirus? *Mol Ther*, 13, 1050-1063.

Bisacchi, D., Benelli, R., Vanzetto, C., Ferrari, N., Tosetti, F. and Albini, A. (2003) Anti-angiogenesis and angioprevention: mechanisms, problems and perspectives. *Cancer Detect Prev*, 27, 229-238.

Bykov, V.J., Issaeva, N., Shilov, A., Hultcrantz, M., Pugacheva, E., Chumakov, P., Bergman, J., Wiman, K.G. and Selivanova, G. (2002) Restoration of the tumor suppressor function to mutant p53 by a low-molecular-weight compound. *Nat Med*, 8, 282-288.

Chen, L.F., Mu, Y. and Greene, W.C. (2002) Acetylation of RelA at discrete sites regulates distinct nuclear functions of NF-kappaB. *Embo J*, 21, 6539-6548.

Cockrell, A.S. and Kafri, T. (2007) Gene delivery by lentivirus vectors. *Mol Biotechnol*, 36, 184-204.

D'Acquisto, F., Sautebin, L., Iuvone, T., Di Rosa, M. and Carnuccio, R. (1998) Prostaglandins prevent inducible nitric oxide synthase protein expression by inhibiting nuclear factor-kappaB activation in J774 macrophages. *FEBS Lett*, 440, 76-80.

Dell'Eva, R., Pfeffer, U., Indraccolo, S., Albini, A. and Noonan, D. (2002) Inhibition of tumor angiogenesis by angiostatin: from recombinant protein to gene therapy. *Endothelium*, 9, 3-10.

Deshaies, R.J. and Joazeiro, C.A. (2009) RING domain E3 ubiquitin ligases. *Annu Rev Biochem*, 78, 399-434.

Dickens, M.P., Fitzgerald, R. and Fischer, P.M. Small-molecule inhibitors of MDM2 as new anticancer therapeutics. *Semin Cancer Biol*, 20, 10-18.

Folkman, J. (1971) Tumor angiogenesis: therapeutic implications. *N Engl J Med*, 285, 1182-1186.

Foster, B.A., Coffey, H.A., Morin, M.J. and Rastinejad, F. (1999) Pharmacological rescue of mutant p53 conformation and function. *Science*, 286, 2507-2510.

Gao, X., Kim, K.S. and Liu, D. (2007) Nonviral gene delivery: what we know and what is next. *Aaps J*, 9, E92-104.

Granville, C.A., Memmott, R.M., Gills, J.J. and Dennis, P.A. (2006) Handicapping the race to develop inhibitors of the phosphoinositide 3-kinase/Akt/mammalian target of rapamycin pathway. *Clin Cancer Res*, 12, 679-689.

Guertin, D.A. and Sabatini, D.M. (2007) Defining the role of mTOR in cancer. *Cancer Cell*, 12, 9-22.

Gura, T. (2002) Therapeutic antibodies: magic bullets hit the target. *Nature*, 417, 584-586.

Han, E.K., Leverson, J.D., McGonigal, T., Shah, O.J., Woods, K.W., Hunter, T., Giranda, V.L. and Luo, Y. (2007) Akt inhibitor A-443654 induces rapid Akt Ser-473 phosphorylation independent of mTORC1 inhibition. *Oncogene*, 26, 5655-5661.

Hartung, G., Hofheinz, R.D., Dencausse, Y., Sturm, J., Kopp-Schneider, A., Dietrich, G., Fackler-Schwalbe, I., Bornbusch, D., Gonnermann, M., Wojatschek, C., Lindemann, W., Eschenburg, H., Jost, K., Edler, L., Hochhaus, A. and Queisser, W. (2005)

Adjuvant therapy with edrecolomab versus observation in stage II colon cancer: a multicenter randomized phase III study. *Onkologie*, 28, 347-350.

Hennessy, B.T., Smith, D.L., Ram, P.T., Lu, Y. and Mills, G.B. (2005) Exploiting the PI3K/AKT pathway for cancer drug discovery. *Nat Rev Drug Discov*, 4, 988-1004.

Imai, K. and Takaoka, A. (2006) Comparing antibody and small-molecule therapies for cancer. *Nat Rev Cancer*, 6, 714-727.

Issaeva, N., Bozko, P., Enge, M., Protopopova, M., Verhoef, L.G., Masucci, M., Pramanik, A. and Selivanova, G. (2004) Small molecule RITA binds to p53, blocks p53-HDM-2 interaction and activates p53 function in tumors. *Nat Med*, 10, 1321-1328.

Jiang, B.H. and Liu, L.Z. (2008) PI3K/PTEN signaling in tumorigenesis and angiogenesis. *Biochim Biophys Acta*, 1784, 150-158.

Jin, X., Gossett, D.R., Wang, S., Yang, D., Cao, Y., Chen, J., Guo, R., Reynolds, R.K. and Lin, J. (2004) Inhibition of AKT survival pathway by a small molecule inhibitor in human endometrial cancer cells. *Br J Cancer*, 91, 1808-1812.

Karin, M., Yamamoto, Y. and Wang, Q.M. (2004) The IKK NF-kappa B system: a treasure trove for drug development. *Nat Rev Drug Discov*, 3, 17-26.

Kohler, G. and Milstein, C. (1975) Continuous cultures of fused cells secreting antibody of predefined specificity. *Nature*, 256, 495-497.

Kruse, J.P. and Gu, W. (2009) Modes of p53 regulation. *Cell*, 137, 609-622.

Ku, G.Y. andIson, D.H. (2010) Esophagogastric cancer: targeted agents. *Cancer Treat Rev*, 36, 235-248.

Lai, C.M., Lai, Y.K. and Rakoczy, P.E. (2002) Adenovirus and adeno-associated virus vectors. *DNA Cell Biol*, 21, 895-913.

Lefkowitz, E.J., Wang, C. and Upton, C. (2006) Poxviruses: past, present and future. *Virus Res*, 117, 105-118.

Lin, X., Huang, H., Li, S., Li, H., Li, Y., Cao, Y., Zhang, D., Xia, Y., Guo, Y., Huang, W. and Jiang, W. (2007) A phase I clinical trial of an adenovirus-mediated endostatin gene (E10A) in patients with solid tumors. *Cancer Biol Ther*, 6, 648-653.

Lo, H.W. Nuclear mode of the EGFR signaling network: biology, prognostic value, and therapeutic implications. *Discov Med*, 10, 44-51.

Martelli, A.M., Tazzari, P.L., Tabellini, G., Bortul, R., Billi, A.M., Manzoli, L., Ruggeri, A., Conte, R. and Cocco, L. (2003) A new selective AKT pharmacological inhibitor reduces resistance to chemotherapeutic drugs, TRAIL, all-trans-retinoic acid, and ionizing radiation of human leukemia cells. *Leukemia*, 17, 1794-1805.

Mendez, M.J., Green, L.L., Corvalan, J.R., Jia, X.C., Maynard-Currie, C.E., Yang, X.D., Gallo, M.L., Louie, D.M., Lee, D.V., Erickson, K.L., Luna, J., Roy, C.M., Abderrahim, H., Kirschenbaum, F., Noguchi, M., Smith, D.H., Fukushima, A., Hales, J.F., Klapholz, S., Finer, M.H., Davis, C.G., Zsebo, K.M. and Jakobovits, A. (1997) Functional transplant of megabase human immunoglobulin loci recapitulates human antibody response in mice. *Nat Genet*, 15, 146-156.

Moy, B., Kirkpatrick, P., Kar, S. and Goss, P. (2007) Lapatinib. *Nat Rev Drug Discov*, 6, 431-432.

O'Reilly, M.S., Boehm, T., Shing, Y., Fukai, N., Vasios, G., Lane, W.S., Flynn, E., Birkhead, J.R., Olsen, B.R. and Folkman, J. (1997) Endostatin: an endogenous inhibitor of angiogenesis and tumor growth. *Cell*, 88, 277-285.

O'Reilly, M.S., Holmgren, L., Shing, Y., Chen, C., Rosenthal, R.A., Moses, M., Lane, W.S., Cao, Y., Sage, E.H. and Folkman, J. (1994) Angiostatin: a novel angiogenesis inhibitor that mediates the suppression of metastases by a Lewis lung carcinoma. *Cell*, 79, 315-328.

Ohlfest, J.R., Freese, A.B. and Largaespada, D.A. (2005) Nonviral vectors for cancer gene therapy: prospects for integrating vectors and combination therapies. *Curr Gene Ther*, 5, 629-641.

Park, D. and Dilda, P.J. Mitochondria as targets in angiogenesis inhibition. *Mol Aspects Med*, 31, 113-131.

Reichert, J.M., Rosensweig, C.J., Faden, L.B. and Dewitz, M.C. (2005) Monoclonal antibody successes in the clinic. *Nat Biotechnol*, 23, 1073-1078.

Sebolt-Leopold, J.S., Dudley, D.T., Herrera, R., Van Becelaere, K., Wiland, A., Gowan, R.C., Tecle, H., Barrett, S.D., Bridges, A., Przybranowski, S., Leopold, W.R. and Saltiel, A.R. (1999) Blockade of the MAP kinase pathway suppresses growth of colon tumors in vivo. *Nat Med*, 5, 810-816.

Sebolt-Leopold, J.S. and Herrera, R. (2004) Targeting the mitogen-activated protein kinase cascade to treat cancer. *Nat Rev Cancer*, 4, 937-947.

Secchiero, P., di Iasio, M.G., Gonelli, A. and Zauli, G. (2008) The MDM2 inhibitor Nutlins as an innovative therapeutic tool for the treatment of haematological malignancies. *Curr Pharm Des*, 14, 2100-2110.

Shen, Y. and Nemunaitis, J. (2006) Herpes simplex virus 1 (HSV-1) for cancer treatment. *Cancer Gene Ther*, 13, 975-992.

Swain, S.M. (2011). Chemotherapy: updates and new perspectives. *Oncologist*, 16 Suppl 1, 30-39.

Tang, H.J., Jin, X., Wang, S., Yang, D., Cao, Y., Chen, J., Gossett, D.R. and Lin, J. (2006) A small molecule compound inhibits AKT pathway in ovarian cancer cell lines. *Gynecol Oncol*, 100, 308-317.

Thomas, J.P., Arzoomanian, R.Z., Alberti, D., Marnocha, R., Lee, F., Friedl, A., Tutsch, K., Dresen, A., Geiger, P., Pluda, J., Fogler, W., Schiller, J.H. and Wilding, G. (2003) Phase I pharmacokinetic and pharmacodynamic study of recombinant human endostatin in patients with advanced solid tumors. *J Clin Oncol*, 21, 223-231.

Tomita, N., Ogihara, T. and Morishita, R. (2003) Transcription factors as molecular targets: molecular mechanisms of decoy ODN and their design. *Curr Drug Targets*, 4, 603-608.

Vousden, K.H. and Lu, X. (2002) Live or let die: the cell's response to p53. *Nat Rev Cancer*, 2, 594-604.

Vousden, K.H. and Prives, C. (2009) Blinded by the Light: The Growing Complexity of p53. *Cell*, 137, 413-431.

Warren, J.L., Yabroff, K.R., Meekins, A., Topor, M., Lamont, E.B. and Brown, M.L. (2008) Evaluation of trends in the cost of initial cancer treatment. *J Natl Cancer Inst*, 100, 888-897.

Willett, C.G., Boucher, Y., di Tomaso, E., Duda, D.G., Munn, L.L., Tong, R.T., Chung, D.C., Sahani, D.V., Kalva, S.P., Kozin, S.V., Mino, M., Cohen, K.S., Scadden, D.T., Hartford, A.C., Fischman, A.J., Clark, J.W., Ryan, D.P., Zhu, A.X., Blaszkowsky, L.S., Chen, H.X., Shellito, P.C., Lauwers, G.Y. and Jain, R.K. (2004) Direct evidence that the VEGF-specific antibody bevacizumab has antivascular effects in human rectal cancer. *Nat Med*, 10, 145-147.

Zhang, J., Grindley, J.C., Yin, T., Jayasinghe, S., He, X.C., Ross, J.T., Haug, J.S., Rupp, D., Porter-Westpfahl, K.S., Wiedemann, L.M., Wu, H. and Li, L. (2006) PTEN maintains haematopoietic stem cells and acts in lineage choice and leukaemia prevention. *Nature*, 441, 518-522.

11

Gene Therapy Strategy for Tumour Hypoxia

Hiroshi Harada
Group of Radiation and Tumour Biology,
Career-Path Promotion Unit for Young Life Scientists,
Kyoto University
Japan

1. Introduction

A characteristic feature of solid tumours is the presence of cells under very low oxygen tensions, hypoxia. These cells, so called hypoxic tumour cells, express a transcription factor, hypoxia-inducible factor 1 (HIF-1), which induces the expression of more than one hundred genes related to angiogenesis, invasion, metastasis, and resistance to conventional treatments such as chemotherapy and radiotherapy. However, because hypoxia is unique to locally advanced malignant tumours, it provides the opportunity to develop tumour-specific targeting strategies. Such an approach has been applied to gene therapy; for example, hypoxia-activated gene therapy using HIF-1-dependent promoters resulted in the selective expression of therapeutic genes and anti-tumour effects with minimum side effects in normal tissues. Here, I review recent advances in the development of cancer gene therapy strategies targeting hypoxic/HIF-1-active tumour cells.

2. A tumour-specific microenvironment, hypoxia, as a therapeutic target

Most human tumours are highly heterogeneous and involve diverse microenvironments. A typical microenvironment seen in solid tumours is hypoxia, low-oxygen conditions under physiological level (Thomlinson & Gray, 1955; Vaupel, Kallinowski, & Okunieff, 1989). Tumour hypoxia is a concern in cancer therapy because it increases the metastatic and angiogenic potential of cancer cells (Erler et al., 2006; Forsythe et al., 1996; Yang et al., 2008) and can render cancer cells resistant to radiation and chemotherapy (Brown & Wilson, 2004; Teicher, 1994; Thomlinson & Gray, 1955).

2.1 What is tumour hypoxia and how does it occur in solid tumours?

A typical feature of cancer cells is an extraordinarily accelerated proliferation caused by the activation of oncogenes and/or disruption of tumour suppressor genes (Hanahan & Weinberg, 2000). It leads to an imbalance in the supply and consumption of O_2 in a solid tumour. This disequilibrium along with the inadequate diffusion of molecular oxygen can cause a dynamic gradient of O_2 content in a solid tumour (Thomlinson & Gray, 1955; Vaupel et al., 1989). Tumour cells proliferate and grow actively only if supplied with enough oxygen and nutrients from tumour blood vessels; therefore, malignant solid tumours grow as a conglomerate of so-called "tumour cords" in each of which a blood vessel is sequentially surrounded with well-oxygenated viable cells (normoxic cells), dormant cells under low oxygen conditions (hypoxic cells), and dead cells (necrotic cells) Fig. 1(Hall, 1994). Because of the distance that O_2 can diffuse, hypoxic cells exist 70-100 µm from a tumour blood vessel in a tumour cord (Hall, 1994). Hypoxic conditions are usually defined as < 2% O_2, and anoxic conditions (severe hypoxia) as < 0.02% O_2.

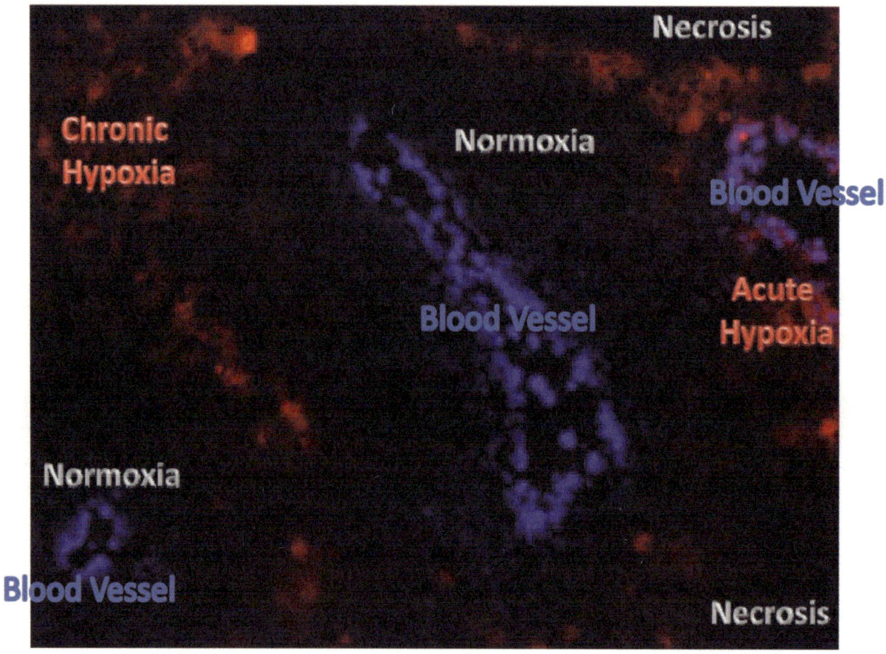

Fig. 1. Spatial relationship between blood vessels and hypoxia in a malignant solid tumour. Chronic hypoxic regions (red) exist 70-100 µm from tumour blood vessels. Acute/cycling hypoxia caused by fluctuations in tumour blood flow occurs proximal to tumour blood vessels.

In addition to areas of chronic hypoxia, malignant tumours contain cancer cells which are temporally exposed to low oxygen conditions for minutes to hours and then reoxygenated (Brown, 1979). This phenomenon, called "acute hypoxia", frequently reoccurs during tumour growth, leading to "cycling hypoxia". The occurrence of acute and cycling hypoxia is attributed to the fact that tumour blood vessels are quite immature and tortuous; and therefore, tumour blood flow fluctuates dramatically during tumour growth (Brown & Wilson, 2004).

2.2 Chemo-resistance of cancer cells under hypoxic conditions

Cancer cells are known to become chemo-resistant in hypoxic regions of locally advanced solid tumours through multiple mechanisms (Kizaka-Kondoh, Inoue, Harada, & Hiraoka, 2003; Teicher, 1994). First, because hypoxic regions occur far from functional vasculatures, the diffusion and delivery of most anticancer drugs are not extensive enough to have a cytotoxic effect (Durand, 1994; Hicks et al., 2006; Tannock, 1998). Second, the cytotoxicity of some anticancer drugs is known to depend on molecular oxygen. For example, bleomycin is reported to chelate metal ions, produce a pseudoenzyme that reacts with oxygen and generates superoxide and hydroxide free radicals, and then cleave DNA. Therefore, the cytotoxic effect of the drug dramatically decreases in the absence of O_2 (Batchelder, Wilson, Hay, & Denny, 1996; Teicher, Lazo, & Sartorelli, 1981). Third, alkylating agents and antimetabolites are also less effective under hypoxic conditions. These kinds of drugs are the most effective against highly proliferating cancer cells, and therefore, hypoxic tumour cells, which are known to be dormant/less proliferating, can tolerate them (Tannock, 1968). Fourth, hypoxia upregulates the expression of genes involved in drug resistance, including the gene for p-glycoprotein (Comerford et al., 2002; Wartenberg et al., 2003). Finally, there is evidence that hypoxia can enhance genetic instability in tumour cells (N. Chan et al., 2008), thus allowing a more rapid development of drug resistance.

2.3 Radio-resistance of cancer cells under hypoxic conditions

Ionizing radiation produces DNA damage, such as DNA double/single strand breaks, DNA base damage, and DNA-DNA and DNA-protein crosslinks (Hall, 1994). The presence or absence of molecular oxygen influences the damage and death of cancer cells (Brown & Wilson, 2004; Thomlinson & Gray, 1955). This phenomenon, the so-called oxygen effect, was first identified in 1912 with the observation that the skin reaction to a radium applicator dramatically decreased when the applicator was pushed tightly onto the skin and consequently decreased blood flow there. The breakthrough linking the effect of oxygen with radioresistance of cancer cells was made by Thomlinson and Gray in 1955 (Thomlinson & Gray, 1955). They proposed that oxygen levels decreased in a solid tumour through successive layers of cancer cells distal to blood vessels, and cancer cells a distance of about 10 cell diameters from vessels are viable but radioresistant. Actually, cancer cells become 2-3 times more radioresistant under hypoxic conditions than normoxic conditions (Brown & Wilson, 2004).

The hypoxia-mediated radioresistance is attributed to both chemical and biological mechanisms. Ionizing radiation induces ionization in or close to the genomic DNA of target cells and produces radicals (Brown & Wilson, 2004). The DNA radicals are subjected to oxidation in the presence of oxygen, leading to fixation of the damage. In the absence of oxygen, however, the DNA radicals are reduced by compounds containing sulfhydryl groups (SH groups), which restore the DNA to its original form. Therefore, DNA damage, especially irreparable double stranded breaks, is significantly less severe in the absence of molecular oxygen. Biological mechanisms are also important. It has been elucidated that hypoxic stimuli trigger changes in both the "DNA damage repair pathway" (Bindra, Crosby, & Glazer, 2007) and the "cell death/survival signaling pathway". Moreover, recent advances in molecular and cellular biology revealed an important role for a transcription factor, hypoxia-inducible factor 1 (HIF-1), in tumour radioresistance (*see* Section 3 for details) (Harada & Hiraoka, 2010).

2.4 Increase in metastatic and angiogenic potential under hypoxic conditions

In addition to mediating resistance to conventional treatments, hypoxia is known to increase the metastatic and angiogenic potential of tumour cells. Cancer patients with relatively more hypoxic regions have a tendency to suffer from distant metastasis as well as local recurrence regardless of whether the initial treatment is surgery or radiation therapy (Brizel et al., 1996). Recent molecular biological analyses have revealed that hypoxia stimulates the expression of a number of genes involved in metastatic cascades, such as lysyl oxidase and the chemokine receptor, *CXCR4*, osteopoetin (D. A. Chan & Giaccia, 2007; Erler et al., 2006;

Rofstad, 2000). Also, cancer cells under hypoxic conditions trigger angiogenesis in order to improve surrounding conditions and obtain enough oxygen and nutrients for their survival (Folkman, 1971). HIF-1 is known to play a pivotal role in the hypoxia-mediated increase in both the metastatic and angiogenic potential of cancer cells.

3. Hypoxia-inducible factor 1 (HIF-1)

Molecular and cellular biological research has identified HIF-1 as an important transcription factor in hypoxia-mediated angiogenesis, metastasis, and resistance to chemo/radiotherapy.

3.1 Regulation of HIF-1 expression and activity

HIF-1 is a heterodimeric transcription factor composed of alpha (HIF-1α) and beta (HIF-1β/ARNT) subunits (Wang, Jiang, Rue, & Semenza, 1995). Its hypoxia-dependent activity is mainly regulated through the stabilization and modification of the HIF-1α subunit (Fig. 2).

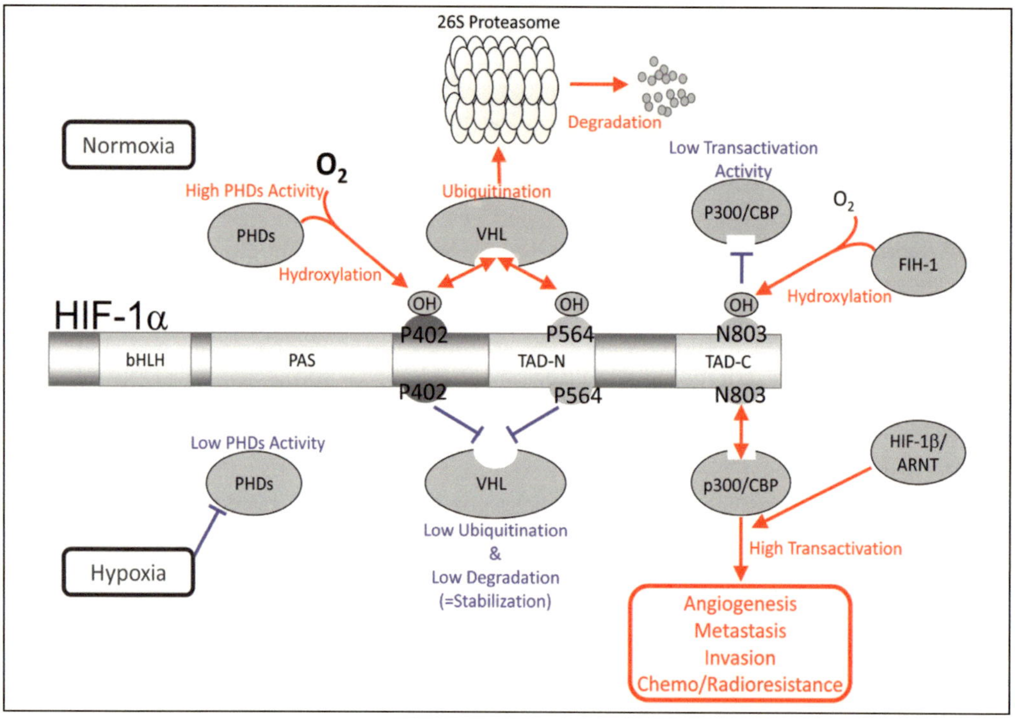

Fig. 2. Molecular mechanism behind the activation of HIF-1 under Hypoxic conditions.

The best-characterized regulatory mechanism is that modulating HIF-1α's stability. Under well-oxygenated normoxic conditions, prolyl hydroxylation (by prolyl hydroxylases [PHDs]) and subsequent ubiquitination (by von-Hippel Lindau (VHL)-containing E3 ubiquitin-protein ligase) of the oxygen-dependent degradation (ODD) domain of HIF-1α leads to rapid degradation of HIF-1α with a half life of 5-8 min. Consequently, HIF-1 is inactive under normoxic conditions (Berra, Roux, Richard, & Pouyssegur, 2001; Hirota & Semenza, 2005; Jaakkola et al., 2001; Maxwell et al., 1999; Semenza, 2001). On the other hand, under oxygen-deprived hypoxic conditions, HIF-1α becomes stable because oxygen-depletion directly decreases the PHDs' activity (Jaakkola et al., 2001). Then, HIF-1α interacts with HIF-1β, forms a heterodimer, HIF-1 (Wang et al., 1995), binds to its cognate DNA sequence, the hypoxic-responsive element (HRE), and finally induces the expression of various genes related to angiogenesis, metastasis, glycolysis and so on (D. A. Chan & Giaccia, 2007; Erler et al., 2006; Forsythe et al., 1996; Kim, Gao, & Dang, 2007; Rofstad, 2000). In addition to the regulation of HIF-1α's stability, another post-translational modification of HIF-1α is known to function in the regulation of the transactivational activity of HIF-1. Under normoxic conditions, factor inhibiting HIF-1 (FIH-1) becomes active and hydroxylates an asparagine residue (N803) of HIF-1α (Hirota & Semenza, 2005; Mahon, Hirota, & Semenza, 2001; Semenza, 2001). The asparaginyl hydroxylation blocks the interaction of HIF-1α with the transcriptional co-factor p300 and CBP, resulting in the suppression of HIF-1's transactivational activity. Because oxygen is a substrate of FIH-1 as well as PHDs, HIF-1's transactivational activity is restored under oxygen-deprived hypoxic conditions.

3.2 Function of HIF-1 in cancer cells

In cancer cells, HIF-1 plays pivotal roles in the adaptation to (metabolic reprograming), evasion from (invasion and metastasis), and improvement of (angiogenesis) severe hypoxic conditions (D. A. Chan & Giaccia, 2007; Erler et al., 2006; Forsythe et al., 1996; Semenza, 2007, 2008). Concerning angiogenesis in locally advanced malignant tumours, an up-regulation of HIF-1 activity caused by intratumoural hypoxia is associated with the overexpression of vascular endothelial growth factor (VEGF), a glycoprotein responsible for angiogenesis and vasculogenesis (Forsythe et al., 1996). Concerning the metabolic reprogramming of cancer cells, HIF-1 induces the expression of genes encoding glucose transporters and glycolytic enzymes to facilitate glycolysis (Semenza, 2009; Wood et al., 1998). At the same time, HIF-1-dependent genes decrease both mitochondrial metabolism (Fukuda et al., 2007; Semenza, 2007) and mitochondrial mass (Semenza, 2008; H. Zhang et al., 2008). These functions of HIF-1 are responsible for both the efficient production of ATP even under oxygen-deprived conditions and the decrease in the cytotoxic reactive oxygen species (ROS) produced through incomplete oxidative phosphorylation under hypoxic conditions (Fukuda et al., 2007; Semenza, 2007, 2009). Concerning invasion and metastasis, HIF-1 is known to trigger various pathways including epithelial-mesenchymal transition (EMT) and expression of the Met protooncogene and lysyl oxidase, which function in tumour metastasis (Erler et al., 2006; Pennacchietti et al., 2003).

3.3 Function of HIF-1 in tumour radioresistance

Preclinical studies have found that inhibition of intratumour HIF-1 activity by a pharmacological HIF-1 inhibitor, YC-1, or by a dominant negative mutant of HIF-1α and the knockdown of HIF-1α expression by short hairpin RNA or short interfering RNA significantly delayed tumour growth after radiation (Harada et al., 2009; Moeller, Cao, Li, & Dewhirst, 2004; Moeller et al., 2005; X. Zhang et al., 2004). It was also confirmed through clinical studies that HIF-1α expression correlates with a poor prognosis after radiation therapy (Aebersold et al., 2001; Irie, Matsuo, & Nagata, 2004; Ishikawa et al., 2004). These results imply that HIF-1 has a certain biological function to increase tumour radioresistance. Actually, HIF-1-mediated radioresistance has been recently revealed: 1) radiation activates HIF-1 in a solid tumour, 2) HIF-1 induces the expression of VEGF, 3) VEGF protects endothelial cells from the cytotoxic effects of radiation, and 4) the radio-protected tumour blood vessels assure the supply of oxygen and nutrients to tumour cells and promote tumour growth (Harada et al., 2009; Moeller et al., 2004; Zeng et al., 2008).

4. Development of gene therapy strategies targeting tumour hypoxia

Because hypoxic/HIF-1-active cells are known to mediate tumour malignancy and resistance to conventional treatments, and because hypoxia has been recognized as a tumour-specific microenvironment, recent studies have tried to exploit hypoxic cells as targets for cancer therapy (Brown & Wilson, 2004; Harris, 2002; Semenza, 2003). Dachs *et al.* were the first to apply this concept to gene therapy (Dachs, Patterson, et al., 1997). Since they demonstrated the effectiveness of hypoxia-specific gene therapy strategy using the HIF-1/HRE system, extensive efforts have been devoted to developing genetically engineered hypoxia-responsive promoters.

4.1 Development of HIF-1-dependent promoters

Various HREs, such as murin phosphoglycerate kinase-1 (PGK-1) HRE, human enolase (ENO) HRE, murin lactate dehydrogenase (mLDH-A) HRE, human erythropoietin (EPO) HRE, and human VEGF HRE, have been used to develop artificial hypoxia-responsive promoters (Table 1) (Binley, Iqball, Kingsman, Kingsman, & Naylor, 1999; Boast et al., 1999; Dachs, Patterson, et al., 1997; Harada et al., 2007; Rinsch et al., 1997; Shibata, Akiyama, Noda, Sasai, & Hiraoka, 1998; Shibata, Giaccia, & Brown, 2000). The number of HREs and combination with the basal promoter influence the hypoxia/HIF-1-responsiveness of each HRE-containing promoter (Table 1).

Above all, the combination of five repeats of a HRE derived from the human VEGF promoter and the human cytomegarovirus (CMV) minimal promoter (mp), the so-called "the 5HRE promoter", showed intense hypoxia-responsiveness and exhibited a more than 500-fold increase in luciferase activity in response to hypoxic stimuli (Shibata et al., 2000). Moreover, the absolute level of luciferase activity from the 5HRE promoter under hypoxic conditions reached the same level as that from the constitutively active CMV-driven promoter under normoxic conditions (Shibata et al., 2000).

However, the 5HRE promoter still has problems relating to the development of gene therapy. It shows a certain level of unwanted gene expression even when oxygen is available under normoxic conditions (Harada et al., 2007), which would cause high basal expression of therapeutic genes and result in side effects in well-oxygenated normal tissues. In order to decrease leakage under normoxic conditions, I and my colleagues came up with the idea of utilizing the ODD domain of HIF-1α. We fused the coding sequence of the ODD domain to that of luciferase, and inserted the fusion gene downstream of the 5HRE promoter. The resultant *5HREp-ODD-luc* gene showed little leakage under normoxic conditions. Leakage from the conventional *5HREp-luc* gene was 1.4×10^3 (arbitary units), on the other hand, that from the novel *5HREp-ODD-luc* gene was just 1.5×10^1 (arbitary units), almost the same as the background level. Moreover, the oxygen-dependent destabilizing effect of the ODD domain contributed to an increase in the hypoxia-responsiveness to about 4.7×10^4.

The potential of hypoxia/HIF-1-dependent promoters *in vivo* has been proved through immunohistochemical analyses and optical imaging experiments. The human melanoma cell line, Be11, was stably transfected with a plasmid expressing a derivative of EGFP, d2EGFP, under the control of the 5HRE promoter, and transplanted into immunodeficient nude mice

HRE	Basal Promoter	Reporter Gene	Induction Ratio	References
3 × mPGK-1	mPGK-1	CD2	1.4-1.9	Dachs, 1997
3 × mPGK-1	minHSV TK	CD2	2.2-2.33	
3 × mPGK-1	9-27 gene	CD2	2.2-4.1	
mPGK-1	mPGK-1	hEPO	2.7	Rinsch, 1997
hVEGF	hVEGF	luciferase	3.3-8.5	Shibata, 1998
hEPO	SV40	luciferase	2-5	
5 × hVEGF	hVEGF	luciferase	20	
5 × hVEGF	hVEGF+ minE1b	luciferase	44	
3 × hENO	SV40	luciferase	120	Boast, 1999
3 × hENO	SV40	luciferase	63	
2 × mLDHA	SV40	luciferase	81	
4 × mLDHA	SV40	luciferase	65	
4 × hEPO	SV40	luciferase	255	
3 × hENO	SV40	luciferase	146	
3 × mPGK-1+ VEGF 3' UTR	SV40	luciferase	300	
mPGK-1	SV40	β-gal	8.5-50	Binley, 1999
5 or 10 × hVEGF	SV40	luciferase	54-57	Shibata, 2000
5 or 10 × hVEGF+ 5' VEGF UTR	SV40	luciferase	23-27	
5-10 × hVEGF+ 5' VEGF UTR	E1b	luciferase	56-60	
5 × hVEGF+ 5' VEGF UTR	E1b	luciferase	131	
5 × hVEGF+ 5' VEGF UTR+ 3' VEGF UTR	E1b	luciferase	193	
5 × hVEGF	hCMV-mp	luciferase	524	
5 × hVEGF	hCMV-mp	luciferase	47,000	Harada, 2007

Table 1. Genetically engineered hypoxia-responsive promoters.

(Liu et al., 2005). Resultant tumour xenografts showed heterogeneous, partition-dependent and weak green fluorescence. Immunohistochemical analyses confirmed that d2EGFP-positive cells were located at the boundary between well-oxygenated viable regions and necrotic regions, which were stained with a hypoxia marker, pimonidazole (Raleigh et al., 1998). When human cervical cancer cells, HeLa cells, transfected with the *5HREp-luc* or *5HREp-ODD-luc* gene were transplanted into nude mice, the resultant xenografts showed intense bioluminescence after the tumour-bearing leg was ligated and the blood flow to the xenograft decreased (Harada, Kizaka-Kondoh, & Hiraoka, 2005; Harada et al., 2007).

4.2 Hypoxia-targeted gene-directed enzyme/prodrug therapy using a HIF-1-dependent promoter

To exploit tumour hypoxia/HIF-1 active cells as a tumour-specific therapeutic target, several approaches have been examined including (1) hypoxia-targeting using hypoxia/HIF-1-responsive promoters combined with Gene-Directed Enzyme Prodrug

Therapies (GDEPT) (Greco, Marples, Joiner, & Scott, 2003; Liu, Harada, Ogura, Shibata, & Hiraoka, 2007; Ogura et al., 2005; Patterson et al., 2002; Shibata, Giaccia, & Brown, 2002), and (2) hypoxia-specific replication of adenovirus (Hernandez-Alcoceba, Pihalja, Qian, & Clarke, 2002; Post & Van Meir, 2003) (Table 2).

Delivery System	Hypoxia-specific Strategy	Result	Reference
NA (Transfected cancer cell line)	GDEPT: 5 x VEGF-HRE-containing promoter driven NTR gene expression in HT1080 cells and i.p. injection of the anticancer prodrug CB1954.	Significant tumour growth delay	Shibata, 2002
NA (Transfected cancer cell line)	GDEPT: 5 x VEGF-HRE-containing promoter-driven HSV-TK gene expression and i.p. injection of GCV	Tumour growth suppression	Ogura, 2005
NA (Transfected cancer cell line)	GDEPT: PGK-1 HRE/SV40 chimeric promoter-driven P450R gene expression and i.p. injection of the 2-nitroimidazole bioreductive prodrug, RB6145	Enhanced Radiotherapy	Patterson, 2002
Adenovirus	GDEPT: optimized hypoxia response promoter using PGK-1 HRE-driven human cytochrome P450 (CYP2B6) gene expression and i.p. injection of cyclophosphamide	Delay in tumour growth	Binley, 2003
Adenovirus	3XHRE/5XERE-regulated E1A expression and hTERT (AdEHT2) or E2F-1 (AdEHE2F) promoter-regulated E4 expression.	Tumour growth suppression and regression	Hernandez-Alcoceba, 2002
Adenovirus (intratumoural injection)	GDEPT: 5 x VEGF-HRE-containing promoter-driven bacterial cytosine deaminase (BCD) gene expression and i.p. injection of 5-FC.	Tumour growth suppression and enhanced radiotherpy	Liu, 2007
Adenovirus	human VEGF promoter-driven BAX gene expression	induction of apoptosis and suppression of cell growth in vitro	Kaliberov, 2002

Table 2. Gene therapy strategies for tumour hypoxia examined so far.

NA, not applicable; HSV-TK, the herpes simplex virus thymidine kinase; GCV, ganciclovir; GDEPT, Gene-Directed Enzyme Pordrug Therapy; NTR, nitroreductase; CRAD, conditionally replicative adenoviruses; ER, estrogen receptor; ERE, estrogen response element; hTERT, human telomerase reverse transcriptase; CD, cytosine deaminase; VEGF, Vascular Endthelial Growth Factor, 5-FU, 5-fluorouracil; 5-FC, 5-flucytosine;

4.2.1 Gene-directed enzyme prodrug therapy (GDEPT) with HIF-1-dependent promoters

GDEPT involves the delivery to target cells of a foreign gene, which is non-toxic but activates prodrugs to toxic agents and induces anti-tumour effects (Fig. 3 Dachs, Dougherty, Stratford, & Chaplin, 1997; Greco et al., 2003). HIF-1 activity is detected at high levels in hypoxic tumour cells but generally not in normal tissues as mentioned above; therefore, HIF-1-dependent promoters provide a chance to accomplish tumour-specific GDEPT. The target-specificity and therapeutic effects of GDEPT with HIF-1-dpendent promoters have been examined in experimental tumour systems either by administering viral vectors (Binley et al., 2003; Liu et al., 2007) or by using unique tumour xenografts prepared by transplanting cancer cells which express a prodrug-activating enzyme under the control of a HIF-1-dependent promoter (Ogura et al., 2005; Patterson et al., 2002; Shibata et al., 2002). Examples of enzyme/prodrug combinations in GDEPT are the bacterial nitroreductase (NTR)/anticancer prodrug CB1954, the cytochrome P450 reductase (P450R)/RSU1069, the herpes simplex virus thymidine kinase (HSV-TK)/ganciclovir (GCV), and the bacterial cytosine deaminase (BCD)/anti-herpes viral agent 5- fluorocytosine (5-FC).

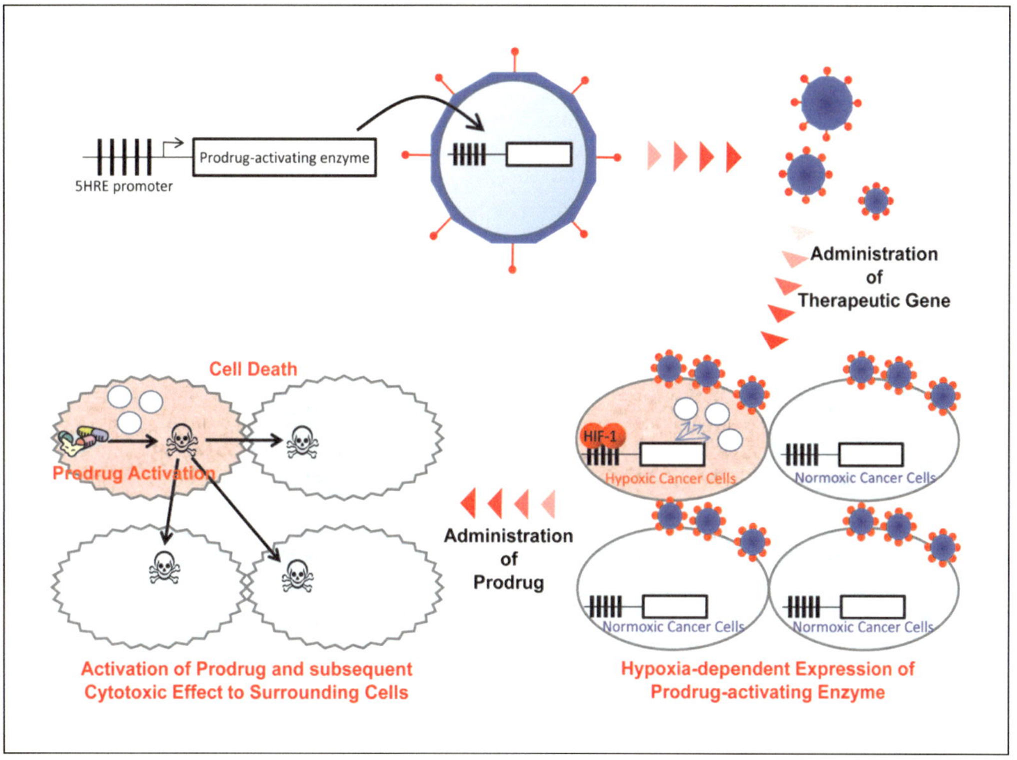

Fig. 3. Concept of GDEPT targeting tumour hypoxia.

Using HREs derived from the VEGF promoter, Shibata *et al.* generated vectors expressing a bacterial NTR gene in a HIF-1-dependent manner, and established stable transfectants of a human fibrosarcoma cell line, HT1080 (Shibata et al., 2002). Hypoxia-induced expression of the NTR protein correlated with increased sensitivity of HT1080 cells to the prodrug CB1954 (Shibata et al., 2002). Growth delay assays with established tumour xenografts derived from the same cells showed that significant antitumour effects were achieved with intraperitoneal injections of CB1954 (Shibata et al., 2002). In addition, respiration of 10% O_2 increased the hypoxic fraction in the tumour xenograft *in vivo* and enhanced the antitumour effects (Shibata et al., 2002).

A one-electron reductase, such as P450R, can be used for prodrug-activation. Patterson *et al.* reported that selective hypoxia-targeting could be accomplished by using an optimized PGK-1 HRE/SV40 chimeric promoter to regulate the expression of P450R. HT1080 cells stably transfected with the gene produced a 3.4-fold increase in P450R activity as a result of anoxic incubation, leading to a 30-fold enhancement of the cytotoxicity of the 2-nitroimidazole bioreductive prodrug, RSU1069 (Patterson et al., 2002).

As for HSV-TK/GCV gene therapy, Ogura *et al.* demonstrated that promoters containing 5 copies of the VEGF HRE assured the expression of the HSV-TK gene in a HIF-active renal cell carcinoma, resulting in GCV-dependent tumour growth suppression (Ogura et al., 2005). An important point of their study is that HIF-dependent HSV-TK/GCV gene therapy can target not only hypoxic but also normoxic renal cell carcinoma (RCC) cells because the VHL gene, which triggers the destruction of HIF-1α and HIF-2α during normoxia, is inactive in 33–57% of sporadic clear-cell RCCs, which accounts for 75% of RCCs.

Binley *et al.* used an optimized hypoxia-responsive promoter (OBHRE) with the PGK-1 HRE and investigated hypoxia-targeted gene expression *in vivo* in the context of an adenoviral vector (Binley et al., 2003). The OBHRE promoter showed limited activity in the liver or spleen such that expression was 1000-fold lower than that driven by the strong CMV/IE promoter (Binley et al., 2003). However, in the context of the tumour microenvironment, the OBHRE promoter achieved expression levels comparable to that of the CMV/IE promoter. Moreover, they showed that an adenovirus expressing the human cytochrome P450 (CYP2B6) regulated by the OBHRE promoter delays tumour growth in response to the prodrug cyclophosphamide (CPA) (Binley et al., 2003).

As for CD/5-FC gene therapy, Liu *et al.* constructed an adenoviral vector in which the 5HRE promoter was responsible for the HIF-1-dependent expression of CD (Liu et al., 2007). Administration of the adenovirus resulted in the expression of CD in hypoxic regions of solid tumours, leading to 5- FC-dependent tumour growth suppression and enhancement of the therapeutic effect of radiation therapy (*See* Section 4.4 for details about the radio-enhancing effect).

In general, GDEPT is thought to have two advantages: amplification of its therapeutic effect and a bystander therapeutic effect. The former is due to the ability of each prodrug-activating enzyme to activate a number of prodrug molecules. The latter advantage results from an extension of the killing effects of the activated/converted drug to surrounding cancer cells, which don't express the therapeutic gene and don't convert the prodrug to the active anticancer drug. Therefore, even if systemic delivery of the therapeutic genes is not effective Fig. 3, tumour eradication may still be achieved.

4.2.2 Other gene therapy strategies targeting tumour hypoixia

4.2.2.1 Gene therapy using a cytotoxic gene and HIF-1-dependent promoter

An alternative GDEPT uses cytotoxic proteins instead of prodrug-activating enzymes expressed in a HIF-1-dependent manner (Table 2). Kaliberov *et al.* prepared an adenovirus, AdVEGFBAX, which expressed an inducer of apoptosis, BAX, under the control of a VEGF promoter (Kaliberov et al., 2002). They confirmed the potential therapeutic application of VEGF promoter–driven cancer-specific expression of the pro-apoptotic Bax gene.

4.2.2.2 Gene therapy using a hypoxia/HIF-dependent oncolytic adenovirus

The lytic cycle of adenoviruses is known to result in the death of infected cells, and thus this property has been exploited as a therapeutic strategy against cancer. Post and Van Meir have developed a hypoxia/HIF-dependent replicative adenovirus (HYPR-Ad) that exhibits HIF-1-dependent E1A expression and conditional cytolysis of hypoxic cells but not normoxic cells (Post & Van Meir, 2003). This is the first evidence that an attenuated oncolytic adenovirus that selectively lyses hypoxic tumour cells can be generated.

4.3 Side effect of hypoxia-targeting gene therapies

To measure the damage to normal tissue after gene therapy targeting tumour hypoxia, Binley *et al.* evaluated the activity of lactate dehydrogenase (LDH) as an indicator of liver dysfunction after their hypoxia-responsive thymidine kinase/ganciclovir (TK/GCV) suicide gene therapy (Binley et al., 2003). Hypoxia-dependent TK expression and subsequent GCV treatment caused no irregularity in LDH levels. On the other hand, constitutive TK expression from a CMV promoter and GCV treatment significantly elevated LDH levels in mice. These results suggest that a hypoxia-responsive promoter would facilitate target specificity and so reduce the side effects on well-oxygenated normal tissues, meaning an increased therapeutic window for cytotoxic cancer gene therapies.

Liu et al observed no obvious side effects after hypoxia-targeting gene therapy with a 5HRE promoter-mediated BCD/5-FC strategy (Liu et al., 2007). On the other hand, after the Ad/EFp-BCD/5-FC treatment, which constitutively expresses BCD regardless of surrounding oxygen conditions, they observed significant weight loss and severe diarrhea (Liu et al., 2007). These results strengthen the argument that we can exploit tumour hypoxia as a tumour-specific target of cancer gene therapy, and that hypoxia/HIF-1-dependent therapeutic gene expression helps to avoid side effects in normal tissues.

4.4 Improvement of the effect of radiotherapy by hypoxia/HIF-1-targeting gene therapies

As tumour hypoxia and HIF-1 activity are responsible for tumour radioresistance (Aebersold et al., 2001; Harada et al., 2009; Irie et al., 2004; Ishikawa et al., 2004; Moeller et al., 2004; Moeller et al., 2005; X. Zhang et al., 2004), the specific targeting of tumour hypoxia and/or HIF-1 activity by gene therapy strategies may improve the efficacy of radiotherapy. Actually, Patterson *et al.* demonstrated that the therapeutic effect of radiation can be enhanced by a hypoxia-targeting gene therapy strategy (Patterson et al., 2002). They transfected HT1080 cells with a hypoxia-regulated expression vector encoding the human P450 reductase (HRE-P450R). Xenografts of HRE-P450R and empty vector transfectants had comparable hypoxic fractions and were refractive to a single dose of radiotherapy of up to 15 Gy. However, combining a prodrug RSU1069 with a reduced dose of radiotherapy (10 Gy) cured 50% of mice bearing HRE-P450R xenografts by 100 days after the treatment. On the other hand, one hundred percent mortality was observed by day 44 in the empty vector control xenografts treated using the same protocol.

Liu *et al.* treated HeLa tumour xenografts with adenovirus-mediated hypoxia-targeting cytosine deaminase gene therapy (Ad/5HREp-BCD/5-FC) and/or radiotherapy (IR), and carried out growth delay assays (Liu et al., 2007). They intentionally chose a low dose of Ad/5HREp-BCD/5-FC, which had minimal effects on the tumour growth rate compared to that after sham-treatment. Combined with IR, the gene therapy strikingly suppressed tumour growth as compared to radiotherapy alone. The period taken for tumour growth to increase two-fold from the initial volume (tumour growth doubling time: TGDT) was 13.2 ± 5.6 days after gene therapy alone, which is not significantly longer than that after sham-treatment (8.2 ± 3.1 days). On the other hand, the combination of gene therapy with radiotherapy prolonged the TGDT to 47.2 ± 16.8 days, which was about 2.4-fold longer than that after radiotherapy alone (19.4 ± 4.8 days). Similar results were observed after fractionated irradiation (3 Gy × 5 fractions). The TGDT after gene therapy alone was 13.0 ± 4.4 days, which is not significantly longer than that after sham treatment (9.8 ± 5.8 days). On the other hand, the TGDT after the fractionated radiotherapy was 17.0 ± 3.7 days, which was significantly delayed by the combination with the gene therapy to 43.3 ± 23.8 days. These results also lead to a conclusion that hypoxia-targeting gene therapy combined with radiotherapy is a promising approach to cancer treatment.

5. Conclusion

Cancer cells under hypoxic conditions/HIF-1-active cancer cells have been recognized as crucial and excellent targets for cancer therapy not only because they mediate tumour malignancy and resistance to conventional treatments but also because they are only seen in malignant tumours, not in normal tissues. Several approaches have been used to target these cell populations; hypoxia-targeting using hypoxia-responsive promoters combined with GDEPT, and hypoxia-specific replication of adenovirus as well as hypoxic cytotoxins and HIF-1 inhibitors. Hypoxia/HIF-1-targeting gene therapy is a promising tumour-specific approach with few side effects in normal tissues, and has the potential to enhance the effect of radiation therapy. Some approaches are now in clinical trials and are expected to lead to breakthroughs in cancer therapy.

6. Acknowledgements

This study was supported by the "Funding Program for Next Generation World-Leading Researchers" from the Japan Society for the Promotion of Science (JSPS), by the "Program for the Promotion of Fundamental Studies in Health Science" from the National Institute of Biomedical Innovation (NIBIO), Japan, by Grants-in-aid for Scientific Research for Young Scientists (B) from the Ministry of Education, Culture, Sports, Science and Technology (MEXT), Japan, and by the Sagawa Foundation for the Promotion of Cancer Research.

7. References

Aebersold, D. M., Burri, P., Beer, K. T., Laissue, J., Djonov, V., Greiner, R. H., et al. (2001). Expression of hypoxia-inducible factor-1alpha: a novel predictive and prognostic parameter in the radiotherapy of oropharyngeal cancer. *Cancer Res, 61*(7), 2911-2916.

Batchelder, R. M., Wilson, W. R., Hay, M. P., & Denny, W. A. (1996). Oxygen dependence of the cytotoxicity of the enediyne anti-tumour antibiotic esperamicin A1. *Br J Cancer Suppl, 27*, S52-56.

Berra, E., Roux, D., Richard, D. E., & Pouyssegur, J. (2001). Hypoxia-inducible factor-1 alpha (HIF-1 alpha) escapes O(2)-driven proteasomal degradation irrespective of its subcellular localization: nucleus or cytoplasm. *EMBO Rep, 2*(7), 615-620.

Bindra, R. S., Crosby, M. E., & Glazer, P. M. (2007). Regulation of DNA repair in hypoxic cancer cells. *Cancer Metastasis Rev, 26*(2), 249-260.

Binley, K., Askham, Z., Martin, L., Spearman, H., Day, D., Kingsman, S., et al. (2003). Hypoxia-mediated tumour targeting. *Gene Ther, 10*(7), 540-549.

Binley, K., Iqball, S., Kingsman, A., Kingsman, S., & Naylor, S. (1999). An adenoviral vector regulated by hypoxia for the treatment of ischaemic disease and cancer. *Gene Ther, 6*(10), 1721-1727.

Boast, K., Binley, K., Iqball, S., Price, T., Spearman, H., Kingsman, S., et al. (1999). Characterization of physiologically regulated vectors for the treatment of ischemic disease. *Hum Gene Ther, 10*(13), 2197-2208.

Brizel, D. M., Scully, S. P., Harrelson, J. M., Layfield, L. J., Bean, J. M., Prosnitz, L. R., et al. (1996). Tumour oxygenation predicts for the likelihood of distant metastases in human soft tissue sarcoma. *Cancer Res, 56*(5), 941-943.

Brown, J. M. (1979). Evidence for acutely hypoxic cells in mouse tumours, and a possible mechanism of reoxygenation. *Br J Radiol, 52*(620), 650-656.

Brown, J. M., & Wilson, W. R. (2004). Exploiting tumour hypoxia in cancer treatment. *Nat Rev Cancer, 4*(6), 437-447.

Chan, D. A., & Giaccia, A. J. (2007). Hypoxia, gene expression, and metastasis. *Cancer Metastasis Rev, 26*(2), 333-339.

Chan, N., Koritzinsky, M., Zhao, H., Bindra, R., Glazer, P. M., Powell, S., et al. (2008). Chronic hypoxia decreases synthesis of homologous recombination proteins to offset chemoresistance and radioresistance. *Cancer Res, 68*(2), 605-614.

Comerford, K. M., Wallace, T. J., Karhausen, J., Louis, N. A., Montalto, M. C., & Colgan, S. P. (2002). Hypoxia-inducible factor-1-dependent regulation of the multidrug resistance (MDR1) gene. *Cancer Res, 62*(12), 3387-3394.

Dachs, G. U., Dougherty, G. J., Stratford, I. J., & Chaplin, D. J. (1997). Targeting gene therapy to cancer: a review. *Oncol Res, 9*(6-7), 313-325.

Dachs, G. U., Patterson, A. V., Firth, J. D., Ratcliffe, P. J., Townsend, K. M., Stratford, I. J., et al. (1997). Targeting gene expression to hypoxic tumour cells. *Nat Med, 3*(5), 515-520.

Durand, R. E. (1994). The influence of microenvironmental factors during cancer therapy. *In Vivo, 8*(5), 691-702.

Erler, J. T., Bennewith, K. L., Nicolau, M., Dornhofer, N., Kong, C., Le, Q. T., et al. (2006). Lysyl oxidase is essential for hypoxia-induced metastasis. *Nature, 440*(7088), 1222-1226.

Folkman, J. (1971). Tumour angiogenesis: therapeutic implications. *N Engl J Med, 285*(21), 1182-1186.

Forsythe, J. A., Jiang, B. H., Iyer, N. V., Agani, F., Leung, S. W., Koos, R. D., et al. (1996). Activation of vascular endothelial growth factor gene transcription by hypoxia-inducible factor 1. *Mol Cell Biol, 16*(9), 4604-4613.

Fukuda, R., Zhang, H., Kim, J. W., Shimoda, L., Dang, C. V., & Semenza, G. L. (2007). HIF-1 regulates cytochrome oxidase subunits to optimize efficiency of respiration in hypoxic cells. *Cell, 129*(1), 111-122.

Greco, O., Marples, B., Joiner, M. C., & Scott, S. D. (2003). How to overcome (and exploit) tumour hypoxia for targeted gene therapy. *J Cell Physiol, 197*(3), 312-325.

Hall, E. J. (Ed.). (1994). *Radiobiology for the Radiologists, Fourth Edition*. Philadelphia: J.B. Lippincott Company.

Hanahan, D., & Weinberg, R. A. (2000). The hallmarks of cancer. *Cell, 100*(1), 57-70.

Harada, H., & Hiraoka, M. (2010). Hypoxia-inducible factor 1 in tumour radioresistance. *Current Signal Transduction Therapy, 5*, 188-196.

Harada, H., Itasaka, S., Zhu, Y., Zeng, L., Xie, X., Morinibu, A., et al. (2009). Treatment regimen determines whether an HIF-1 inhibitor enhances or inhibits the effect of radiation therapy. *Br J Cancer, 100*(5), 747-757.

Harada, H., Kizaka-Kondoh, S., & Hiraoka, M. (2005). Optical imaging of tumour hypoxia and evaluation of efficacy of a hypoxia-targeting drug in living animals. *Mol Imaging, 4*(3), 182-193.

Harada, H., Kizaka-Kondoh, S., Itasaka, S., Shibuya, K., Morinibu, A., Shinomiya, K., et al. (2007). The combination of hypoxia-response enhancers and an oxygen-dependent proteolytic motif enables real-time imaging of absolute HIF-1 activity in tumour xenografts. *Biochem Biophys Res Commun, 360*(4), 791-796.

Harris, A. L. (2002). Hypoxia--a key regulatory factor in tumour growth. *Nat Rev Cancer, 2*(1), 38-47.

Hernandez-Alcoceba, R., Pihalja, M., Qian, D., & Clarke, M. F. (2002). New oncolytic adenoviruses with hypoxia- and estrogen receptor-regulated replication. *Hum Gene Ther, 13*(14), 1737-1750.

Hicks, K. O., Pruijn, F. B., Secomb, T. W., Hay, M. P., Hsu, R., Brown, J. M., et al. (2006). Use of three-dimensional tissue cultures to model extravascular transport and predict in vivo activity of hypoxia-targeted anticancer drugs. *J Natl Cancer Inst, 98*(16), 1118-1128.

Hirota, K., & Semenza, G. L. (2005). Regulation of hypoxia-inducible factor 1 by prolyl and asparaginyl hydroxylases. *Biochem Biophys Res Commun, 338*(1), 610-616.

Irie, N., Matsuo, T., & Nagata, I. (2004). Protocol of radiotherapy for glioblastoma according to the expression of HIF-1. *Brain Tumour Pathol, 21*(1), 1-6.

Ishikawa, H., Sakurai, H., Hasegawa, M., Mitsuhashi, N., Takahashi, M., Masuda, N., et al. (2004). Expression of hypoxic-inducible factor 1alpha predicts metastasis-free survival after radiation therapy alone in stage IIIB cervical squamous cell carcinoma. *Int J Radiat Oncol Biol Phys, 60*(2), 513-521.

Jaakkola, P., Mole, D. R., Tian, Y. M., Wilson, M. I., Gielbert, J., Gaskell, S. J., et al. (2001). Targeting of HIF-alpha to the von Hippel-Lindau ubiquitylation complex by O2-regulated prolyl hydroxylation. *Science, 292*(5516), 468-472.

Kaliberov, S. A., Buchsbaum, D. J., Gillespie, G. Y., Curiel, D. T., Arafat, W. O., Carpenter, M., et al. (2002). Adenovirus-mediated transfer of BAX driven by the vascular endothelial growth factor promoter induces apoptosis in lung cancer cells. *Mol Ther, 6*(2), 190-198.

Kim, J. W., Gao, P., & Dang, C. V. (2007). Effects of hypoxia on tumour metabolism. *Cancer Metastasis Rev, 26*(2), 291-298.

Kizaka-Kondoh, S., Inoue, M., Harada, H., & Hiraoka, M. (2003). Tumour hypoxia: a target for selective cancer therapy. *Cancer Sci, 94*(12), 1021-1028.

Liu, J., Harada, H., Ogura, M., Shibata, T., & Hiraoka, M. (2007). Adenovirus-mediated hypoxia-targeting cytosine deaminase gene therapy enhances radiotherapy in tumour xenografts. *Br J Cancer, 96*(12), 1871-1878.

Liu, J., Qu, R., Ogura, M., Shibata, T., Harada, H., & Hiraoka, M. (2005). Real-time imaging of hypoxia-inducible factor-1 activity in tumour xenografts. *J Radiat Res (Tokyo), 46*(1), 93-102.

Mahon, P. C., Hirota, K., & Semenza, G. L. (2001). FIH-1: a novel protein that interacts with HIF-1alpha and VHL to mediate repression of HIF-1 transcriptional activity. *Genes Dev, 15*(20), 2675-2686.

Maxwell, P. H., Wiesener, M. S., Chang, G. W., Clifford, S. C., Vaux, E. C., Cockman, M. E., et al. (1999). The tumour suppressor protein VHL targets hypoxia-inducible factors for oxygen-dependent proteolysis. *Nature, 399*(6733), 271-275.

Moeller, B. J., Cao, Y., Li, C. Y., & Dewhirst, M. W. (2004). Radiation activates HIF-1 to regulate vascular radiosensitivity in tumours: role of reoxygenation, free radicals, and stress granules. *Cancer Cell, 5*(5), 429-441.

Moeller, B. J., Dreher, M. R., Rabbani, Z. N., Schroeder, T., Cao, Y., Li, C. Y., et al. (2005). Pleiotropic effects of HIF-1 blockade on tumour radiosensitivity. *Cancer Cell, 8*(2), 99-110.

Ogura, M., Shibata, T., Yi, J., Liu, J., Qu, R., Harada, H., et al. (2005). A tumour-specific gene therapy strategy targeting dysregulation of the VHL/HIF pathway in renal cell carcinomas. *Cancer Sci, 96*(5), 288-294.

Patterson, A. V., Williams, K. J., Cowen, R. L., Jaffar, M., Telfer, B. A., Saunders, M., et al. (2002). Oxygen-sensitive enzyme-prodrug gene therapy for the eradication of radiation-resistant solid tumours. *Gene Ther, 9*(14), 946-954.

Pennacchietti, S., Michieli, P., Galluzzo, M., Mazzone, M., Giordano, S., & Comoglio, P. M. (2003). Hypoxia promotes invasive growth by transcriptional activation of the met protooncogene. *Cancer Cell, 3*(4), 347-361.

Post, D. E., & Van Meir, E. G. (2003). A novel hypoxia-inducible factor (HIF) activated oncolytic adenovirus for cancer therapy. *Oncogene, 22*(14), 2065-2072.

Raleigh, J. A., Calkins-Adams, D. P., Rinker, L. H., Ballenger, C. A., Weissler, M. C., Fowler, W. C., Jr., et al. (1998). Hypoxia and vascular endothelial growth factor expression in human squamous cell carcinomas using pimonidazole as a hypoxia marker. *Cancer Res, 58*(17), 3765-3768.

Rinsch, C., Regulier, E., Deglon, N., Dalle, B., Beuzard, Y., & Aebischer, P. (1997). A gene therapy approach to regulated delivery of erythropoietin as a function of oxygen tension. *Hum Gene Ther, 8*(16), 1881-1889.

Rofstad, E. K. (2000). Microenvironment-induced cancer metastasis. *Int J Radiat Biol, 76*(5), 589-605.

Semenza, G. L. (2001). HIF-1, O(2), and the 3 PHDs: how animal cells signal hypoxia to the nucleus. *Cell, 107*(1), 1-3.

Semenza, G. L. (2003). Targeting HIF-1 for cancer therapy. *Nat Rev Cancer, 3*(10), 721-732.

Semenza, G. L. (2007). Oxygen-dependent regulation of mitochondrial respiration by hypoxia-inducible factor 1. *Biochem J, 405*(1), 1-9.

Semenza, G. L. (2008). Mitochondrial autophagy: life and breath of the cell. *Autophagy, 4*(4), 534-536.

Semenza, G. L. (2009). Regulation of cancer cell metabolism by hypoxia-inducible factor 1. *Semin Cancer Biol, 19*(1), 12-16.

Shibata, T., Akiyama, N., Noda, M., Sasai, K., & Hiraoka, M. (1998). Enhancement of gene expression under hypoxic conditions using fragments of the human vascular endothelial growth factor and the erythropoietin genes. *Int J Radiat Oncol Biol Phys, 42*(4), 913-916.

Shibata, T., Giaccia, A. J., & Brown, J. M. (2000). Development of a hypoxia-responsive vector for tumour-specific gene therapy. *Gene Ther, 7*(6), 493-498.

Shibata, T., Giaccia, A. J., & Brown, J. M. (2002). Hypoxia-inducible regulation of a prodrug-activating enzyme for tumour-specific gene therapy. *Neoplasia, 4*(1), 40-48.

Tannock, I. F. (1968). The relation between cell proliferation and the vascular system in a transplanted mouse mammary tumour. *Br J Cancer, 22*(2), 258-273.

Tannock, I. F. (1998). Conventional cancer therapy: promise broken or promise delayed? *Lancet, 351 Suppl 2*, SII9-16.

Teicher, B. A. (1994). Hypoxia and drug resistance. *Cancer Metastasis Rev, 13*(2), 139-168.

Teicher, B. A., Lazo, J. S., & Sartorelli, A. C. (1981). Classification of antineoplastic agents by their selective toxicities toward oxygenated and hypoxic tumour cells. *Cancer Res, 41*(1), 73-81.

Thomlinson, R. H., & Gray, L. H. (1955). The histological structure of some human lung cancers and the possible implications for radiotherapy. *Br J Cancer, 9*(4), 539-549.

Vaupel, P., Kallinowski, F., & Okunieff, P. (1989). Blood flow, oxygen and nutrient supply, and metabolic microenvironment of human tumours: a review. *Cancer Res, 49*(23), 6449-6465.

Wang, G. L., Jiang, B. H., Rue, E. A., & Semenza, G. L. (1995). Hypoxia-inducible factor 1 is a basic-helix-loop-helix-PAS heterodimer regulated by cellular O2 tension. *Proc Natl Acad Sci U S A, 92*(12), 5510-5514.

Wartenberg, M., Ling, F. C., Muschen, M., Klein, F., Acker, H., Gassmann, M., et al. (2003). Regulation of the multidrug resistance transporter P-glycoprotein in multicellular tumour spheroids by hypoxia-inducible factor (HIF-1) and reactive oxygen species. *FASEB J, 17*(3), 503-505.

Wood, S. M., Wiesener, M. S., Yeates, K. M., Okada, N., Pugh, C. W., Maxwell, P. H., et al. (1998). Selection and analysis of a mutant cell line defective in the hypoxia-inducible factor-1 alpha-subunit (HIF-1alpha). Characterization of hif-1alpha-dependent and -independent hypoxia-inducible gene expression. *J Biol Chem, 273*(14), 8360-8368.

Yang, M. H., Wu, M. Z., Chiou, S. H., Chen, P. M., Chang, S. Y., Liu, C. J., et al. (2008). Direct regulation of TWIST by HIF-1alpha promotes metastasis. *Nat Cell Biol, 10*(3), 295-305.

Zeng, L., Ou, G., Itasaka, S., Harada, H., Xie, X., Shibuya, K., et al. (2008). TS-1 enhances the effect of radiotherapy by suppressing radiation-induced hypoxia-inducible factor-1 activation and inducing endothelial cell apoptosis. *Cancer Sci, 99*(11), 2327-2335.

Zhang, H., Bosch-Marce, M., Shimoda, L. A., Tan, Y. S., Baek, J. H., Wesley, J. B., et al. (2008). Mitochondrial autophagy is an HIF-1-dependent adaptive metabolic response to hypoxia. *J Biol Chem, 283*(16), 10892-10903.

Zhang, X., Kon, T., Wang, H., Li, F., Huang, Q., Rabbani, Z. N., et al. (2004). Enhancement of hypoxia-induced tumour cell death in vitro and radiation therapy in vivo by use of small interfering RNA targeted to hypoxia-inducible factor-1alpha. *Cancer Res, 64*(22), 8139-8142.

12

Gene Therapy of Glioblastoma: Anti – Gene Anti IGF-I Strategy

Jerzy Trojan
INSERM U602 , Paul Brousse Hospital, University Paris XI, 94007 Villejuif and Gene Therapy Laboratory, Faculty of Medicine, La Sabana University, Bogota,
France
Colombia

1. Introduction

One of the most trying pathological conditions of the central nervous system is the malignant glial development of the brain. The major malignancy is the glioblastoma multiforme, GBM, which almost uniformly leads to the patient's demise: mortality is still close to 100 %, and median survival 8 - 11 months. All currently used therapies - surgery, radiotherapy, chemotherapy and pharmacology - have not given satisfactory results; the median survival, using an immune- or chemotherapy is 15 months, rarely 18 months (Stupp *et al.*, 2006). The search for new approaches based on gene molecular biology/immunology techniques, is therefore a necessary step. In the presented chapter we highlight to biomedical researchers and physicians not only the importance of the glioblastoma problem but the fact that we are currently successfully progressing in the studies and the treatment of this pathology. The most recent approaches for the treatment of malignant tumors and especially of gliomas are now focusing on the use of different types of inhibitors. More specifically gene therapy approach using anti - gene technology including antisense strategy is considered to target as well growth factors (IGF-I, EGF, VEGF, TGF) as their receptors and related downstream steps of signal transduction pathways (IRS-1, PI3K, AKT, PKC, Bcl-2, GSK3, glycogen synthase GS) (Helene, 1994; Beckner *et al.*, 2005; Trojan *et al.*, 2007a). Among growth factors, IGF-I plays a principal role during development of the brain reappearing in malignant glial differentiation (Pollak *et al.*, 2004). This hypothesis has strongly underlined the usefulness of techniques permitting to target and stop the expression of growth factors present in tumoral development by anti - gene strategies, particularly antisense approach.
The "discovery" of the antisense approach, AS, was made in 1984/1985 (Rubenstein *et al.*, 1984; Weintraub *et al.*, 1985). The AS approach, as a concept, was created to study basic problems of gene regulation, particularly useful in developmental biology investigations, bypassing inherent limitations of functional studies dependent upon natural mutant cells or artificially mutagenized cells (Izant & Weintraub, 1985). Antisense technique was particularly used to target tumor antigens, which arrest of expression was not efficiently stopped using antibodies or other inhibitors (Dias & Stein, 2002). The demonstration of AS technology as a efficient gene therapy tool, simultaneously suppressing the targeted protein

expression, changing a morphologic phenotype of cultured neoplastic cells, and stopping *in vivo* a growth of experimentally established tumors, was done for the first time using AS anti IGF-I approach for glioma treatment (Trojan *et al.*, 1993). We can also consider the 1992/3 years as the beginning of gene therapy of gliomas exploring either strategy of AS anti IGF-I using episomal vector (Trojan *et al.*, 1992), or strategy of retroviral vector with gene encoding TK -HSV (Culver *et al.*, 1992) (only the first approach - AS anti IGF-I - has shown valuable results in ulterior clinical trials). The first clinical cases of glioblastoma were treated with AS strategies - anti IGF-I and anti IGF-I receptor - in 2000/1 (Wongkojornsilp *et al.*, 2001; Andrews *et al.*, 2001). Since the past decade, we observe a significant increase of AS approach for the treatment of tumors and especially of gliomas. Recently, other targets than IGF-I, as TGFbeta and their downstream signal transduction pathway elements as GS among others were proposed for treatment of malignant gliomas using AS technology (Schlingensiepen, R. *et al.*, 2005; Ardourel *et al.*, 2007). The approach of AS TGF-beta, similarly to that of AS IGF-I, has given satisfactory clinical results.

2. Anti - genes

Since twenty years different approaches of the treatment of tumours, including glioblastoma, were considered. For example, the treatment of liver cancer with antibodies to AFP was widely used. Unfortunately these techniques were not specific for the treated tissues. Actually, the "anti-gene" strategies offer new possibilities for cancer therapy. The anti-genes can be classified into three categories, as follows: 1) the antisense molecules (Rubenstein *et al.*, 1984; Weintraub *et al.*, 1985; Galderisi *et al.*, 1999; Stein, 2001; Dias & Stein, 2002; Biroccio *et al.*, 2003; Kalota *et al.*, 2004) targeted to the complementary sequence in mRNA, including antisense RNA, antisense oligodeoxynucleotides and ribozymes; 2) the triple helix-forming oligomers (Dervan, 1992; Helene, 1994; Shevelev *et al.*, 1997) targeted to the double stranded DNA gene; and 3) the sense oligodeoxynucleotides designed to act as decoys to trap regulatory proteins (Morishita *et al.*, 1998). The "antisense" and "triple helix" techniques seem very promising, stopping the protein synthesis at transcription level (Green *et al.*, 1986), and translation level (Derwan, 1992), respectively.
Other recently introduced technologies include those of triple helix, TH (Dervan, 1992; Helene, 1994), as well as potentially useful siRNA (Boado, 2005; Pai *et al.*, 2006) and miRNA (microRNA) (Berezikov *et al.*, 2006). The role of 21-23 mer double-stranded RNA (si RNA) in the silencing of genes is strongly similar to that of the TH DNA mechanism, which also involves 23 mer RNA (Helene, 1994). As to miRNAs, they are noncoding RNA molecules of 21 to 24 nucleotides that can regulate gene expression at the post-transcriptional level. Moreover, miRNA may play a fundamental role in tumorigenesis, controlling cell proliferation and apoptosis; in gliomas, the miRNA (microRNA-21) level has been reported to be elevated (Corsten *et al.*, 2007). Whether or not siRNA technology or miRNA knockdown will supplant the AS oligodeoxynucleotide approaches remains in question at this time, because we do not yet have final clinical results (Dias & Stein, 2002; Pai *et al.*, 2006; Corsten *et al.*, 2007).

2.1 Antisense approach

The "discovery" of antisense approach was done by the groups of F. Jacob and R.M. Harland (Rubinstein *et al.*, 1984; Weintraub *et al.*, 1985). This event has been suggested to physiologically occur as the regulation mechanism of gene expression in cells. Some years ago, regulating activities of untranscribed DNA strand ("antisense" strand) has been suggested (Ring & Roberts, 1994). It has also been widely proven that a lot of genes present an open reading frame on the antisense strand (Merino *et al.,* 1994; Yomo & Urabe, 1994; Campbell *et al.,* 1994). The role of this natural antisense RNA is not yet understood. More recently, it was found that mouse thymidine kinase (Tk) gene expression is regulated by antisense transcription: a putative promoter in intron 3 of the murine Tk will transcribe this antisense RNA. However, concerning natural antisense RNA in prokaryotes, it has been shown that they could play a regulatory role in replication, transcription or translation steps of some genes; it was demonstrated that the translation of the bacterial enzyme transposase was controlled by an antisense RNA (Weintraub *et al.,* 1985).

An antisense RNA, hybridized on its complementary sequence in a mRNA blocks the ribosome progression during the translation of the mRNA. This observation constitutes the "starting point" of the antisense or non-sense approach (Rubinstein *et al.,* 1984) based on antisense RNA or antisense oligonucleotides to modulate artificially and specifically the expression of genes involved in important cellular processes. The mRNA complementary sequence is introduced in the cell either by a plasmid vector (dsDNA) coding for an antisense RNA or by a single stranded oligonucleotide form. The plasmid vector allows the intracellular transcription of antisense RNA which can strongly hybridize to the mRNA and stop the translation. Generally, an effective inhibition demands a high copy number of antisense RNA relative to mRNA . The antisense oligodeoxynucleotides, once in the cell, can stimulate the ribonuclease H after hybridization with target RNA. This enzyme, which is implicated in DNA replication, damages RNA moiety of the hybrids formed in the cell. On the other hand, the antisense oligonucleotide can remain as nondegraded, hybridizing to another messenger and inducing the degradation of this mRNA. In this way, in the presence of RNAse H, the antisense oligonucleotide acts in a catalytic marrow, with the enzyme potentiating the antisense effect (Hélène, 1990).

The chemical stability of plasmid-derived antisense RNA seems much more efficient than that of antisense oligonucleotides delivered directly into cells. The antisense oligonucleotides are exposed to intra- and extracellular nuclease actvity. Antisense oligomers action can be reinforced by association with polycations like polyethyleneimin (PEI), polylysine or cationic lipids (DOTMA, DOTAP) facilitating endocytosis of oligomers (Galderisi *et al.,* 1999). These positively charged molecules are also used for transfection of cells with plasmids encoding antisense RNA.

The first antisense oligonucleotide used in clinical pharmacology was as anti-cytomegalovirus therapy (Vitravene™) (Vitravene Study Group, 2002). The antisense strategy was then largely used in order to analyze gene expression and intron splicing. The phosphorothioates are the most widely studied oligonucleotides, because of their nuclease stability are highly soluble and have excellent antisense activity. These data have led to the introduction of phosphorothioate oligonucleotides into clinical therapeutic trials (melanoma, chronic lymphocytic leukemia, lung cancer and other tumors) (Jansen *et al.,* 2000; Geiger *et al.,* 1998).

A good example of a new generation oligonucleotide is the N3' P5' PN. The PN exhibits highly selective and specific antisense activity *in vitro* and *in vivo*. An 11-mer PN, complementary to junction region of the *bcr-abl* mRNA (thought to be a determinant of the chronic myelogenous leukemia phenotype) efficiently inhibited the growth of treated BV173 cells (Gryaznow *et al.,* 1996). Another exemple of new generation oligonucleotides concerns antisense survivine oligonucleotides, ASODN, which were transfected into gastric cancer

cell line SGC 7901 (Yang *et al.*, 2004). ASODN caused a statistically significant reduction of cell viability and the cell growth was significantly inhibited. A significant loss of survivin mRNA was also presented, and the protein level was significantly decreased. ASODN may provide a novel approach to therapy of gastric cancer.
The antisense technology was used to study several protein actions: the alpha subunit of human chorionic gonadotrophin in choriocarcinoma cells (Cao *et al.*, 1995); the regulating protein E2F-1, in S cellular cycle phase, and its action on genes linked to proliferation (Sala *et al.*, 1994); nerve growth factor (NGF) in skin of transgenic mice, and its relationship with response to mechanical stimuli (Davis *et al.*, 1993). Lately, the antisense strategy is "classically" used to analyze gene expression and intron splicing. The same technology was employed to study the function of the heat shock protein hsp70, overexpressed in mouse fibrosarcoma cells; a direct correlation was found between hsp70 overexpression and tumorigenicity of cells. Cells which express high rates of hsp70 are resistant *in vitro* to cytotoxic cells and macrophages (Jaattela, 1995).
The action of IGF-I - BP-4, insulin-like growth factor I – binding protein 4, has also been studied using antisense strategy. The IGF-I – BP-4 was shown to inhibit the mitogenic effect of exogenous IGF on IIT29 tumor cells (Singh *et al.*, 1994). The same antisense strategy was applied to study p27kipl protein. The quiescent state of cells needs the p27. The inhibition of p27 expression induces the progression of cell cycle and the cyclin D1 promoter activity. Hamster fibroblasts transformed in this way grow faster than non-treated cells, even in serum free medium (Rivard *et al.*, 1996).
In "antisense" anti-tumor experimental therapy different strategies were applied coming from 1992. Among them were strategies based on :

- antisense oncogenes (i.e. Okabe *et al.*, 1993);
- antisense of genes encoding enzymes (i.e. Ahmad *et al.*, 1994);
- antisense of protein related to MHC expression (i.e. Lichtenstein *et al.*, 1992) and
- antisense of genes encoding growth factors (i.e. Trojan *et al*, 1992); the last antisense strategy seems to constitute the most promoting approach in clinical trials. Some examples of gliomas experimental studies are done in Table 1.

microRNA 21 (miR-21)	Antisense oligonucleotide Experimental therapy	Shi et al. Zhonghua Yi 2008;25(5):497
TGF beta and specific. immun. activation	Antisense oligonucleotide (NPs) Experimental therapy	Schneider et al. J Neuroimmun 2008; 195(1-2): 21.
TGF beta and immun. activation	Antisense oligonucleotide Experimental therapy	Vega et al. Future oncol 2008; 4(3): 433
heat shock protein 27 (Hsp27)	Antisense oligonucleotide Experimental therapy	Aloy et al. Int J Radiat Oncol Biol Phys 2008; 70(2): 543.
VEGF	Antisense (vector) Experimental therapy	Lin et al. Cancer Sci 2008; 99(12): 2540
TGF beta 2	Antisense oligodeoxynucleotide Clinical trial	Schlingensiepen et al. Rec Res Cancer Res 2008; 177: 137.
IGF-I	Antisense (vector) Clinical trial	Trojan et al. JAC 2008/09; 1: 1.

MiR221/222	Antisense oligonucleotide Experimental therapy	Zhang et al. Zhonghua Zhong Liu Za Zhi. 2009; 31(10): 72
TGF beta 2	Antisense oligodeoxynucleotide Clinical trial	Hau et al. Expert Rev Anticancer Ther 2009; 9(11):1663.
IGF BP2	Antisense (vector) Experimental therapy	Moore et al. Proc Natl Acad Sci USA 2009; 106(39): 16675
CD133/prominin-1	Antisense oligonucleotide Experimental therapy	Yao et al. Oncol Rep 2009; 22(4): 781.
EGFR	Antisense oligonucleotide Experimental therapy	Loew et al. Anticancrer Agents Med Chem 2009; 9(6): 703.
TGF beta	Antisense oligodeoxynucleotide Clinical trial	Vallieres IDrugs 2009; 12(7): 445.
microRNA-21	Antisense oligonucleotide Experimental therapy	Li et al. Brain Res 2009; 25(1286): 13.
miR221/222	Antisense oligonucleotide Experimental therapy	Zhang et al. Int J Oncol 2009; 34(6): 1653.
VEGF	Antisense (vector) Experimental therapy	Yang et al. J Neurooncol 2010; Aug 26 Epub
miR-21	Antisense oligonucleotide Experimental therapy	Zhou et al. Oncol Rep 2010; 24(1):195.
c-Met	Antisense oligonucleotide Experimental therapy	Chu et al. Oncol Rep 2010; 24(1):189.
AKT2	Antisense oligonucleotide Experimental therapy	Zhang et al. Oncol Rep 2010; 24(1):65.
EGFR	Antisense oligonucleotide Experimental therapy	Li et al. Oncol Rep 2010; 23(6): 1585.
PED/PEA-15 (ERK1/2-interacting protein)	Antisense oligonucleotide Experimental therapy	Botta et al. Hum Gene Ther 2010; 21(9): 1067.
miR-21 & 5FU	Antisense oligonucleotide Experimental therapy	Ren et al. J Biomater Sci Polym Ed 2010; 21(3): 303.
miR-21	Antisense oligonucleotide Experimental therapy	Zhou et al. Lab Invest. 2010; 90(2): 144.
EGFR	Antisense oligonucleotide Experimental therapy	Kang et al. J Biomed Mater Res A 2010; 93(2): 585
TGFbeta & T cell therapy	Antisense oligodeoxynucleotide Clinical trial	Dietrich et al. Curr Opin Oncol 2010; 22(6):604
IGF-I	Antisense (vector) Clinical trial	Trojan et al. Biomed & Pharmacother 2010; 64(8): 576.

Table 1. Examples of experimental and clinical gene therapies of gliomas using antisense technology (selection from the 2008s).

2.2 Triple helix approach

Since the 1990's, in parallel with antisense strategy, another approach – triple helix strategy is starting to be successfully introduced in experimental and clinical gene therapy trials (Scaggiante *et al.*, 1994; Postel *et al.*, 1991; Thomas *et al.*, 1995). The triple helix (TH) technology is the new approach, which belongs together with antisense approach to anti-gene strategies *sensu lato*, i.e. the techniques targeting the expression of respective up-regulated gene. The TH technology was "discovered" by groups of P.B. Derwan (Derwan, 1992) and of C. Helene (Helene, 1994). Its action is well defined by gene inhibition at the translation level. In brief, the short specific oligonucleotides (so called triple-helix forming oligonucleotides, TFOs) are delivered to cells both by cell transfection with chemical carriers and via vector plasmid that can drive the synthesis of TFO RNA. TFOs link to genomic double-strand DNA, form triple-helix structure with target gene and strongly inhibit its expression at transcriptional level. A triple-helical structure on DNA is considered to block transit of RNA polymerase. TFOs are usually targeted against polypurine/polypyrimidine sequences located in control regions (promoters) of the genes of interest (Derwan, 1992).

The examples of the inhibitory activity of triplex-forming oligonucleotides on target genes involved in tumorigenesis are now available (i.e. Giovannangeli & Hélène, 1997; Vasquez & Wilson, 1998). Most of the TFOs are targeted to polypurine-polypyrimidine sequences located in control regions of the gene of interest and are cell delivered via transfection with various chemical carriers. An alternative way to introduce TFOs in cells is to use a plasmid vector that can drive the synthesis of an RNA triplex-forming oligonucleotide inside the cells. This TFO generated in situ is therefore protected from degradation by nucleases and could reach its DNA target without being trapped in lysosomal vesicles. Obviously, it could be transfected in cells via either standard cell transfection procedures or via ways similarly used in virus-based gene therapy. An application of this triplex-based approach has been used for the inhibition of the IGF-I which plays a major role in tumorigenesis (Shevelev *et al.*, 1997).

Triple helix strategy was also applied to the ras oncogenes which are the most frequently activated oncogenes in human cancer. In vitro transcription of human Ha-ras was inhibited by triplex-forming oligonucleotides targeted to sequences recognized by the Sp I tran-cription factor (Mayfield *et al.*, 1994). Growth factors are known to play a role in tumorigenesis, and thereby represent relevant targets for antigene therapies. The synthesis of human tumor necrosis factor (TNF), which acts as an autocrine growth factor in various tumor cell lines including neuroblastoma and glioblastoma, has been blocked by triplex-forming oligonucleotide treatment (Aggarwal *et al.*, 1996

2.3 Biotechnological limitations

Human gene therapy is defined as a medical intervention based on the administration of genetic material in order to modify or manipulate the expression of a gene product or to alter the biological properties of living cells. Cells may be modified *ex vivo* for subsequent administration or altered *in vivo* by gene therapy products given directly to the subject. Example that falls under this definition includes use of antisense oligonucleotides to block gene transcription or use of sequence-specific oligonucleotides to correct a genetic mutation (Miller & Simek, 2000).

The specificity of antisense mechanism of action should be verified by: a proof of cellular uptake, the use of multiple control oligonucleotide sequences and direct measurement of target mRNA or protein levels. Anyway, phosphorothioate oligonucleotides are in general able to produce a wide spectrum of nonspecific effects, especially at high concentration. Fortunatelly non-antisense effects can be therapeutically useful although their unpredictability can confound research applications of these biologically active molecules in human gene therapy (Lebedeva & Stein, 2002).

Antisense oligonucleotides have been widely employed as a method to decrease tumor cell viability and chemoresistance and to induce apoptosis *in vitro* and *in vivo*. The "weakness" of oligonucleotides is not only their sensitivity to nuclease digestion, which affects their half-life in culture and *in vivo*, but also their inappropriate intracellular compartmentalization. It seems that the most reliable way to choose an antisense sequence is the "mRNA walking" method (i.e. in bcl-2 antisense) (Lebedeva & Stein, 2002).

Undesirable properties have been identified for phosphorothioate oligodeoxynucleotides. When dosed at high levels it is possible to identify toxicities in rodents and primates. However, at doses currently under evaluation in the clinic, phosphorothioate oligodeoxynucleotides have been well tolerated. Extensive medicinal chemistry efforts have been successfully focused on identifying improved antisense oligonucleotides. Oligonucleotide modifications have been identified that exhibit increased resistance to serum and cellular nucleases, enabling use of oligonucleotides that do not have phosphorothioate linkages (Benett *et* al., 2000). The tissue distribution of oligonucleotides may be altered with either chemical modifications or formulations. The modified oligonucleotides have been described that potentially exhibited less toxicity than first-generation phosphorothioate oligodeoxynucleotides. Because experience with these modified oligonucleotides is rather limited, it remains to be seen whether they will have a distinct toxicity profile. The data also suggest that oral delivery of antisense oligonucleotides may be feasible, which would increase the utility of the technology. Identification of second- and third-generation oligonucleotides should ameliorate therapies for patients (Benett *et al.*, 2000).

3. IGF-I and tumorigenicity

There is a convergence between ontogenesis and cancerogenesis and the same specific antigens (oncoproteins) are present in embryo/fetal tissues and in corresponding neoplastic developing tissues. The development of the brain is related to appearance of specific antigens. These disappear in mature brain and reappear in the development of neoplastic nervous tissue development. Gene expression during neoplastic brain development concerns oncoproteins (such as alpha-fetoptrotein, as well as serum albumin) (Trojan *et al.*, 1984), growth factors and their respective receptors (i.e. IGF-I, EGF, FGF, VEGF, TGF-alpha and -beta) (Baserga, 1994). Their down stream proteins and glycogen signalling elements including glycogen synthase (GS), are also involved (Patel *et al.*, 2004; Trojan *et al.*, 2007). In 1992 Trojan and his co-workers have demonstrated that an Insulin-like growth factor 1, IGF-I, is present in glioma cells but absent in neuroblastoma cells (Trojan *et al.*, 1992). Using teratocarcinoma model, Trojan and his co-workers have shown that neoplastic hepatocytes express IGF-I and IGF-II, and neuroblastic cells express IGF-II (Trojan *et al.*, 1994). These observations permitted to study separetly, using IGF-I and IGF-II as the oncoprotein markers, different groups of diseases: of glial, neural and digestive tube and hepatocyte origin.

IGF-I is a 70-amino acid polypeptide involved in cell and tissue differentiation (Daughaday *et al.*, 1972; Froesch *et al.*, 1985; Baserga, 1994; Trojan *et al.*, 1994) coded by IGF-I gene (Sussenbach *et al.*, 1992). IGF-I plays an important role in growth as a mediator of growth hormone, GH, and a locally acting stimulator (Froesch *et al.*, 1985; Le Roith *et al.*, 2001). The action of IGF-I on cellular metabolism depends on binding proteins, IGFBP, which prolong the half life of this factor and modify its interaction with receptor (i.e. Rosen, 1999). IGF-I acts via specific IGF-I receptor and subsequent activation of a protein tyrosine phosphorylic signal transduction cascade, similar to that of insulin action (Werner and Le Roith, 2000). Through its binding to IGF-I-R, which activates a protein tyrosine phosphorylic signal transduction cascade, PI3K/AKT/GSK3, similar to that of insulin action (Adams et al., 2000), IGF-I has been reported to block the apoptosis pathway (IRS/PI3K/AKT/Bcl or GSK3 or Ca^{++} or caspases). Such a blockade occurs at the cytoplasmic and nuclear levels in a variety of cell lines, including neuronal and glial cells (D'Mello *et al.*, 1993; Baserga, 1994; Mason *et al.*, 2000, Chrysis *et al.*, 2001). The anti-inflammatory and anti-apoptotic effects of IGF-I are established through an increase of phosphatidylinosotol 3' kinase (PI3 kinase) activity and a maintain of Bcl-2 survival proteins. PI3 kinase is directly related to insulin receptor substrate (IRS-1), the latter following the tyrosine kinase (IGF-I receptor) (D'Ambrosio *et al.*, 1996). IGF-I being known as a factor protecting cells from apoptosis, different researchers have tried to stop apoptotic effect using the approach of antisense IGF-I receptor (Resnicoff *et al.*, 1994). The block of IGF-I synthesis, induces apoptotic and also immunogenic phenomenons (Upegui-Gonzalez *et al.*, 1998).
The human IGF-I gene is located within a region of over 85 kb on the chromosome 12 - 12p22 (Daughaday and Rotwein, 1989; Sussenbach *et al.*, 1992). Deregulated expression of growth factors and/or their receptors, and especially of IGF-I, is associated as well with growth as with pathology of different diseases, including tumors (Trojan *et al.*, 1993; Baserga, 1994; Rubin and Baserga, 1995). Since last Symposium "IGFs and Cancer", held in Halle in Germany (15-17.09.2000), IGF-I is considered as a diagnostic marker and a biological modulator in different types of tumors, especially in brain tumors (Zumkeller & Westphal, 2001).

4. Methodology

Described methodology established for an experimental preclinical research was applied for clinical research.

4.1 Plasmids

The episome based plasmid pMT-Anti IGF-I was constructed as previously described (Trojan *et al.*, 1992). The vector pMT-EP, under the control of the metallothionein, MT-I, inducible promotor was used as its base. The casette contains the Epstein-Barr Virus origin of replication and the gene encoding nuclear antigen I which together drive extrachromosomal replication. Down-stream of the insertion site is a poly A termination signal followed by the hygromycin B and ampilicin resistance genes. Comparatively, the same plasmid was prepared containing either CMV or HS (heat shock) promotors. The vector expressing IGF-I triple helix (pMT-AG triple helix) was constructed as previously described (Shevelev *et al.*, 1997). This cassette consists of a 23 bp DNA fragment cloned into the vector pMT-EP which transcribes a third RNA strand forming a triple helix structure within the target region of the human IGF-I gene, between its transcription and translation

initiation sites. The vector pMT-EP with either the lac-Z reporter gene, or cDNA expressing IGF-II antisense RNA as insert was used in control experiments (Trojan *et al.*, 1994).
Vectors encoding MHC-I or B-7 antisense cDNA were constructed in the laboratory of J. Ilan (CWRU, Cleveland) using pMT-EP containing the neomycine (G418) resistance gene instead of the hygromycin B resistance gene, and the MHC-I or B7 insert in antisense orientation in place of the IGF-I gene sequence.

4.2 Cell culture

Human primary glioma cell lines (Anthony *et al.*, 1998; Trojan *et al.*, 2003), were cultured in DMEM+F12 (v/v) (GIBCO-BRL) supplemented with 10 % FCS, 2mM glutamine, 100 U/ml penicillin and 100 µg/ml streptomycin, at 37° C and 5 % C02. Hygromycin B (Boehringer Mannheim) at a concentration of 0,005 mg/ml was added 48 hours after transfection to select for transfected cells. Then the concentration of hygromycin for cell culture was determined as previously described (Anthony *et al.*, 1998). B-104 rat neuroblastoma cell line (obtained from ATCC) was used as a negative control (Trojan *et al.*, 1992).
Primary cell cultures of human glioma were derived from tumors of glioblastoma patients during surgical resection in the University Hospital of Cleveland, OH, Hopital Val-de-Grace, Paris and the Medical University Hospital of Bydgoszcz (5 to 6 cases from every hospital). Surgical sections approximately 3x3 mm X 1-2 cm in length were placed in DMEM containing high glucose concentration, 100 U/ml penicillin and 100 U/ml streptomycin. Specimens were then transferred to phosphate buffered saline (PBS) containing no Ca2+ or Mg2+ and dissected into 1-2 mm fragments. The tissue was then centrifuged at 1500 rpm x 5 min. The pellet was resuspended in DMEM containing 20 % FCS supplemented with 2mM glutamine, 100 U/ml penicillin, 100 microg/ml streptomycin and 10 ng/ml EGF. Cell suspensions were adjusted to a concentration of 2 million cells / well in 6-well plates and incubated at 37 C and 5 % C02 in culture medium containing 10 ng/ml EGF (Sigma) (GIBCO). After two days, dead cells were removed and incubation was continued in DMEM containing 10% FCS, and no EGF, for three additional days. The medium was then changed to DMEM minus FCS and incubation was continued x 48 hours. Following this first week, cells were maintained in 5% FCS / DMEM / 10% C02 / 37° C until stable transfection was established (approximately 4 weeks).

4.3 Transfection

Cultures of cells, 60-80 % confluent, were transfected in 6-well plates utilizing a ratio of 1 µg plasmid DNA per 400 000 cells. The FuGENE 6 Transfection Reagent (Boehringer Mannheim) was used according to the supplier's instructions. To determine the efficiency of transfection, the process was carried out using the pMT-EP construct containing lac-Z as a reporter gene. Cell cultures were washed in PBS and incubated at 37° C in the presence of the staining solution which contained 5mM K3Fe(CN)6, 2mM MgC12, 0,8 mg/ml X-gal made in PBS. The selected IGF-I « antisense » or « triple helix » cell clones (expressing MHC-I and B7) were co-transfected with vectors either encoding MHC-I or B7 antisense cDNA , in the presence of 0,4 mg/ml of G-418 .

4.4 Northern blot

Content of IGF-I antisense RNA was determined in 50 % confluent cell cultures. Cells were deprived of serum and cultured overnight in DMEM containing 0,1 % BSA ; 60 µM Zn S04

(Sigma) was then added x 5 hours to induce the MTI promoter. The cells were then prepared for Northern blot. Labeling of human IGF-I cDNA and chicken beta actin cDNA and hybridizations were done according to Maniatis and procedures previously described (Trojan *et al*, 1992, 2003); the 770 bp human IGF-I cDNA and 500 bp rat IGF-I cDNA used as probes were a gift from J. llan (CWRU, Cleveland). The Northern blot was used also to verify expression of IGF-I in solid glioblastomas.

4.5 Histology

The removed human samples of tumours were fixed in 4% para-formaldehyde, and paraffin embedded sections were stained for IGF-I by immunoperoxidase technique (Vectastain ABC kit, Vector Laboratories, Burlingame, CA, USA).

4.6 Immunocytochemistry and flow cytometry analysis (FACS)

Immunocytochemical localization of IGF-I protein was done by the immunoperoxidase technique (Vectastain ABC kit, Vector Laboratories, Burlingame, CA, USA). Cells were fixed in 4 % paraformaldehyde. Polyclonal antibodies against rat and mouse IGF-I and against human IGF-I were purchased from Valbiotech (Paris, France).
For FACS, paraformaldehyde-fixed cells were treated as described earlier (Trojan *et al.*, 1996). Stained cells were analyzed for MHC-I, MHC-II and B7 antigens, as well as for CD antigens of PBL cells, in a FACSCAN flow cytometer (Becton Dickinson).

4.7 Fluorescein cell - death detection

Apoptosis was determined by dUTP-fluorescein terminal transferase-labeling of nicked DNA (TUNEL apoptosis assay). The « In situ Cell Death Detection Kit, fluorescein » (Boehringer Mannheim) was used according to supplier's instructions.

4.8 Preparation of cell membranes

Human glioma cells membranes were prepared according to the method of M.A. Matlib with modifications (Matlib *et al.*, 1988). The Na+-Ca2+ exchange system in vascular smooth muscle cell membrane vesicles isolated from cultured cells and from tissue is similar. Homogenization of tissues was performed on ice by Polytron homogenizer in 20 mM MOPS, 250 mM sucrose, 0.05% BSA, 0.25 mM PMSF, pH 7.5. Homogenates were centrifuged for 10 min at 1000 x g, and the supernatant was recentrifuged for 15 min at 10000 x g. Microsome membranes were sedimented from the supernatant by centrifugation for 60 min at 100000 x g. The pellet was resuspended in 20 mM MOPS, pH 7.5, layered on top of 0.8 M sucrose in 20 mM MOPS and centrifuged in SW-27 bucket rotor (60 min x 24000 rpm). The pellet was collected from the interphase and recentrifuged under the same conditions. Finally, the membrane pellet was resuspended in 20 mM MOPS, pH 7.5, frozen in liquid nitrogen and stored at -70°C. For treatment of glioblastoma patients, the membrane pellet resuspended in MOPS, was, one hour befor vaccination, ressuspended in PBS (0.9% NaCl, pH 7.5) in ratio 1: 100.

4.9 Vaccination of glioblastoma patients

Human glioma cell lines were transfected with the "triple helix" pMT–AG TH plasmid vector. Clones of transfected cells (down-regulated for IGF-I and expressing MHC-I and B7 molecules) were selected after two months - coming from a day of transfection. Before injection the cells were irradiated. The first injection was done using the membranes only of so prepared 1 mln cells - injected subcutaneously into the left arm of operated glioblastoma patients (The next 3 weeks permitted to prepare a sufficient number of 5 million cells for the second injection, and then for the third injection). The blood was collected before the first vaccination, and then 3 weeks after the first and the second injection. Peripheral blood lymphocyte (PBL) typing was performed using mouse monoclonal antibodies directed against the superficial cell antigens.

The samples of monoclonal antibodies were used for flow cytometer analysis as follows: conjugated to FITC - (a) CD45, (b) CD 4, (c) CD3, (d) CD25, (e) CD45RO, (f) CD19, (g) CD8, (h) CD8CD11b+, (i) control antibody IgG1, and those conjugated to PE – (a) CD14, (b) CD8, (c) CD16+CD6, (d) CD4(CD8), (e) CD4(CD8), (f)CD5, (g) CD8CD11b-, (h) CD8CD28, (i) IgG2.

5. Results

The approval for the gene therapy clinical trial (based on NIH clinical study n°1602, Bethesda, Maryland, 24. 11. 1993) was administrated by the Bioethical Commission of the L. Rydygier Medical University, Bromberg (Bydgoszcz), Poland (n° KB/176/2001, 28. 06. 2002) and registered by international Wiley Gene Therapy Clinical Trial database n° 635 and 636 (J. Gene Med., updated 2002), and by NATO Science program (LST 980517).

Primary glioma cell cultures were established from biopsies of human GBM (Trojan *et al.*, 1996). The established cell lines were transfected with "antisense" or "triple helix" IGF-I vector. The cells were down regulated in IGF-I and presented both MHC-I and B7.1 molecules. The IGF-I antisense cells or "vaccine" were irradiated before injection into status post-surgically resected glioblastoma patients. The significant changes observed were primarily after the first vaccination (Fig. 1). The phenotypic changes in peripheral blood lymphocytes were as follows. There was an increase in the percentage of CD8+T cells with a characteristic CD8+CD11b- and CD8CD28+ phenotype after each of three vaccinations, the alteration that may reflect the enhanced activation of T cytotoxic cells in blood (Fig. 2). Additionally, an increased percentage of the lymphocytes positive for superficial interleukine-2 receptor (CD25) was observed. No changes in other CD molecules were demonstrated (Trojan *et al.*, 2003, 2007). In our work in progress (new protocol) 4th and 5th injections of IGF-I TH cells in glioblastoma patients have been introduced. After the 4th injection the blood of treated patients showed a progressive increase in CD8 and NK cells, as compared with the 1st and 2nd injections, which underlines the *in vivo* immune effect of injected IGF-I TH cells. An increase in CD25 after the 2nd and 3rd injections was also observed. Then, after the 4th and 5th injections this progression slowed down. The only side effect observed was a post-vaccination fever of 38°C, corresponding probably to a cellular immune response (induction of T lymphocytes). These alterations may reflect the enhanced activation of cytotoxic T cells (Trojan *et al.*, 2007a).

The promising results were obtained in six Phase-I patients at University Hospitals of Cleveland, USA, in two patients in Bangkock Thailand and in four patients at the University Hospital of Bromberg (Bydgoszcz), Poland. In these Phase I trials, no unacceptable complications in patients were observed from the treatment. The only complicating finding was transit increase in temperature to 38-38.5 ^{0}C lasting 24-48 hours (confirming the presence of immune anti-tumour response). This usually occurred by 12 hours and in 8 of the 12 GBM patients that were treated. In the patients treated in the United States study, and in those investigated in Bromberg, Poland, tumour burden at time of treatment was advanced. One patient who was treated at University Hospitals of Cleveland, had lived 24

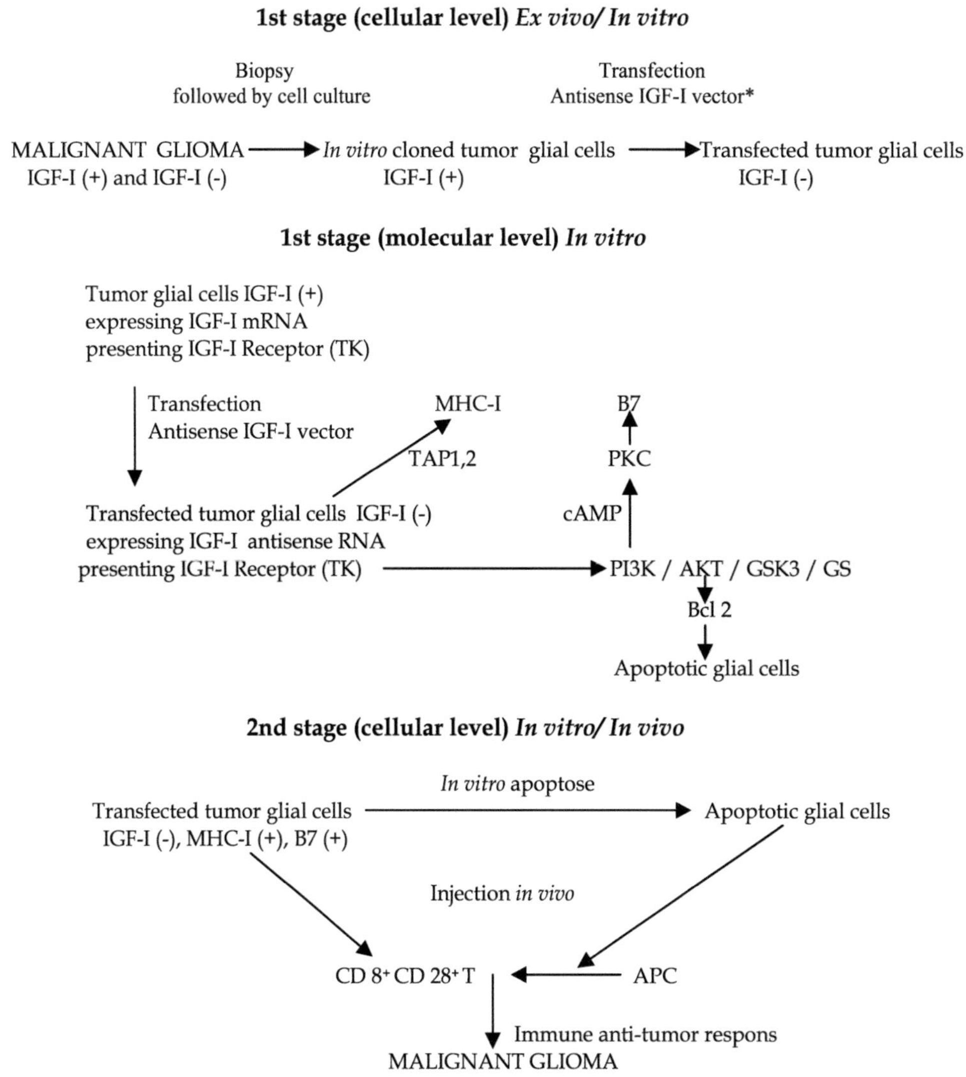

Fig. 1. Schema of IGF-I antisense therapy. The tumor cells are cloned *in vitro* to obtain a cell line positive for IGF-I. *After transfection of the cell line with a vector containing IGF-I cDNA in antisens orientation, the cells express IGF-I antisens RNA, and become negatively stained for IGF-I and positively for MHC-I and B7. Moreover they become apoptotic. Both phenomenons, immune and apoptotic, are related to signal transduction pathway (*the presented pathway is common for different growth factors as EGF, VEGF, TGF-beta or PDGF).* The injected transfected cells including apoptotic cells, together with APC cells induced *in vivo*, activate T lymphocytes (CTL $CD8^+CD28^+$); activated CTL produce immune anti tumot response (Beckner *et al.*, 2005; Fontenau *et al.*, 2002; Ly *et al.*, 2001; Trojan *et al.*, 2007a, 2010). Abréviations : TAP 1,2 (transporter associated with antigen processing antigen); TK (tyrosine kinase); PI3K (phosphatidyinositol 3 kinase); PDK1 (phosphoinositide-dependent kinase 1); AKT (PKB, protein kinase B); Bcl 2 (key molecule of apoptose); GSK3 (glycogene synthetase kinase 3); GS (glycogene synthetase); MAPK (MAP kinase – mitogen activated protein kinase); PKC (protein kinase C).

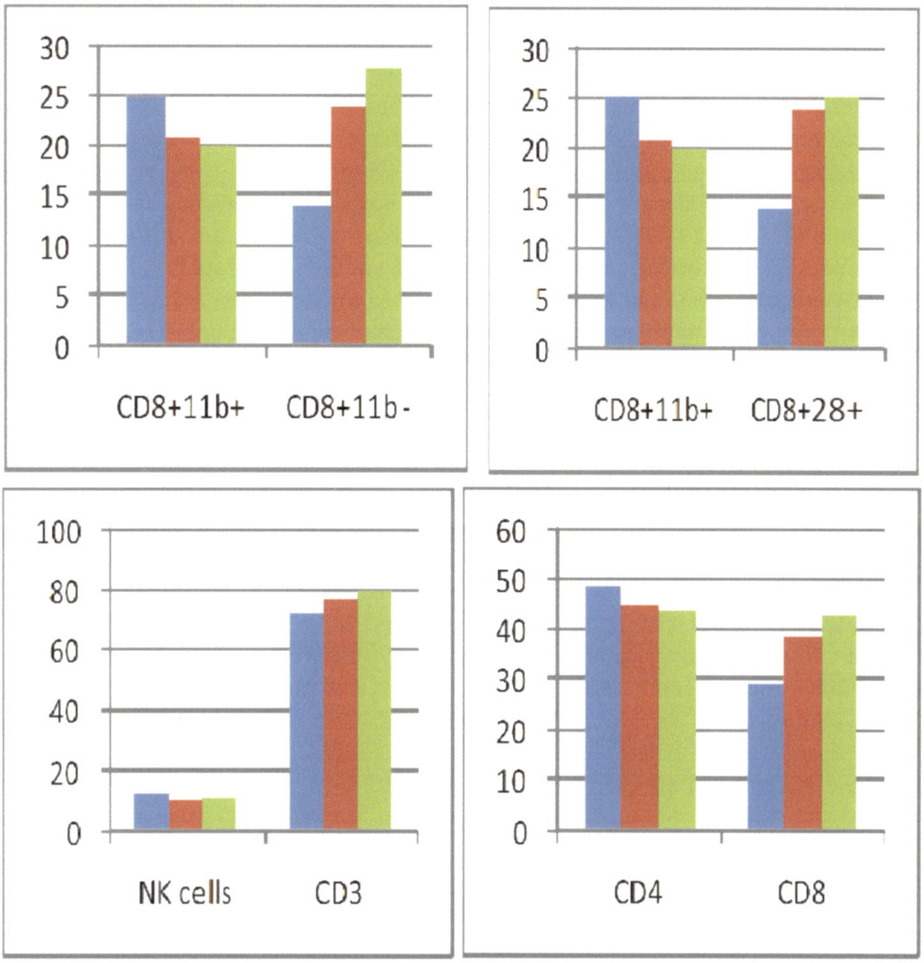

Fig. 2. Flow cytometric peripheral blood lymphocyte CD marker patterns following cellular anti - gene anti IGF-I therapy in glioblastoma multiforme. CD molecules were labelled in peripheral blood lymphocytes (PBL) obtained from prevaccinated and "vaccinated " cancer patients. Each of the first column (blue) corresponds to data obtained before vaccinations; each second and third column corresponds to data obtained after two successive cellular vaccinations. Two cases of glioblastoma were examined (every column represents the median value of two cases). The successive vaccinations consited of injections of $1.5x10^6$ to $2.0x10^6$ transfected cells. Interval between successive injections was four weeks. PBL were analyzed by flow cytometry analysis using FACScan Becton Dickinson cytometer. Double direct immunotyping with pairs of monoclonal antibodies conjugated with FITC and PE were used. Lymphocyte gate was defined according to the CD45 back gating. Data are expressed as percent of positive cells when compared to the isotype control. Difference in percentage of CD8+ CD11b- and CD8+ CD28+ subpopulations before and after vaccination was strongly significant with a range of p from 0.001 to 0.02 according to the Student's t test, and weakly significant concerning the decreasing CD8+ CD11b+ subpopulation from the relevant patients. Difference in percentage of NK, CD3, CD4 sub-populations before and after vaccinations was not significant.

months from time of diagnosis. He had been treated with conventional courses of combination chemotherapy followed by stem cell transplantation, prior to treatment with vaccine. Among five other patients treated in USA (University Hospitals of Cleveland), two of the treated patients forming a group of maximum median OS have both survived 19 months. The therapy done in USA has shown that the number of cell vaccinations (between one and four) was not related to to the median OS. Other group of three patients treated in USA, have not responded as positively to the therapy. The patient had advanced disease with cerebral oedema at the time of first treatment with vaccine, and also were receiving treatment with high dose of decadron or related steroids to reduce the effect of CNS oedema. This of course has caused further jeopardy to the immune system, and can explain the relatively negative results in three treated cases (not published data). In two of the four patients with GBM treated in Bromberg (NATO Science Programme - U.S./France/Poland), life from time of diagnosis to time of demise was 19 and 24 months. In two control treated patients, life was an average of 9,5-10 months (Trojan *et al.*, 2010). The significant clinical results were published in 2006/2007, when it was shown that using AS approach following radio- and chemotherapy, the median survival of patients reached 21 months (Trojan *et al.*, 2007a, 2007b). In 2010 we have communicated, that this relatively high median survival of glioblastoma patients could be explained by immune response related to the increase of CD28 molecules in PBL cells shown after every of two successive "vaccinations". Moreover this phenomenon was observed also in other studied tumours (four cases of liver, colon, ovary, uterus and prostate cancers (Trojan *et al.*, 2010). Histopathologic examination of resected glioblastoma tumours showed that subjects had developed peritumour necrosis and tissue bordering the necrotic tumour showed infiltration by lymphocytes consisting of both $CD8^+$ T and $CD4^+$ T cells (Wongkajornsilp *et al.*, 2011). There was no difference before or after the vaccination in the CD3, CD16+CD56, CD19, CD5, CD45 and CD14 levels.

6. Discussion

The immunosuppression phenomenon was largely described in cancer patients (Brooks *et al.*, 1981; Roszman *et al.*, 1991). TGF-beta was identified as factor suppressing T lymphocytes in tumors (Couldwell *et al.*, 1991). Surgery seems to diminish the immunosuppressive effect (Sawamura & de Tribolet, 1990). Immune response could be increased by different approaches as the injections of interferon, IL-2, activated lymphocytes, monoclonal antibodies or irradiated cells (i.e. Apuzzo & Mitchell, 1981) or using approach of IGF-I antisense treatment (Trojan *et al.*, 1993; Ly *et al.*, 2001).

Previous results have shown that tumor cells of glioma, transfected with IGF-I antisense expression vector had no longer induced tumor formation, when injected into host recipients as compared to unmanipulated cells (Trojan *et al.*, 1993). The mechanisms leading to this tumor inhibition in host animals could be drawn:

Tumor cells treated by IGF-I antisense become immunogenic to the isogenic recipients whose immune system was triggered via the novo expression of MHC-I presenting antigen as well as B7 costimulation molecule (Trojan *et al.*, 1996). The effects of antisense IGF-I and targetting to IGF-I on tumor growth could also be discussed at the molecular basis in considering the balance between survival versus death signals. Thus the role of insulin-like growth factor must also be analyzed for its inhibitotry effects on prototypical proinflammatory cytokine tumor necrosis factor alpha (TNF alpha) (Upegui-Gonzalez *et al.*, 2001). TNF alpha is a pleiotropic cytokine that promotes inflammation and signals of death.

The IGF-I antisense transfected cells, when co-transfected with vectors encoding MHC-I and/or and B-7 antisense cDNA, however maintained their previous IGF-I « antisense » morphology, the number of apoptotic cells in the cultures of the double co-transfected IGF-I antisense glioma cells decreased from 60-70 to 20-30 % (Ly *et al.,* 2001). The observation suggests that a relation could exist between immunogenicity and apoptosis in IGF-I transfected cells. They also indicate that both antigens, B-7 and MHC-I, are necessary to « render » the IGF-I antisense or triple-helix glioma cells immunogenic. The role of both B-7 and MHC-I antigens in the induction of T cell immunity against tumors has been extensively investigated (Chen *et al.,* 1992). As far as B-7 appeararance in IGF-I antisense transfected cells is considered, the absence of IGF-I synthesis would be expected to lead to a higher activation of the receptor of IGF-I (tyrosine kinase). This in turn could lead to induction in the expression of B7 antigen; enhancement in B7 co-stimulation through a cAMP mechanism linked to tyrosine kinase of the CD 28 receptor has been previously reported (Schwartz, 1992). As to the MHC-I expression, down-regulation of MHC-I due to action of IGF-I has been reported for experiments with rat thyroid cells (Saji *et al,* 1992). This would be in agreement with results reported here concerning the inverse correlation between IGF-I and MHC-I protein expression in glioma cells.

In tumor cells, the absence of IGF-I, when induced by IGF-I antisense technology, is associated with massive apoptosis. A qualitative relationship between the level of IGF-I receptor and tumorigenesis in nude mice, which correlates to the extent of apoptosis has been shown (Resnicoff *et al.,* 1996). When the function of IGF-I receptor is decreased, glioma cells undergo massive apoptosis. It was concluded for the IGF-I-R result, that this receptor activated by its ligand plays a protective role against programmed cell death. This protection was even more striking *in vivo* than *in vitro* (Resnicoff *et al.,* 1996). Another possible interpretation could be that an immune response occurring in the animals inhibits tumorigenesis. This is probably because nude mice do have a residual immune system containing both natural killer cells and B lymphocyte. The observation that C6 glioma cells transfected with IGF-I-R anti-gene approach express MHC-I (Szpechcinski *et al.,* 2004) seems to confirm that both apoptosis and an immune mechanism occur in the inhibition of tumour genesis. These IGF-I-R antisense and triple helix transfected C6 cells also express protease nexin I, which may reduce the tumourigenic potential of the C6 glioma cells injected into nude mice (Rininsland *et al.,* 1997, Shevelev *et al.,* 1997).

A further elucidation of the relationship between the immune process, related to MHC-I or HLA system (Blanchet *et al.,* 1996), and the apoptotic process is under investigation. Recently it was demonstrated that dendritic cells which are involved in tumor-immunogenicity mechanisms by activation of lymphocytes CD8 in the context of MHC-I, recognize apoptotic cells (Matthew *et al,* 1998). The last data could suggest the following mechanism of IGF-I anti - gene therapy : suppression of IGF-I – induction of MHC-I and B7 – Induction of apoptosis – involving of APC cells – induction of CD8 T cells. The relationship between two phenomenons, immunogenicity and apoptosis is crucial for the discussion of mechanism of IGF-I antisense gene therapy. Moreover, this point is capital for the selection of cell clones used in gene therapy of glioblastoma in clinical trial.

The first clinical results obtained with glioblastoma using anti – gene anti IGF-I therapy are very promising. Comparatively, the most recent chemotherapy, proposing temozolomid combined with radiotherapy, has shown in recurrent glioma patients the median progression-free survival as 10 weeks, and median overall survival as 30 weeks, respectively (Stupp *et al.,* 2005). However, median survival is the most important consideration to be taken into account (Stupp reported a 14.6 months median survival). In some cases of glioblastoma a strong association between methylation of the promoter region of the gene for 06-methylguanin-DNA methyltransferase (MGMT) and a benefit from temozolomid has been demonstrated (Hegi *et al.*, 2005). Patients whose tumours had methylation of the MGMT gene, and who received chemo-radiation, had a 2-year survival rate of 46% compared with a 2-year survival rate of less than 2% in patients whose tumours had an actively unmethylated MGMT gene. On the contrary, other studies do not support the correlation of MGMT promoter methylation. Both temozolomide/MGMT and IGF-I anti-gene approaches strongly support the strategy of individualized therapy. In the case of the IGF-I anti-gene approach the verification of MHC-I and B7 in the "vaccine" of every patient is the *sine qua non* condition for success in obtaining maximum survival.

Obviously, IGF-I was not the only growth factor target as an anti-gene approach for glioblastoma treatment. The recently studied TGF-β2 antisense compound (AP 12009) gave satisfactory results in preclinical investigations, and was introduced in a clinical phase I/II study in malignant tumours, including glioblastoma (Kaminska et al., 2005, Schlingensiepen et al., 2006). The important data have been presented in international trial since 2004: in three phase I/II dose escalation studies of GBM patients, the median overall survival time (mOS) from start of the first chemotherapy after recurrence was 44 weeks. The mOS for a patient subgroup that received temozolomide as chemotherapy before AP-12009 was 46.1 weeks. In 2007 the mOS group was 28.6 months (and 75% were still alive), and in the control group, survival was 20.2 months (and 42% remained alive). In another clinical AS TGF-beta study, a phase I clinical trial of GBM was performed using autologous tumor cells modified by a AS TGF-beta2 vector (Fakhrai et al., 1996). Six patients with progressive GBM were enrolled in the trial. Patients received 2-7 subcutaneous injections of transfected tumor cells. There were indications of humoral and cellular immunity induced by the vaccine. Two patients had partial regressions and two had stable disease following therapy. The oMS was 68 weeks. mOS of the responding patients was 78 weeks (Fakhrai et al., 1996).

The *in vitro* and *in vivo* "antisense" results obtained with IGF-I and its receptor seem more significant than those obtained with other growth factors. That is probably due to a special role playing by IGF-I among other growth factors (Pollak *et al.*, 2004; Trojan *et al.*, 2007a) – thus IGF-I via IGF-I-R, not only increases cell proliferation but "supervises" mitogenic action of other growth factors (EGF, PDGF etc.) by its autocrine-paracrine stimulation, becoming somewhat of growth factors director. As to a clinical trial of glioblastoma using the antisense IGF-I-R strategy (Andrews *et al.*, 2001) 12 patients with recurrent glioblastoma and anaplastic astrocytoma were treated using an antisense oligonucleotide directed against IGF-I-R (implantation into the rectus sheath of irradiated autologous glioma cells encapsulated in diffusion chambers, after incubation with antisense IGF-I-R). Three patients were re-treated later using the same dose of oligodeoxynucleotides. Treatment was associated with incidences of vein thrombosis, but also with a rather high rate of clinical and radiological improvements. Two complete responses and four partial responses were achieved. Two patients were alive at 168 and 134 weeks after antisense therapy. Histological analysis of tumours resected from patients with disease progression revealed lymphocytic infiltration and necrosis (Andrews *et al.*, 2001). It seems that this therapy could be more efficient if the cell "vaccines" used were prepared after cloning of IGF-I-R antisense cells for MHC-I expression (Szpechcinski *et al.*, 2004). Currently, regarding IGF-I, about 400 articles are published a year, and since 2001, more than 2000 publications deal with a relationship existing between growth factors and gliomas. In this context, the treatment of gliomas using different technologies targeting growth factors and their down stream elements, has produced a burst in use of the antisense approach, presenting almost 100 publications a year since 2005.

7. Conclusion

The presented chapter on gene therapy of GBM draws attention to the latest studies in the area of antisense cancer therapy (in relation with apoptotic and immune phenomena as well as signal transduction pathway) being among the most promising strategy of treatment of this malignant brain tumour. Although the number of "antisense" clinical trials is much lower than that of experimental preclinical therapies (Table 1), we would like to underline that every experimental therapy is a potential clinical trial, the later often depending on hospital/administrative logistics. The current clinical strategies of glioma treatment are generally a combination of chemotherapy with therapies using different types of inhibitors (imatinib, gefitinb) including antibodies (i.e. avastin) targeting growth factors and their receptors (i.e. Stupp *et al.* 2005; Reardon *et al.* 2006; Wen *et al.* 2006). The most recent therapies are now focusing on antisense technology used alone or combined also with pharmacological treatment (Dietrich *et al.* 2010). A pharmacologic strategy - the use of temozolomide, introduced by Dr R. Stupp, has offered a new hope for the treatment of this tumour. However, even though the median survival has reached almost two years, we are still far from victory (Hegi *et al.*, 2005; Gorlia *et al.*, 2008). Among the new strategies in efforts to successfully treat GBM, the use of AS approach targeting IGF-I, TGF-beta or VEGF, their receptors and their down stream transduction signalling elements (Trojan *et al.*, 2007a; Pan et al., 2007; Hau *et al.*, 2009), appears to offer hope for a promising solution.

8. References

Adams, T.E., Epa, V.C., Garrett, T.P. & Ward CV. (2000). Structure and function of the type I insulin- like growth factor receptor. *Cellular and Molecular Life Science,* Vol. 57, pp. 1050-1093.

Aggarwal, B., Schwarz, L., Hogan, M. & Rando, R. (1996). Triple helix-forming oligodeoxyribonucleotides targeted to the human tumor necrosis factor (TNF) gene inhibit TNF production and block the TNF dependent growth of human glioblastoma tumor cells. *Cancer Research, Vol.* 56, pp. 5156-5164.

Ahmad, S., Mineta, T., Martuza, R.L. & Glazer, R.I. (1994). Antisense expression of protei kinase alpha inhibits the growth and tumorigenicity of human glioblastoma cells. *Neurosurgery,* Vol. 35, No. 5, pp. 904-908.

Andrews, D. W., Resnicoff, M., Flanders, A. E., Kenyon, L., Curtis, M., Merli, G., Baserga, R., Iliakis, G. & Aiken, R. D. (2001). Results of a pilot study involving the use of an antisense oligodeoxynucleotide directed against the insulin-like growth factor type I receptor in malignant astrocytomas. *Journal of Clinical Oncology,* Vol. 19, pp. 2189-2200.

Anthony, D.D., Pan, Y., Wu, S., Shen, F. & Guo, Y. (1998) Ex vivo and in vivo IGF-I antisense RNA strategies for treatement of cancers in humans. *Advances in Experimental Medicine and Biology,* Vol. 45, pp. 27-34.

Apuzzo, M.L.J. & Mitchell, M.S. (1981). Immunonological aspects of intrinsic glial tumors. *Journal of Neurosurgery,* Vol. 55, pp. 1-18.

Ardourel, M.-Y., Blin, M., Moret, J.-L., Dufour, T., Duc, H.T., Hevor, T., Trojan, J. & Cloix, J.-F. (2007). A new putative target for antisense gene therapy of glioma: glycogen synthetase. *Cancer Biology and Therapy*, Vol. 6, No. 5, pp. 719-723.

Baserga, R. (1994). Oncogenes and strategy of growth factors. *Cell,* Vol. 79, pp. : 927-930.

Beckner, M. E., Gobbel, G. T., Abounader, R., Burovic, F., Agostino, N. R., Laterra, J. & Pollack, I. F. (2005). Glycolytic glioma cells with active glycogen synthase are sensitive to PTEN and inhibitors of PI3K and gluconeogenesis. *Laboratory Investigation,* Vol. 85, pp. 1457-1470.

Bennett, C.F., Butler, M., Cook, P.D., Geary, R.S., Levin, A.A., Mehta, R., Teng, C.L., Desmukh, H., Tillman, L. & Hardee, G. (2000). Antisense oligonucleotides - based therapeutics. In: *Gene therapy,* N.S. Templeton, D.D. Lasic, pp. 305-332, Marcel Dekker, New York

Berezikov, E., Thuemmler, F., van Laake, L.W., Kondova, I., Bontrop, R., Cuppen, E. & Plasterk, R.H. (2006). Diversity of microRNAs in human and chimpanzee brain. *Nature Genetics*, Vol. 38, No 12, pp. 1375-1377.

Biroccio, A., Leonetti, C. & Zupi, G. (2003). The future of antisense therapy: combination with anticancer reatments. *Oncogene*, Vol. 22, pp. 6579-6588.

Blanchet, O., Bourge, J.F., Zinszner, H., Israel, A., Kourilsky, P., Dausset, J., Degos, L. & Paul P. (1992). Altered binding of regulatory factors to HLA class I enhancer sequence in human tumor cell lines lacking class I antigen expression. *Proceedings of National Academy of Science USA,* Vol. 89, No 8, pp. 3488-3492.

Boado, R.J. (2005). RNA interference and nonviral targeted gene therapy of experimental brain cancer. *NeuroRx, Vol.* 2, No. 1, pp. 139-150.

Brooks, W.H., Latta, R.B. & Mahaley, M:S. (1981). Immunobiology of primary intracranial tumors. *Journal of Neurosurgery,* Vol. 54, pp. 331-337.

Campbell, M.J., Woodside, J.V., Secker-Walker, J., Titcomb, A. & Leathem, A.J. (2001). IGF status is altered by tamoxifen in patients with breast cancer. *Molecular Pathology,* Vol. 54, No. 5, pp. 307-310.

Cao, H., Lei, Z.M. & Rao, C.V. (1995). Consequences antisense human chorionic gonadotrophin-alpha subunit cDNA expression in human choriocarcinoma JAR cells. *Journal of Molecular Endocrinology,* Vol.14, No. 3, pp. 337- 347.

Chen, L., Ashe, S., Brady, W.A., Hellstrom, K.E., Ledbetter, I.A., Mc Growan, P. & Linsley PS. (1992). Costimulation of anti-tumor immunity by the B7 counter receptor for the T lymphocyte molecules CD28 and CTLA-4. *Cell,* Vol. 71, pp. 1093-1102.

Chrysis, D., Calikoglu, A. S., Ye, P. & D'Ercole, A. J. (2001). Insulin-like growth factor-I overexpression attenuates cerebellar apoptosis by altering the expression of Bcl family proteins in a developmentally specific manner. Journal of Neuroscience. Vol. 21, pp. 1481-1489.

Corsten, M.F., Miranda, R., Kasmieh, R., Krishevsky, A.M., Weisslederer, R. & Shak, R. (2007). MicroRNA-21 knockdown disrupts glioma growth in vivo and displays synergistic cytotoxicity with neural precursor cell delivered S-TRAIL in human gliomas. *Cancer Research,* Vol. 67, No. 19, pp. 8994-9000.

Couldwell, W.T., Dore-Duffy, P., Apuzzo, M.L.J. & Antel, H. (1991). Malignant glioma modulation of immune function: relative contribution of different soluble factors. *Journal of Neuroimmunology,* Vol. 31, pp. 89-96.

Culver, K. W., Rarn, Z. & Wallbridge, S. (1992). In vivo gene transfer with retroviral vector-producer cells for treatment of experimental brain tumors. *Science,* 256, pp. 1550-1552.

D'Ambrosio, C., Ferber, A., Resnicoff, M. & Baserga R. (1996). A soluble insulin-like growth factor receptor that induces apoptosis of tumor cells in vivo and inhibitstumorigenesis. *Cancer Research,* Vol. 56, pp. 4013-4020.

Daughaday, W.H., Hall, K., Raben, M.S., Salmon, W.D., Van den Brande, J.L. & Wyk, J.I. (1972). Somatomedin: proposed designation for sulphation factor. *Nature, Vol.* 235, pp. 107.

Daughaday, W.H. & Rotwein, P. (1989). Insulin-like growth factorsI and II. Peptide, messenger ribonucleic acid and gene structures, serum, and tissue concentrations. *Endocrinology Review,* Vol. 10, No. 1, pp. 68-91.

Davis, B.M., Lewin, G.R., Mendell, L.M., Jones, M.E. & Albers, K.M. (1993). Altered expression of nerve growth factor in the skin of transgenic mice leads to changes in response to mechanical stimuli. *Neurosciences,* Vol. 56, No. 4, pp. 789-792.

Dervan P. (1992). Reagents for the site-specific cleavage of megabase DNA. *Nature,* Vol. 359, pp. 87-88.

Dias, N. & Stein, C.A. (2002). Basic concepts and antisense oligonucleotides mechanisms. Molecular Cancer Therapeutics, Vol. 1, pp. 347-355.

Dietrich, P.Y., Dutoit, V., Tran Thang, N.N. & Walker, P.R. (2010). T cell immunotherapy for malignant glioma: toward a combined approach. *Current Opinion in Oncology,* Vol. 22, No. 6, pp. 604-610.

D'Mello, S., Galli, C., Ciotti, T. & Calissano P. (1993). Induction of apoptosis in cerebellar granule neurons by low potassium: inhibition of death by IGF-I and cAMP. *Proceedings of National Academy of Science USA,* Vol. 90, No. 23, pp. 10989-10993.

Fakhrai, H., Dorigo, O., Shawler, D.L., Lin, H., Mercola, D., Black, K.L., Royston, Y. & Sobol, R.E. (1996). Eradication of established intracranial rat gliomas by transforming growth factor beta antisense gene therapy. *Proceedings of National Academy of Science USA,* Vol. 93, No. 7, pp. 2909-2914.

Fonteneau, J.F., Larsson, M. & Bhardwaj, N. (2002). Interactions between dead cells and dendritic in the induction of antiviral CTL responses. *Current Opinion in Immunology,* Vol. 14, pp. 471- 477.

Froesch, C. S., Schwander, J. & Zapf, J. (1985). Actions of insulin-like growth factors. *Annual Review of Physiology,* Vol. 47, pp. 443-467.

Galderisi, U., Cascino, A. & Giordano, A. (1999). Antisense oligonucleotides as therapeutic agents. *Journal of Cell Physiology,* Vol. 181, pp. 251-257.

Geiger, T., Muller, M., Dean, N.M. & Fabbro. D. (1998). Antitumor activity of a PKC-antisense oligonucleotide in combination with standard chemotherapeutic agents against various human tumors transplanted into nude mice. *Anticancer Drug, Vol.* 13, No. 35–45. Giovannangeli C. & Hélène C. (1997). Progress in developments of triplex-based strategies. *Antisense Nucleic Acid Drug Development,* Vol. 7, pp. 413-421.

Gorlia, T., van den Bent, M.J., Hegi, M.E., Mirimanoff, R.O., Weller, M., Cairncross, J.G., Eisenhauer, E., Belanger, K., Brandes, A.A., Allgeier, A., Lacombe, D. & Stupp R. (2008). Nomograms for predicting survival of patients with newly diagnosed lioblastoma: prognostic factor analysis of EORTC and NCIC trial 26981 22981/CE.3. *Lancet Oncology,* Vol. 9, No. 1, pp. 29-38.

Green, P.J., Pines, O. & Inouye, M. (1986). The role of antisense RNA in gene regulation. *Annual Review of Biochemistry,* Vol. 55, pp. 569-597.

Gryaznov, S., Skorski, T., Cucco, C., Nieborowska-Skorska, M., Chiu, C. Y., Lloyd, D., Chen, J.K., Koziolkiewicz, M. & Calabretta, B. (1996). Oligonucleotide N3'->P5'phosphoramidates as antisense agents. *Nucleic Acids Research,* Vol. 24, pp. 1508–1514.

Hau, P., Jachimczak, P. & Bogdahn, U. (2009). Treatment of malignant gliomas with TGF-beta2 antisense olgonucleotides. *Expert Review Anticancer Therapy,* Vol. 9, No. 11, pp. 1663-1674.

Hegi, M. E., Diserens, A. C., Gorlia, T., Hamou, M. F., de Tribolet, N., Weller, M., Kros, J. M., Hainfellner, J. A., Mason, W., Mariani, L., Bromberg, J. E., Hau, P., Mirimanoff, R. O., Cairncross, J. G., Janzer, R. C. & Stupp, R. (2005). MGMT gene silencing and benefit from temozolomide in glioblastoma. *New England Journal of Medicine,* Vol. 352, pp. 997-1003.

Hélène C. (1994). Control of oncogene expression by antisense nucleic acids. *European J ournal of Cancer,* Vol. 30, No. A, pp. 1721-1726.

Izant, J.G. & Weintraub, H. (1985). Constitutive and conditional suppression of exogenous and endogenous genes by antisense RNA. *Science,* Vol. 229, pp. 345-352.

Jaattela, M. (1995): Over-expression of hsp70 confers tumorigenicity to mouse fibrosarcoma cells. *International Journal of Cancer,* Vol. 60, No. 5, pp. 689-693.

Jansen, B., Wacheck, V., Heere-Ress, E., Schlagbauer-Wadl, H., Hoeller, C., Lucas, T., Hoermann, M., Hollenstein, U., Wolff, K. & Pehamberger, H. (2000). Chemosensitization of malignant melanoma by BCL2 antisense therapy. *Lancet, Vol.* 356, pp. 1728 –1733.

Kalota, A., Shetzline, S. E. & Gewirtz, A. M. (2004). Progress in the development of nucleic acid therapeutics for cancer. *Cancer Biology and Therapy,* Vol. 3, pp. 4-12.

Kaminska, B., Wesolowska, A. & Danilkiewicz, M. (2005). TGF beta signalling and its role in tumour pathogenesis. *Acta Biochimica Polonica,* Vol. 52, pp. 329-337.

Le Roith, D., Bondy, C., Yakar, S., Liu, J. & Butler, A. (2001). The somatomedin hypothesis. *Endocrinology Review.* Vol. 22, No. 1, pp. 53-74.

Lebedeva, I.V. & Stein, C.A. Antisense downregulation of the apoptosis - related bcl-2 and bcl-xl proteins: a new approach to cancer therapy, In: *Gene therapy of cancer,* E.C. Lattime & SL Gerson, pp. 315-330, Academic Press, New York

Lichtenstein, A., Fady, C., Gera, J.F., Gardner, A., Chazin, V.R., Kelley, D. & Berenson, J. (1992). Effects of beta-2 microglobulin anti-sense oligonucleotides on sensitivity of HER2/neu oncogene-expressing and non expressing target cells to lymphocyte-mediated lysis. *Cell Immunology,* Vol. 141, No. 1, pp. 219-232.

Ly, A., Duc, H.T., Kalamarides, M., Trojan, L.A., Pan, Y., Shevelev, A., François, J.-C., Noël, T., Kane, A., Henin, D., Anthony. D.D. & Trojan J. (2001). Human glioma cells transformed by IGF-I triple-helix technology show immune and apoptotic characteristics determining cell selection for gene therapy of glioblastoma. *Journal of Clinical Pathology (Mol. Pathol.),* Vol. 54, No. 4, pp. 230-239.

Mason, J. L., Ye, P., Suzuki, K., D'Ercole, A. J. & Matsushima, G. K. (2000). Insulin-like growth factor-1 inhibits mature oligodendrocyte apoptosis during primary demyelination. *Journal of Neuroscience,* Vol. 20 pp. 5703-5708.

Matlib, M.A., Kihara, M., Farrell, C. & Dage, R.C. (1988). The Na+-Ca2+ exchange system in vascular smooth muscle cell membrane vesicles isolated from cultured cells and from tissue is similar. *Biochimical and Biophysical Acta,* Vol. 939, No. 1, pp. 173-177.

Matthew, L., Saiter, B. & Bhardwag, N. (1998). Dendritic cells acquire antigen from apoptotic cells and induce class I restricted CTL. *Nature,* Vol. 392, pp. 86-89.

Mayfield,C., Ebbinghaus, S., Gee, I., Jones, D., Rodu, B., Squibb, M. & Miller, D. (1994). Triplex formation by the human Ha-ras promoter inhibits Spl binding and in vitro transcription. *Journal of Biological Chemistry,* Vol. 69, pp. 18232-18238.

Merino, E., Balbas, P., Puente, J.L. & Bolivar F. (1994). Antisense overlapping open reading frames in genes from bacteria to humans. *Nucleic Acids Research,* Vol. 22, No. 10, pp. 19-77.

Miller, A.E. & Simek, S.L. (2000). Regulatory aspects of gene therapy, In: *Gene therapy,* NS Templeton, DD Lasic, pp. 371-382, Marcel Dekker, New York

Morishita, R., Higaki, J., Tomita, N. & Ogihara, T. (1998). Application of transcription factor "decoy" strategy as means of gene therapy and study of gene expression in cardiovascular disease. *Circ Research, Vol.* 82, pp. 1023-1028.

Okabe, M., Kunieda, Y., Miyagishima, T., Kobayashi, M., Kurosawa, M., Itaya, T., Sakurada, K. & Miyazaki, T. (1993). BCR/ABL oncoprotein-targeted antitumor activity of antisense oligodeoxynucleotides complementary to bcr/abl mRNA and herbimycin A, an antagonist of protein tyrosine kinase: inhibitory effects on in vitro growth of Ph1- positive leukemia cells and BCR/ABL oncoprotein-associated transformed cells. *Leukemia Lymphoma,* Vol. 10, No. 4-5, pp. 307-316.Pai, S.I., Lin, Y.Y., Macaes, B., Meneshian, A., Hung, C.F. & Wu, T.C. (2006). Prospects of RNA interference therapy for cancer. *Gene Therapy,* Vol. 13, N0. 6, pp. 464-477.

Pan , Q., Luo, X. & Chegini, N. (2007). Blocking neuropilin-1 function has an additive effect with anti- VEGF to inhibit tumor growth. *Cancer Cell,* Vol. 11, No. 1, pp. 53-67.

Patel, S., Doble, B. & Woodgett, J.R. (2004). Glycogen synthase kinase-3 in insulin and Wnt signalling: a double-edged sword?. Biochemical Society Transversal, Vol. 32, pp. 803-808.

Pollak, M. N., Schernhammer, E. S. & Hankinson, S. E. (2004). Insulin-like growth factors and neoplasia. *Nature Review* Cancer,Vol. 4, pp. 505-518.

Postel, E.H., Flint, S.J., Kessler, D.J. & Hogan, M.E. (1991). Evidence that a triplex-forming oligodeoxyribonucleotide binds to the c-myc promoter in HeLa cells, thereby reducing c-myc mRNA levels. *Proceedings of National Academy of Science USA, Vol.* 88, pp. 8227-8831.

Reardon, D. A., Quinn, J. A., Vredenburgh, J. J., Gururangan, S., Friedman, A. H., Desjardins, A., Sathornsumetee, S., Herndon, J. E., 2nd, Dowell, J. M., McLendon, R. E., Provenzale, J. M., Sampson, J. H., Smith, R. P., Swaisland, A. J., Ochs, J. S., Lyons, P., Tourt-Uhlig, S., Bigner, D.D., Friedman, H. S. & Rich, J. N. (2006). Phase 1 trial of gefitinib plus sirolimus in adults with recurrent malignant glioma. *Clinical Cancer Research,* Vol. 12, pp. 860-868.

Resnicoff, M., Sell, C., Rubini, M., Coppola, D., Ambrose, D., Baserga, R. & Rubin, R. (1994). Rat glioblastoma cells expressing an antisens RNA to the insulin-like growth factor receptor are non tumorigenic and induce regression of wild-type tumors. *Cancer Research,* Vol. 54, pp. 2218-2222.

Resnicoff, M., Li, W., Basak, S., Herlyn, D., Baserga, R. & Rubin, R. (1996). Inhibition of rat C6 glioblastoma tumor growth by expression of insulin-like growth factor I receptor antisense mRNA. *Cancer Immunology and Immunotherapy*, Vol. 42, pp. 64-68.

Ring, B.Z. & Roberts, J.W. (1994). Function of a nontranscribed DNA strand site in transcription elongation. *Cell*, Vol. 78, No. 2, pp. 317-324.

Rininsland, F., Johnson, T. R., Chernicky, C. L., Schulze, E., Burfeind, P. & Ilan, J. (1997). Suppression of insulin-like growth factor type I receptor by a triple-helix strategy inhibits IGF-I transcription and tumorigenic potential of rat C6 glioblastoma cells. *Proceedings of National Academy of Science USA*, Vol. 94, pp. 5854-5859.

Rivard, N., Allemain, G., Bartek, J. & Pouysségur, J. (1996). Abrogation of p27kipl by cDNA antisense suppresses quiescence in fibroblasts. *Journal of Biological Chemistry*, Vol. 271, No. 31, pp. 18337-18341.

Rosen, C.J. (1999). Serum insulin-like growth factors and insulin-like growth factor binding proteins: clinical implications. *Clinical Chemistry, Vol.* 45, No. 8, pp. 1384- 1390.

Roszman, T., Elliot, L. & Brooks, W. (1991). Modulation of T-cell function by gliomas. *Immunology today*, Vol. 12, pp. 370-374.

Rubin, R. & Baserga, R. (1995). Biology of disease. Insulin-like growth factor I receptor. Its role in cell proliferation, apoptosis and tumorigenicity. *Laboratory Investigatio*, Vol. 73, pp. 311-331.

Rubenstein, J.L., Nicolas, J.F. & Jacob, F. (1984). L'ARN non sens (nsARN) : un outil pour inactiver spécifiquement l'expression d'un gène donné in vivo [Nonsense RNA: a tool for specifically inhibiting the expression of a gene in vivo]. *Copmtes Rendus Academie des Sciences Paris*, Vol. 299, No. 8, pp. 271-274.

Saji, M., Moriarty, J., Ban, T., Singer, D. & Kohn, L. (1992). Major Histocompatibility Complex class I gene expression in rat thyroid cells is regulated by hormones, methimazole and iodide as well as interferon. *Journal of Clinical Endocrinology and Metabolism*, Vol. 75, No. 3, pp. 871-878.

Sala, A., Nicolaides, N.C., Engelhard, A., Bellon, T., Lawe, D.C., Arnold, A., Grana, X., Giordano, A. & Calabretta, B. (1994). Correlation between E2F-1requirement in the S phase and E2F-1 transactivation of cell cycle-related genes in human cells. *Cancer Research*, Vol. 54, No. 6, pp. 1402-1406.

Sawamura, Y. & deTribolet, N. (1990). Immunotherapy of brain tumors. *Journal of Neurosurgical Science, Vol.* 34, pp. 265-278.

Scaggiante, B., Morassutti, C., Tolazzi, G., Michelutti, A., Baccarani, M. & Quadrifoglio, E. (1994). Effect of unmodified triple helix-forming oligodeoxyribonucleotide targeted to human multidrug-resistance gene mdrl in MDR cancer cells. *FEBS Letters*, Vol. 352, pp. 380-384.

Schlingensiepen, R., Goldbtunner, M., Szyrah, M.N., Stauder, G., Jachimczak, P., Bogdahn, U., Schulmeyer, F., Hau, P. & Schlingensiepen, K.H. (2005). Intracerebral and intrathecal infusion of the TGF-beta2-soecific antisense phosphorothioata oligonucleotide AP 12009 in rabbits and primates: toxicology and safety. *Oligonucleotides* Vol. 15, No. 2, pp. 94-104.

Schlingensiepen, K. H., Schlingensiepen, R., Steinbrecher, A., Hau, P., Bogdahn, U., Fischer-Blass, B. & Jachimczak, P. (2006). Targeted tumor therapy with the TGF-beta2 antisense compound AP 12009. *Cytokine Growth Factor Review*, Vol. 17, pp. 129-139.

Schwartz, R.H. (1992). Costimulation of T Iymphocytes: the role ofCD28, CTLA-4 and B7/BBI in interleukin-2 production and immunotherapy. *Cell*, Vol. 71, pp. 1065-1068.

Shevelev, A., Burfeind, P., Schulze, E., Rininsland. F., Johnson, T., Trojan, J., Chernicky, C., Hélène, C., Ilan, Ju & Ilan, J. (1997). Potential triple helix-mediated inhibition of IGF-I gene expression significantly reduces tumorigenicity of glioblastoma in an animal model. *Cancer Gene Therapy*, 1997, Vol. 4, No. 2, pp. 105-112. Singh, P., Dai, B., Dhruva, B. & Widen, S.G. (1994). Episomal of sense and antisense insulin like growth factor (IGF)-binding protein-4 complementary DNA alters the mitogenic response of a human colon cancer cell line (HT-289) by mechanisms that are independent of and dependent upon IGF-I. *Cancer Research*, Vol. 54, No. 24, pp. 6563-6570. Stein, C. A. (2001). The experimental use of antisense oligonucleotides: a guide for the perplexed. *Journal of Clinical Investigation*, Vol. 108, pp. 641-644.

Stupp, R., Hegi, M. E., van den Bent, M. J., Mason, W. P., Weller, M., Mirimanoff, R. O. & Cairncross, J. G. (2006). Changing paradigms--an update on the multidisciplinary management of malignant glioma. *Oncologist*, Vol. 11, pp. 165-180.

Sussenbach, J.S., Steenbergh, P.H. & Holthuizen, P. (1992). Structure and expression of the human insulin-like growth factor genes. *Growth Regulation,*Vol. 2, No. 1, pp. 1-9. Szpechcinski, A., Trzos, R., Jarocki, P., Trojan, L. A., Oficjalska, K., Junkiert, A., Wei, M. X., Mazurek, M., Czapiewska, J. L., Niklinski, J., Kopinski, P., Chyczewski, L., Kasacka, I. & Trojan, J. (2004). Presence of MHC-I in rat glioma cells expressing antisense IGF-I-receptor RNA. *Annales Academiae Medicae Bialostocensis (Roc. Akad. Med. Bial.),* Vol. 49, No. 1, pp. 98-104.

Thomas, T., Faaland, C., Gallo, M. & Thomas, T. (1995). Suppression of c-myc oncogene Expression by a polyamine-complexed triplex forming oligonucleotide in MCF-7 breast cancer cells. *Nucleic Acids Research,* Vol. 23, pp. 3594-3599.

Trojan, J., Uriel, J., Deugnier, M.A., Gaillard, J. (1984). Immunocytochemical quantitative study of alphafetoprotein in normal and neoplastic neural development. *Developmental Neuroscience,* Vol. 6, pp. 251-259.

Trojan, J., Blossey, B., Johnson, T., Rudin, S., Tykocinski, M. & Ilan J. (1992). Loss of tumorigenicity of rat glioblastoma directed by episome-based antisens cDNA transcription of insulin-like growth factor I. *Procedings of National Academy of Science U S A*, Vol. 89, pp. 4874-4878.

Trojan, J., Johnson, T.R., Rudin, S.D., Ilan, Ju., Tykocinski, M.L. & Ilan, J. (1993). Treatment and prevention of rat glioblastoma by immunogenic C6 cells expressing antisense insulin-like growth factor I RNA. *Science*, Vol. 259, pp. 94-97.

Trojan, J., Johnson, T., Rudin, S., Blossey, B., Kelley, K., Shevelev, A., Abdul-Karim, F., Anthony, D., Tykocinski, M., Ilan, Ju. & Ilan, J. (1994) Gene therapy of murine T eratocarcinoma: separate functions for insulin-like growth factors I and II in immunogenicity and differentiation. *Proceedings of National Academy of Science USA* Vol. 91, pp. 6088-6092.

Trojan, J., Duc, H.T., Upegui-Gonzalez, L., Hor, F., Guo, Y., Anthony, D.D. & Ilan, J. (1996). Presence of MHCI and B-7 molecules in rat and human glioma cells expressing antisense IGF-I mRNA. *Neuroscience Letters,* Vol. 212, pp. 9-12.

Trojan, J., Cloix, J.-F., Ardourel, M.-Y., Chatel, M. & Anthony, D. (2007a). IGF-I biology and targeting in malignant glioma. *Neuroscience*, Vol. 145, No 3, pp. 795-812.

Trojan, J., Ly, A., Wei, M.X., Kopinski, P., Ardourel, M.-Y., Pan, Y., Trojan. L.A., Dufour, D., Shevelev, A., Andres, C., Chatel, M., Kasprzak, H., Anthony. D.D., Duc, H.T.(2010). Antisense anti-IGF-I cellular therapy of malignant tumours: immune response in cancer patients· *Biomedicine & Pharmacotherapy*, Vol. 64, No. 8, pp. 576-578.

Trojan, L.A., Kopinski, P., Mazurek, A., Chyczewski, L., Ly, A., Jarocki, P., Niklinski, J., Shevelev, A., Trzos, R., Pan, Y., Gitis, D.J., Bierwagen, M., Czapiewska, J.L., Wei, M.X., Michalkiewicz, J., Henin, D., Popiela, T., Evrard, F., Kasprzak, H., Anthony, D.D. & Trojan, J. (2003). IGF-I triple helix gene therapy of rat and human gliomas. *Annales Academiae Medicae Bialostocensis (Roc Akad Med Bial)*, Vol. 48, pp. 18-27.

Trojan LA., Ly A, Kopinski, P., Ardourel, M.-Y., Dufour, T., Duc, H.T., Kasprzak, H., Cloix, J.-F.,Wei, M.X., Chyczewski, L., Pan, Y., Chatel, M., Anthony, D.D. & Trojan, J. (2007b). Antisense and triple helix anti IGF-I tumours vaccines - gene therapy of gliomas. *International Journal of Cancer Prevention*, Vol. 2, No. 4, pp. 227-243.

Upegui-Gonzalez, L.C., Duc, H.T., Buisson, Y., Arborio, M., Lafarge-Frayssinet, C., Jasmin, C., Guo, Y. & Trojan, J. (1998). Use of antisense strategy in the treatment of the hepatocarcinoma. *Advances in Experimental Medicine and Biology,* Vol. 451, pp. 35-42.

Vasquez KM. & Wilson IH. (1998). Triplex-directed modification of genes and gene activity. *Trends in Biochemical Science,* Vol. 23, pp. 4-9.

Vitravene Study Group. (2002) A randomized controlled clinical trial of intravitreous fomivirsen for treatment of newly diagnosed peripheral cytomegalovirus retinitis in patients with AIDS. *American Journal of Ophthalmology,* Vol. 133, No. 4, pp. 467-474.

Weintraub, H., Izant, J.G. & Harland, R.M. (1985). Antisense RNA as a molecular tool for genetic analysis. *Trends in Genetics,* Vol. 1, No. 1, pp. 23-25.

Wen, P. Y., Yung, W. K., Lamborn, K. R., Dahia, P. L., Wang, Y., Peng, B., Abrey, L. E., Raizer, J.,Cloughesy, T. F., Fink, K., Gilbert, M., Chang, S., Junck, L., Schiff, D., Lieberman, F., Fine, H. A., et al. & Prados, M. D. (2006). Phase I/II study of imatinib mesylate for recurrent malignant gliomas: North American Brain Tumor Consortium Study 99-08. *Clinical Cancer Research,* Vol. 12, pp. 4899-4907.

Werner, H. & Le Roith, D. (2000). New concepts in regulation and function of the insulin-like growth factors: implications for understanding normal growth and neoplasia.*Cellular and Molecular Life Science,* Vol. 57, pp. 932-942.

Wongkajornsilp, A., Ouyprasertkul, M., Sangruchi. T., Huabprasert S, Pan, Y. & Anthony, D.D. (2001).The analysis of peri-tumour necrosis following the subcutaneous implantation of autologous tumor cells transfected with an episome transcribing an antisense IGF-I RNA in a glioblastoma multiforme subject. *J Med Assoc Thai,* Vol. 4, No. 3, pp. 740-747.

Yang, J.H., Zhang, Y.C. & Qian, H.Q. (2004). Surviving antisense oligodeoxynucleotide inhibits growth of gastric cancer cells. *World Journal of Gastroenterology, Vol.* 10, No. 8, pp. 1121-1124.

Yomo, T. & Urabe, I. (1994). A frame-specific syrnmetry of complementary strands of DNA suggests the existence of genes on the antisense strand. Journal of MolecularEvolution, Vol. 38, No. 2, pp. 113-120.

Zumkeller, W. & Westphal, M. (2001). The IGF/IGFBP system in CNS malignancy. Molecular Pathology, Vol. 54, pp. 227-229.

13

Mechanism of Hypoxia-Inducible Factor-1alpha Over- Expression and Molecular-Target Therapy for Hepatocellular Carcinoma

Dengfu Yao, Min Yao, Shanshan Li and Zhizhen Dong
Research Center of Clinical Medicine, Affiliated Hospital of Nantong University, 20 West Temple Road, China

1. Introduction

Hepatocellular carcinoma (HCC) is one of the most common and rapidly fatal malignancies worldwide and has been ranked the second highest cancer killer in China since the 1990s, particularly in the eastern and southern areas, including the inshore area of the Yangtze River (1). Multiple risk factors are associated with HCC disease etiology, with the highest incidence in patients with chronic hepatitis B virus (HBV) and hepatitis C virus (HCV), although other factors such as genetic makeup and environmental exposure are involved (2~4). As a common malignant, solid tumor, HCC is characterized by fast infiltrating growth, early metastasis, high-grade malignancy, and poor therapeutic efficacy. It is a highly vascular tumor dependent on neovascularization and one of the most common and rapidly developing malignancies (5, 6). HCC treatment options are severely limited by the frequent presence of metastases (7～10, Fig.1).

Multistep malignance of HCC progression with multigene alterations mostly accompany with chronic hepatitis and liver cirrhosis (11, 12). Hypoxia inducible factor-1 (HIF-1) is a basic-Helix–Loop–Helix Per-Arnt-Sim protein (bHLH-PAS) consisting of α and β subunits and a key transcription factor regulating cellular responses to hypoxia (13, 14), and can regulate neovascularization, activate expressions of many hypoxia-response genes, leading to closely associate with HCC ecosystem for tumor growth, infiltration, metastasis and prognosis (15~17). HIF-1α is an oxygen-dependent protein, which is degraded by poly ubiquitination and proteasomal degradation via the Von-Hippel-Lindau tumor suppressor protein under normoxic conditions (4, 18, 19). Here we briefly review the expression of rat hepatic HIF-1α and its gene during the malignant transformation of hepatocytes, the hepatic expression and circulating level of HIF-1α in patients with liver diseases for prospectively elucidating the relationship between HIF-1α level and the pathological features as well as the diagnosis and metastasis of HCC, and the effect of miRNA silencing HIF-1α gene on inhibition of $HepG_2$ cell proliferation.

2. HIF-1alpha expression and HCC development

Hepatocarcinogenesis is a complex process requiring multiple factors and multiple steps. Chemical carcinogens can induce cancer development in liver cells in a short time, with

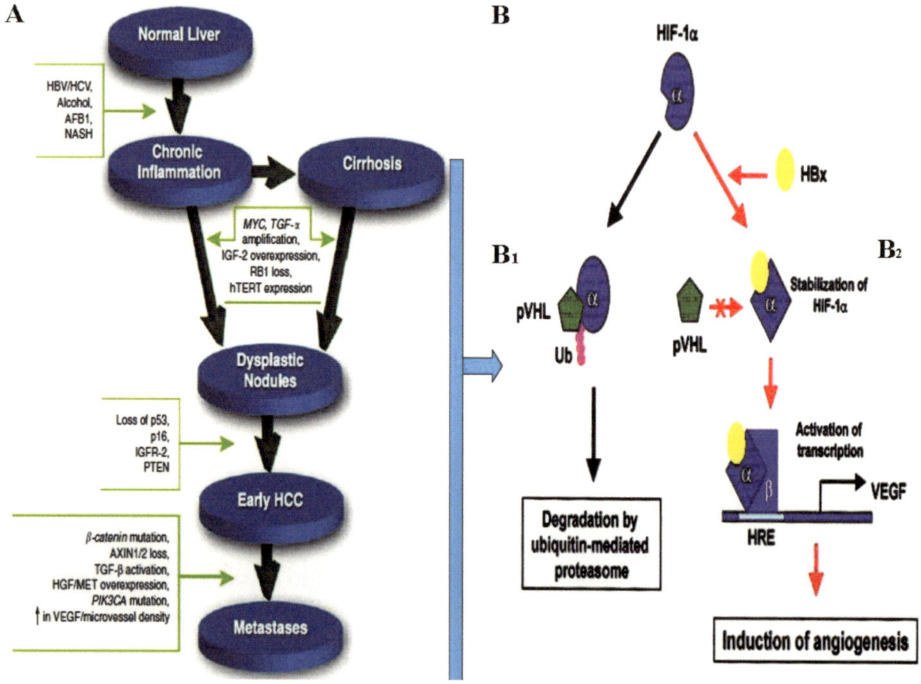

Fig. 1. HCC development and the role of hepatic HIF-1α. A, Model for the development of hepatocyte malignant transformation and the role of HIF-1α during liver tumorigenesis. The gradual replacement of cells during normal physiologic turnover is accomplished by the proliferation of the differentiated liver cells, in response to various forms of liver injury to canceration. In contrast, when parenchymal cells are unable to proliferate (e.g., in response to hepatocyte toxins), rare cells associated with the bile ducts known as oval cells expand and then differentiate to restore liver mass. The alterations of many genes result in hepatocyte and oval cell proliferation and the development of HCC. B, The role of hepatic HIF-1α. Regulation of the α-subunit is mediated by the oxygen dependent degradation domain (ODD), which contains two regulatory proline residues. Transcriptional activity of HIF-1 is facilitated by a N- vs. C-terminal transactivation domains (TAD-N vs. TAD-C) in HIF-1α. B1, Under normoxia O2 is available and hydroxylation via FIH-1 and PHDs proceeds. FIH-1 hydroxylates Asn 803 in the C-TAD of HIF-1α. This modification causes CBP/p300 to dissociate from HIF-1α, thus repressing HIF-1 transcriptional activity. PHDs hydroxylate Pro 402 and Pro 564 within the ODD of HIF-1α thereby making it available for the binding of pVHL. pVHL forms a E3-ubiquitin ligase complex with co-factors which subsequently facilitates poly-ubiquitination of HIF-1α and thus degradation by the 26S proteasome. B2, Scheme of the proposed role of HBx in the HIF-1-mediated angiogenesis of HCC. HBx interacts and stabilizes HIF-1 through inhibition of the interaction between pVHL and HIF-1 and the ubiquitin (Ub)-dependent degradation. Subsequently, HBx activates the HIF-1-dependent transcription and leads to angiogenesis. Under hypoxia O2 is limited and PHDs as well as FIH are inactive. In turn HIF-1α accumulates associates with the β-subunit and upon recruitment of the co-factor p300 forms the transcriptionally active HIF-1 complex. Activation of genes that contain HIF-responsive elements (HRE) in their promotor region follows

large-scale RNA transcription. The total RNA content gradually increases, and in the precancerous lesion, this can be significantly different from normal tissues. Angiogenesis is necessary for solid tumors larger than 1×1 mm, or the tumor remains dormant and does not metastasize. As soon as the angiogenesis stage arrives, potent metastasis is exhibited at once. The expression of HIF-1α plays important roles in angiogenesis, tumor growth, invasion, and metastasis in different cancers. We have investigated the expression of HIF-1α and its gene at the early stage of hepatocarcinogenesis, and provided the first evidence to show that HIF-1α is activated in preneoplastic hepatocytes during the early stage of carcinogenesis and long before the development of HCC.

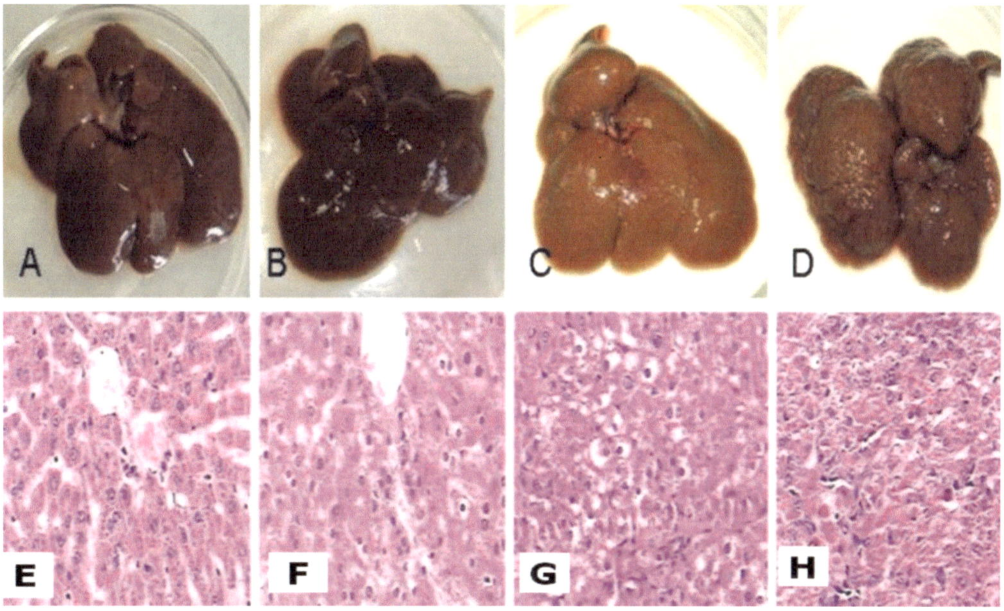

Fig. 2. Appearance of rat liver and morphological changes of rat hepatocytes during 2-FAA-induced hepatocarcinogenesis. A-D: liver appearance of control rats, at the early, middle, and late stages during the malignant transformation of hepatocytes ; E-H: corresponding histopathological images confirming normal tissue, hepatocyte degeneration, precancerous, changes and HCC (original magnification ×100), respectively.

Forty-eight male Sprague-Dawley rats, 6 weeks old, weighing 150-160 g, were purchased from the Experimental Animal Center, Nantong University, China. All animals were treated according to the guidelines of Nantong University for the Care and Use of Laboratory Animals. The rats were randomly divided into 8 groups with 6 rats per cage. One group was selected as controls while the others made up the experimental groups. Among the 7 experimental groups one served as a substitute for accidental deaths. All rats were fed with general grain, except that the grain of the hepatoma model rats contained 0.05% 2-fluorenyl-acetamide (2-FAA, Sigma Chemical Co., USA). All rats were housed under bio-clean conditions. One control rat and one experimental rat were sacrificed every 2 weeks. All surgical procedures were conducted under deep ether anesthesia. Four ml of blood was drawn from the heart and anticoagulated with EDTA-K2. Plasma and karyocytes were separated and kept at -80 °C for further analysis. After washing off the blood, one liver sample was fixed in 10% neutral buffered formalin and embedded in paraffin for pathological examination and immunohistochemical staining, and the rest were kept at -80 °C until use.

The changes of liver appearance and the pathohistology of hepatocytes during 2-FAA-induced rat HCC development are shown in Fig. 2. Apparent morphological changes (Fig. 2A-D) were confirmed pathohistologically examination (Fig. 2E-H). No pathological changes of rat hepatocytes were found in normal controls (Fig. 2E). During 2-FAA-induced hepatocarcinogenesis, granule-like degeneration in the cytoplasm of hepatocytes occurred at the early stage of hepatocarcinogenesis, with a few large and dysmorphic nuclei (degeneration group, n=18, Fig. 2F). An increase in the number of cell layers of hepatic plates was observed at the middle stage, at which there were more than 3 cell layers in some foci. Thickened chromatin in the nucleus was found, and the ratio of nucleus versus cytoplasm was elevated (precancerous group, n=9, Fig. 2G). At the late stage, the normal structure of liver tissue was completely destroyed, hepatocytes were rearranged to be nest-like and crudely cord-like, cellular nuclei were moderate in size and chromatinthickened, the ratio of nucleus versus cytoplasm was elevated, and the liver tissues were confirmed as highly differentiated (cancerous group, n=9, Fig. 2H).

Immunohistochemical staining confirmed positive expression of HIF-1α as clear and brown particles, mainly located in the cytosol and nuclei, with no staining of the plasma membrane (Fig. 3). The positive staining was mostly located in the border of hepatic terminal portal venules or near the central veins (Fig. 2A). With carcinogenesis, the rate of HIF-1α-positive expression increased and there was significantly higher intensity in the degeneration, precancerous, and cancerous groups than in the normal control (Table 1, $P < 0.05$), with a dynamically changing HIF-1α expression intensity.

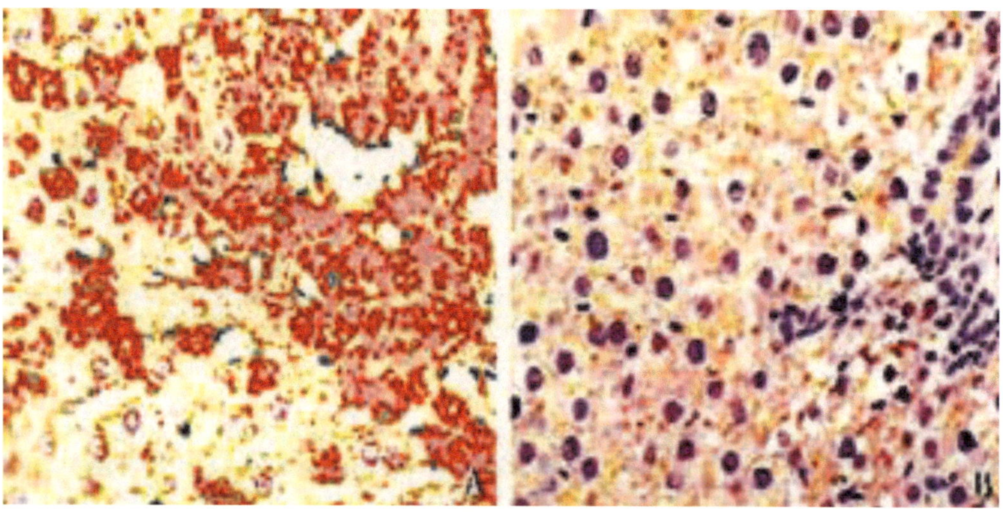

Fig. 3. Immunohistochemical staining with anti-HIF-1α in rat HCC. A: HIF-1α-positive expression in cytoplasm and cell membrane (S-P, original magnification ×200) in HCC focus from rat hepatoma; B: HIF-1α-negative expression, brown particles in cytoplasm and cell membrane (S-P, original magnification ×200) in control rats.

Group	n	Positive (%)	Intensity of HIF-1α			
			-	+	++	+++
Control	6	0 (0.0)	6	0	0	0
Degeneration	18	14(77.8)	4	9	5	0
Precancerous	9	8(88.9)*	1	2	5	1
Cancerous	9	9(100)*	0	1	2	6

<0.01, compared with the control group.

Table 1. Comparative analysis of hepatic HIF-1α expression intensity at different stages of rat hepatocarcinogenesis

Reverse-transcribed HIF-1α cDNA from hepatic HIF-1α mRNA during the malignant alteration of rat hepatocytes was amplified by nested-PCR, and the sizes of amplified fragments were identical to the original designed ones, i.e., the size of the PCR product was 500 bp in the 1st PCR and 210 bp in the 2nd PCR (Fig. 4). The amplified fragments (210 bp) of the rat HIF-1α gene from the degeneration, the precancerous, and the cancerous livers were purified and confirmed by DNA sequencing. The alignments of their nucleotide sequences at the different stages of hepatocarcinogenesis by sequencing, and no alteration of the amplified gene fragment was found during the malignant alteration of rat hepatocytes.

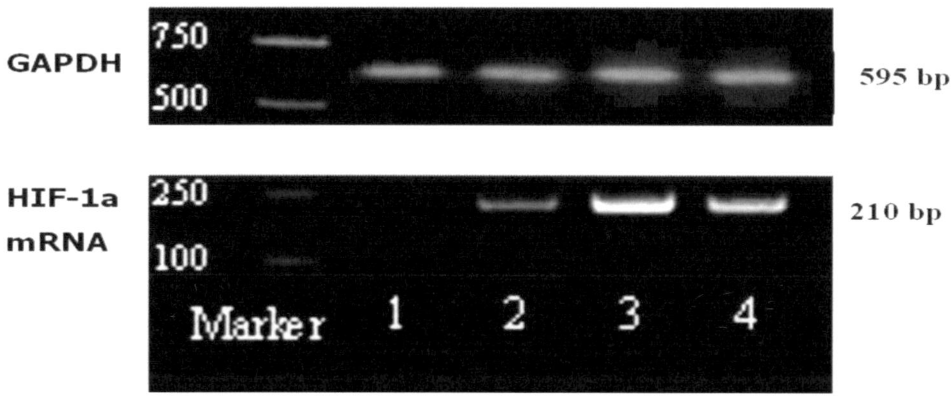

Fig. 4. Amplification and alteration of HIF-1α gene from rat hepatoma tissues. In order to obverse the alteration of HIF-1α at RNA level, HIF-1α mRNAs were synthesized to HIF-1α cDNA with random hexamers and moloney murine leukemia virus reverse-transcriptase, and detected with different primer pairs by nested PCR (210bp). The amplified positive fragments of HIF-1α gene were distinctly found in rat hepatoma tissues. HIF-1α mRNA in rat liver (Lanes. 1-4). Lane 1: control rat; lane 2: Degeneration rat; lane 3: precancerous rat; lane 4: HCC rat; marker: DNA molecular weight marker.

The levels of total RNA and HIF-1α mRNA expression in rat liver tissues during the malignant alteration of hepatocytes are shown in Table 2. The expression of total RNA and HIF-1α mRNA with histological alteration of hepatocytes was observed in the rats after treatment with 2-FAA, progressing from granule-like degeneration to precancerous lesions to HCC. The levels increased markedly in the cancerous group and the precancerous lesion group, and the incidence of amplified HIF-1α mRNA dynamically increased as hepatocytes changed from normal to granule-like denaturation to precancerous and cancerous lesions. Induction of HIF-1α mRNA expression was detected in all the liver tissues of the cancerous group and parts of the precancerous lesion and degeneration group, i.e., 44.4% in the hepatocyte degeneration group, 77.8% in the precancerous lesion group, and 88.9% in the HCC group. It was significantly higher in the cancerous group than in the degeneration and the control groups, and the precancerous lesion group was also significantly higher than the normal control.

Group	n	Total RNA (μg/mg liver)	HIF-1α mRNA (%)
Control	6	1.58±0.49	0 (0.0)
Degeneration	18	1.91±0.60	8 (44.4)
Precancerous	9	2.00±0.21*	7 (77.8)*
Cancerous	9	2.86±0.60*	8 (88.9)*

*$P<0.05$, compared with the control group.

Table 2. Dynamic alterations of total RNA and amplification of HIF-1α mRNA in liver tissues at different stages of rat hepatocarcinogenesis

Nested PCR results revealed that HIF-1α mRNA was induced in hepatoma, precancerous and degenerative tissues, but was not expressed in normal tissues. During the course of cancer development, the levels of HIF1α mRNA in precancerous tissues were higher than in normal and degenerating tissues, and the levels of HIF-1α mRNA in HCC tissues were even higher than in precancerous tissues. The activation of HIF-1α gene transcription may participate in the signal transmission of cancer development. In the early stage, the expression of HIF-1α mRNA and HIF-1α was at low levels. In the advanced stage of cancer development, the expression of HIF-1α mRNA and HIF-1α was at high levels. The preneoplastic hepatic lesions showed increased levels of HIF-1α and HIF-1α mRNA compared with the normal liver. So the upregulation of hepatic HIF-1α protein synthesis and HIF-1α mRNA levels strongly suggest that HIF-1α participates in the development of HCC. The expression of HIF-1α gradually increased along with the histological changes, it was significantly higher in premalignant tissues than in the control group, and it may be related to the activation of signal pathways.

The quantitative data of hepatic and circulating HIF-1α expression are shown in Table 3. The HIF-1α levels showed a tendency to increase with the histopathological changes: cancerous group > precancerous lesion group > hepatocyte degeneration group > control group. The levels were markedly higher in the cancerous and precancerous lesion groups than in the hepatocyte degeneration and normal control groups. As a result of its low molecular weight, HIF-1α is easily released into the blood, leading to a higher concentration there. Blood levels in the precancerous lesion group were higher than in the hepatocyte degeneration and normal control groups ($P<0.05$). The HIF-1α blood levels in the cancerous group were markedly higher than in any other group ($P<0.05$). An apparent positive correlation between the levels in blood and liver samples was found ($r=0.474$, $P = 0.030$). The expression level of HIF-1α gradually increased both in liver cells and blood. The increasing tendency of hepatic and circulating HIF-1α was synchronized, suggesting that the increasing expression of HIF-1α is closely related to the malignant transformation of hepatocytes.

Group	n	HIF-1α in blood (μg/mg NP)	HIF-1α in liver (μg/mg)
Control	6	206.3±18.6	9.8±2.9
Degeneration	18	277.2±96.1	12.6±3.2
Precancerous	9	401.6±178.8*	16.9±2.2*
Cancerous	9	445.9±138.9*	23.5±8.7*

*$P<0.05$, compared with the control group.

Table 3. Quantitative analysis of HIF-1α dynamic expression in circulation and liver tissues at different stages of rat hepatocarcinogenesis

Increasing evidence suggests that HIF-1 activation occurs in the early stages of carcinogenesis. HIF-1α genes are overexpressed in morphologically normal single cells, forming multicellular foci or microcysts similar to overt HCC. HIF-1α was also shown to be expressed in a few cells in ductal hyperplastic areas adjacent to invasive cancer, and their malignant counterparts. Furthermore, HIF-1α genes were shown to be overexpressed in hyperplastic and dysplastic lesions during multistage carcinogenesis. Recent new findings from several laboratories have implicated constitutive activation of the transcription factor NF-κB as one of the early key events involved in neoplastic progression of chronic liver disease. Further studies will permit us to analyze mechanism of human hepatocarcinogenesis and to know how to target HIF-1α sites or RNA interference-mediated suppression of HIF-1α expression for HCC therapy. However, the combination of the pathological features of HIF-1α expression and some of the biomarkers with high sensitivity and specificity for early HCC seems to be more practical so far.

3. Expression difference in human HCC tissues

The self-controlled HCC and para-cancerous specimens (2 cm to cancer) were collected from 35 patients who underwent operations for liver cancer at the Affiliated Hospital of Nantong University. The specimens were immediately frozen in liquid nitrogen and kept at -85°C until required. The patients included 28 men and 7 women, ranging in age from 22 to 70 years. Prior written informed consent was obtained from all patients according to the World Medical Association Declaration of Helsinki, and the study received ethics board approval from the Affiliated Hospital of Nantong University. The histological types of all HCC specimens were graded in differentiation degrees as follows: well, 9; moderate, 12; and poor, 14. Of these specimens, 20 showed single tumor tubercles and the rest multiple; 14 were stage II, 13 were stage III, and 8 were stage IV. Each specimen was analyzed by total RNA abstraction and pathologic examination.

The expressions and cellular distribution of HIF-1α in HCC tissues and comparative analysis with their para-cancerous tissues are shown in Fig. 5. The positive HIF-1α was brown and granule-like, mainly presented in cytoplasm and few in nucleus, with obvious differences of HIF-1α positive expression intensity among different areas of tissues. HIF-1α staining in paracancerous tissues was showing significantly in the compressed hepatic cords and central veins. The intensity of HIF-1α expressions was significantly higher in paracancerous tissues than that in HCC, mainly due to more necrosis in the latter, representing that there is a very close relationship between high intensity of HIF-1α expressions and active proliferation or hypoxia microenvironment in paracancerous tissues. The distribution of positive cells was well-distributed and higher in adjacent areas of necrosis and tumor infiltration in HCC (Fig.5A), whereas it was showing significantly in the compressed hepatic cords and the border of central veins in the para-cancerous tissues (Fig.5B). Moreover, the HIF-1α positive staining was significantly higher (P=0.017) in the para- cancerous group (100%, 35 of 35) than in the corresponding HCC group (80%, 28 of 35). The intensity of hepatic HIF-1α expression was also higher in the para-cancerous tissues than in the HCC tissues (Z =4.728, P< 0.001, Table 4).

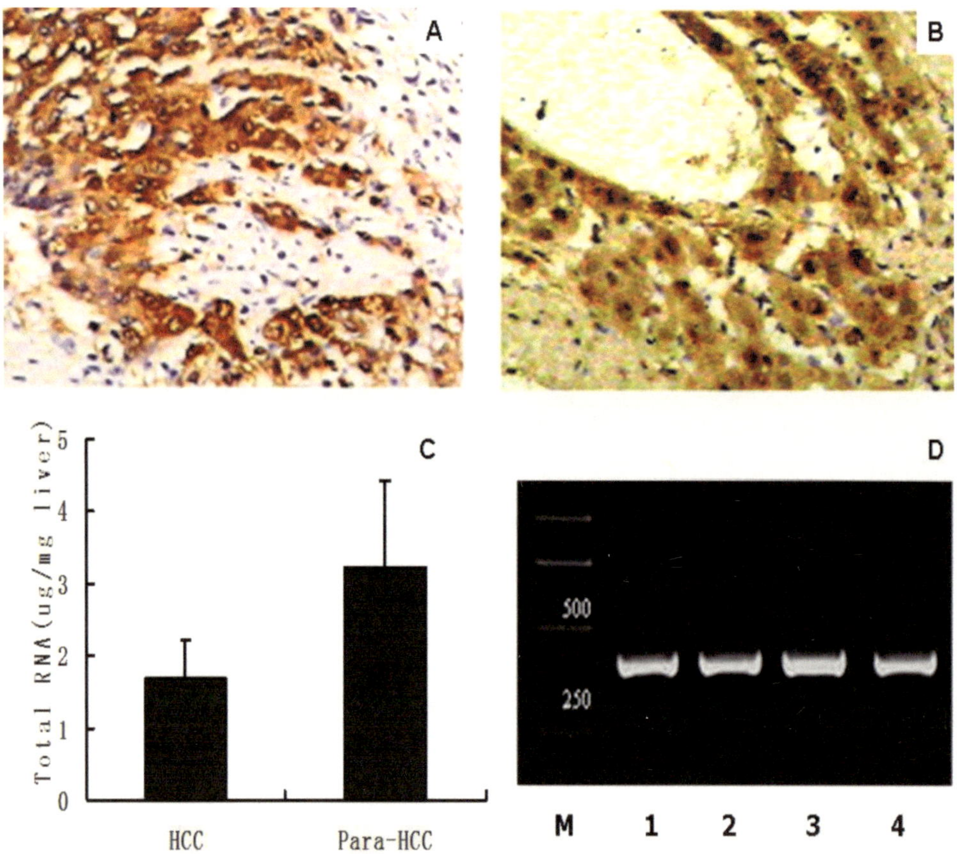

Fig. 5. Immunohistochemical staining of HIF-1α, total RNA levels and amplification of HIF-1α mRNA in HCC or their paracancerous tissues. Hepatic HIF-1α expression with brown particles in cytoplasm and cell membrane, A, the HCC tissue; B, the para-cancerous tissue (S-P, original magnification × 200). C, the levels of total RNA expression in HCC or their paracancerous tissues; D, the HIF-1α mRNA was synthesized to HIF-1α cDNA and amplified by nested PCR (349 bp), Line 1, 2, the amplified fragment of HIF-1αmRNA in HCC tissues; Line 3, 4, the amplified fragment of HIF-1αmRNA in para-cancerous tissues; M, DNA marker with molecular weight standard. HCC, the hepatocellular carcinoma tissues; Para-HCC, the para-cancerous tissues.

HCC is mostly characterized by uncontrolled growth of tumor cells. Increasing oxygen consumption results in hypoxic microenvironment. HIF-1α expression is significantly high in adjacent areas of necrosis and tumor infiltration. Many factors, such as hypoxia, oncogenes activation, inactivation of tumor suppressors, growth factors, inflammatory factors, can up-regulate HIF-1α expressions, directly or indirectly promoting more than 2 %

human genes transcriptions, which are all related to oxygen and energy metabolism. Productive nucleic acids metabolism, abnormal gene expressions, development of HCC are closely associated with surrounding vessels state and hypoxic conditions (20).

Group	n	Positive (%)	*P* value*	HIF-1α intensity				Z value	*P* value*
				−	+	++	+++		
HCC	35	28 (80.0)	0.017	7	21	7	0	4.728	0.000
Para-HCC	35	35 (100)		0	10	18	7		

**P* value *vs* the paracancerous tissue group; HCC, the hepatocellular carcinoma tissues.

Table 4. The comparative analysis of HIF-1α expression intensity in HCC or their paracancerous tissues

```
          2452                                                                        2521
HIF-1a    ctcatccaag aagccctaac gtgttatctg tcgctttgag tcaaagaact acagttcctg aggaagaact
HCC       ---------- ---------- ---------- ---------- ---------- ---------- ----------
Para-HCC  ---------- ---------- ---------- ---------- ---------- ---------- ----------

          2522                                                                        2591
HIF-1a    aaatccaaag atactagctt tgcagaatgc tcagagaaag cgaaaaatgg aacatgatgg ttcacttttt
HCC       ---------- ---------- ---------- ---------- ---------- ---------- ----------
Para-HCC  ---------- ---------- ---------- ---------- ---------- ---------- ----------

          2592                                                                        2661
HIF-1a    caagcagtag gaattggaac attattacag cagccagacg atcatgcagc tactacatca ctttcttgga
HCC       ---------- ---------- ---------- ---------- ---------- ---------- ----------
Para-HCC  ---------- ---------- ---------- ---------- ---------- ---------- ----------

          2662                                                                        2731
HIF-1a    aacgtgtaaa aggatgcaaa tctagtgaac agaatggaat ggagcaaaag acaattattt taataccctc
HCC       ---------- ---------- ---------- ---------- ---------- ---------- ----------
Para-HCC  ---------- ---------- ---------- ---------- ---------- ---------- ----------

          2732                                                                       2800
HIF-1a    tgatttagca tgtagactgc tggggcaatc aatggatgaa agtggattac cacagctgac cagttatga
HCC       ---------- ---------- ---------- ---------- ---------- ---------- ---------
Para-HCC  ---------- ---------- ---------- ---------- ---------- ---------- ---------
```

Fig. 6. Alignment of the amplified fragments of HIF-1α gene and homology analysis of their sequences. The HIF-1α mRNA from cancerous tissue and para-cancerous tissue of HCC patients was synthesized to HIF-1α cDNA and amplified by nested PCR (349 bp) and confirmed by sequencing. No mutation was found between HCC tissues and para-cancerous tissue. HIF-1α: the cited sequence (349 bp, nt 2452-2800) of human HIF-1α genome (NM_001530); HCC, the amplified fragment of HIF-1α genome from HCC tissues; Para-HCC, the amplified fragment of HIF-1α genome from their paracancerous tissues.

Hepatic total RNA was purified from human HCC or their para- cancerous tissues, the specific concentrations of total RNA were 12.4 ± 7.3 μg/mg wet liver in the HCC group, and 53.8 ± 52.0 μg/mg wet liver in the para-cancerous group (Fig.5C), with significant difference between them (t = 3.05, P < 0.01). The final amplified fragment of hepatic HIF-1α gene was 349 bp (Fig.5D), and the incidence was 85.7% in the HCC group and 100 % in the para-cancerous group (P > 0.05). The amplified fragments of HIF-1α gene were confirmed by sequencing, with consistent completely with the cited sequence of human HIF-1α gene (Fig.6). The level of total RNA was obviously higher in paracancerous tissues than in HCC, indicating HIF-1αmRNA involved in cell proliferation, neovascularization and metastasis and could be a prime target for gene therapy.

4. Expression of circulating HIF-1α in HCC

One hundred thirty-one of HCC patients, 30 of chronic hepatitis, 22 of acute hepatitis, and 37 of cirrhosis were diagnosed at the Affiliated Hospital of Nantong University, Nantong, China, and 27 healthy people obtained from the Nantong Central Blood Bank as controls (Table 5). All cases were diagnosed by blood biochemical tests, with negative hepatitis viral markers (HBsAg, and anti-HCV antibody), normal alanine aminotransferase (ALT) levels, and B-ultrasonic examination. All samples (5 mL of peripheral blood) were collected in the morning and sera were separated at once. The serum AFP concentrations exceeded 50 μg/L were taken as a positive result. The diagnosis of HCC and viral hepatitis was based on the criteria proposed by Chinese National Collaborative Cancer Research Group (21) and at the Chinese National Viral Hepatitis Meeting (22), respectively.

Group	n	Sex M/F	Age (Year)	HBsAg (+/-)	AFP (μg/L)		
					≤20	21-399	≥400
HCC	131	109/22	33-85	100/31	20	57	54
LC	37	16/21	20-82	23/14	24	11	2
CH	30	25/5	18-63	22/8	18	11	1
AH	22	17/5	24-80	10/12	18	4	0
NC	27	12/15	26-69	0/27	27	0	0

HCC, hepatocellular carcinoma; LC, liver cirrhosis; CH, chronic hepatitis; AH, acute hepatitis; NC, normal control.

Table 5. Patients' data in the present study

The levels of circulating HIF-1α expression in 220 patients with liver diseases are shown in Table 6. The circulating HIF-1α level was increased, especially in patients with chronic liver diseases. If the cutoff value of serum HIF-1α level was >50 μg/L, the incidence of HIF-1α abnormality was 100 % in HCC, 89.2% in LC, 66.7 % in CH, none in AH or NC, respectively; And the cutoff values rise to 100 μg/L, the abnormality of circulating HIF-1α level was 90.8% in HCC and 27.0% in LC, none in CH or AH or NC, respectively. The level of serum

HIF-1α in HCC patients was significantly higher ($P < 0.001$) than those in cases with benign liver diseases.

The prognosis of HCC is poor, and early detection is of the utmost importance. Treatment options are severely limited by the frequent presence of metastases. Although the mechanisms of hepatocarcinogenesis have not been elucidated, a long-lasting inflammation induced by hepatitis virus infection is a definite risk for neoplastic degeneration and accumulation of genetic alterations. The fragments of circulating HIF-1α could be detected in all patients with HCC with extrahepatic metastasis; like circulating IGF-II, these results argue for growth factor–dependent HCC development and could provide novel markers of severity and prognosis for HCC. The present data indicate that the expression levels of serum HIF-1α, Ang-2, and VEGF could be detected only in the peripheral blood of patients with HCC.

Group	n	HIF-1α (μg/L)		>50 μg/L	>100 μg/L
		Ranges	Mean ± SD	n (%)	n (%)
HCC	131	57.5~208.5	136.3 ± 28.8	131(100)	119(90.8)
LC	37	39.1~123.4	84.6 ± 25.9*	33(89.2)	10(27.0)*
CH	30	38.0~96.4	58.8 ± 14.5*[a]	20(66.7)*	0(0)*
AH	22	33.1~48.8	37.6 ± 5.3*[bc]	0(0)*	0(0)*
NC	27	20.3~31.9	24.1 ± 3.3*[de]	0(0)*	0(0)*

*$P < 0.001$, *vs* the HCC group ; [a]$P < 0.001$, *vs* the liver cirrhosis group ($q = 4.39$) ; [b]$P < 0.01$ *vs* the chronic hepatitis group ($q = 3.17$) ; [c]$P < 0.001$, *vs* the liver cirrhosis group ($q = 7.31$) ; [d] $P < 0.001$, *vs* the chronic hepatitis group ($q = 5.47$) ; [e]$P < 0.001$, *vs* the liver cirrhosis group ($q = 9.99$) ; HCC, hepatocellular carcinoma; LC, liver cirrhosis; CH, chronic hepatitis; AH, acute hepatitis; NC, normal control.

Table 6. Quantitative analysis of circulating HIF-1α level (mean ± SD) in patients with liver diseases

The evaluation of serum HIF-1α and AFP levels for HCC diagnosis using the ROC curves is shown in Fig.7. The advantage of analyzing two markers over the whole range of sensitivities and specificities using the area (0.854 in AFP, 0.909 in HIF-1α) under ROC curves indicated that the abnormality of serum HIF-1α level could be a useful seroloical marker for HCC diagnosis.

5. Quantitative detection of VEGF and Ang-2

The levels of serum VEGF and Ang-2 were detected and the concentrations were calculated using a standard curve generated with specific standards. Inter and intra-assay variances were lower than 10%. The levels of circulating VEGF and Ang-2 expression in patients with chronic liver diseases are shown in Table 7. Like circulating HIF-1α expression, the circulating VEGF and Ang-2 levels were increased in patients with chronic liver diseases, especially in HCC patients. If the cutoff value with >280 μg/L for VEGF and >35 μg/L for

Ang-2, the incidence of VEGF and Ang-2 were 87.0 % and 94.7 % abnormality in HCC, 12.7 % and 2.9 % in LC, 13.3 % and 0% in CH, both none in NC, respectively.

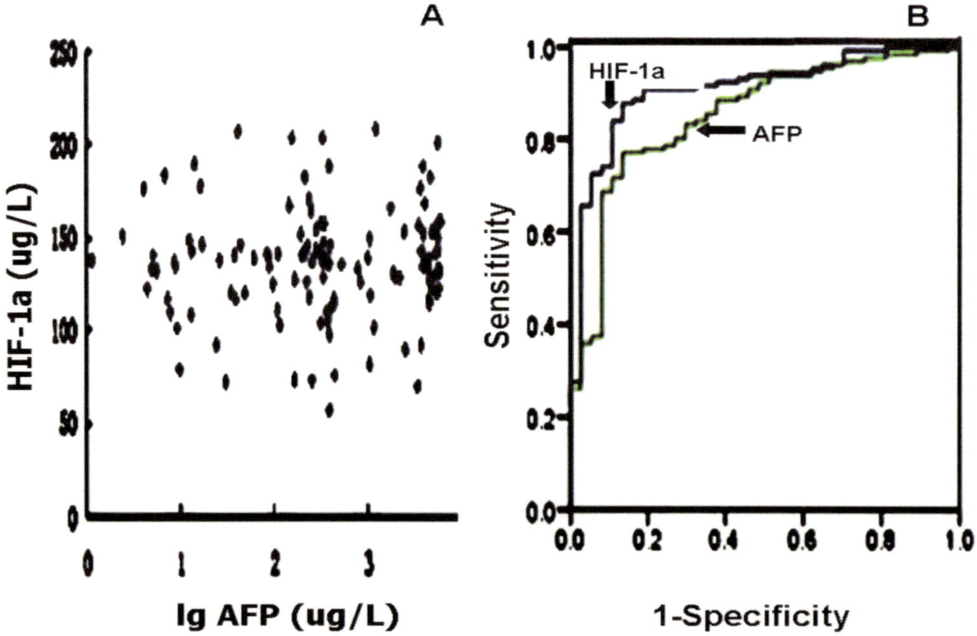

Fig. 7. The relationship between circulating HIF-1α and AFP levels and receiver operating characteristic (ROC) curves. A, the scatter diagram of circulating HIF-1α and AFP levels in HCC patients, and no significant relationship was found between circulating HIF-1α and AFP levels; B, ROC curves for circulating HIF-1α and AFP investigated markers for HCC. Sensitivity = true-positive rate; specificity = false-positive rate; and the area under ROC curves was 0.854 for AFP and 0.909 for HIF-1α. Sensitivity and specificity were calculated according to the following formulas: Sensitivity = a/(a+c); and Specificity = d/ (b+d), where a = true-positive cases, b = false-positive cases, c = false- negative cases, and d = true-negative cases. ROC curves were constructed by calculating the sensitivities and specificities at several cutoff points, and indicated that both of circulating HIF-1α and AFP level be useful molecular markers for HCC diagnosis.

HCC is known to contain aberantly vascularized regions characterized by severe hypoxia. Hypoxia can stimulate cell proliferation, induce angiogenesis, accelerate invasion and is also responsible for treatment resistance in HCC. Activation of oncogenes or inactivation of tumor suppressors can change signaling pathway and up-regulate HIF-1α expression, leading to HIF-1α activation. Under hypoxic conditions it can be stabilized, binding to the specific sites of hypoxia-response target genes, regulating proliferation on transcriptional level and activating expression of many hypoxia-response genes, which are closely relevant with energy metabolism, angiogenesis, infiltration, metastasis and prognosis. The frequency of circulating HIF-1α and its diagnostic value increased with distal metastases of HCC hepatocytes. The pathological characteristics of serum HIF-1α associated with the levels of circulating VEGF and Ang-2 expression, the size of tumor and extra-hepatic metastasis, and but not to patients' gender, age, and AFP level.

Group	n	VEGF (μg/L)	>280 μg/L	Ang-2 (μg/L)	>35 μg/L
		Mean ± SD	n (%)	Mean ± SD	n (%)
HCC	131	462.7±119.2	114(87.0)	40.8±3.5	124(94.7)
LC	37	216.3±54.5*	6(16.2)*	25.5±5.8*	1(2.7)*
CH	30	160.9±98.2*	4(13.3)*	20.9±7.1*	0(0)*
NC	27	140.9±54.5*	0(0)*	17.4±2.6*	0(0)*

*$P < 0.001$, *vs* the HCC group ; HCC, hepatocellular carcinoma; LC, liver cirrhosis; CH, chronic hepatitis; NC, normal control.

Table 7. The levels of circulating VEGF and Ang-2 expression in patients with chronic liver diseases

6. Clinicopathological features of HIF-1α expression

The clinicopathological characteristics of circulating HIF-1α expression in HCC patients are shown in Table 8. Significant difference was found between high HIF-1α expression and tumor size (P=0.007) or HCC with extra-hepatic metastasis (P< 0.001), but not with patients' gender, age, or AFP level. There was a very close relationship between circulating HIF-1α level and VEGF ($r=0.937$, $P<0.001$) or Ang-2 ($r= 0.933$, $P < 0.001$), suggesting that high expression of HIF-1α associated with HCC metastasis and poor prognosis.

Clinical pathological features of HIF-1α expression indicated that HIF-1α expression intensity and positive rate was lower in HCC than in paracancerous tissues, which were in accordance with total RNA. HIF-1α positive rate was associated with tumor diameter, because they were usually singles, enveloped, well-differentiated, more diplonts and less heteromorphism when tumors were small. With tumors swelling, the biological characteristics have changed, developed into the opposite. Therefore, the invasion is strengthened, and tumor blood supply can not satisfy growth demand. HBx and HIF-1α are presented in cytoplasm in HCC. Moreover, HBx can up-regulate HIF-1α under normoxia or hypoxia, reinforce HIF-1α transcriptional activity via MAPK pathway, increase HIF-1α protein levels, induce neovascularization and contribute to metastasis. No correlation was found between HIF-1α and HBsAg positive in HCC and further studies whether it associates with HBV replication are required.

7. Effect of miRNA silencing HIF-1α gene on HCC

In order to investigate the effect of miRNA silencing HIF-1α gene on inhibition of $HepG_2$ cell proliferation. Recently, we constructed the eukaryotic expression plasmids of HIF-1αmiRNA and report gene containing hypoxia-reponse element. After $HepG_2$ cells transfection with plasmid, the expression of HIF-1α gene and protein were determined by real time-PCR or Western blotting. The expressions of HIF-1α, VEGF, and Ang-2 were quantitatively detected by ELISA. The alterations of cell cycles and apoptosis rate were quantitatively measured by flow cytometry or Annexin V-FITC/PI double dyeing assay.

At 72h After $HepG_2$ cell transfection with HIF-1αmiRNA, the down- regulation of HIF-1α was 87% at mRNA or 56% at protein level, and the decreasing of target gene was 46% in the report gene, 54% in VEGF and 36% in Ang-2, respectively. The apoptotic ratio of $HepG_2$ cells was 22.46 ± 0.61% ($P < 0.01$), and the cell cycle changed greatly at the ratio of G_1 (61.49±1.12%) and S phase (22.40± 0.58%, $P < 0.01$). After the cells combined with doxorubicin, the apoptotic ratio increased to 36.99 ± 0.88%. The ratio of G_1 and S phase were upregulated to 65.68 ± 0.91% and 19.47 ± 1.34%. HIF-1αmiRNA or / and doxorubicin can regulate the growth cycle, promote apoptotic and inhibit proliferation of $HepG_2$ cells.

Group		n	HIF-1α(μg/L)	*t* value	*P* value
HCC		131	136.3 ± 28.8		
Sex	Male	109	137.4 ± 28.7	1.009	0.315
	Female	22	130.7 ± 29.0		
Age	≥ 50y	98	133.7 ± 30.1	1.702	0.091
	<50y	33	143.2 ± 24.0		
Tumor size	≥ 5.0 cm	53	144.4 ± 26.3*	2.721	0.007
	<5.0 cm	78	130.8 ± 29.2		
AFP(μg/L)	≥ 400.0	53	136.9 ± 25.8	0.201	0.841
	< 400.0	78	135.9 ± 30.7		
HBsAg	Positive	100	137.9 ± 29.6	1.712	0.089
	Negative	31	129.2 ± 25.5		
EHT	Yes	49	152.5 ± 21.5**	5.522	0.000
	No	82	126.6 ± 28.3		

*$P < 0.01$, *vs* the tumor size less than 5㎝ group; **$P < 0.001$, *vs* the non- extrahepatic metastasis group; HCC, hepatocellular carcinoma; EHT, Extra- hepatic metastasis.

Table 8. The pathological characteristics of HIF-1α levels (mean ± SD) in sera of HCC patients.

8. Perspectives

HCCs exhibit numerous genetic abnormalities as well as epigenetic alterations including modulation of DNA methylation (23, 24). Molecular factors are involved in the process of HCC development and metastasis (25~27). Recent findings from several laboratories have implicated constitutive activation of the transcription factor NFkappa B as one of the early key events involving in neoplastic progression of the liver. Further studies will permit us to analyze mechanism of human hepatocarcinogenesis and pay attention to these areas (28~31). However, the hepatic HIF-1α expression is associated with development and prognosis of HCC, and circulating HIF-1α level is a useful molecular marker in HCC diagnosis, and monitor prognosis (32~36). HIF-1α expression in hepatic tissues plays an important role in development and prognosis of HCC. HIF-1α, as an initial hypoxia moderator, should be a promising molecular-target for the development of anti-HCC agents (37~40). The intensity of HIF-1α expressions was significantly higher in paracancerous tissues than in HCC, mainly due to more necrosis in the latter, representing that there is a very close relationship between high intensity of HIF-1α expressions and active metabolism or hypoxia microenvironment in paracancerous tissues and HIF-1α could be a molecular-target for gene therapy (41, 42).

9. Acknowledgments

Our studies were supported in part by Grants-in-Aid from the Natural Science Foundation (BK2008187), and from the Medical Science (H200925) of Jiangsu Province, China.

10. References

[1] Tang ZY. Small hepatocellular carcinoma: current status and prospects. Hepatobiliary Pancreat Dis Int. 2002; 1(3): 349-353.

[2] Raza SA, Clifford GM, Franceschi S. Worldwide variation in the relative importance of hepatitis B and hepatitic C viruses in hepatocellular carcinoma: a systematic review. Br J Cancer 2007, 96: 1127-1134.

[3] Hui KM. Human hepatocellular carcinoma: Expression profiles-based molecular interpretations and clinical applications. Cancer Lett 2009, 286: 96-102.

[4] Feo F, Frau M, Tomasi ML, Brozzetti S, Pascale RM. Genetic and epigenetic control of molecular alterations in hepatocellular carcinoma. Exp Biol Med (Maywood). 2009; 234(7): 726-736.

[5] Liu LP, Liang HF, Chen XP, Zhang WG, Yang SL, Xu T, et al. The role of NF-kappaB in Hepatitis b virus X protein-mediated upregulation of VEGF and MMPs. Cancer Invest. 2010; 28(5): 443-451.

[6] Dong ZZ, Yao DF, Wu W, Yao M, Yu HB, Shen JJ, et al. Delayed hepatocarcinogenesis through antiangiogenic intervention in the nuclear factor-kappa B activation pathway in rats. Hepatobiliary Pancreat Dis Int. 2010; 9(2): 169-174.

[7] Yao DF, Dong ZZ, Yao M. Specific molecular markers in hepatocellular carcinoma. Hepatobiliary Pancreat Dis Int. 2007; 6(3): 241-247.

[8] Whittaker S, Marais R, Zhu AX. The role of signaling pathways in the development and treatment of hepatocellular carcinoma. Oncogene. 2010; 29(36): 4989–5005.

[9] Schmid T, Zhou J, Brüne B. HIF-1 and p53: communication of transcription factors under hypoxia. J Cell Mol Med, 2004; 8(4): 423-431.

[10] Moon EJ, Jeong CH, Jeong JW, Kim KR, Yu DY, Murakami S, et al. Hepatitis B virus X protein induces angiogenesis by stabilizing hypoxia-inducible factor- 1alpha. FASEB J, 2004; 18(2): 382-384.

[11] Xie H, Song J, Liu K, Ji H, Shen H, Hu S, et al. The expression of hypoxia- inducible factor-1alpha in hepatitis B virus-related hepatocellular carcinoma: correlation with patients' prognosis and hepatitis B virus X protein. Dig Dis Sci 2008; 53: 3225-3233

[12] Daskalow K, Pfander D, Weichert W, Rohwer N, Thelen A, Neuhaus P, et al. Distinct temporospatial expression patterns of glycolysis-related proteins in human hepatocellular carcinoma. Histochem Cell Biol 2009; 132: 21-31

[13] Mabjeesh NJ, Amir S. Hypoxia-inducible factor (HIF) in human tumorigenesis. Histol Histopathol 2007, 22(5): 559-572.

[14] Patiar S, Harris AL. Role of hypoxia-inducible factor-1alpha as a cancer therapy target. Endocr Relat Cancer 2006, 13: S61-75

[15] Weidemann A, Johnson RS. Biology of HIF-1alpha. Cell Death Differ 2008, 15: 621-627.

[16] Liao D, Johnson RS. Hypoxia: a key regulator of angiogenesis in cancer. Cancer Metastasis Rev 2007, 26: 281-290.

[17] Copple BL, Bustamante JJ, Welch TP, Kim ND, Moon JO. Hypoxia-inducible factor-dependent production of profibrotic mediators by hypoxic hepatocytes. Liver Int 2009; 29: 1010-1021

[18] Semenza GL. Regulation of oxygen homeostasis by hypoxia-inducible factor 1. Physiology (Bethesda) 2009; 24: 97-106

[19] Brahimi-Horn C, Mazure N, Pouyssegur J. Signalling via the hypoxia- inducible factor-1alpha requires multiple posttranslational modifications. Cell Signal 2005; 17: 1-9

[20] Yao DF, Jiang H, Yao M, Li YM, Gu WJ, Shen YC, et al. Quantitative analysis of hepatic hypoxia-inducible factor-1alpha and its abnormal gene expression during the formation of hepatocellular carcinoma. Hepatobiliary Pancreat Dis Int 2009; 8: 407-413

[21] The Liver Cancer Committee of Chinese Anticancer Association. Diagnostic criteria of primary hepatocellular carcinoma. Zhonghua Ganzang Bing Zazhi. 2000; 8: 135. [in Chinese]

[22] The Group of Viral Hepatitis Research. The prevention and cure scheme of viral hepatitis. Zhonghua Ganzang Bing Zazhi. 2000; 8: 324-329. [in Chinese]

[23] Qian J, Yao D, Dong Z, Wu W, Qiu L, Yao N, et al. Characteristics of hepatic igf-ii expression and monitored levels of circulating igf-ii mRNA in metastasis of hepatocellular carcinoma. Am J Clin Pathol. 2010; 134(5): 799-806.

[24] Yao D, Jiang D, Huang Z, Lu J, Tao Q, Yu Z, Meng X. Abnormal expression of hepatoma specific gamma-glutamyl transferase and alteration of gamma- glutamyl transferase gene methylation status in patients with hepatocellular carcinoma. Cancer. 2000; 88(4): 761-769.

[25] Yoo YG, Kong G, Lee MO. Metastasis-associated protein 1 enhances stability of hypoxia-inducible factor-1alpha protein by recruiting histone deacetylase 1. EMBO J 2006; 25: 1231-1241

[26] Ripoli M, D'Aprile A, Quarato G, Sarasin-Filipowicz M, Gouttenoire J, Scrima R, et al. Hepatitis C virus-linked mitochondrial dysfunction promotes hypoxia- inducible factor 1alpha-mediated glycolytic adaptation. J Virol 2010; 84: 647-660

[27] Cummins EP, Berra E, Comerford KM, Ginouves A, Fitzgerald KT, Seeballuck F, et al. Prolyl hydroxylase-1 negatively regulates IkappaB kinase-beta, giving insight into

hypoxia-induced NFkappaB activity. Proc Natl Acad Sci USA 2006; 103: 18154-18159

[28] Walmsley SR, Print C, Farahi N, Peyssonnaux C, Johnson RS, Cramer T, et al. Hypoxia-induced neutrophil survival is mediated by HIF-1alpha-dependent NF-kappaB activity. J Exp Med 2005; 201: 105-115

[29] Shin DH, Li SH, Yang SW, Lee BL, Lee MK, Park JW. Inhibitor of nuclear factor-kappaB alpha derepresses hypoxia-inducible factor-1 during moderate hypoxia by sequestering factor inhibiting hypoxia-inducible factor from hypoxia-inducible factor 1alpha. FEBS J 2009; 276: 3470-3480 [PMID: 19456861]

[30] van Uden P, Kenneth NS, Rocha S. Regulation of hypoxia-inducible factor- 1alpha by NF-kappaB. Biochem J 2008; 412: 477-484

[31] Buchler P, Reber HA, Tomlinson JS, Hankinson O, Kallifatidis G, Friess H, et al. Transcriptional regulation of urokinase-type plasminogen activator receptor by hypoxia-inducible factor 1 is crucial for invasion of pancreatic and liver cancer. Neoplasia 2009; 11: 196-206

[32] Hamaguchi T, Iizuka N, Tsunedomi R, Hamamoto Y, Miyamoto T, Iida M, et al. Glycolysis module activated by hypoxia-inducible factor 1alpha is related to the aggressive phenotype of hepatocellular carcinoma. Int J Oncol 2008; 33: 725-731

[33] Forooghian F, Das B. Anti-angiogenic effects of ribonucleic acid interference targeting vascular endothelial growth factor and hypoxia- inducible factor-1alpha. Am J Ophthalmol 2007; 144: 761-768

[34] Nasimuzzaman M, Waris G, Mikolon D, Stupack DG, Siddiqui A. Hepatitis C virus stabilizes hypoxia-inducible factor 1alpha and stimulates the synthesis of vascular endothelial growth factor. J Virol 2007; 81: 10249-10257

[35] Dong ZZ, Yao DF, Yao M, Qiu LW, Zong L, Wu W, et al. Clinical impact of plasma TGF-beta1 and circulating TGF-beta1 mRNA in diagnosis of hepatocellular carcinoma. Hepatobiliary Pancreat Dis Int. 2008; 7(3): 288- 295.

[36] Lee TK, Poon RT, Yuen AP, Ling MT, Wang XH, Wong YC, et al. Regulation of angiogenesis by Id-1 through hypoxia-inducible factor-1alpha-mediated vascular endothelial growth factor up-regulation in hepatocellular carcinoma. Clin Cancer Res 2006; 12: 6910-6919

[37] Zhu H, Chen XP, Luo SF, Guan J, Zhang WG, Zhang BX. Involvement of hypoxia-inducible factor-1-alpha in multidrug resistance induced by hypoxia in HepG2 cells. J Exp Clin Cancer Res 2005; 24: 565-574

[38] Wada H, Nagano H, Yamamoto H, Yang Y, Kondo M, Ota H, et al. Expression pattern of angiogenic factors and prognosis after hepatic resection in hepatocellular carcinoma: importance of angiopoietin-2 and hypoxia- induced factor-1 alpha. Liver Int 2006; 26: 414-423

[39] Yao DF, Wu XH, Zhu Y, Shi GS, Dong ZZ, Yao DB, et al. Quantitative analysis of vascular endothelial growth factor, microvascular density and their clinicopathologic features in human hepatocellular carcinoma. Hepatobiliary Pancreat Dis Int. 2005; 4(2): 220-226.

[40] Wu W, Yao DF, Yuan YM, Fan JW, Lu XF, Li XH, et al. Combined serum hepatoma-specific alpha-fetoprotein and circulating alpha- fetoprotein-mRNA in diagnosis of hepatocellular carcinoma. Hepatobiliary Pancreat Dis Int. 2006; 5(4): 538-544.

[41] Kulshreshtha R, Davuluri RV, Calin GA, Ivan M. A microRNA component of the hypoxic response. Cell Death Differ 2008; 15: 667-671

[42] Takahashi Y, Nishikawa M, Takakura Y. Inhibition of tumor cell growth in the liver by RNA interference-mediated suppression of HIF-1α expression in tumor cells and hepatocytes. Gene Ther 2008, 15: 572-582.

14

Cancer Gene Therapy via NKG2D and FAS Pathways

Yanzhang Wei, Jinhua Li and Hari Shankar R. Kotturi
Clemson University
USA

1. Introduction

NKG2D (natural-killer group 2, member D) belongs to a sub-family of C type lectin-like receptors. NKG2D is a homodimeric, type II transmembrane glycoprotein (Wolan et al., 2001). The *NKG2D* gene is located in the NK gene complex which is on chromosome 6 in the mouse (Ho et al., 1998) and chromosome 12 in human (Glienke et al., 1998). Like most activating receptors, NKG2D is a multi-subunit receptor complex. Signaling in NKG2D is mediated by specialized signaling adaptors. In mouse NKG2D associates with two distinct adaptors: DAP-10 and DAP-12/KARAP (Diefenbach et al., 2002a), while in human NKG2D exclusively uses DAP-10 (Rosen et al., 2004). Non-covalent interactions are responsible for these associations (Diefenbach et al., 2002b). One NKG2D homodimer associates with two DAP-10 dimers to form a hexameric complex (Garrity et al., 2005). Two distinct NKG2D isoforms (NKG2D-S and NKG2D-L) are expressed in mouse as a result of alternative exon usage and are responsible for differential adaptor associations. The short (NKG2D-S) and long (NKG2D-L) isoforms differ by their 13 NH_2-terminal amino acids. While DAP-10 associates with both NKG2D isoforms, the extended cytoplasmic domain of NKG2D-L prevents the association with DAP-12 (Diefenbach et al., 2002a; Rosen et al., 2004). NKG2D-L is constitutively expressed in resting NK cells. In contrast, the abundance of NKG2D-S increases considerably upon NK cell stimulation with cytokines (Rabinovich et al., 2006).
NKG2D has the ability to interact with a significant number of distinct ligands with affinities ranging from 4 to 800nM (Carayannopoulos et al., 2002a; O'Callaghan et al., 2001; Li et al., 2001). Both chains of the NKG2D homodimer contribute to the interaction with the different monomeric ligands, making contacts with either the α1 or α2 domain of the ligand. Thus, the symmetric, homodimeric NKG2D receptor binds asymmetric ligands, and the contribution of the individual NKG2D chains is unequal (Radaev et al., 2002; Mc Farland et al., 2003). It is surprising that mouse and human NKG2D, which are only 69% identical in their ectodomains, can recognize most ligands of the other species (Mc Farland et al., 2003).

1.1 Expression of NKG2D receptor

The NKG2D receptor is constitutively expressed on most innate immune effector cells of lymphoid origin, including NK cells, most TCR γδ T cells (Jamieson et al., 2002), and a large fraction of NKT cells (Jamieson et al., 2002; Gumperz et al., 2002). Functional NKG2D is also found on murine interferon producing killer dendritic cells (IKDC) which are of myeloid origin (Taieb et al., 2006) interferon producing killer dendritic cells (IKDC) which are of myeloid origin (Taib et al., 2006; Chan et al., 2006). On adaptive immune system cells, NKG2D is constitutively expressed on all human CD8+ T cells and on activated and memory (but not on naive) CD8+ αß T cells in the mouse (Jamieson et al., 2002). NKG2D is not normally expressed on CD4+ T cells (Table 1).

	Human	Mouse
NK cells	All NK cells	All NK cells
TCRαβ T cells	Naïve, activated and memory CD8+ T cells Subpopulation of Synovial and circulating CD4+ T cells in rheumatoid arthritis patients	Activated and memory CD8+ T cells Not express on naïve CD8+ T cells Not express on CD4+ T cells
TCRγδ T cells	Most blood and IEL TCRγδ T cells	25% of splenic TCRγδ T cells Large fraction of NKT cells
NKT cells	ND	
DC	ND	IKDC subset
Macrophages	ND	Only mRNA

Table 1. Pattern of NKG2D receptor expression in human and in mouse. IEL: intestinal intraepithelial lymphocytes. IKDC: interferon producing killer dendritic cells. ND: not determined. (Coudert and Held, 2006).

1.2 Function of NKG2D receptor

Human NKG2D signals exclusively via DAP-10, while mouse NKG2D associates with both DAP-10 and DAP-12. Upon NKG2D engagement, DAP-12 recruits ZAP-70 and Syk protein tyrosine kinases with the help of its immunoreceptor tyrosine-based activation motif (ITAM) (Lanier et al., 1998). It has been observed that mouse deficient for DAP-12 retained significant NKG2D-dependent NK cell mediated killing (Diefenbach et al., 2002a; Zompi et al., 2003). Moreover, NK cells from Syk/ZAP-70 deficient mouse also retained significant lytic activity. In contrast, DAP-10 lacks an ITAM but instead contains a YINM motif. Upon engagement of human NKG2D, the recruitment of the p85 subunit of phosphatidylinositol 3- kinase (PI3-K) (Wu et al., 1999) and of Grb2 to DAP-10 occurs (Chang et al., 1999). Both p85 and Grb2 have to be recruited to DAP-10 for full calcium flux and cell-mediated cytotoxicity (Upshaw et al., 2006). The residual lytic activity observed in DAP-12 deficient mice was abrogated when pharmacological blockade of Src family kinases and PI3-K, which act down-stream of DAP-10, were used (Colucci et al., 2002), indicating that DAP-10 is crucial for NK cell cytotoxicity. The NKG2D/DAP-10 complex triggers granule release and cytotoxicity following NKG2D crosslinking in human NK cells (Billadeau et al., 2003). Thus, ITAM-independent, DAP-10- dependent signaling triggers NKG2D-dependent cytotoxic function in NK cells.

Besides NK cells, NKG2D receptors are constitutively expressed in human CD8+ T cells and upon activation in mouse CD8+ T cells. Since T cells generally lack DAP-12 expression, NKG2D signaling occurs exclusively via DAP-10 in humans and in mice. In T cells, NKG2D serves as co-stimulatory and in some instances, as primary activation function. In CD8+ T cells NKG2D engagement enhances T cell activation rather than induces activation (Groh et al., 2001; Maasho et al., 2005). Prolonged exposure of T cells derived from human intestinal epithelium to high amounts of IL-15 changes NKG2D function and expression by up-regulating DAP-10 (Roberts et al., 2001).

1.3 NKG2D ligands

NKG2D ligands are structurally similar to MHC class I molecules. The number of NKG2D ligands currently known stands at seven both in humans and mice. In humans these ligands are grouped into two families: the MHC-class-I-polypeptide related sequence A (MICA) and MICB protein family and the other family including cytomegalovirus UL16-binding protein (ULBP; also known as RAET1 proteins) consisting of five members (ULBP1–ULBP4 and RAET1G) (Bahram et al., 1994; Chalupny et al., 2003; Bacon et al., 2004). NKG2D ligands are variable in both their amino acid sequence and domain structure. MICA, for example, only shares 20–25% sequence identity with ULBP molecules (Radosavljevic et al., 2002). In mice there are five retinoic acid early transcript 1 (RAE1) proteins and the minor histocompatibility protein H60 and MULT (Diefenbach et al., 2003).

All ligands share an MHC-class-I-like α1α2 domain that binds to NKG2D. The MICA and MICB proteins also have an additional α3 domain. The RAE1 proteins in mice and ULBP1, ULBP2 and ULBP3 in humans are glycosylphosphatidylinositol (GPI)- anchored receptors. By contrast, MICA, MICB, ULBP4, RAET1G, H60 and MULT1 possess transmembrane domains and cytoplasmic tails (Eagle and Trowsdale, 2007). The *ULBP* genes are clustered in the telomeric region of human chromosome 6; a corresponding region with NKG2D ligands is found on mouse chromosome 10. The *MICA* and *MICB* genes are localized within the human HLA locus on chromosome 6, which also harbors orthologous MHC class I related *Rae* genes (Radosavlievic et al., 2002). Some NKG2D ligands are polymorphic, over 70 distinct alleles have been identified in MIC genes (Radosavljevic et al., 2002). Even though the number of NKG2D ligands in humans and mice are same, phylogenetic analysis shows that these ligands have almost certainly diversified independently from each other (Raulet et al., 2003).

1.4 NKG2D ligand expression

The expression of NKG2D ligands are induced by a wide variety of stimuli referred as "cellular stress", which includes tumorigenesis (Gasser et al., 2005), infection by a variety of pathogens (Lodoen et al., 2006), classic cell-stress stimuli such as heat shock (Venkataraman et al., 2007) and, also, as a result of Toll-like receptor (TLR) signaling (Nedvetzki et al., 2007). The aberrant expression of NKG2D ligands has also been linked with autoimmune diseases, including rheumatoid arthritis, coeliac disease and autoimmune diabetes (Hue et al., 2004). Not much is know about the precise mechanisms that lead to upregulation of NKG2D ligands. In cancer, NKG2D ligand expression has been associated with activation of the DNA-damage response pathways by genotoxic stress (Gasser et al., 2005). The triggers for switching on of NKG2D-ligand expression during infection have not yet been well defined (Eagle and Trowsdale, 2007).

1.5 NKG2D ligands and tumor

A large fraction of tumor cells express NKG2D ligands constitutively. MICA/B expression is detected on many types of epithelial tumor cell lines of different tissue origins (Bauer et al., 1999; Jinushi et al., 2003; Groh et al., 1999; Groh et al., 1998). In contrast, ULBPs are preferentially expressed on T cell leukemia cell lines (Pende et al., 2002) as well as on freshly isolated lymphoid leukemia cells. RAE-1 and H60 are up-regulated in skin treated with carcinogens (Girardi et al., 2001) and are found on skin, renal and lung carcinoma cell lines (Girardi et al., 2001; Smyth et al., 2002). The murine NKG2D ligands H60 and RAE-1 are also found on numerous hematopoietic tumor cell lines (Lowin-Kropf et al., 2002). In some cases, NKG2D ligand up-regulation has been observed to be associated with transformation, having both oncogene and tumor suppressor roles. Embryonic fibroblasts deficient for JunB show an enhanced expression of RAE-1ϵ and MULT1. JunB exerts tumor suppressor activity through the negative regulation of c-jun function (Deng et al., 1993). The chronic activity of the DNA damage response pathways have also been implicated to be responsible for the constitutive expression of NKG2D ligands such as RAE-1, MULT1 in mouse lymphoid tumor cell lines (Gasser et al., 2005).

1.6 MULT1 ligand

Murine ULBP-like transcript 1 (MULT1) is a ligand of NKG2D receptor. NKG2D receptors present on the effector cells recognize and bind to MULT1 on target cells. The cDNA sequence of MULT1 consists of a full length open reading frame (ORF) of 1.1 Kb and encoding a protein with a molecular weight of 37.1 KD. MULT1 protein is a type I transmembrane protein with an N-terminal signal sequence of 25 aa, two class I MHC like α domains (89 aa and 91 aa, respectively), a transmembrane domain 17 aa and a cytoplasmic domain of 109 aa. Compare to other NKG2D ligands MULT1 lacks α3- like domain and the GPI trans amidation site (Diefenbach et al., 2003).

MULT1 protein is a glycoprotein with two ectodomains containing four N-glycosylation sites and one O-glycosylation site. Sequence alignments of MULT1 with other known mouse NKG2D ligands such as H60, Rae1ß and other known human NKG2D ligands such as MICA, ULBP1 and MHC-1, reveals that MULT1 protein is distantly related to known NKG2D ligands, which are in turn distantly related to MHC class I proteins. The sequence identity of MULT1 with known human ligands like MICA and ULBP1, are 16.7% and 29.9% respectively, thus MULT1 is closely related to the members of human ULBP family (Diefenbach et al., 2003).

1.6.1 Expression of MULT1 ligand

MULT1 mRNA is detected in a wide variety of tissues such as thymus, spleen, lymph nodes, and to a lesser extent liver and heart, but is not detected in kidney or brain. However, surface expression of MULT1 is not detected in lymph node, liver or kidney cells, suggesting that MULT1 may be regulated post-transcriptionally (Diefenbach et al., 2003).

MULT1 mRNA expression has been observed in multiple tumor cell lines like YAC-1, WEH17.1, A20, P815, S49.1, BW5147 and TRAMP-C1. In WEHI7.1, S49.1 and BW5147 T cell lymphomas, and the P815 mastocytoma, MULT1 is the only known NKG2D ligand expressed in the cells. Other cell lines such as A20 B cell lymphoma and TRAMP-C1 prostate carcinoma coexpress MULT1 and RAE1 ligands (Diefenbach et al., 2003). The finding that MULT1, like RAE1 and H60 family members, is expressed by multiple tumor cell lines suggests that MULT1 contributes to immune surveillance in tumors (Diefenbach et al., 2002b).

1.6.2 Function of MULT1 ligand

High-level expression of NKG2D ligand on a tumor cell helps the tumor cell to overcome class 1-mediated inhibition of NK cells resulting in its cell lysis (Carayannopoulos et al., 2002). Tumor cells expressing high levels of MULT1 are highly susceptible to NK mediated lysis and strongly induce IFN-γ production in freshly isolated, as well as IL-2 expanded, NK cells. MULT1 also induces the production of nitric oxide in activated macrophages. When ectopically expressed by tumor cells, MULT1 induces a very potent antitumor response *in vivo* resulting in strong rejection of the transduced tumor cells in syngeneic B6 mice. Interestingly, the MULT1-transduced tumor cells have been observed to prime the mice, rendering them immune to the tumor antigens of the parental tumor cell (Diefenbach et al., 2003). Tumor cells expressing different NKG2D ligands such as MULT1, RAE1ß and/or H60 can induce protective immunity against multiple tumor cell lines such as RMA, B16-BL6 and EL4 (Hayakawa et al., 2002).

MULT1 protein has a K_D of 6 nM and K_{off} of ~0.006 S^{-1} which is several times lower than RAE1є and H60 (K_D ~ 10-30 nM). MULT1 has a $t_{1/2}$ of ~ 2 min, longer than either H60 (~ 20 s) or RAE1 α-δ (~ 5s). These results indicate that MULT1 binds NKG2D with the highest affinity of all known ligands and has a half life longer than all known NKG2D ligands (Carayannopoulos et al., 2002a). Thus, three distinct MHC class 1-like molecules in the mouse, H60, RAE1є and MULT1 bind NKG2D with high affinity despite low mutual sequence identity (<20%).

Evolutionary advantage of selecting such a complicated receptor ligand system is two-fold. First, the functional consequences of NKG2D engagement are pleiotropic, involving T cell co-stimulation, NK cell activation, macrophage stimulation, and possibly regulation of fetal development (Diefenbach et al., 2000; Groh et al., 2001). Precise execution of these diverse functions requires multiple genes with distinct promoter/enhancer sequences, posttranslational controls, and even kinetics of binding. Second, microbes exert enormous selective pressure to diversify immune-related functions, albeit at differing rates (Klein et al., 1993; Khakoo et al., 2000). Recent evidence suggests that human CMV interferes with the NKG2D system using the *UL16* gene product to bind ULBP1 and ULBP2 (Cosman et al., 2001) also, mouse CMV gp40 downregulates H60 (Krmpotic et al., 2002). Pathogen-encoded factors such as these might have selected for NKG2D-binding partners which retain receptor specificity but lack susceptibility to interference or subversion (e.g., ULBP3, which does not bind to UL16), resulting in the current repertoire of dissimilar NKG2D ligands (Carayannopoulos et al., 2002).

1.7 Escape mechanism by tumors

Tumors have developed many distinct mechanisms that would allow them to escape the detection by NKG2D expressing effector cells. As cancer progresses, immune pressure on the tumor may lead to selection of cells devoid of NKG2D ligands. It has been observed in cancer patients that most primary tumors seem to express NKG2D ligands, whereas more advanced tumors and metastases express very low level ligand (Vetter et al., 2004; Raffaghello et al., 2005). This leads to selection of variants with low levels of NKG2D ligands.

NKG2D ligand cleavage has been observed in some tumors. Metalloproteinases can cleave MICA/B off the cell surface of tumor cells (Doubrovina et al., 2003) reducing their cell surface levels and limiting recognition by NKG2D-expressing effector cells. In addition, soluble NKG2D ligands such as MICA in the serum, upon binding to NKG2D, induce the internalization and lysosomal degradation of the NKG2D receptor on CD8+ T cells and NK cells (Doubrovina et al., 2003; Jinushi et al., 2003), reducing the efficiency of NKG2D recognition.

TGF-ß, a major immunosuppressive cytokine produced by tumor cells also decreases the surface expression of MICA, effecting tumor cell recognition by CD8+ T and NK cells (Friese

et al., 2004). *In vitro* experiments have shown that NK cells cultured in the presence of TGF-ß down-regulated NKG2D receptor expression (Lee et al., 2004). It has been reported that IFN-γ can render certain susceptible target cells resistant to NK cell responses *in vitro* and *in vivo*. This has been attributed to an up-regulation of MHC class I molecules, which are recognized by inhibitory NK cell receptors (Bui et al., 2006).
Research has also shown that sustained NKG2D ligand encounters can promote NK cell dysfunction *in vitro* and *in vivo*. The enforced constitutive expression of NKG2D ligands such as RAE-1ß, RAE-1ϵ and MICA as transgenes in mice impair NKG2D functions *in vivo* (Wiemann et al., 2005). This observed NKG2D dysfunction also raises the possibility that CD8+ T cells and human NK cells may similarly be susceptible to inactivation.

1.8 NKG2D ligands diversity

Even though NKG2D ligands are not functionally equivalent, their roles are redundant to some extent (Komatsu et al., 1999). The evolutionary advantage for the presence of diverse NKG2D ligands can be explained with 3 possible reasons: 1) escaping immune recognition, 2) evading tumor responses and 3) tissue specific function (Eagle and Trowsdale, 2007).

1.8.1 Escaping immune recognition

In nature, both host and pathogen are under natural selection pressure to diversify and refine their defense strategies in response to improvements made by their competitor. It has been observed that viruses, such as human cytomegalovirus (HCMV), MCMV, Influenza A, and Epstein-Barr virus, induce NKG2D ligands in infected cells (Draghi et al., 2007; Pappworth et al., 2007). As an escape mechanism HCMV deploys immunoevasin proteins such as UL16 that can bind to MICB, ULBP1, ULBP2 and RAET1G and prevent the expression of NKG2D ligands, helping the virus to escape immune recognition (Cosman et al., 2001; Chalupny et al., 2003; Bacon et al., 2004). Since viruses have evolved mechanisms to evade immune system, the host responds by developing variants of NKG2D ligands by gene duplication and going beyond the reach of the virus (Zhou et al., 2005; Chalupny et al., 2006).

1.8.2 Evading tumor responses

One of the main functions of NKG2D is to participate in antitumour immune response and immune surveillance (Diefenbach et al., 2001; Smyth et al., 2005). Tumors have evolved many mechanisms that would allow them to avoid NKG2D-mediated immune attack. Some of these mechanisms are shedding soluble NKG2D ligands like MIC from their cell surface or down regulating MICA expression, producing TGF-β, effectively anergizing NKG2D-mediated immune recognition, and switching off the expression of NKG2D ligands as they progress (Groh et al., 2002; Vetter et al., 2004). Possessing multiple NKG2D ligands under the control of different cancer-related stress-response would provide the host with a fail-safe alert mechanism. Since expression of an individual NKG2D ligand may be lost as part of a cancer immunoediting process, the advantage of having more than one NKG2D ligand is that it would be much more difficult for the cancer to switch off multiple NKG2D ligands at once and help a host in detecting tumors (Eagle and Trowsdale, 2007).

1.8.3 Tissue specific functions

In humans, MICA and RAET1G proteins are expressed constitutively in the polarized epithelial-cell layer of the gut where they are likely to come in contact with pathogens (Groh

et al., 1996). MICA and ULBP1–ULBP3 are expressed by normal airway epithelial cells (Borchers et al., 2006). RAE1 transcripts were reported in mouse embryonic tissues such as embryonic brain (Nomura et al., 1996). MICA has a specialized role in the gut, whereas ULBP4 may have a related but equally specialized role in the skin (Groh et al., 1996).
NKG2D ligands, like RAE-1 or MICA/B are not expressed in most tissues in healthy adult mice and humans (Nomura et al., 1996; Groh et al., 1996). ULBP1-3 mRNA is expressed in various healthy tissues (Cosman et al., 2001) and ULBP4 mRNA expression is detected in the skin (Jan Chalupny et al., 2003). Likewise, MULT1 mRNA is expressed in a wide variety of tissues such as thymus, spleen, lymph node, liver and heart (Carayannopoulos et al., 2002b; Diefenbach et al., 2003). RAE-1ß and RAE-1δ mRNA expression is detected in the early embryos, particularly in the brain (Nomura et al., 2006). Bone marrow cells express low levels of RAE-1 and H60 but not MULT1 (Ogasawara et al., 2003). Some NKG2D ligands are constitutively expressed in a restricted number of normal cells, indicating that they may have evolved unique tissue-specific functions that are not necessarily relate to their role in immune surveillance. Hence, it seems that NKG2D-ligand diversity may have allowed for the evolution of individual ligands with functional specialties that are specific for different cell types and tissues (Eagle and Trowsdale, 2007).

1.9 NKG2D dependent immunotherapy

As NKG2D receptor recognizes ligands that are constitutively expressed on many transformed but not on most normal cells, this provides an opportunity for their use in immunotherapy of cancer. Many different therapeutic strategies are being developed using NKG2D receptor-ligand interactions (Coudert and Held, 2006). Chimeric anti-tumor mAb/NKG2D-ligand, with the antibody portion of the chimeric protein specific to tumor cell targeting, while the NKG2D ligand re-directs NKG2D-expressing effector cells to the site of tumor have been generated. An anti-CEA (carcinoembryonic antigen)/MICA chimera and H60/anti-CEA specifically bind CEA+ human tumor cells and enhanced the *in vitro* lysis by NK cells in a NKG2D-dependent manner (Zhou et al., 2005). NKG2D receptor fused to the cytoplasmic portion of CD3ζ has been expressed in splenic T cells. This chimeric NKG2D receptor/CD3ζ protein confers primary activation function to T cells in response to NKG2D ligand-bearing tumor cells *in vitro* and induces memory response to NKG2D ligand-negative tumor cells (Zhang et al., 2005).
Cytokines, such as IL-21, IL-12 and IFN-α, exert anti-tumor effects by up-regulating NKG2D cell surface expression have been used in some tumor models with positive results. Mice treated with IL-21 have been observed to reject tumors cells more efficiently than control mice. IL-21 up-regulated NK cell mediated NKG2D-dependent tumor cell lysis *in vitro* and the rejection of grafted tumor cells *in vivo* (Takaki et al., 2005). Similar results were observed with IL-12 and IFN-α (Zhang et al., 2005).
Irradiation or alkylating compounds commonly used in chemotherapy treatment of cancer activate the DNA damage response pathway and can induce the expression of NKG2D ligands in mouse and human cells. ULBP3 and MICA are up-regulated by transretinoic acid in patients with chronic B cell lymphocytic leukemia (B-CLL) (Poggi et al., 2004). These treatments rendered tumor cells susceptible to killing by autologous NKG2D expressing effector cells and can be used as part of the combination therapy regime with any of the above discussed approaches (Coudert and Held, 2006).
NKG2D recognition of multiple stress-inducible host proteins is of considerable research interest since this system has potential to be manipulated for therapeutic purposes. Tumor

cells expressing NKG2D ligands have been shown to be susceptible to NK cell mediated lysis, to induce a very potent antitumor response, and to provide protective immunity *in vivo* (Carayannopoulos et al., 2002a; Carayannopoulos et al., 2002b; Diefenbach et al., 2003; Kotturi et al., 2008; Eagle and Trowsdale, 2007). NKG2D recognition system has potential as a promising entry point to induce and/or improve immune responses against cancer for the following reasons. First, NKG2D ligands are generally poorly and only transiently expressed on healthy tissues, while they are constitutively expressed at significant levels on tumor cells. Second, NKG2D ligands are expressed on a broad variety of tumor cells of distinct tissue origins. Third, in situations where NKG2D ligands are poorly expressed, it may be possible to enhance their expression using radiation and/or chemotherapies. Fourth, NKG2D is expressed on all NK cells and also on a substantial fraction of T lymphocytes, providing a large number of potential effector cells. Fifth, cytokines may be used to improve NKG2D function. Finally, NKG2D-mediated adoptive immunotherapy should, in principal, be applicable to all individuals as the NKG2D receptor is monomorphic (Coudert and Held, 2006).

A great deal has yet to be understood about the involvement of NKG2D ligands in disease. A lot is known about the function of MICA; however, investigation of the expression and function of other NKG2D ligands with transmembrane domains and cytoplasmic tails is needed. A better understanding of the differences in the functional properties of NKG2D ligands and the pathways that regulate NKG2D ligand expression could help us develop better therapeutic interventions that could induce NKG2D-mediated immune responses and more efficient therapeutic strategies in the future (Eagle and Trowsdale, 2007).

1.10 Fas/CD95

CD95/APO-1/Fas receptor is a member of the tumor necrosis factor (TNF) superfamily of receptors. Its main function in signaling is the induction of apoptosis (Schulze-Osthoff et al., 1998). CD95/Fas receptor is expressed on various human cells, including myeloid cells, T lymphoblastoid cells, and diploid fibroblasts. Fas is a 48-kDa type I transmembrane receptor of 319 amino acids with a single transmembrane domain of 17 amino acids, an N-terminal cysteine-rich extracellular domain and a C-terminal cytoplasmic domain containing 145 amino acids relatively abundant in charged amino acids. The cytoplasmic portion of Fas contains a domain called "*death domain*" of about 85 amino acids. The "*death domain*" is very crucial as it plays a role in transmitting the death signal from the cell's surface to intracellular pathways and mediates signaling through protein-protein interactions (Nagata, 1997). The tertiary structure of the Fas death domain consists of six antiparallel, amphipathic α helices. Helices $\alpha1$ and $\alpha2$ are centrally located and flanked on each side by $\alpha3/\alpha4$ and $\alpha5/\alpha6$. This leads to an unusual topology in which the loops connecting $\alpha1/\alpha2$ and $\alpha4/\alpha5$ cross over each other. The presence of a high number of charged amino acids in the death domain is responsible for interactions between death domains (Mollinedo and Gajate, 2006). CD95 receptors are expressed on the surface of cells as preassociated homotrimers (Siegel et al., 2000). These interactions were found to be mediated by a domain in the N-terminus, within the first of the cysteine-rich domains called PLAD (preligand binding assembly domain) (Siegel et al., 2000). CD95 receptors only function as trimers (Kischkel et al., 1995).

CD95 contains a protein–protein interaction domain in its cytoplasmic region termed the death domain (DD) (Peter et al., 1999). When the preassociated receptor is ligated, CD95 becomes competent to form the death-inducing signaling complex (DISC). In the DISC, the adaptor molecule Fas-associated DD containing protein (FADD) binds to CD95 through homotypic interaction of its DD with the DD of CD95 (Kischkel et al., 1995). In addition to its DD, FADD contains another protein–protein interaction domain at its N-terminus, termed the death effector domain (DED). This domain recruits caspases containing these DED domains to the DISC. Both the DD and DED enable proteins containing the same domains to interact with one another. FADD interacts with procaspase-8 through its DED (Boldin et al., 1996). Thus, activation of Fas results in receptor aggregation and formation of DISC (Kischkel et al., 1995), containing trimerized Fas, FADD and procaspase-8. The apoptotic caspases perform different roles. The effector caspases, which include caspases 3, 7, and 6 are responsible for most of the cleavage of proteins characteristic of apoptosis and are responsible for cleavage of proteins which induce the major morphological changes observed during programmed cell death (Ernshaw et al., 1999). Caspase-8 is a main initiator caspase and transduces the first signals of apoptosis in CD95 signaling and is expressed as two isoforms, caspase-8/a and -8/b, which are both recruited to the activated CD95 receptor (Scaffidi et al., 1997). Two molecules (FADD and caspase-8) are the key components of the CD95 DISC. Once procaspase-8 associates with FADD, the high local concentration of procaspase-8 leads to its autoproteolytic cleavage and activation (Salvesan and Dixit, 1999). Following the autoproteolytic cleavage of the enzyme, caspase-8 is released from the DISC as an active heterotetramer (Peter and Krammer, 2003).

1.11 Fas ligand (FasL)

FasL belongs to the TNF family and can be found as a 40-kDa membrane-bound or a 26-kDa soluble protein (Nagata, 1997). Rat FasL has no signal sequence at the N-terminus, but has a domain of hydrophobic amino acids in the middle of the molecule, indication that it is a type 11 membrane protein with the COOH-terminal region outside the cell. Mouse and human FasL are 76.9% identical at the amino acid sequence level and are functionally interchangeable. A stretch of about 150 amino acids in the extracellular region of FasL show significant homology to the corresponding region of other members of the TNF family which includes TNF, lymphotoxin (LT), CD40 ligand, CD27 ligand, CD30 ligand and OX40 ligand. A single FasL gene is located on human and mouse chromosome 1 in the neighborhood of the OX40 ligand gene. Fas/FasL system is the major regulator of apoptosis at the cell membrane in mammalian cells through a receptor/ligand interaction (Mollinedo and Gajate, 2006).

1.11.1 Expression of fasL

FasL has been found to be expressed on cells of the lymphoid/myeloid lineage, including activated T cells and natural killer (NK) cells, where it plays an important role in immune homeostasis, T cell and NK cell-mediated toxicity (Brunner et al., 2003). FasL is also found to be expressed in sites such as the eye (Griffith et al., 1995) and testis (Bellgrau et al., 1995) contributing to immune privilege by inducing apoptosis of infiltrating proinflammatory immunocytes (Houston and O'Connell, 2004). FasL expression has also been observed in a variety of tumor cells indicating a possibility that FasL could mediate immune privilege in human tumors by inducing apoptosis of anti-tumor lymphocytes and also, stimulate proliferation of tumor cells (Houston and O'Connell, 2004). Tumor expression of FasL was first demonstrated in the colon carcinoma cell line SW620, where it could induce apoptosis of Fas-sensitive lymphoid cells *in vitro* (O'Connell et al., 1996). A functional FasL expression has also been reported on numerous tumors of varying origin including colon (Okada et al., 2000), gastric (Zheng et al., 2003), lung (Niehans et al., 1997) carcinoma, and astrocytoma (Saas et al., 1997). Tumor cells expressing FasL demonstrated the ability to kill Fas-sensitive target cells when co-cultured *in vitro*. Apoptosis of tumor-infiltrating lymphocytes (TILs) has also been detected *in situ* within FasL-expressing human tumors such as esophageal carcinoma (Houston and O'Connell, 2004; Okada et al., 2000; Zheng et al., 2003; Niehans et al., 1997).

FasL expression was found to be higher in metastatic tumors than in primary ones. In breast and cervical tumors, high FasL expression was significantly associated with lymph node metastases (Kase et al., 2003) whereas, stronger FasL expression was found in liver metastases of colon cancer relative to the primary tumor (Houston and O'Connell, 2004).

1.11.2 Inhibition of apoptosis

One of the hallmarks of cancer is resistance to apoptosis (Hanahan and Weinberg, 2000). Most cancer cells are relatively resistant to apoptosis mediated through Fas. Fas-mediated apoptosis can be inhibited at different points in the apoptotic signaling pathway. Cells may secrete soluble 'decoy' receptors, such as sFasL or DcR3, which can bind to FasL and inhibit FasL-induced apoptosis (Pitti et al., 1998). FADD-like interleukin-1ß-converting enzyme inhibitory protein (cFLIP) binds to the DISC and prevents the activation of caspase-8 (Irmler et al., 1997). Reduced expression of FADD (Tourneur et al., 2003) or caspase-8 (Fulda et al., 2001) can also inhibit Fas signaling. IAPs present in the cytosol can bind to and inhibit caspases and upregulation of Bcl-2 or Bcl-xL can render type II cells resistant to Fas-mediated apoptosis. Cytochrome c and inhibitor-of-apoptosis protein (IAP) can inhibit apoptosis (Igney and Krammer, 2002). Thus, because of their insensitivity to Fas-mediated apoptosis, tumor cells can express FasL without undergoing apoptosis (Houston et al., 2003). It has been observed that resistance to Fas-mediated apoptosis protects tumor cells not only from tumor-expressed FasL but also from FasL expressed as a cytotoxic mediator by infiltrating anti-tumor T cells and NK cells (Houston and O'Connell, 2004).

1.12 Immunotherapy

Death receptors are members of the tumor necrosis factor (TNF) receptor gene superfamily, consisting of more than 20 proteins with a broad range of biological function, including regulation of cell death, survival, differentiation or immune regulation (Debatin and Krammer, 2004). Death receptors share regions of high homology including cysteine-rich extracellular domains and a cytoplasmic domain of about 80 amino acids called death domain (DD), which plays a crucial role in transmitting the death signal from the cells surface to intracellular signaling pathways (Mollinedo and Gajate, 2006).

The death receptors which have potential to induce apoptosis are Fas, TNF receptor 1 (TNFR1), TNF-related apoptosis-inducing ligand receptor 1 (TRAIL-R1), TRAIL-R2, death receptor 4 (DR4) and death receptor 5 (DR5). Due to their potential to induce apoptosis, ligands such as TNF, Fas ligand (FasL) and TRAIL are interesting candidates for antitumor therapy (Shankar and Srivastava, 2004; Mollinedo and Gajate, 2006). However, ligands of the TNF family and their cognate receptors have been found to play a key role in liver pathogenesis and have become a major challenge for the clinical application of death receptor-targeted therapy (Hohenberger and Tunn, 2003; Ogasawara et al., 1993; Nesterov et al., 2002).

Conventional chemotherapy is based on the perception that malignant cells have uncontrolled proliferation. The rather modest impact of antiproliferative drugs in the clinic is not surprising since many tumors have a low growth capacity. In addition, exposure of normal tissues that have a high rate of cellular proliferation, such as the bone marrow, the gastrointestinal epithelial cells and the cells of the hair follicles, to anti-proliferative drugs leads to major toxicities. The effectiveness of anticancer drugs reflects the ability of tumor cells to detect and respond to the perturbation induced by the drug (Mashima and Tsuruo, 2005). The failure of some tumor cells to die following drug treatment and their resistance to drugs is due to their resistance to apoptosis as tumors cells have defects in triggering their own death by apoptosis (Mollinedo and Gajate, 2006). If liver toxicity could be circumvented, Fas would be a worthy anticancer target due to its potent proapoptotic activity and widespread expression in tumor cells (Mollinedo and Gajate, 2006).

1.13 Adenovirus and cancer gene therapy

Different viral vectors like lentivirus, retrovirus, pox virus, herpes simplex virus-1, vaccinia virus, adeno-associated virus (AAV) and adenovirus have been used for experimental cancer gene therapy (Young et al., 2006). These viral vectors have been used individually and in combination with conventional therapies to treat cancers that are refractory to just conventional therapy (surgery, radiation, and chemotherapy). Of all the vectors used, adenoviruses are one of the most widely accepted viral agents for cancer gene therapy. The features of adenovirus that make them well suited for gene therapy are: its capacity for gene transfer (up to 7-8 Kb), *in vivo* stability, inability to integrate into host genome, ability to transduce dividing and non dividing cells, a well characterized genome and relative ease of production, purification and manipulation. From a clinical point of view, adenovirus is endemic in the human population and its natural pathogenicity is associated with mild respiratory infections, and therefore, manifests a well defined safety profile (Gomes and Tong, 2006; Young et al., 2006).

Adenovirus was first isolated and cultured from human tonsils and adenoid tissues (Garnett et al., 2002). Currently, 51 human adenovirus serotypes have been identified and grouped into six subgroups (A-F) of which the most widely studied serotype are group C types 2 and 5. Adenovirus is a non-enveloped icosohedral particle which carries a 36 Kb double stranded DNA genome. The capsid consists of three main components: hexon, penton and fiber. Hexon is the most abundant structural protein which appears to play a role in coating the virus. The pentameric structure called penton is known to mediate viral internalization. The fiber protrudes from the penton bases and appears to play a role in viral attachment to the cellular receptor namely coxsackie adenovirus receptor (CAR). Attachment via knob-CAR interactions is followed by interactions between cellular integrins and an arginine-glycine aspartic acid motif (RGD-motif) located at the penton base. This binding leads to the formation of endosomes, viral internalization, disassembly and the release of viral nucleic acid. Thereafter viral DNA is transported to the nucleus where the genes are expressed and viral replication occurs. The adenoviral genome can be divided into immediately early (*E1A*), early (*E1B, E2, E3, E4*), intermediate (*IX, IVa2*) and late genes. The early genes are expressed prior to viral replication consisting of mainly regulatory proteins that prepare the host cell for virus DNA replication and block antiviral mechanisms. The late viral genes encode for viral structural proteins. Importantly, E3 region encodes a variety of proteins involved in immune response evasion. Adenoviruses with deletions in E1 and/or E3 regions have been developed to provide cloning sites for transgene insertion (Gomes and Tong, 2006).

1.14 Conditional replicative and oncolytic adenovirus for cancer therapy

Research has shown that adenovirus can be safely used for gene delivery. Adenoviruses have been modified by replacing early genes, E1A and E1B or E3 with the gene of interest. Since the E1 unit is essential for viral replication, the recombinant vector is replicative defective and its replication requires helper functions provided by a packaging cell line with complementing E1 genes. However, these recombinant constructs have been useful mainly at local/ regional stage. Their therapeutic limitation has been the incomplete infection of tumor cells, transient expression of the transgene, and a lack of systemic efficacy. Recently, conditional replicative oncolytic adenoviruses have been shown to replicate and kill tumor cells without harming normal cells. The tumor specificity of these viruses has been manifested through the incorporation of tissue or tumor specific promoters that limit viral gene (Tong, 2006; Gomes and Tong, 2006).
A recent study indicates that the use of adenoviral vectors for clinical gene therapy is widespread. As of July 2006, adenoviral vectors are used in 26% of the 1,192 current worldwide gene therapy clinical trials. Of the 301 clinical trials involving the use of Ad vectors, 76% are for the treatment of cancer followed by vascular disease and monogenic disorders at 14% and 7%, respectively (http://www.wiley.co.uk/ genetherapy /clinical/) (Campos and Barry. 2007).
Adenoviral gene therapy approaches have shown promising results in clinical trials. Adenovirus mediated delivery of NTR (nitroreductase enzyme) from *E. Coli* by direct intratumoural injection in patients with primary or secondary liver cancer showed appropriate levels of NTR expression in tumor cells. The early clinical trial data of the NTR/CB1954 system in patients with liver cancer or prostate cancer are extremely encouraging (Palmer et al., 2004). Adenoviral delivery of TRAIL (tumor necrosis factor-related apoptosis-inducing ligand) showed significant anti-tumor efficacy in animal models of aggressive primary and metastatic cancer (Ma et al., 2005). Clinical trials of a recombinant adenovirus expressing interleukin-12 (IL-12) in patients with advanced digestive tumors have produced evidence of antitumor effects (Sangro et al., 2004).

2. Hypothesis and objectives

2.1 Hypothesis

A novel fusion protein consisting of MULT1 extracellular domain and Fas transmembrane and intracellular domains (MULT1E/FasTI) when expressed on a cell, would activate NKG2D expressing cells such as NK cells from its MULT1E extracellular region, upon binding of MULT1E to NKG2D receptor on NK cells. At the same time the engagement of the fusion protein with NKG2D receptor would send death signals into the cells that express the fusion protein and induce apoptosis of the cell (Fig.1).

2.2 Objectives

The work presented here is a two pronged approach of using a novel fusion protein consisting of MULT1 extracellular domain and Fas transmembrane and intracellular domains for cancer therapy. First, the construction and expression of MULT1E/FasTI fusion protein is examined. Second, *in vitro* and *in vivo* activity of the fusion protein is tested.

Finally, the adenoviral vector mediated delivery and *in vivo* therapeutic effect of the novel fusion protein is evaluated.

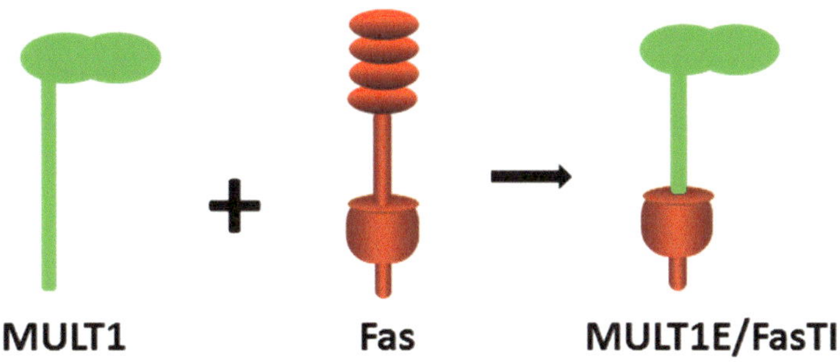

Fig. 1. Schematic representation of proposed mechanism of novel fusion protein MULT1E /FasTI.

3. Construction and evaluation of fusion protein MULT1E/FasTI

3.1 Plasmid construction of pMULT1E/FasTI

Thymus glands from 4-day old newborn C57BL/6J mice were removed and stored in liquid nitrogen. The glands were homogenized using a tissue homogenizer and total RNA was extracted using TRIzol reagent (Invitrogen, Carlsbad, CA). Primers were designed for amplification of the extracellular domain of MULT1 (Genebank accession # NM_029975) from 236bp to 868bp. The sequence of the 5′ primer is CCCAAGCTTATGGAGCTG ACTGCCAGTAACAAGGTCC and that of the 3′ primer is CGGGATCCGGTACTGAAA GATCCTGCAGGCTCCAG. At the 5′ end of the upstream primer, a HindIII enzyme site was created and at the 5′ end of downstream primer, a BamHI site was created. cDNA was synthesized from the extracted total RNA using an RT-PCR kit (Promega, Madison, WI). The fragment was excised and gel purified using a Qiagen gel purification kit (Valencia, CA). Double enzyme digestion was performed on the purified fragment using HindIII and BamHI. The enzyme digested fragment was then ligated into a pcDNA3.1 (+) vector (Invitrogen, CA). The full MULT1 cDNA sequence in the new vector, pMULT1E, was confirmed by DNA sequencing.

The cDNA clone of the Fas receptor in pDNR-LIB (ATCC # 10088798) was purchased from American Type Collection Centre (ATCC, Manassas, VA). A pair of primers was designed for amplification of the transmembrane and intracellular domains of Fas from 524 bp to 1013bp (Genebank accession# BC061160). The 5′ primer used was CGGGATCCCCC AGAA ATCGCCTATGGTTGTTGTTGACC and the 3′ primer was CGGAATTCTCACTCCAGACA TTGTCCTTCATTTTC. At the 5′ end of upstream primer, a BamHI enzyme site was created and at the 5′ end of downstream primer, an EcoRI enzyme site was created. DNA PCR was performed to amplify the Fas transmembrane and intracellular domains from pDNR-LIB. The gel purified fragment was treated with BamHI and EcoRI enzymes and ligated into the pcDNA3.1 (+)/Zeo vector to create pFasTI. The DNA sequence of the transmembrane and intracellular domains of Fas in vector pFasTI was confirmed by DNA sequencing.

The cDNA fragment encoding the MULT1 extracellular domain was cut out from pMULT1E by HindIII and BamHI enzyme digestion and ligated into the pFasTI. The resulting vector was named pMULT1E/FasTI (Fig.2) and used for transfection.

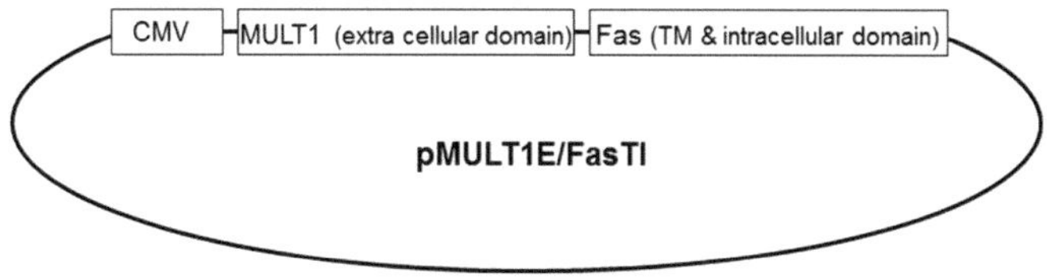

Fig. 2. Construction of the MULT1E/FasTI plasmid.

3.2 Expression of pMULT1E/FasTI

Lung carcinoma TC-1 tumor cells were transfected with pMULT1E/FasTI. Three clones that were zeocin resistant were selected and labeled as L-5, L-7 and L-10. An *in vitro* cell growth study showed that all the clones grew at a similar rate as TC-1 cells. The cells of these clones were stained with anti-mouse MULT1 antibody and analyzed by fluorescence-activated cell sorting (FACS). The result showed that TC-1 cells and clone L-7 cells were negative, whereas clones L-5 and L-10 cells were strongly positive (Fig. 3). To confirm that MULT1E of the fusion protein can indeed bind to NKG2D, the cells were incubated with NKG2D/Fc, a recombinant fusion protein, and then stained with anti-mouse NKG2D antibody conjugated with fluorescein isothiocyanate (FITC). TC-1 cells and clone L-7 cells were dimly positive, whereas clones L-5 and L-10 cells were strongly positive (Fig. 4) with L-10 cells the strongest. The results indicate that clones L-5 and L-10 are MULT1E/FasTI-positive clones, whereas TC-1 and clone L-7 are negative for the fusion protein, but express some endogenous MULT1 protein.

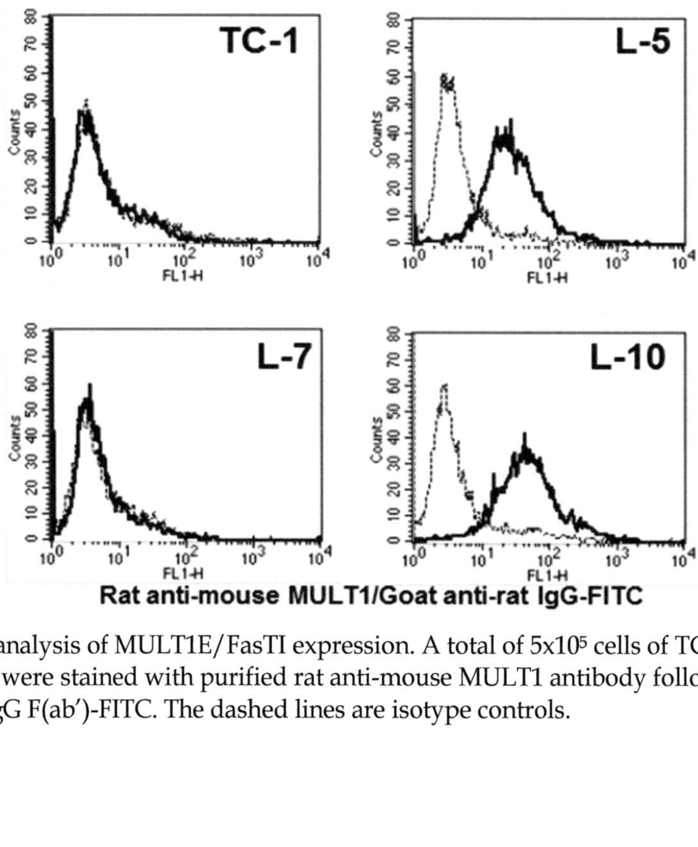

Fig. 3. FACS analysis of MULT1E/FasTI expression. A total of 5x10^5 cells of TC-1 and clones L5, L7 or L10 were stained with purified rat anti-mouse MULT1 antibody followed by goat anti-mouse IgG F(ab')-FITC. The dashed lines are isotype controls.

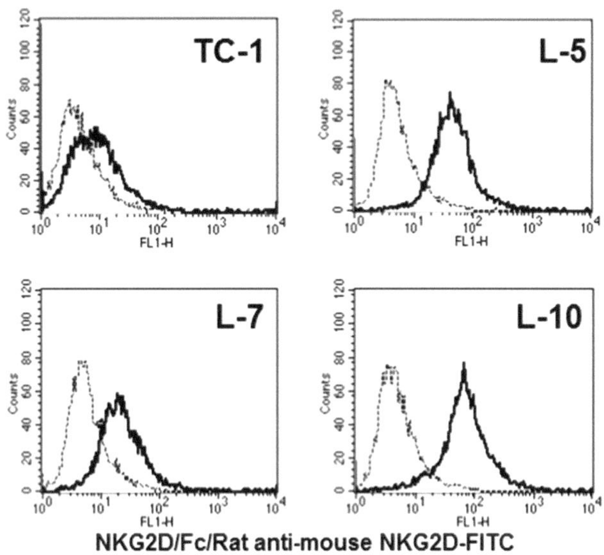

Fig. 4. FACS analysis of MULT1E/FasTI expression. A total of 1x10⁶ cells of TC-1 and clones L-5, L-7 or L-10 were first treated with NKG2D/Fc and then stained with anti-mouse NKG2D antibody conjugated with FITC. The cells were analyzed on FACS Calibur with CellQuest software. Dashed lines are controls without NKG2D/Fc incubation.

3.3 Fusion protein MULT1E/FasTI induces apoptosis of cells

To confirm the concept that when bound to its ligand NKG2D fusion protein MULT1E/FasTI can send death signals through its Fas portion into the cells, TC-1 cells and clones L-5, L-7, L-10 were treated with recombinant protein NKG2D/Fc and analyzed by Annexin V staining and caspase-3 activation assay. The treatment of NKG2D/Fc increased both Annexin V-positive cells and Annexin V/propidium iodide (PI) double-positive cells in clones L-5 and L-10, but not in TC-1 cells or clone L-7 (Fig. 5). After the NKG2D/Fc treatment, not only apoptotic cells (Annexin V-positive cells and Annexin V/PI double-positive cells), but also the necrotic cells (PI-positive/Annexin V-negative cells) in clone L-5 and L-10 were significantly higher than those of TC-1 or clone L-7 (Fig. 6A and 6B). Similarly, caspase-3 activities in cells of clones L-5 and L-10 were significantly higher than those of TC-1 or clone L-7 (Fig. 6C). The treatment of NKG2D/Fc induced more apoptotic cells in clone L-10 than clone L-5 (Fig. 6A and 6C).

3.4 Cells expressing MULT1E/FasTI activate NK cells

It is critical to know whether fusion protein MULT1E/FasTI can activate NKG2D-expressing cells, such as NK cells. Cells from TC-1 or clones L-5, L-7 and L-10 were co-cultured with NK cells isolated from mouse spleen. Intracellular interferon-γ (IFN- γ) was detected by FACS analysis (Fig. 7A). The percentage of the NK cells that express IFN- γ was significantly increased in wells that contained cells of clone L-5 or L-10 compared to those co-cultured with TC-1 ($P<0.05$). Although the percentage of NK cells expressing IFN-γ in wells that contained cells of clone L-7 increased slightly compared to those co-cultured with TC-1 cells, it was not statistically significant (Fig. 7B).

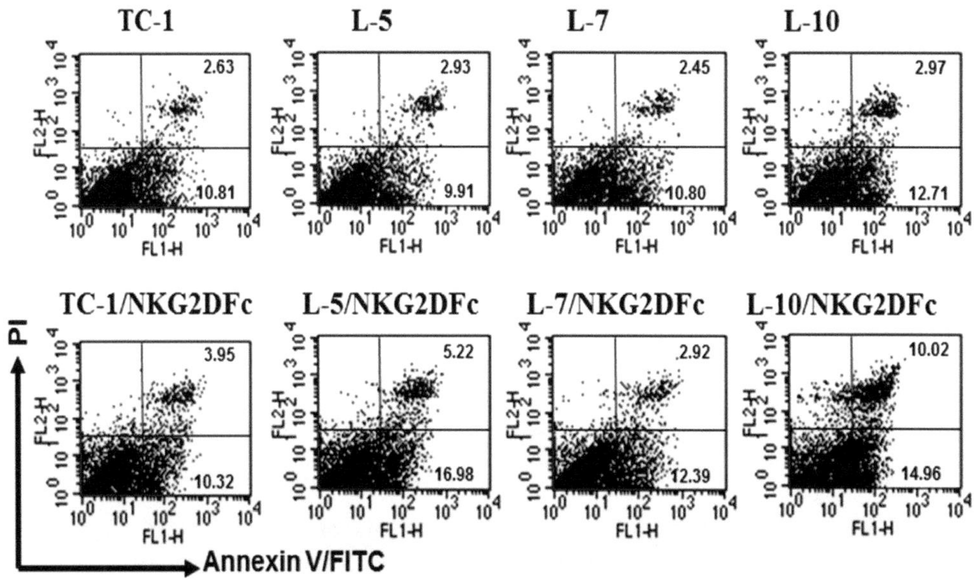

Fig. 5. MULT1E/FasTI induces apoptosis. A total of 1x10⁶ cells of TC-1 and clones L-5, L-7 and L-10 were treated with 1 µg/ml NKG2D/Fc for 16 h. The cells were then analyzed for apoptosis and necrosis using Annexin V staining and PI. This figure is an example of the FACS data.

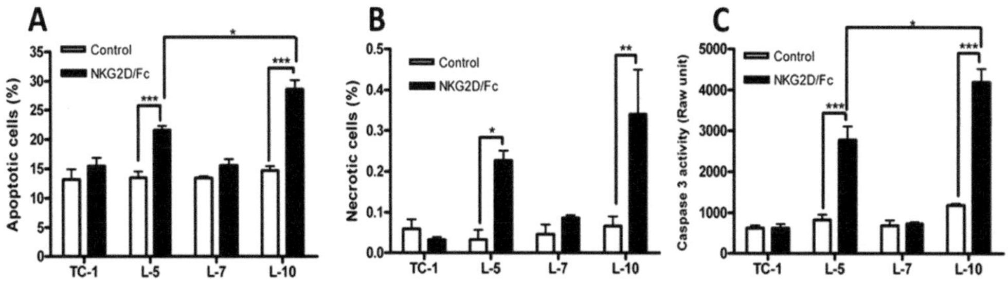

Fig. 6. MULT1E/FasTI induces apoptosis. A total of 1x10⁶ cells of TC-1 and clones L-5, L-7 and L-10 were treated with 1 µg/ml NKG2D/Fc for 16 h. The cells were then analyzed for apoptosis and necrosis using Annexin V staining (A, B) or caspase-3 assay (C). The statistical analyses were conducted between the controls (open bars) and NKG2D/Fc-treated cells (solid bars) using two-way analysis of variance (ANOVA). The difference between NKG2D/Fc-treated L-5 cells and NKG2D/Fc-treated L-10 cells was also compared using Student's t-test. $^*P<0.05$; $^{**}P<0.01$ and $^{***}P<0.001$.

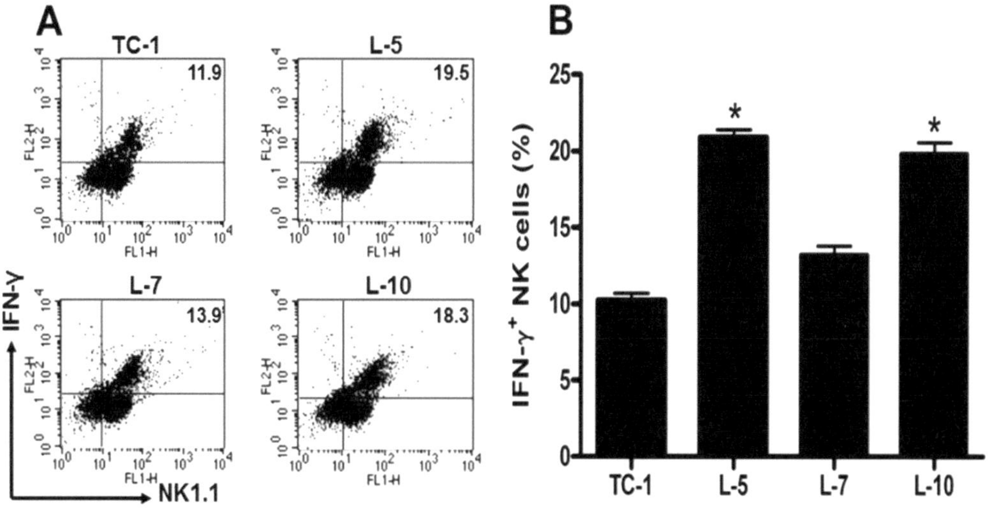

Fig. 7. MULT1E/FasTI activates natural killer (NK) cells. A total of 1x10⁶ cells of TC-1 and clones L-5, L-7 and L-10 were co-cultured with NK cells for 3 h. The cells were stained with anti-NK1.1-FITC and were then permeabilized and fixed, and stained with antimouse IFN-γ-PE. The cells were analyzed on FACS Calibur with CellQuest software. (A) represents an example of the FACS data and (B) is the summery of the data from three separate experiments. *P<0.05.

3.5 *In vivo* antitumor effect of fusion protein MULT1E/FasTI

The *in vivo* therapeutic effect of the fusion protein was evaluated in a subcutaneous tumor model as well as a pulmonary metastasis model. Two hundred thousand cells of TC-1 and clones L-5, L-7 and L-10 in 0.2 ml Hank's balanced salt solution (HBSS) were injected subcutaneously into 6- to 8-week-old mice and tumor size was measured twice weekly with a caliper and tumor volume was calculated. The tumor growth of clone L-7 was slightly, but not significantly (P>0.05) slower when compared to that of TC-1 cells. At day 18, the growth of clones L-5 and L-10 was significantly slower (P<0.01, P<0.01) when compared to that of TC-1 cells. At day 24, the difference of tumor growth between TC-1 and clone L-10 was even more significant (P<0.001), whereas the difference of tumor growth between TC-1 and clone L-5 remained the same (P<0.01; Fig. 8). An even better antitumor effect of the fusion protein was observed in the pulmonary metastasis model. Four weeks after i.v. tumor cell injection, the mice were euthanized and lungs were excised (Fig. 9A). The total weight of the lungs with the tumors was measured (Fig. 9B) and the tumor nodules on the surface of the lungs were counted (Fig. 9C). The lungs isolated from mice injected with TC-1 cells were fully covered with tumors and weighed an average 0.82 g. All the four lungs have more than 200 tumor nodules each. The lungs isolated from mice injected with clone L-7 cells are covered with many tumors as well and weighed averagely 0.48 g. There are 118, 89, 67, 125 tumor nodules on the lungs. The lungs isolated from mice injected with clones L-5 and L-10 were almost tumor free and weighed much less (0.15 and 0.14 g, respectively) than those of mice injected with either TC-1 cells or clone L-7 cells. The average weight of lungs from normal mice was 0.14 g.

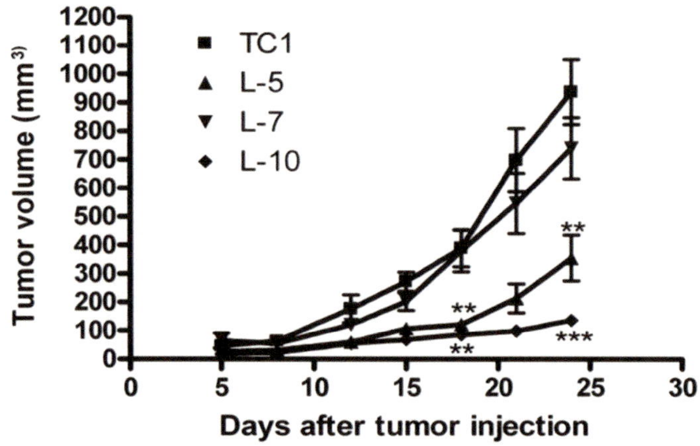

Fig. 8. Subcutaneous tumor study. A total of $2x10^5$ tumor cells of TC-1 or clones L-5, L-7 and L-10 in 0.2 ml HBSS were subcutaneously injected into C57BL/6J mice (four mice per group). Tumor growth was measured and presented as $1/2LW^2$. **P<0.01; ***P<0.001.

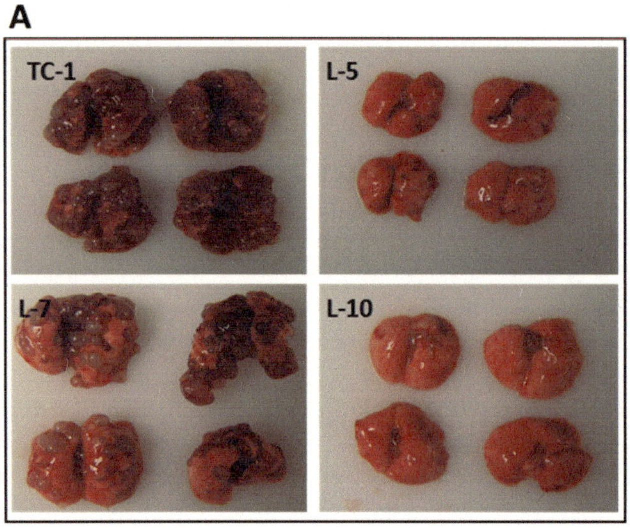

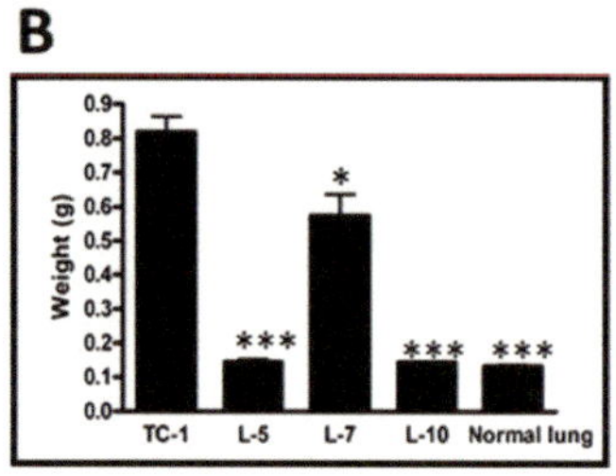

C

Clones	Pulmonary Metastases
TC-1	>200, >200, >200, >200
L-5	0, 0, 1, 1
L-7	118, 89, 67, 125
L-10	0, 0, 0, 2

Fig. 9. Pulmonary metastatic tumor study. A total of $2x10^5$ tumor cells of TC-1 or clones L-5, L-7 and L-10 in 0.5 ml HBSS were i.v. injected into C57BL/6J mice (four mice per group). Four weeks after tumor cell injection, mice were killed and their lungs were dissected (A). The lungs were weighted (B) and the tumor nodules on the lungs were counted (C). *P<0.05; ***P<0.001.

3.6 Construction of adenoviral vectors

In order to effectively deliver the fusion protein into cells, especially tumor cells, adenovirus vectors were chosen. Ad-MULT1E/FasTI, Ad-MULT1E and Ad-Lac-Z adenovirus were generated using the ViraPower Adenoviral Expression System (Invitrogen, Carlsbad, CA) according to the manufacturer's instructions. The full-length cDNAs of MULT1E/FasTI or

MULT1E (Section 3.1) were cloned into the pCR ®8/GW/TOPO® vector. The pCR ®8/GW/TOPO® vector with MULT1E/FasTI or MULT1E inserts were used as entry clone vectors and transferred into the destination vector pAd/CMV/V5-DEST (Invitrogen, Carlsbad, CA) using the Gateway LR Clonase II enzyme mix according to the manufacturer's directions (Invitrogen, Carlsbad, CA) to generate pAd/CMV/MULT1E/FasTI/V5 and pAd/CMV/MULT1E/V5. The vectors were linearized with *PacI* enzyme and transfected into 293A cells using Lipofectamine™ 2000 reagent as per manufacturer's directions. The 293A cells were maintained in DMEM medium until a cytophathic effect was apparent 5–7 days post-transfection. Cells were collected and lysed by subjecting them to four freeze/thaw cycles. The cell debris was pelleted at 3000 x g for 15 min and the supernatant was collected and stored at -80 °C as crude viral lysate. Fifty microliters of crude viral lysate were added into each 293A cell culture dish and incubated for 2-3 days until an 80-100% cytophathic effect was observed. Two recombinant adenoviruses (Ad-MULT1E/FasTI and Ad-MULT1E) were harvested and purified using the Adeno-X ™ virus Mini Purification Kit according to the manufacturer's directions (Clontech, Mountain View, CA) and stored at -80 °C. Ad-Lac-Z was purchased directly from the manufacturer (Clontech) and amplified as per the above method. Titers of Ad-MULT1E/FasTI, Ad-MULT1E and Ad-Lac-Z stocks were determined using an Adeno-X ™ Rapid Titer Kit as per manufacturer's directions (Clontech).

3.7 Adenoviral vector effectively delivers MULT1E/FasTI into cultured TC-1 cells

Three adenoviral vectors were constructed: 1) Ad-MULT1E/FasTI containing the full fusion protein sequence of MULT1E extracellular domain and FasTI transmembrane and intracellular domains; 2) Ad-MULT1E containing only the MULT1E extracellular domain; 3) Ad-Lac-Z containing the Lac-Z gene as control adenoviral vector. The adenoviral vectors were linearized using *Pac*1 and transfected into 293A cells to generate adenoviral stocks. The titer of these adenoviral stocks are in the range of 10^{10} PFU/ml.

TC-1 tumor cells were infected with Ad-MULT1E/FasTI viral particles with different multiplicities of infection (MOI): 500, 250, 100, 25, and 0 for 24 hours. The fusion gene expression was detected by RT-PCR (Fig. 10) and FACS analysis (Fig. 11). Both assays not only demonstrate the fusion gene expression in the infected cells, but also show a clear dose dependent expression manner.

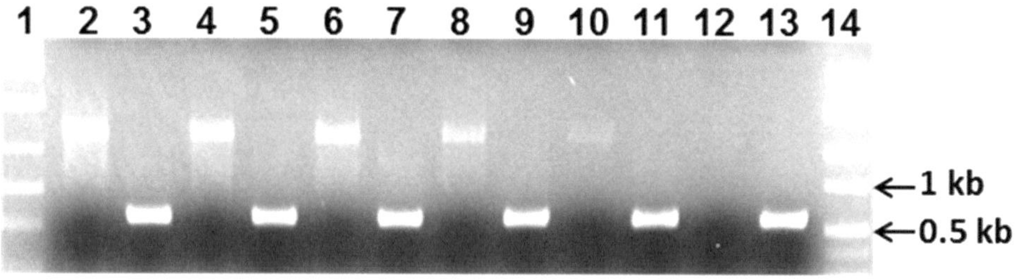

Fig. 10. RT-PCR analysis of AD-MULT1E/FasTI expression at different MOIs. RNAs were isolated from infected cells and RT-PCR was performed. Lanes 2, 4, 6, 8, 10 and 12 are 1134bp RT-PCR product of total RNA from TC1 cells infected with Ad-MULT1E/ FasTI at MOIs 500, 250, 100, 50, 25 and 0, amplified with MULT1E forward and Fas reverse primers; Lanes 3, 5, 7, 9, 11 and 13 are ß-actin controls; and lanes 1 and 14 are 1 kb markers.

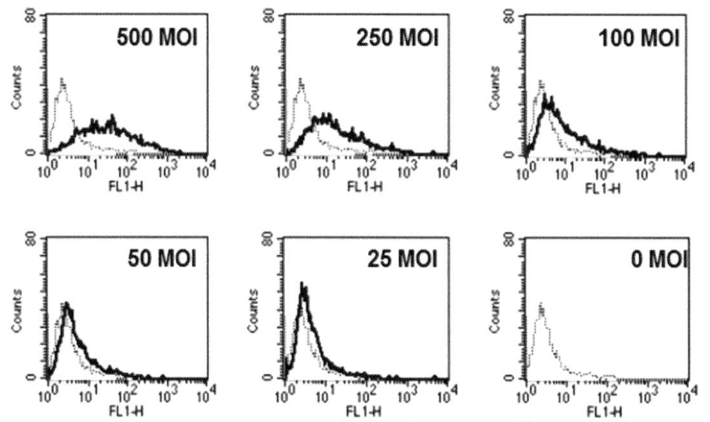

Fig. 11. FACS analyses of AD-MULT1E/FasTI expression at different MOIs. 5 x 10^5 TC1 cells were harvested from each group that were infected with Ad-MULT1E/FasTI at MOIs 500, 250, 100, 50, 25, 0 and stained with purified rat anti-mouse MULT1 antibody followed by goat anti IgG F(ab')-FITC. Dashed lines represent un-infected TC-1 cells.

3.8 MULT1E/FasTI delivered by adenoviral vector induces apoptosis in TC-1 cells

To confirm the activity of adenoviral vector delivered MULT1E/FasTI fusion protein in TC-1 cells, recombinant NKG2D/Fc ligand was added to the infected cells. As MULT1E binds to its ligand NKG2D, the binding would send apoptotic signal through its FasTI region into TC-1 cells (Kotturi et al., 2008). When TC-1 cells were infected with 100 MOI of Ad-MULT1E/FasTI and treated with NKG2D/Fc, their caspase 3 activity was significantly higher ($p<0.001$) than the cells that were also infected by Ad-MULT1E/FasTI but not treated with NKG2D/Fc. Ad-MULT1E or Ad-Lac-Z infection showed slightly increased caspase 3 activity ($p>0.05$) compared with non-infected TC-1 cells (Fig. 12A). The caspase activity in Ad-MULT1E/FasTI infected and NKG2D treated TC-1 cells is adenoviral particle dose

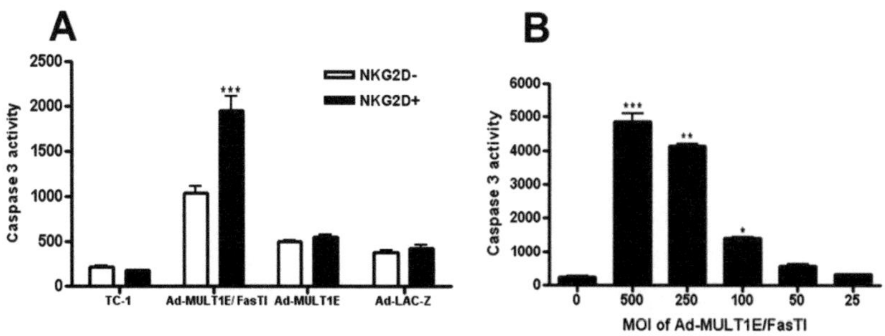

Fig. 12. Ad-MULT1E/FasTI infection induces apoptosis *in vitro*. A) TC-1 (5x10^5) cells were infected with Ad-MULT1E/FasTI, Ad-MULT1E and Ad-Lac-Z at 100 MOI. Twenty-four hour after infection, cells were treated with 1μg/ml NKG2D/Fc for 16 hrs. The cells were then analyzed for apoptosis by caspase-3 assay. B) TC-1 (5x10^5) cells were infected with Ad-MULT1E/FasTI at different MOIs: 500, 250, 100, 50, 25. Twenty-four hour after infection, cells were treated with 1μg/ml NKG2D/Fc for 16 hrs. The cells were then analyzed for apoptosis by caspase-3 assay. The data represented are summaries of three separate experiments. *$p< 0.05$; **$p< 0.01$ and ***$p< 0.001$.

dependent: 500 MOI infection generated the highest caspase activity, while a 25 MOI infection did not show any increased caspase 3 activity compared with un-infected TC-1 cells (Fig. 12B).

3.9 Intratumor delivery of MULT1E/FasTI by adenoviral vector

To observe the antitumor activity of MULT1E/FasTI delivered by adenoviral vector, subcutaneous TC-1 tumors were grown in C57BL/6J mice. When the tumor reached about a size of 40 mm^3, Ad-MULT1E/FasTI, Ad-MULT1E or Ad-Lac-Z at a dose of $1x10^9$ pfu/tumor in 0.05ml HBSS was injected into the tumors. Control mice received HBSS only. The injections were repeated every other day for 4 times. The size of the tumors was measured every two days. At day 22 after tumor cell injection, the mice were sacrificed and the tumors were collected and measured. Although tumors received Ad-MULT1E or Ad-Lac-Z grew slightly slower than tumors received only HBSS, tumors received Ad-MULT1E/FasTI showed the slowest growth rate (Fig. 13A). The end point tumor measurement confirmed the conclusion that Ad-MULT1E/FasTI treatment significantly slowed the tumor growth (P<0.01, Fig. 13B).

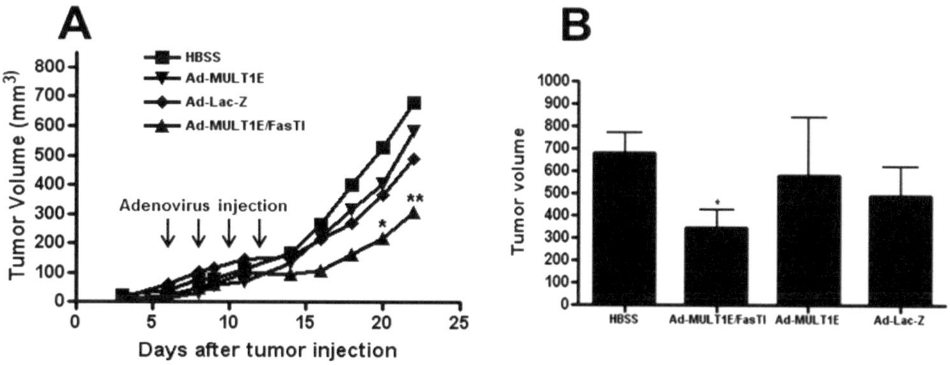

Fig. 13. MULT1E/FasTI delivered by adenoviral vector inhibits *in vivo* tumor growth. TC-1 cells (2 x 10^5) in 0.2ml HBSS were subcutaneously injected into flanks of C57BL/6J mice (n = 6). One week after tumor cell injection, various viral vectors at a dose of 1 x 10^9 pfu/tumor were intratumorally injected on every other day for a total of 4 injections. Control animals received injections of 50μl HBSS. Tumor growth was measured and presented as $1/2LW^2$ (A). At the end of this experiment, the mice were sacrificed and tumors were harvested and measured (B). *P< 0.05

3.10 MULT1E/FasTI delivered by adenoviral vector induces apoptosis in tumor

In order to confirm that MULT1E/FasTI delivered by adenoviral vector slows tumor growth by inducing tumor cell to undergo apoptosis, two days after last adenoviral particle injection, some mice were i.v. injected with FLIVO™ *in vivo* apoptosis detection reagent. Thirty minutes later, the tumor tissues were collected and 7 μm frozen sections were produced. The slides were examined under fluorescent microscope and the green fluorescent cells were counted. The number of apoptotic cells in tumors receiving Ad-MULT1E/FasTI is significantly higher than that of tumors receiving either Ad-MULT1E or Ad-Lac-Z. There are no significantly more apoptotic cells in tumors receiving Ad-MULT1E or Ad-Lac-Z when compared with tumors that received just HBSS (Fig. 14).

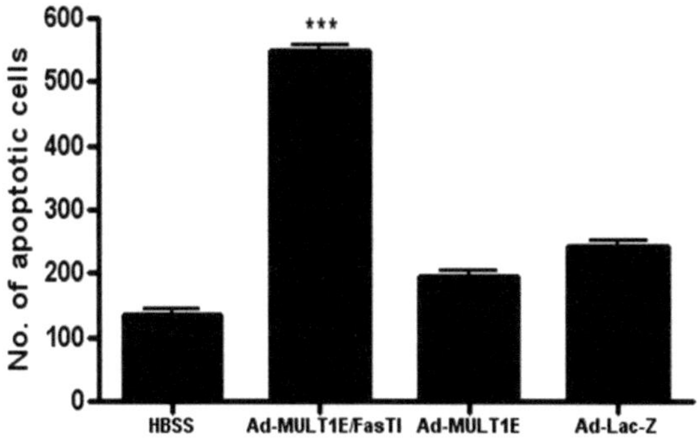

Fig. 14. MULT1E/FasTI delivered by adenoviral vector induces apoptosis *in vivo*. Two days after the last intratumor virus injection, 100μl of FLIVO™ *in vivo* apoptosis detection reagent (green) was injected into mice. Thirty minutes later, the mice were sacrificed and tumors collected. Frozen sections were made from the tumor tissues and examined under fluorescent microscope. The data presented are the sum of apoptotic cells from 12 random fields of each section. *** P < 0001

4. Conclusion

Tumor cells have developed multiple mechanisms to subvert and suppress immune responses by regulating cell-surface expression of Fas (Ivanov et al., 2003) and Fas ligand (Zheng et al., 2003) and shedding NKG2D ligands such as MULT1 (Raffaghello et al., 2004), resulting in escape from killing by infiltrating antitumor NK cells and T cells (Elsasser-Beile et al., 2003). As NKG2D ligand surface levels critically determine the susceptibility to NKG2D-mediated NK cell lysis, stable expression of NKG2D ligands on tumors would help increase NK cell lysis of tumors (Diefenbach and Raulet, 2001). In this study, we enhanced the cell-surface expression of MULT1, one of the mouse NKG2D ligands, by anchoring the extracellular domain of MULT1 on tumor cells using a transmembrane sequence of Fas. We also introduced the DD of Fas in the intracellular domain of the fusion protein MULT1E/FasTI, hoping to develop a bifunctional chimeric protein that can send an apoptosis signal to the tumor cells and at the same time activate NKG2D-expressing immune cells such as NK cells.

We cloned the cDNA encoding the extracellular domain of MULT1 gene from thymus of new born mice and ligated it to the transmembrane and intracellular domains of mouse *fas* cDNA. The resulting fusion cDNA was inserted into a mammalian cell expressing vector under the control of CMV promoter. The vector was then transfected into mouse TC-1 lung epithelial cancer cells, and stable cell lines expressing the fusion protein were established. The transcription of the novel fusion protein MULT1E/FasTI in the transfected cells was confirmed by RT–PCR and its expression was characterized by surface FACS analysis.

One of the key features of the designed fusion protein is to send apoptosis signals into the cells expressing the fusion protein, upon binding to its ligand, NKG2D. Although we do not have direct evidence supporting that the binding of NKG2D can form DISC inside tumor cells, a clear apoptosis signal is sent to the cells as indicated by the increased caspase-3 activity and increased Annexin V-positive cells after treatment with recombinant NKG2D/Fc. Our data shows that fusion protein MULT1E/FasTI, when expressed on cells, not only sends apoptotic signals into cells expressing it, but also activates immune cells that

express receptors for MULT1 like NK cells. When co-culutred with NK cells isolated from spleen, the fusion proteins expressing clones activated NK cells by producing IFN-γ.
This study shows that fusion protein MULT1E/FasTI has antitumor activity *in vivo*. We used a subcutaneous tumor model and a pulmonary metastatic tumor model in this study. In the subcutaneous tumor study, MULT1E/FasTI expressing clones formed smaller tumors compared to controls; and in the pulmonary metastasis study, mice completely rejected tumor cells expressing the fusion protein. We showed that the fusion protein had a much stronger antitumor effect in the pulmonary metastasis setting than in the subcutaneous setting. This is in agreement with a study demonstrating that NK cells are more effective against blood borne metastasis (Smyth et al., 2002). Previous studies have shown that tumor cells ectopically expressing NKG2D ligands such as MULT1 are potently rejected by NKG2D-expressing lymphocytes (Diefenbach et al., 2001). Our data shows that adding Fas to the MULT1 has a clear additional antitumor effect.
A significant challenge facing cancer gene therapy is how to specifically deliver tumor-killing genes into tumor cells efficiently. The recent development of adenovirus as gene delivery vectors opens a new window for cancer gene therapy (Cohen and Rudin, 2001; Ries and Korn, 2002). We used adenoviruses to deliver the fusion protein MULT1E/FasTI into tumor cells. The findings of this study demonstrate the therapeutic effect of adenovirus-mediated gene therapy of novel fusion protein MULT1E/FasTI. The most encouraging finding from a preclinical viewpoint is that mice receiving treatment with Ad-MULTE/FasTI showed more apoptosis *in vivo*, formed smaller tumors, and survived longer.
NK cell function is regulated by a balance between activating and inhibiting receptor signals (Trinchieri, 1989; Diefenbach and Raulet, 2001). Several types of inhibitory NK cell receptors recognize MHC class I molecules on target cells and prevent NK cell cytotoxicity toward normal cells (Yokoyama et al., 1995). The expression of ligands for activating receptor on target cells tips the balance toward activation of NK cells and induces NK cell cytotoxicity by formation of NK cell lytic synapse. NK cell cytotoxicity involves the secretion of cytolytic effector molecules known as lytic granules. The induction of NK cell effector functions, such as cytotoxicity, requires the contact between the NK cell and its target cell. The events that occur following the interaction between a cytolytic cell and its target cell, and the formation of the NK cell lytic synapse can be divided into three main stages: 1) initiation stage, 2) effector stage, and 3) termination stage. Initiation stage includes adhesion and initial signaling for cell activation. Effector stage involves actin reorganization, receptor clustering, raft formation, polarization of the microtubule-organizing centre (MTOC) and lytic granule fusion with the plasma membrane. Termination stage includes a period of inactivity and detachment.
Fas receptor activation can occur through different mechanisms. Binding of homotrimers of FasL to Fas can homotrimerize Fas receptor (Papoff et al., 1999; Siegel et al., 2000). A death domain-independent oligomerization domain in the extracellular region of the Fas, mapping to the N-terminal 49 amino acids, can also mediate homo- and heterooligomerization of the death receptor (Papoff et al., 1999). Apoptosis can be triggered in the absence of FasL by overexpression of the Fas cytoplasmic domain or Fas lacking the N-terminal 42 amino acids (Papoff et al., 1999), suggesting that the extracellular oligomerization domain of Fas is not required to initiate signaling and that self-association of the death domain is necessary and sufficient to induce cell death. The intracellular death domains of death receptors show a high tendency to self-associate, and when overexpressed by gene transfer in eukaryotic cells, trigger apoptotic signaling (Boldin et al., 1996). These findings indicate that the Fas receptor

plays an active role in its own clustering and that its oligomerization can be achieved in the absence of FasL.

We hypothesize that, when NKG2D expressing cells such as NK cells come in contact with TC-1 cells expressing the MULT1E/FasTI fusion protein, an NK cell lytic synapse would be formed as a result of the receptor-ligand interaction between NK cells and fusion protein expressing target cells. At this NK cell lytic synapse, activated NKG2D receptors bind to MULT1 ligands, cluster together and form lipid rafts. Formation of lipid rafts consisting of receptor-ligand complexes would result in activation of NK cells and NK cell cytotoxicity with the release of lytic granules consisting of granzymes and IFN-γ at the immunological synapse. Binding of NKG2D to the MULT1E region of the fusion protein causes clustering of the fusion protein, and through death domain interactions would trigger formation of microaggregates resulting in larger clusters of FasTI, formation of DISC, caspase-8 activation and apoptosis in cell. Hence, our fusion protein approach is a two pronged approach for activating NK cells as well as inducing apoptosis, when the fusion protein binds to NKG2D receptors. Even though we do not have evidence of the formation of lytic synapses with NK cells and DISC formation in fusion protein expressing cells, our IFN-γ assay using NK cells and caspase-3 ELISA assay confirm the functionality of both MULT1E and FasTI regions in our fusion protein and the dual role of MULT1E/FasTI.

In summary, a bi-functional chimeric protein containing the extracellular domain of MULT1 and the transmembrane and intracellular domains of Fas is created. It may provide a potential avenue for new cancer therapies and supports further investigation of therapeutic strategies using other NKG2D ligands combined with Fas transmembrane and intracellular domains for treating cancer. When combined with adenovirus gene delivery vectors, especially the oncolytic adenovirus vectors, the fusion protein will provide a robust anti-cancer agent.

5. References

Bacon L *et al.* (2004).Two human ULBP/RAET1 molecules with transmembrane regions are ligands for NKG2D. *J Immunol,* Vol. 173, pp. 1078-1084.

Bahram S, Bresnahan M, Geraghty DE, & Spies TA. (1994). Second lineage of mammalian major histocompatibility complex class I genes. *Proc Natl Acad ScI USA,* Vol. 91, pp. 6259-6263.

Bauer S, Groh V, Wu J, Steinle A, Phillips J H, Lanier LL, & Spies T. (1999). Activation of NK cells and T cells by NKG2D, a receptor for stress-inducible MICA. *Science,* Vol. 285, pp. 727-729.

Bellgrau D, Gold D, Selawry H, Moore J, Franzusoff A, & Duke RC. (1995). A role for CD95 ligand in preventing graft rejection. *Nature,* Vol. 377, pp. 630-632.

Billadeau DD, Upshaw JL, Schoon RA, Dick CJ, & Leibson PJ. (2003).NKG2D DAP10 triggers human NK cell-mediated killing via a Syk-independent regulatory pathway. *Nat Immunol,* Vol. 4, pp. 557-564.

Boldin MP, Goncharov TM, Goltsev YV, & Wallach D. (1996). Involvement of MACH, a novel MORT1/FADD-interacting protease, in Fas/APO-1- and TNF receptor-induced cell death. *Cell,* Vol. 85, pp. 803-815.

Borchers MT, Harris NL, Wesselkamper SC, Vitucci M, & Cosman D. (2006). NKG2D ligands are expressed on stressed human airway epithelial cells. *Am J Physiol Lung Cell Mol Physiol,* Vol. 291, pp. 222- 231.

Brunner T, Wasem C, Torgler R, Cima I, Jakob S, & Corazza N. (2003). Fas (CD95/Apo-1) ligand regulation in T cell homeostasis, cell-mediated cytotoxicity and immune pathology. *Semin Immunol,* Vol. 15, pp. 167-176.

Bui JD, Carayannopoulos LN, Lanier LL,Yokoyama WM, Schreiber RD. Busche A, Goldmann T, Naumann U, Steinle A, & Brandau S. (2006). Natural killer cell-mediated rejection of experimental human lung cancer by genetic overexpression of major histocompatibility complex class I chain-related gene A. *Hum Gene Ther,* Vol. 17, pp. 135–146.

Campos SK, & Barry MA. (2007). Current advances and future challenges in adenoviral vector biology and targeting. *Curr Gene Therapy,* Vol. 7, pp. 189-204.

Carayannopoulos LN, Naidenko OV, Fremont DH, & Yokoyama WM. (2002). Cutting edge: murine UL16-binding protein-like transcript 1: a newly described transcript encoding a high-affinity ligand for murine NKG2D. *J Immunol,* Vol. 169, pp. 4079-4083.

Carayannopoulos LN, Naidenko OV, Kinder J, Ho EL, Fremont DH, & Yokoyama WM. (2002a). Ligands for murine NKG2D display heterogeneous binding behavior. *Eur J Immunol,* Vol. 32, pp. 597-605.

Chalupny NJ, Rein-Weston A, Dosch S, Cosman D. (2006). Down-regulation of the NKG2D ligand MICA by the human cytomegalovirus glycoprotein UL142. *Biochem Biophys Res Commun,* Vol. 346, pp. 175-181.

Chalupny N, Sutherland C, Lawrence W, Rein-Weston A, & Cosman D. (2003). ULBP4 is a novel ligand for human NKG2D. *Biochem Biophys Res Commun,* Vol. 305, pp. 129-135.

Chan CW, Crafton E, Fan HN, Flook J, Yoshimura K, Skarica M *et al.* (2006). Interferon-producing killer dendritic cells provide a link between innate and adaptive immunity. *Nat Med,* Vol. 12, pp. 207-213.

Chang C, Dietrich J, Harpur AG, Lindquist JA, Haude A, Loke YW *et al.* (1999). Cutting edge: KAP10, a novel transmembrane adapter protein genetically linked to DAP12 but with unique signaling properties. *J Immunol,* Vol. 163, pp. 4651-4654.

Cohen EE, & Rudin CM. ONYX-015: (2001). Onyx Pharmaceuticals. *Curr Opin Investig Drugs,* Vol. 2, pp. 1770-1775.

Colucci F, Schweighoffer E, Tomasello E, Turner M, Ortaldo JR, Vivier E *et al.* (2002). Natural cytotoxicity uncoupled from the Syk and ZAP-70 intracellular kinases. *Nat Immunol,* Vol. 3, pp. 288-294.

Cosman, D, Müllberg J, Sutherland CL, Chin W, Armitage R, Fanslow W, Kubin M, & Chalupny NJ. (2001). ULBPs, novel MHC class I-related molecules, bind to CMV glycoprotein UL16 and stimulate NK cytotoxicity through the NKG2D receptor. *Immunity,* Vol. 14, pp. 123-133.

Coudert JD, & Held W. (2006). The role of the NKG2D receptor for tumor immnity. *Sem Can Biol,* Vol. 16, pp. 333-343.

Debatin KM, Krammer PH. Death receptors in chemotherapy and cancer. *Oncogene* 2004; 23: 2950-2966.

Deng T, & Karin M. (1993). JunB differs from c-Jun in its DNA-binding and dimerization domains, and represses c-Jun by formation of inactive heterodimers. *Genes Dev,* Vol. 7, pp. 479-490.

Diefenbach A, Hsia JK, Hsiung MY, & Raulet DH. (2003). A novel ligand for the NKG2D receptor activates NK cells and macrophages and induces tumor immunity. *Eur J Immunol,* Vol. 33, pp. 381-391.

Diefenbach A, Jamieson AM, Liu SD, Shastri N, & Raulet DH. (2000). Ligands for the murine NKG2D receptor: expression by tumor cells and activation of NK cells and macrophages. *Nat Immunol,* Vol. 1, pp. 119-126.

Diefenbach A, & Raulet DH. (2001). Strategies for target cell recognition by natural killer cells. *Immunol Rev,* Vol. 181, pp. 170-184.

Diefenbach A, Tomasello E, Lucas M, Jamieson AM, Hsia JK, Vivier E, & Raulet DH. (2002a). Selective associations with signaling molecules determines stimulatory versus costimulatory activity of NKG2D. *Nat Immunol,* Vol. 3, pp. 1142-1149.

Diefenbach A, & Raulet DH. (2002b). The innate immune response to tumors and its role in the induction of T cell immunity. *Immunol Rev,* Vol. 188, pp. 19-21.

Doubrovina ES, Doubrovin MM, Vider E, Sisson RB, O'Reilly RJ, Dupont B *et al.* (2003). Evasion from NK cell immunity by MHC class I chain-related molecules expressing colon adenocarcinoma. *J Immunol,* Vol. 171, pp. 6891-6899.

Draghi M *et al.* (2007). NKp46 and NKG2D recognition of infected dendritic cells is necessary for NK cell activation in the human response to influenza infection. *J Immunol,* Vol. 178, pp. 2688-2698.

Eagle RA, & Trowsdale J. (2007). Promiscuity and the single receptor: NKG2D. *Nat Rev Immunol,* Vol. 7, pp. 737-44.

Earnshaw WC, Martins LM, & Kaufmann SH. (1999). Mammalian caspases: structure, activation, substrates, and functions during apoptosis. *Annu Rev Biochem,* Vol. 68, pp. 383-424.

Elsasser-Beile U, Gierschner D, Welchner T, & Wetterauer U. (2003). Different expression of Fas and Fas ligand in tumor infiltrating and peripheral lymphocytes of patients with renal cell carcinomas. *Anticancer Res,* Vol. 23, pp. 433-437.

Friese MA, Wischhusen J, Wick W, Weiler M, Eisele G, Steinle A *et al.* (2004). RNA interference targeting transforming growth factor-beta enhances NKG2D-mediated antiglioma immune response, inhibits glioma cell migration and invasiveness, and abrogates tumorigenicity *in vivo*. *Cancer Res,* Vol. 64, pp. 7596-603.

Fulda S, Kufer MU, Meyer E, van Valen F, Dockhorn-Dworniczak B, & Debatin KM. (2001). Sensitization for death receptor or drug-induced apoptosis by re-expression of caspase-8 through demethylation or gene transfer. *Oncogene,* Vol. 20, pp. 5865-5877.

Garnett CT, Erdman D, Xu W, & Gooding LR. (2002). Prevalence and quantitation of species C adenovirus DNA in human mucosal lymphocytes. *J Virol,* Vol. 76, pp. 10608-10616.

Garrity D, Call ME, Feng J, & Wucherpfennig KW. (2005). The activating NKG2D receptor assembles in the membrane with two signaling dimers into a hexameric structure. *Proc Natl Acad Sci USA,* Vol. 102, pp. 7641-7646.

Gasser S, Orsulic S, Brown EJ, & Raulet DH. (2005). The DNA damage pathway regulates innate immune system ligands of the NKG2D receptor. *Nature,* Vol. 436, pp. 1186-1190.

Girardi M, Oppenheim DE, Steele CR, Lewis JM, Glusac E, Filler R *et al.* (2001). Regulation of cutaneous malignancy by gammadelta T cells. *Science,* Vol. 294, pp. 605-609.

Glienke J, Sobanov Y, Brostjan C, Steffens C, Nguyen C, Lehrach H *et al.* (1998). The genomic organization of NKG2C, E, F, and D receptor genes in the human natural killer gene complex. *Immunogenetics,* Vol. 48, pp. 163-173.

Gomes EM, & Tong AW. (2006). Anti-Tumor Properties of CD40 Ligand when Delivered as a Transgene by the Conditional Replicative Oncolytic Adenovirus AdEH to Breast Cancer Cells. PhD disseetation. Baylor University.

Griffith TS, Brunner T, Fletcher SM, Green DR, & Ferguson TA. (1995). Fas ligand-induced apoptosis as a mechanism of immune privilege. *Science,* Vol. 270, pp. 1189-1192.

Groh V, Bahram S, Bauer S, Herman A, Beauchamp M, & Spies T. (1996). Cell stress-regulated human major histocompatibility complex class I gene expressed in gastrointestinal epithelium. *Proc Natl Acad Sci USA,* Vol. 93, pp. 12445-12450.

Groh V, Rhinehart R, Randolph-Habecker J, Topp MS, Riddell SR, & Spies T. (2001). Costimulation of CD8 alphabeta T cells by NKG2D via engagement by MIC induced on virus-infected cells. *Nat Immunol,* Vol. 2, pp. 255-260.

Groh V, Rhinehart R, Secrist H, Bauer S, Grabstein KH, & Spies T. (1999). Broad tumor-associated expression and recognition by tumor-derived gamma delta T cells of MICA and MICB. *Proc Natl Acad Sci USA,* Vol. 96, pp. 6879-6884.

Groh V, Steinle A, Bauer S, & Spies T. (1998). Recognition of stress-induced MHC molecules by intestinal epithelial gammadelta T cells. *Science,* Vol. 279, pp. 1737-1740.

Groh V, Wu J, Yee C, & Spies T. (2002). Tumor-derived soluble MIC ligands impair expression of NKG2D and T-cell activation. *Nature,* Vol. 419, pp. 734-738.

Gumperz JE, Miyake S, Yamamura T, & Brenner MB. (2002). Functionally distinct subsets of CD1d-restricted natural killer T cells revealed by CD1d tetramer staining. *J Exp Med,* Vol. 195, pp. 625-636.

Hanahan D, & Weinberg RA. (2000). The hallmarks of cancer. *Cell,* Vol. 100, pp. 57-70.

Hayakawa Y, Kelly JM, Westwood J, Darcy PK, Diefenbach A, Raulet DH, & Smyth MJ. (2002). Tumor rejection mediated by NKG2D receptor-ligand interaction is strictly dependent on perforin. *J Immunol,* Vol. 169, pp. 5377-5381.

Ho EL, Heusel JW, Brown MG, Matsumoto K, Scalzo AA, & Yokoyama WM. (1998). Murine Nkg2d and Cd94 are clustered within the natural killer complex and are expressed independently in natural killer cells. *Proc Natl Acad Sci USA,* Vol. 95, pp. 6320-6325.

Hohenberger P, & Tunn PU. (2003). Isolated limb perfusion with rhTNFalpha and melphalan for locally recurrent childhood synovial sarcoma of the limb. *J Pediatr Hematol Oncol,* Vol. 25, pp. 905-909.

Houston A, & O' Connell J. (2004). The Fas signalling pathway and its role in the pathogenesis of cancer. *Cur Opinion Phar,* Vol. 4, pp. 321-326.

Houston A, Waldron-Lynch FD, Bennett MW, Roche D, O'Sullivan GC, Shanahan F, & O'Connell J. (2003). Fas ligand expressed in colon cancer is not associated with increased apoptosis of tumor cells *in vivo. Int J Cancer,* Vol. 107, pp. 209-214.

Hue S *et al.* (2004). A direct role for NKG2D/MICA interaction in villous atrophy during celiac disease. *Immunity,* Vol. 21, pp. 367-377.

Igney FH, & Krammer PH. (2002). Death and anti-death: tumour resistance to apoptosis. *Nat Rev Cancer,* Vol. 2, pp. 277-288.

Irmler M, Thome M, Hahne M, Schneider P, Hofmann K, Steiner V, Bodmer JL, Schroter M, Burns K, Mattmann C, *et al.* (1997). Inhibition of death receptor signals by cellular FLIP. *Nature,* Vol. 388, pp. 190-195.

Ivanov VN, Bergami PL, Maulit G, Sato TA, Sassoon D, & Ronai Z. (2003). FAP-1 association with Fas (Apo-1) inhibits Fas expression on the cell surface. *Mol Cell Biol,* Vol. 23, pp. 3623-3635.

Jamieson AM, Diefenbach A, McMahon CW, Xiong N, Carlyle JR, & Raulet DH. (2002). The role of the NKG2D immunoreceptor in immune cell activation and natural killing. *Immunity,* Vol. 17, pp. 19-29.

Jan Chalupny N, Sutherland CL, LawrenceWA, Rein-Weston A, (2003). Cosman D. ULBP4 is a novel ligand for human NKG2D. *Biochem Biophys Res Commun,* Vol. 305, pp. 129-135.

Jinushi M, Takehara T, Tatsumi T, Kanto T, Groh V, Spies T *et al.* (2003). Expression and role of MICA and MICB in human hepatocellular carcinomas and their regulation by retinoic acid. *Int J Cancer,* Vol. 104, pp. 354-361.

Kase H, Aoki Y, & Tanaka K. (2003). Fas ligand expression in cervical adenocarcinoma. Relevance to lymph node metastasis and tumor progression. *Gynecol Oncol,* Vol. 90, pp. 70-74.

Khakoo SIR. Rajalingam BP, Shum K, Weidenbach L, Flodin DG, Muir F, Canavez SL, Cooper NM, Valiante LL, Lanier, & Parham P. (2000). Rapid evolution of NK cell receptor systems demonstrated by comparison of chimpanzees and humans. *Immunity,* Vol. 12, pp. 687-694.

Kischkel FC, Hellbardt S, Behrmann I, Germer M, Pawlita M, Krammer PH, & Peter ME. (1995). Cytotoxicity-dependent APO-1 (Fas/CD95)-associated proteins form a death-inducing signaling complex (DISC) with the receptor. *EMBO J,* Vol. 14, pp. 5579-5588.

Klein JY, Satta C, O'Huigin, & Takahata N. (1993). The molecular descent of the major histocompatibility complex. *Annu Rev Immunol,* Vol. 11, pp. 269-276.

Komatsu-Wakui M *et al.* (1999). *MICA* polymorphism in Japanese and a *MICA-MICB* null haplotype. *Immunogenetics,* Vol. 49, pp. 620-628.

Kotturi HSR, Li J, Branham –O" Connor M, Stickel SL, Yu X, Wagner TE, & Wei Y. (2008). Tumor cells expressing a fusion protein of MULT1 and Fas are rejected *in vivo* by apoptosis and NK cell activation. *Gene Ther,* Vol. 15, pp. 1302-1310.

Kotturi HSR, Li J, Branham-O'Connor M, Yu X, Wagner TE, Wei Y. (2010). In vitro and in vivo delivery of a novel anticancer fusion protein MULT1E/FasTI via adenoviral vectors. *Can Gene Ther,* Vol. 17, pp. 164-170.

Krmpotic A, Busch DH, Bubic I, Gebhardt F, Hengel H, Hasan M, Scalzo AA, Koszinowski UH, & Jonjic S. (2002). MCMV glycoprotein gp40 confers virus resistance to CD8+ T cells and NK cells *in vivo. Nat Immunol,* Vol. 3, pp. 529-535.

Lanier LL, Corliss BC, Wu J, Leong C, & Phillips JH. (1998). Immunoreceptor DAP12 bearing a tyrosine-based activation motif is involved in activating NK cells. *Nature,* Vol. 391, pp. 703-707.

Lee JC, Lee KM, Kim DW, & Heo DS. (2004). Elevated TGF β1 secretion and down-modulation of NKG2D underlies impaired NK cytotoxicity in cancer patients. *J Immunol,* Vol. 172, pp. 7335-7340.

Li P, Morris DL, Willcox BE, Steinle A, Spies T, & Strong RK. (2001). Complex structure of the activating immunoreceptor NKG2D and its MHC class I-like ligand MICA. *Nat Immunol,* Vol. 2, pp. 443-451.

Lodoen MB, & Lanier LL. (2006). Natural killer cells as an initial defense against pathogens. *Curr Opin Immunol,* Vol. 18, pp. 391-398.
Lowin-Kropf B, Kunz B, Schneider P, & Held W. (2002). A role for the src family kinase Fyn in NK cell activation and the formation of the repertoire of Ly49 receptors. *Eur J Immunol,* Vol. 32, pp. 773-782.
Ma H, Liu Y, Liu S, Kung HF, Sun X, Zheng D *et al.* (2005). Recombinant adeno-associated virus-mediated TRAIL gene therapy suppresses liver metastatic tumours. *Int J Cancer,* Vol. 116, pp. 314-321.
Maasho K, Opoku-Anane J, Marusina AI, Coligan JE, & Borrego F. (2005). NKG2D is a costimulatory receptor for human naive CD8+ T cells. *J Immunol,* Vol. 174, pp. 4480-4484.
Mashima T, & Tsuruo T. (2005). Defects of the apoptotic pathway as therapeutic target against cancer. *Drug Resist Updat,* Vol. 8, pp. 339-343.
McFarland BJ, Kortemme T, Yu SF, Baker D, & Strong RK. (2003). Symmetry recognizing asymmetry: analysis of the interactions between the C-type lectin-like immunoreceptor NKG2D andMHCclass I-like ligands. *Structure,* Vol. 11, pp. 411-422.
Mollinedo F, & Gajate C. (1997). Fas/CD95 death receptor and lipid rafts: New targets for apoptosis-directed cancer therapy. *Drug Res Upda* 2006; 9: 51-73.
Nagata S. Apoptosis by death factor. *Cell,* Vol. 88, pp. 355-365.
Nedvetzki S *et al.* (2007). Reciprocal regulation of natural killer cells and macrophages associated with distinct immune synapses. *Blood,* Vol. 109, pp. 3776-3785.
Nesterov A, Ivashchenko Y, & Kraft AS. (2002). Tumor necrosis factorrelated apoptosis-inducing ligand (TRAIL) triggers apoptosis in normal prostate epithelial cells. *Oncogene,* Vol. 21, pp. 1135-1140.
Niehans GA, Brunner T, Frizelle SP, Liston JC, Salerno CT, Knapp DJ *et al.* (1997). Human lung carcinomas express Fas ligand. *Cancer Res,* Vol. 57, pp. 1007-1012.
Nomura M *et al.* (1996). Genomic structures and characterization of Rae1 family members encoding GPI-anchored cell surface proteins and expressed predominantly in embryonic mouse brain. *J Biochem,* Vol. 120, pp. 987-995.
O'Callaghan CA, Cerwenka A, Willcox BE, Lanier LL, & Bjorkman PJ. (2001). Molecular competition for NKG2D: H60 and RAE1 compete unequally for NKG2D with dominance of H60. *Immunity,* Vol. 15, pp. 201-211.
O'Connell J, O'Sullivan GC, Collins JK, & Shanahan F. (1996). The Fas counterattack. Fas-mediated T cell killing by colon cancer cells expressing Fas ligand. *J Exp Med,* Vol. 184, pp. 1075-1082.
Ogasawara J, Watanabe-Fukunaga R, Adachi M, Matsuzawa A, Kasugai T, Kitamura Y, Itoh N, Suda T, & Nagata S. (1993). Lethal effect of the anti-Fas antibody in mice. *Nature,* Vol. 364, pp. 806- 809.
Ogasawara K, Benjamin J, Takaki R, Phillips JH, Lanier LL *et al.* (2003). Impairment of NK cell function by NKG2D modulation in NOD mice. *Immunity,* Vol. 18, pp. 41-51.
Okada K, Komuta K, Hashimoto S, Matsuzaki S, Kanematsu T, & Koji T. (2000). Frequency of apoptosis of tumor-infiltrating lymphocytes induced by Fas counterattack in human colorectal carcinoma and its correlation with prognosis. *Clin Cancer Res,* Vol. 6, pp. 3560-3564.

Palmer DH, Mautner V, Mirza D, Oliff S, Gerritsen W, van der Sijp JRM *et al.* (2004). Virus-directed enzyme prodrug therapy: intratumoral administration of a replication-deficient adenovirus encoding nitroreductase to patients with resectable liver cancer. *J Clin Oncol,* Vol. 22, pp. 1546-1552.

Papoff G, Hausler P, Eramo A, Pagano MG, Di Leve G, Signore A, & Ruberti G. (1999). Identification and characterization of a ligandindependent oligomerization domain in the extracellular region of the CD95 death receptor. *J Biol Chem,* Vol. 274, pp. 38241-38250.

Pappworth IY, Wang EC, & Rowe M. (2007). The switch from latent to productive infection in Epstein–Barr virus-infected B cells is associated with sensitization to NK cell killing. *J Virol,* Vol. 81, pp. 474-482.

Pende D, Rivera P, Marcenaro S, Chang CC, Biassoni R, Conte R *et al.* (2002). Major histocompatibility complex class I-related chain A and UL16- binding protein expression on tumor cell lines of different histotypes: analysis of tumor susceptibility to NKG2D-dependent natural killer cell cytotoxicity. *Cancer Res,* Vol. 62, pp. 6178-6186.

Peter ME, & Krammer PH. (2003). The CD95(APO-1/Fas) DISC and beyond. *Cell Death Differ,* Vol. 10, pp. 26-35.

Peter ME, Scaffidi C, Medema JP, Kischkel F, & Krammer PH. (1999). The death receptors. Results Problem. *Cell Differ,* Vol. 23, pp. 25-63.

Pitti RM, Marsters SA, Lawrence DA, Roy M, Kischkel FC, Dowd P *et al.* (1998). Genomic amplification of a decoy receptor for Fas ligand in lung and colon cancer. *Nature,* Vol. 396, pp. 699-703.

Poggi A, Venturino C, Catellani S, Clavio M, Miglino M, Gobbi M *et al.* (2004). Vδ1 T lymphocytes from B-CLL patients recognize ULBP3 expressed on leukemic B cells and up-regulated by *trans*-retinoic acid. *Cancer Res,* Vol. 64, pp. 9172-9179.

Rabinovich B, Li J, Wolfson M, Lawrence W, Beers C, Chalupny J *et al.* (2006). NKG2D splice variants: a reexamination of adaptor molecule associations. *Immunogenetics,* Vol. 58, pp. 81-88.

Radaev S, Kattah M, Zou Z, Colonna M, & Sun PD. (2002). Making sense of the diverse ligand recognition by NKG2D. *J Immunol,* Vol. 169, pp. 6279-6285.

Radosavljevic M, Cuillerier B, Wilson MJ, Clement O, Wicker S, Gilfillan S *et al.* (2002). A cluster of ten novel MHC class I related genes on human chromosome 6q24.2–q25.3. *Genomics,* Vol. 79, pp. 114-123.

Raffaghello L, Prigione I, Airoldi I, Camoriano M, Levreri I, Gambini C *et al.* (2004). Downregulation and/or release of NKG2D ligands as immune evasion strategy of human neuroblastoma. *Neoplasia,* Vol. 6, pp. 558-568.

Raffaghello L, Prigione I, Airoldi I, Camoriano M, Morandi F, Bocca P *et al.* (2005). Mechanisms of immune evasion of human neuroblastoma. *Cancer Lett,* Vol. 228, pp. 155-161.

Raulet DH, Vance RE, & McMahon CW. (2001). Regulation of the natural killer cell receptor repertoire. *Annu Rev Immunol,* Vol. 19, pp. 291-330.

Raulet DH. (2003). Roles of the NKG2D immunoreceptor and its ligands. *Nature Rev Immunol,* Vol. 3, pp. 781-790.

Ries S, & Korn WM. (2002). ONYX-015: mechanisms of action and clinical potential of a replication-selective adenovirus. *Br J Cancer,* Vol. 86, pp. 5-11.

Roberts AI, Lee L, Schwarz E, Groh V, Spies T, Ebert EC *et al.* (2001). NKG2D receptors induced by IL-15 costimulate CD28-negative effector CTL in the tissue microenvironment. *J Immunol,* Vol. 167, pp. 5527-5530.

Rosen DB, Araki M, Hamerman JA, Chen T, Yamamura T, & Lanier LL. (2004). A Structural basis for the association of DAP12 with mouse, but not human, NKG2D. *J Immunol,* Vol. 173, pp. 2470-2478.

Saas P, Walker PR, Hahne M, Quiquerez AL, Schnuriger V, Perrin G, French L, Van Meir EG, de Tribolet N, Tschopp J *et al.* (1997). Fas ligand expression by astrocytoma in vivo: maintaining immune privilege in the brain? *J Clin Invest,* Vol. 99, pp. 1173-1178.

Salvesen GS, & Dixit VM. (1999). Caspase activation: the induced-proximity model. *Proc Natl Acad Sci USA,* Vol. 96, pp. 10964-10967.

Sangro B, Mazzolini G, Ruiz J, Herraiz M, Quiroga J, Herrero I *et al.* (2004). Phase I trial of intratumoral injection of an adenovirus encoding interleukin-12 for advanced digestive tumours. *J Clin Oncol,* Vol. 22, pp. 1389-1397.

Scaffidi C, Medema JP, Krammer PH, & Peter ME. (1997). FLICE is predominantly expressed as two functionally active isoforms, caspase-8/a and caspase-8/b. *J Biol Chem,* Vol. 272, pp. 26953-26958.

Schulze-Osthoff K, Ferrari D, Los M, Wesselborg S, & Peter ME. (1998). Apoptosis signaling by death receptors. *Eur J Biochem,* Vol. 254, pp. 439-459.

Shankar S, & Srivastava RK. (2004). Enhancement of therapeutic potential of TRAIL by cancer therapy and irradiation: mechanisms and clinical implications. *Drug Resist Updat,* Vol. 7, pp. 139-156.

Siegel RM, Chan FK, Chun HJ, & Lenardo MJ. (2000). The multifaceted role of Fas signaling in immune cell homeostasis and autoimmunity. *Nat Immunol,* Vol. 1, pp. 469-474.

Smyth MJ, Hayakawa Y, Takeda K, & Yagita H. (2002). New aspects of natural killer cell surveillance and therapy of cancer. *Nature Reviews Cancer,* Vol. 2, pp. 850-851.

Smyth MJ *et al.* (2005). NKG2D function protects the host from tumor initiation. *J Exp Med,* Vol. 202, pp. 583-588.

Taieb J, Chaput N, Menard C, Apetoh L, Ullrich E, Bonmort M *et al.* (2006). A novel dendritic cell subset involved in tumor immunosurveillance. *Nat Med* Vol. 12, pp. 214-219.

Takaki R, HayakawaY, Nelson A, Sivakumar PV, Hughes S, Smyth MJ *et al.* (2005). Tumor cells to specific lysis by natural killer cells. *Clin Cancer Res,* Vol. 11, pp. 7516-7552.

Tong AW. (2006). Oncolytic viral therapy for human cancer: challenges revisited. *Drug Development Research,* Vol. 66, pp. 260-277.

Tourneur L, Mistou S, Michiels FM, Devauchelle V, Renia L, Feunteun J, & Chiocchia G. (2003). Loss of FADD protein expression results in a biased Fas-signaling pathway and correlates with the development of tumoral status in thyroid follicular cells. *Oncogene,* Vol. 22, pp. 2795-2804.

Trinchieri G. (1989). Biology of natural killer cells. *Adv Immunol,* Vol. 47, pp. 187-376.

Upshaw JL, Arneson LN, Schoon RA, Dick CJ, Billadeau DD, & Leibson PJ. (2006). NKG2D-mediated signaling requires aDAP10-bound Grb2–Vav1 intermediate and phosphatidylinositol-3-kinase in human natural killer cells. *Nat Immunol,* Vol. 7, pp. 524-532.

Venkataraman GM, Suciu D, Groh V, Boss JM, & Spies T. (2007). Promoter region architecture and transcriptional regulation of the genes for the MHC class Irelated chain A and B ligands of NKG2D. *J Immunol,* Vol. 178, pp. 961-969.

Vetter CS, Lieb W, Brocker EB, & Becker JC. (2004). Loss of nonclassical MHC molecules MIC-A/B expression during progression of uveal melanoma. *Br J Cancer,* Vol. 91, pp. 1495-1499.

Wiemann K, Mittrucker HW, Feger U, Welte SA, Yokoyama WM, Spies T *et al.* (2005). Systemic NKG2D down-regulation impairs NK and CD8 T cell responses in vivo. *J Immunol,* Vol. 175, pp. 720-729.

Wolan DW, Teyton L, Rudolph MG, Villmow B, Bauer S, Busch DH *et al.* (2001). Crystal structure of the murine NK cell-activating receptor NKG2D at 1.95 A. *Nat Immunol,* Vol. 2, pp. 248-254.

Wu J, Song Y, Bakker AB, Bauer S, Spies T, Lanier LL *et al.* (1999). An activating immunoreceptor complex formed by NKG2D and DAP10. *Science,* Vol. 285, pp. 730-732.

Yokoyama WM, Daniels BF, Seaman WE, Hunziker R, Margulies DH, Smith HR *et al.* (1995). A family of murine NK cell receptors specific for target cell MHC class I molecules. *Semin Immunol,* Vol. 7, pp. 89-101.

Young LS, Searle PF, Onion D, & Mautner V. (2006). Viral gene therapy strategies: from basic science to clinical application. *J Pathol,* Vol. 208, pp. 299-318.

Zhang T, Lemoi BA, & Sentman CL. (2005). Chimeric NK-receptor-bearing T cells mediate antitumor immunotherapy. *Blood,* Vol. 106, pp. 1544-1551.

Zheng HC, Sun JM, Wei ZL, Yang XF, Zhang YC, (2003). Xin Y. Expression of Fas ligand and caspase-3 contributes to formation of immune escape in gastric cancer. *World J Gastroenterol,* Vol. 9, pp. 1415-1420.

Zhou H, Luo Y, Lo JF, Kaplan CD, Mizutani M, Mizutani N *et al.* (2005). DNA-based vaccines activate innate and adaptive antitumor immunity by engaging the NKG2D receptor. *Proc Natl Acad Sci USA,* Vol. 102, pp. 10846-10851.

Zompi S, Hamerman JA, Ogasawara K, Schweighoffer E, Tybulewicz VL, Di JP *et al.* NKG2D triggers cytotoxicity in mouse NK cells lacking DAP12 or Syk family kinases. *Nat Immunol* 2003; 4: 565-572.

15

Emergence of IFN-lambda as a Potential Antitumor Agent

Ahmed Lasfar[1] and Karine A. Cohen-Solal[2]
[1]*University of Medicine and Dentistry of New Jersey - New Jersey Medical School, University Hospital Cancer Center*
[2]*University of Medicine and Dentistry of New Jersey - Robert Wood Johnson Medical School, the Cancer Institute of New Jersey, USA*

1. Introduction

Despite the early discovery of interferon (IFN) in 1957, some members of the IFN family were just identified during the recent years. Interferon was discovered and characterized by Isaacs & Lindenmann during their study of viral infection and the biology of interference (Isaacs and Lindenmann, 1957). The authors used chick membranes infected with influenza viruses, and found that those cells released into the medium a substance which rendered other cells resistant to viral infection. The authors named this substance interferon. Subsequent studies demonstrated that interferon is not a virus particle but a protein released by the cells during viral infection.

Early studies have defined three different subfamilies of interferons, depending on their cell origin (Stewart et al., 1973). IFN-α was characterized from virus-infected leukocytes, IFN-β from fibroblasts and IFN-γ produced by transformed lymphocytes, which was first designated as an immune interferon. Other properties such as hydrophobicity, antigenicity and heat/pH sensitivity were also investigated to distinguish between IFN molecules. By probing on several hydrophobic adsorbents, one group demonstrated that the fibroblast interferon is more hydrophobic than leukocyte interferon (Jankowski et al., 1975). Rabbit antiserum prepared against the leukocyte IFN was found to contain two populations of neutralizing antibodies specific for leukocytes and fibroblasts populations and the authors concluded that two antigenic species of IFN were present (Havell et al., 1975). However, this rabbit antiserum preparation was shown to be less active against immune interferon (IFN-γ), which was also found to be relatively unstable at pH 2 and at 56 degrees (Valle et al., 1975). In the last 30 years, IFN-α, β and γ were purified and receptor binding assays using radio-labeled ligands were performed. The data clearly indicated that IFN-α and IFN-β interacted with the same binding site, which was distinct from IFN-γ (Littman et al., 1985; Merlin et al., 1985). Subsequently, characterization of the IFN receptor, followed by the production of IFN knockout mice, clearly showed that IFN-α/β signal through a receptor that is completely distinct from IFN-γ receptor (Ding et al., 1993; Muller et al., 1994). As a result of all these studies, IFNs were classified as two types. Type I IFN family is composed of several members, which include IFN-α, IFN-β and other related IFNs such as IFN-ω, IFN-ε and IFN-κ. The type II IFN family only includes IFN-γ (Pestka, 2007). In 2003, another

IFN family (type III) was identified and its members designated as IFN-λ (Kotenko et al., 2003; Sheppard et al., 2003) (Figure 1).
The new IFN members identified in human were designated as IFN-λs, by Kotenko's group (Kotenko et al., 2003), or IL-28A, IL-28B and IL-29 by Sheppard and coll. (Sheppard et al., 2003). IFN-λs demonstrate structural features that are similar to the IL-10-related cytokine family II [CRFII] but possess antiviral activity (Langer et al., 2004; Pestka et al., 2004). In 2005, the International Community of Interferon and Cytokine Research designated IFN-λs as type III IFNs, which include three distinct IFN-λ proteins, called IFN-λ1 (IL-29), IFN-λ2 (IL-28A) and IFN-λ3 (IL-28B). The genes encoding all three type III IFNs are clustered on human chromosome 19. The IFN-λ3 gene is transcribed in the opposite direction to the IFN-λ1 and IFN-λ2 genes. The coding region of each of the genes is divided into five exons (exon 1-5). The overall intron/exon structure of the IFN-λ genes correlates well with the common conserved architecture of the genes encoding IL-10-related cytokines (Kotenko, 2002). It is thought that the human IFN-λs genes derived from a common predecessor fairly recently. This is based on the fact that there is a great deal of homology between human IFN-λs It is also suggested that during the divergence of the IFN-λ1 and IFN-λ2 genes, occurred a more recent duplication event in which a fragment containing the IFN-λ1 and IFN-λ2 genes was copied and integrated back into the genome in a head-to-head orientation with the IFN-λ1-IFN-λ2 segment. It is speculated that this duplication may have created the IFN-λ3 gene, which is nearly identical to the IFN-λ2 gene in terms of the upstream and downstream flanking sequences and coding region. Therefore, the promoters of the genes for IFN-λ2 and IFN-λ3 share a great similarity and have many common elements with the IFN-λ1 promoter (Kotenko et al., 2003; Sheppard et al., 2003). Based on this, it is suggested that the IFN-λ genes are regulated in a similar fashion.
The members of this new IFN family were found to interact through unique receptors that are distinct from type I and type II IFN receptors. The receptor for type III IFN is composed of the unique IFN-λR1 chain and the IL-10R2 chain, which is shared with IL-10, IL-22 and IL-26 receptor complexes. Although type III IFNs bind to a specific receptor, the downstream signaling is similar to that induced by type I IFNs. Both type I and type III IFNs stimulate common signaling pathways, consisting of the activation of JAK1 and TYK2 kinases and leading to the activation of the IFN-stimulated gene factor 3 (ISGF3) transcription complex. ISGF3 is composed of STAT1 and STAT2, and the interferon regulatory factor IRF9 (ISGF3-γ or p48).
This complex translocates into the nucleus and interacts with a specific DNA sequence designated IFN stimulated response element (ISRE), present upstream of the genes stimulated by the IFNs. The Type II IFN activates cell signaling through another pathway. After the interaction with IFNGR, JAK1 and JAK2 are activated and phosphorylate STAT1, which dimerizes, translocates into the nucleus, binds to the gamma activated sequence (GAS) and induces gene expression.
Although there are three genes encoding highly homologous but distinct human IFN-λ proteins (IFN-λ1, IFN-λ2, and IFN-λ3), our search of the mouse genome revealed the existence of only two genes, representing mouse *IFN-λ2* and *IFN-λ3* gene orthologues, located in chromosome 7 and encoding intact proteins. The mouse *IFN-λ1* gene orthologue is a pseudogene containing some variations in addition to a stop codon in the first exon and does not code for an active protein (Lasfar et al., 2006). We have cloned the mouse IFN-λs

(mIFN-λ2 and mIFN-λ3) and IFN-λ receptor (mIFN-λR1) orthologues and found them to be quite similar to their human counterparts. Experiments showed that similar to their human counterparts, mIFN-λ2 and mIFN-λ3 signal through the IFN-λ receptor complex, activate ISGF3, and are capable of inducing antiviral protection and MHC class I antigen expression in several cell types. The results showed that murine type III IFNs (IFN-λs) engage a unique receptor complex, composed of IFN-λR1 and IL-10R2 subunits, to induce signaling and biological activities similar to those of type I IFNs. Interestingly, in contrast to type I and type II IFNs, type III IFNs demonstrate less specie specificity. This characteristic of type III IFN may be of prime importance in the development of a xenogenic model.

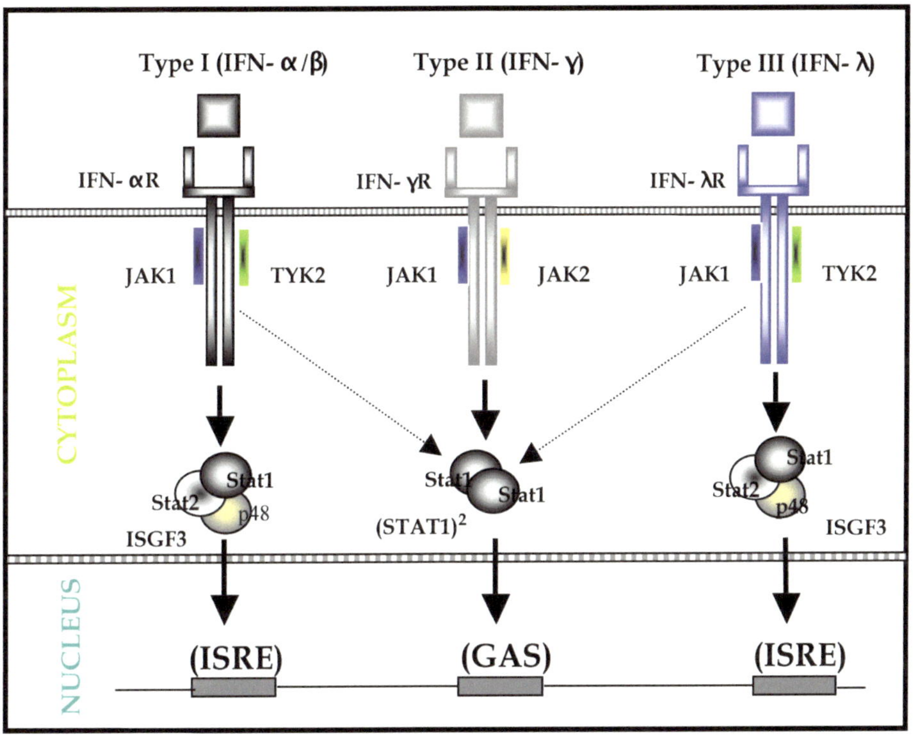

Fig. 1. Interferons, interferon receptors and cell signaling.

2. Characteristics of the IFN- λ receptor

2.1 The human IFN-λ receptor (hIFN-λR1)

The human IFN-λR1 (hIFN-λR1) consists of 520 amino acids, including a signal peptide of 20 amino acids. In SDS-PAGE (Sodium Dodecyl Sulfate PolyAcrylamide Gel Electrophoresis), the IFN-λR1 protein was estimated at around 70 kD, much higher than the theoretical molecular weight calculated at 56 KD, implying the existence of post-translational modifications (Witte et al., 2009). Although the extracellular domain presents 4 putative N-linked glycosylation sites and 1 O-linked glycosylation site, effective IFN-λR1 glycosylation has not been definitely established. The intracellular domain of IFN-λR1 contains three tyrosine residues. Tyrosines 343 and 517 are essential for STAT2 and STAT5 activation (Dumoutier et al., 2004). The existence of splice variants of IFN-λR1 has been reported. Shepard and coll. suggested the presence of one splice variant lacking a part of exon VII (Sheppard et al., 2003). However, we did not confirm yet the existence of these splice variants. Another splice variant lacking exon VI was first described in 2003 (Dumoutier et al., 2004), and its existence has been recently confirmed. This variant was designated sIFN-λR1 for soluble IFN-λR1 or sIL-28R1 for soluble IL-28R1 (Witte et al., 2009). The cloning and protein expression analysis of the soluble IFN-λR1, sIFN-λR1, were performed and the ligand binding studies showed the aptitude of this soluble receptor to inhibit the IFN-λ response. However, high concentrations of sIFN-lR1 were used and only partial inhibition was achieved, suggesting that the described form of sIFN-λR1 may not play an important role in the regulation of IFN-λ response. However, we cannot rule out the induction of other post-translational modifications of the IFN-λR1 that may modulate the activity of sIFN-λR1 by increasing its inhibitory effects on circulating IFN-λs in normal or pathologic situations. Witte and coll. (Witte et al., 2009) showed the presence of sIFN-λR1 in all cells expressing IFN-λR1, with high levels in immune cells such as B, T and NK cells and suggested a correlation between the level of sIFN-λR1 and the lack of response to IFN-λ.

2.2 The mouse IFN-λ receptor and comparison to the human counterpart

After the identification of the human IFN-λ system, we cloned the mouse IFN-λR1 (mIFN-λR1) chain and found it around 67% similar to its human counterpart. The mIFN-λR1 is encoded on mouse chromosome 4D3. Although the mouse and human IFN-λR1 sequences are very similar, only two of three tyrosine residues of the human receptor intracellular domain are conserved in the mouse orthologue. In addition, the mouse receptor contains three additional tyrosine residues. There is also a stretch of negatively charged residues close to the end of the human receptor intracellular domain. This region in the mouse receptor is significantly altered by a short insertion and substitutions of several amino acid residues, resulting in a longer and more negatively charged region in the mouse receptor (18 of 20 amino acids are negatively charged). Two tyrosines, Tyr^{343} and Tyr^{517}, of hIFN-λR1 can independently mediate STAT2 activation by IFN-λs. Interestingly, the Tyr^{341}-based motif of mIFN-λR1 (YLERP) shows similarities with that surrounding Tyr^{343} of hIFN-λR1 (YIEPP). In addition, the COOH-terminal amino acid sequence of mIFN-λR1 containing Tyr^{533} (YLVRstop) is very similar to the COOH-terminal amino acid sequence of hIFN-λR1 containing Tyr^{517} (YMARstop). Therefore, both the mouse and human IFN-λR1 chains contain similar docking sites for STAT2 recruitment and activation, YΦEXP and YΦXRstop (where Φ is hydrophobic). Thus, Tyr^{341}- and Tyr^{533}-based motifs on mIFN-λR1 are also likely to mediate STAT2 recruitment and, therefore, mediate ISGF3 activation, which is responsible for most of the IFN-λ-induced biological activities. Interestingly, by using hamster cells transfected with chimeric human IFN-λR1/γR1 and IL-10R2 expression vectors, we demonstrated that the cells were responsive to both human and mouse IFN-λs, as measured by STAT1 activation in electromobility shift assay and up-regulation of MHC class I antigen expression (Lasfar et al., 2006). However, expression of murine IFN-λR1/γR1 alone rendered hamster cells responsive to both human and mouse IFN-λs, implying that hamster IL-10R2 can dimerize with murine IFN-λR1 to mediate signaling in response to either human or mouse IFN-λs. As controls, we did not detect any response of parental hamster cells to either human or mouse IFN-λ (Lasfar et al., 2006). Therefore, the mouse and human IFN-λs are not specie specific.

3. Distribution of IFN-λR1 and responsiveness to IFN- λ

The functional IFN-λR is formed by two chains, IFN-λR1 (also called IL-28R1) and IL-10R2. IFN-λR1 is unique for the IFN-λs and its tissue distribution is highly restricted. In contrast to IFN-λR1, IL-10R2 is shared by IL-10, IL-22 and IL-26 and ubiquitously expressed in all tissues. Unlike IFN-α, only few cell types respond to IFN-λ (Figure 2) . In contrast to the epithelial-like cells, fibroblasts and endothelial cells were completely unresponsive to IFN-λ (Lasfar et al., 2006). Although the hematopoeitic system is not the primary target of IFN-λ, the response of some subpopulations to IFN-λ is not excluded. In mice, we found that IFN-λ induces STAT1 activation in both plasmacytoid and myeloid dentritic cells (Abushahba et al., 2010). These results are in accordance with Mennechet and Uze (Mennechet and Uze, 2006), who proposed the acquisition of an IFNλ response by the monocytes after their differentiation into dentritic cells. Therefore, the response to IFN-λ may be controlled by the induction of the IFN-λR1 expression. Recently, Witte and coll. found different levels of IFN-λR1 in different tissues (Witte et al., 2009). The highest levels were found in the gastrointestinal tract and lung. The brain showed the lowest level. The IFN-λR1 expression

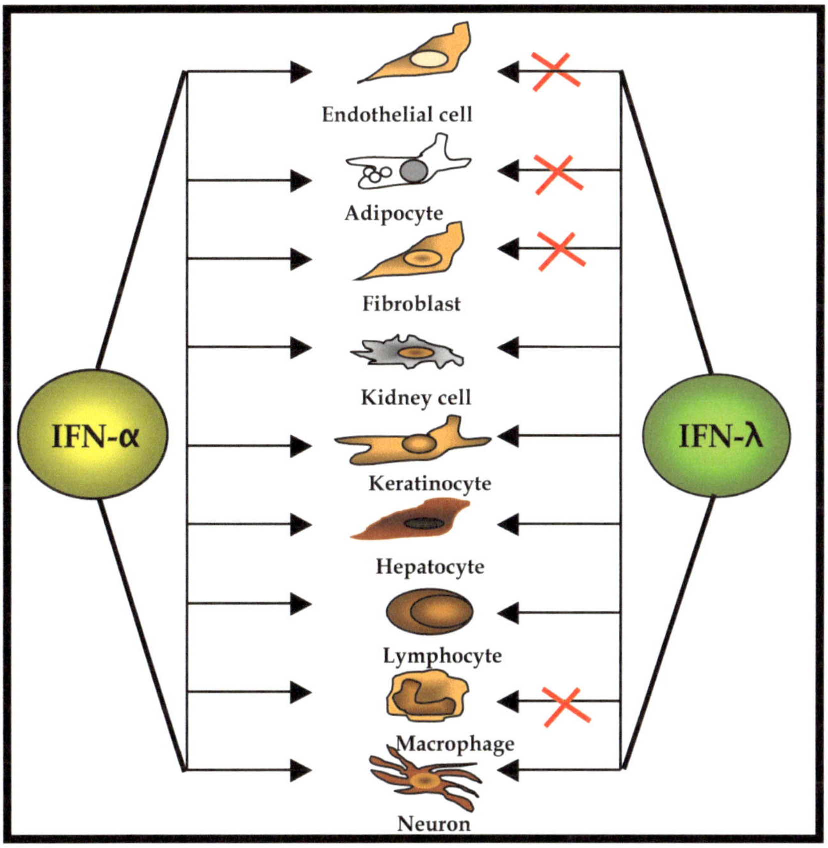

Fig. 2. Cellular targets for type I and type III IFNs. Cells from different origins were tested for IFN-α and IFN-λ response by measuring the IFN induced-cell signaling (Stat activation) and biological activity (MHC class I antigen stimulation).

was also analyzed in different cell types. The expression of cell populations isolated from human skin showed a high expression of IFN-λR1 in keratinocytes and melanocytes. However, dermal fibroblasts, endothelial cells and sub-dermal adipocytes did not express significant amounts of IFN-λR1. Significant expression of IFN-λR1 was detected in primary human hepatocytes in comparison with the condrocytes, isolated from the hyaline cartilage of the knee joint (Witte et al., 2009; Wolk et al., 2008). Although the expression of IFN-λR1 was significantly high in lymphoid tissues, the IFN-λ response was very weak, implying the presence of specific mechanisms on the lymphoid tissues that may inhibit the IFN-λ response. For example, IFN-λR1 levels in B cells are three fold those detected in keratinocytes, which exhibit one of the highest response to IFN-λ. Witte and coll. proposed the potential role of sIFN-λR1, highly released by the immune cells, in this weak response to IFN-λ (Witte et al., 2009).
Although all the IFN-λs interact with the same receptor, IFN-λR1, the binding characteristics for each ligand are still under investigation. In the future, it will be important to analyze the IFN-λ activity in the light of the IFN-λ binding to the cells and understand particularly the role of IFN- λ3, which possesses the highest activity as compared with the other IFN-λs (Dellgren et al., 2009). Analysis of the ligand binding in combination with the activity induced by IFN-λ will be also important in understanding the role of IFN-λ in epithelial cells, particularly in comparison with the immune cells expressing IFN-λR1. Besides several carcinomas, originating from epithelial cells, which respond to IFN- λ, other tumors not arising from epithelial cells may become more sensitive to IFN-λ. It was reported that multiple myeloma cells, which originate from B cell plasmocytes, showed high binding and response to IFN-λ (Novak et al., 2008). Studying the IFN-λ binding in transformed cells versus normal cells may be very helpful for tumor targeting and for the establishment of the optimum dose of IFN- λ to be used for the *in vivo* treatment. IFN-λ can also be used as a drug carrier, to specifically target a drug to tumors expressing high IFN-λ binding sites.

4. Biological and clinical activities of IFN-λ

4.1 Comparative studies between type I and type III IFN (IFN- λs)

To date, every cell line responding to IFN-λ also responded to type I IFNs. However, the cell signaling induced by type III IFNs appeared to be significantly weaker as compared to type I IFNs. Interestingly, the intensity of cell signaling induced by IFN-λ, as assessed by STAT activation, is not always correlated with the level of biological activity, as determined by MHC class I expression (Figure 3).
Antiviral studies performed *in vitro* and *in vivo* have shown that both IFN-α and IFN-λ contribute to the overall host antiviral defense system (Ank et al., 2008; Ank et al., 2006; Kotenko et al., 2003; Kugel et al., 2009; Mordstein et al., 2008; Sheppard et al., 2003). It has been demonstrated that IFN-λ induces antiviral activity against VSV (vesicular stomatitis virus) and EMCV (encephalomyocarditis) in many cell types (Kotenko et al., 2003; Li et al., 2009; Sheppard et al., 2003; Uze and Monneron, 2007). Several studies demonstrated that type III IFNs can also inhibit replication of Hepatitis C Virus (HCV) and Hepatitis B Virus (HBV) *in vitro* (Hong et al., 2007; Lazaro et al., 2007; Marcello et al., 2006; Robek et al., 2005; Uze and Monneron, 2007). These studies were important since they underlined the fact that IFN-λ could be used as an alternative to IFN-α for HCV patients who are resistant to IFN-α treatment. Just recently, it has been reported that IFN-λ has the ability to inhibit human immunodeficiency virus type 1 (HIV-1) infection of blood monocyte-derived macrophages

that expressed IFN-λ receptors (Hou et al., 2009). However, in most other cases, the antiviral potency of IFN-λ against several viruses seems to be lower than that of IFN-α (Kotenko et al., 2003; Li et al., 2009; Marcello et al., 2006; Meager et al., 2005; Mordstein et al., 2008; Sheppard et al., 2003). In addition, IFN-λ and IFN-α may induce distinct signal transduction and gene regulation kinetics (Maher et al., 2008; Marcello et al., 2006).

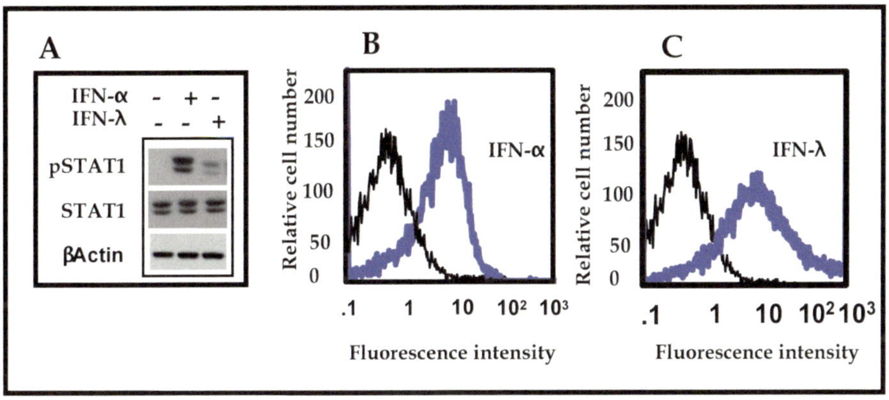

Fig. 3. Intensity of the IFN signaling and biological activity induced by IFN-α and IFN-λ. B16 melanoma cells were treated with IFN-α or IFN-λ followed by STAT1 activation (A) and MHC class I antigen expression (B and C) analysis.

Moreover, Type I IFN-α activates a plethora of innate and adaptive immune mechanisms that help eliminate tumors and viral infections. IFN-α immunoregulatory functions include major histocompatibility complex (MHC) class I expression in normal and tumor cells, activation of NK cells, dendritic cells (DCs) and macrophages, resulting in the promotion of adaptive immune responses against tumors and virally infected cells (Biron, 2001; Le Bon and Tough, 2002). The role of IFN-λ in the immune system is currently being investigated by several groups. So far, data suggests that IFN-λ exerts immunomodulatory effects that overlap those of type I IFN. It has been recently demonstrated that human IFN-λ1 (IL-29) modulates the human cytokine response (Jordan et al., 2007a). IFN-λ1 treatment of whole peripheral blood mononuclear cells (PBMC) up-regulated the expression of IL-6, IL-8, and IL-10 but not IL-1 or TNF. This IFN-λ-induced cytokine production was inhibited by IL-10. By examination of purified cell populations, it was also shown that IFN-λ1 activated monocytes and macrophages, rather than lymphocytes, resulting in the secretion of the above panel of cytokines, suggesting that IFN-λ1 may be an important activator of innate immune responses particularly at the site of viral infections (Jordan et al., 2007a). IFN-λ1 was also shown to possess immunoregulatory functions on T helper 2 (Th2) responses by markedly inhibiting IL-13. However, only moderate effect was observed on IL-4 and IL-15, the other important cytokines in the Th2 response. (Dai et al., 2009; Jordan et al., 2007b; Srinivas et al., 2008). This immunoregulatory function was enhanced through the expression of IFN-λR1 on $CD4^+$ T cells (Dai et al., 2009). These findings correlate with data suggesting that IFN-λ may have an immunoprotective role against asthma, the allergy disease caused by an exaggerated Th2 response (Bullens et al., 2008; Johnston, 2007; Li et al., 2009).
Similar to IFN-α, IFN-λ produced by DCs, in response to Toll-like receptor (TLR) stimulation, was found to have specific effects on DC differentiation and maturation (Coccia et al., 2004), which include only partial maturation of DCs, upregulation of MHC class I and

II molecules, and no induction of co-stimulatory molecules (Li et al., 2009; Mennechet and Uze, 2006). During their differentiation from monocytes, DCs acquire IFN-λ responsiveness through the expression of IFN-λR1. Interestingly, DCs treated with IFN-λ promoted the generation of tolerogenic DCs and the IL-2 dependent proliferation of Foxp3-expressing $CD4^{+}CD25^{+}$ regulatory T cells (Tregs) (Mennechet and Uze, 2006). More recently, Morrow and coll. have demonstrated through DNA vaccination with plasmids encoding IFN-λ3 (IL-28B) and IL-12, that IFN-λ3, just like IL-12, is able to enhance adaptive immunity. However, in contrast to IL-12, IFN-λ3 reduces regulatory T-cell populations. They also showed that unlike IL-12, IFN-λ3 is able to increase the percentage of splenic $CD8^{+}$ T cells in vaccinated animals and that IFN-λ3 can completely protect mice from death following a lethal influenza challenge (Morrow et al., 2009). These studies altogether highlight the strong candidacy of IFN-λ as a potential novel immunotherapeutic agent.

In addition to antiviral and immunomodulatory activities, type I IFNs demonstrate antiproliferative activities in most cell lines, while this activity seems to be restricted with IFN-λs (Li et al., 2009; Meager et al., 2005). Type I IFNs have been shown to induce apoptosis in tumor cells. Yet, the molecular mechanisms mediating cell death in response to these IFNs remain to be fully explained. By binding to their corresponding cellular receptor complexes, IFNs induce a quick and potent signaling which leads to the expression of more than 300 IFN-stimulated genes (ISGs) (Der et al., 1998; Doyle et al., 2006; Marcello et al., 2006). Many ISGs encode proteins that have been implicated in apoptosis (Clemens, 2003; Kalvakolanu, 2004). Unlike IFN-α, IFN-λs do not inhibit the proliferation of several cell lines including Daudi cells (a B-lymphoblastoid cell line from Burkitt's lymphoma), which strongly respond to type I IFNs in an antiproliferative assay (Kotenko et al., 2003; Meager et al., 2005; Sheppard et al., 2003; Uze and Monneron, 2007). However, it was demonstrated that IFN-λs do inhibit the proliferation of few tumor cell lines, such as the LN319 human glioblastoma cell line (Meager et al., 2005) and of cells constitutively expressing high levels of IFN-λR1 (Dumoutier et al., 2004). The antiproliferative effects of IFN-λ have been demonstrated in various tumor cell lines that express ectopic or endogenous IFN-λ receptors (Brand et al., 2005; Meager et al., 2005; Zitzmann et al., 2006). Therefore, the ability of IFN-λs to induce antiproliferative activity in cells depends on the level of IFN-λR1 expression.

It has been reported that IFN-λ signaling in colorectal adenocarcinoma HT29 cells led to caspase activation, externalization of phosphatidylserine (PS), and DNA fragmentation, resulting in subsequent apoptosis (Li et al., 2008). This study provided evidence for the first time that type III IFNs, alone or in combination with other stimuli, have the potential to induce apoptosis. Moreover, another recent study revealed that IFN-α and IFN-λ differ in their antiproliferative effects and this was correlated with a difference in the duration of JAK/STAT signaling activity between the two IFNs and prolonged ISG expression upon IFN-λ treatment (Maher et al., 2008). Using the human keratinocyte HaCaT cell line that expresses receptors for both IFN-α and IFN-λ, they found that IFN-λ induced a more pronounced growth inhibitory effect than IFN-α. IFN-λ was also more efficient than IFN-α in inducing an antiproliferative effect that overlapped with the activation of apoptosis. Prolonged duration of IFN-λ-induced STAT activation and ISG expression could account for the enhanced antiproliferative and pro-apoptotic effects observed in HaCaT cells, effects not seen upon treatment with high doses of IFN-α (Maher et al., 2008). Interestingly, a study has shown that IFN-λ can induce the growth of multiple myeloma cells and antagonize the dexamethasone-induced cell death in these cells (Novak et al., 2008). IFN-λ-mediated cell growth of multiple myeloma cells was MAPK dependent (Novak et al., 2008). High level of

IFN-λ was found in the malignant bone marrow microenvironment, implying that IFN-λ may play a direct role on multiple myeloma development.

4.2 Role of endogenous IFN-λ in viral protection

The availability of IFN-λR1 knock-out mice allowed to investigate the role of type III IFNs *in vivo*. By using those mice, Mordstein and coll. showed for the first time the contribution of IFN-λ in the innate immunity against the influenza virus (Mordstein et al., 2008). Later, they found that IFN-λ played an important role in the defense against other pathogens that infect the respiratory tract, such as the respiratory syncitial virus, the metapneumovirus and the severe acute respiratory syndrome (SARS) coronavirus. However, the lassa fever virus which replicates in the liver, was not affected by the lack of IFN-λR1 (Mordstein et al., 2010). Although this study clearly demonstrated that IFN-λ played an important role in protecting the respiratory and gastrointestinal tracts against virus infection, in comparison with type I IFN, the protection provided by type III IFN remains limited. However, in combination, type I and type III may provide a better viral protection. When the response to both type I and type III is deficient, the mice are not able to clear the SARS coronavirus from the intestine as compared with mice in which type I or type III remains functional, implying that IFN-λ may strengthen the antiviral activity by acting as a first line of defense for the mucosa (Mordstein et al., 2008, 2010).

4.3 Clinical application of IFN-λ

The first use of IFN-λ in the clinic has started for hepatitis C. The phase 1b study has been conducted in patients with chronic genotype 1 hepatitis C virus infection ((HCV) (Muir et al., 2010)). Pegylated IFN-λ1 in combination or not with ribavirin (RBV, which belongs to a class of antiviral medications called the nucleoside analogues) has been used in this study to assess the efficacy and the potential cytotoxicity. The study was performed in 3 parts. The first part evaluated the pegylated IFN-λ as single agent for relapsed patients after IFN-α-based treatment. The second part concerned the combination of pegylated IFN-λ and RBV in treatment-relapse patients. The third part evaluated pegylated IFN-λ in combination with RBV in treatment-naïve patients. In addition, different doses (from 0.5 to 3 microg/kg) of pegylated IFN-λ were used. Fifty-six patients were enrolled. 24, 25 and 7 patients were used respectively for part 1 to 3. The data showed an antiviral activity in all doses of pegylated IFN-λ tested. 29% of treatment-naïve patients achieved rapid virological response. As expected, due to the limited IFN-λR1 distribution, the treatment was well tolerated with few adverse effects. Minimal flu-like symptoms and limited hematologic suppression were reported. In summary, the authors concluded that weekly PEG-IFN-λ with or without daily RBV for 4 weeks is associated with a clear antiviral activity in patients with chronic HCV. However, this study lacks a direct comparison between IFN-λ and IFN-α and the influence of viral and patient genotypes. Now it is well accepted that the response to IFN-α or the natural clearance of HCV infection is depending on single nucleotide polymorphisms (SNPs), upstream of IFN-λ3, that could be used as biomarkers to help determine the treatment outcome (Kelly et al., 2011). The first genome-wide association studies (GWAS) in HCV infection were reported by Ge and coll. They evaluated the treatment outcome in a group of 1671 patients of mixed ethnicity, receiving pegylated-IFN-α and ribavirin. An association was discovered between sustained viral response (SVR) to treatment and a cluster of seven SNPs linked to the IFN-λ3 gene, with the most significant SNP (rs12979860) demonstrating high statistical significance (Ge et al., 2009). Many other studies have replicated these findings, demonstrating the high link between IFN-λ3 and treatment outcome (Labie and Gilgenkrantz, 2010; Mangia et al., 2010; McCarthy et al., 2010; Montes-Cano et al., 2010; Mosbruger et al., 2010; Rauch et al., 2010; Suppiah et al., 2009; Tanaka et al., 2009). However the mechanisms explaining this link remain to be determined. It is not clear yet if this SNP is associated with a constitutive production of IFN-λ that may play a role in HCV clearance and the success of IFN-α treatment. These results also suggest the therapeutic potential of the IFN-α and IFN-λ combination therapy as demonstrated for the hepatocellular carcinoma (HCC) mouse model (Lasfar et al., 2008).

5. Emergence of IFN-λ as a new antitumor agent

5.1 First report in animal model

Although they engage distinct receptors, IFN-α and IFN-λ induce similar cell signaling (Figure 1). Since IFN-α is widely used in clinic to treat cancer, we have investigated the potential antitumor activity of IFN-λ by using the mouse B16 melanoma model. We have chosen this cancer model because melanoma is a very aggressive cancer and one of the therapeutic agents frequently used in the treatment of melanoma is IFN-α. Significant improvements in relapse-free and overall survival, with postoperative adjuvant IFN-α therapy, have been reported by large and randomized studies (Kirkwood et al., 1996, 2001; Moschos et al., 2005). However, the beneficial effect of IFN-α was only obtained when the patients received high doses (20 MIU/m2 intravenously five times per week). Studies with low doses of IFN-α have not shown significant increase in overall survival (Cascinelli et al., 2001; Kleeberg et al., 2004). Usually, the dose for optimal antitumor activity is higher than the maximally tolerated dose. This dose-dilemma profoundly affects the acceptance of IFN-α treatment by both the clinicians and the patients. The adverse effects associated with high doses of IFN-α include myelosuppression and nervous system disorders. These effects often compromise the beneficial antitumor effect, with premature discontinuation of the treatment or the reduction of the dose of IFN-α. Since virtually all the cells of the body respond to IFN-α, it is not surprising that the patients develop numerous side effects. Making a dissection between the beneficial and harmful effects of IFN-α is a very challenging task, which requires more investigation of the interferon system. To investigate the antitumor effect of IFN-λ in melanoma, we used a gene therapy approach, consisting on the delivery of the IFN-λ gene to tumor cells. Gene transfer into tumor cells is a very useful approach to test the effectiveness of cytokines in animal cancer models. This approach does not require a production and the purification of the protein. The secretion of constant amounts of various cytokines by transduced tumor cells at the site of tumor growth could elicit more effective antitumor responses by acting directly on the tumor microenvironment. Another advantage of the cytokine gene transfer into tumor cells versus systemic administration is the potential of inducing the antitumor effect without eliciting the side effects associated with the systemic administration of high doses of cytokines.

To investigate the potential antitumoral role of IFN-λ, we first evaluated the response of B16 melanoma cells to IFN-λ, by analyzing STAT1 activation and MHC class I antigen expression. In comparison with IFN-α, we have found that IFN-λ induces weak STAT1 phosphorylation but strong stimulation of MHC class I antigen expression, indicating a difference between IFN-α and IFN-λ in the link intensity of cell signaling/biological activity (Figure 3). This result warrants further investigation, by comparing the response to IFN-α and IFN-λ. As shown in this figure, although IFN-λ induces weak STAT1 activation, the biological activity can be very strong. By using gene transfer as illustrated in Figure 4, we next engineered B16 cells, which constitutively produced mIFN-λ (B16.IFN-λ cells). In response to their secretion of IFN-λ, B16.IFN-λ cells exhibited constitutively high levels of MHC class I antigen expression. All the C57BL/6 syngeneic mice injected with parental B16 cells developed tumors. However, the constitutive production of mIFN-λ by B16.IFN-λ cells markedly affected tumorigenicity of the cells. B16.IFN-λ cells were either rejected by the host or grew at a slower rate than control parental B16 cells. The antitumor effect of IFN-λ was dose dependent. B16.IFN-λ cells also inhibited the growth of parental B16 cells when both cell types were injected together (Lasfar et al., 2006). We also used B16.IFN-λ Res. cells which in addition to their constitutive IFN-λ secretion, are completely resistant to IFN-λ as demonstrated by the lack of IFN-λ-induced MHC class I antigen expression (Table 1). Interestingly, similar to B16.IFN-λ cells, we have found a reduction of the tumorigenicity of B16.IFN-λ Res. cells, implying the involvement of host antitumor mechanisms induced by IFN-λ.

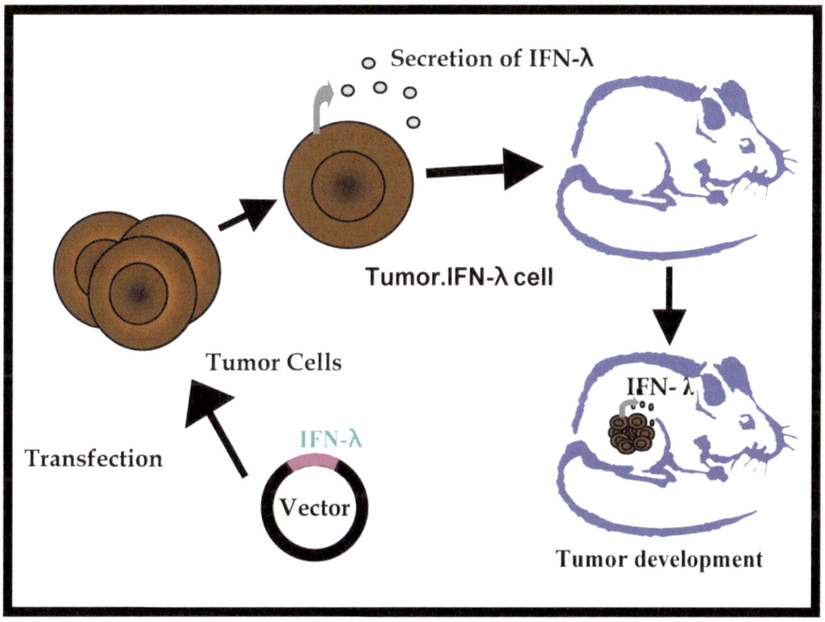

Fig. 4. IFN-λ gene transfer. Tumor cells were engineered to constitutively produce IFN-λ. Immunocompetent syngeneic mice were injected subcutaneously with the engineered tumor cells and monitored for tumor development.

Following our report on the characterization of the mouse IFN-λ system and the potent antitumor activity of IFN-λ in the B16 mouse melanoma model, independent groups confirmed the role of IFN-λ as antitumoral agent in melanoma and other tumor models. To demonstrate the antitumor activity of IFN-λ, Sato and coll. (Sato et al., 2006) used the mouse melanoma B16F0 and B16F10 and the Colon26 cell lines transfected with IFN-λ2 cDNA. The IFN-λ-transduced B16F0 cells showed an increased activity of caspase 3/7, an induction of p21 and a dephosphoryation of Rb, which triggered a cell cycle arrest and apoptosis. These events obtained *in vitro*, were apparently associated with a tumor growth delay, observed *in vivo* after the injection of the B16F0 cells, transduced with IFN-λ. A delay in tumor growth was also observed after the administration of the Colon26 cells transduced with IFN-λ. By using the B16F10 cell line, which represents metastatic mouse melanoma cells, the authors showed that the overexpression of IFN-λ significantly inhibited lung metastasis. In another study, to evaluate the antitumor activity of IFN-λ, Numasaki and coll. (Numasaki et al., 2007) first transduced the mouse fibrosarcoma cells, MCA2005, with the retroviral vector PA317IL-28 (IFN-λ2). Following the injection of the engineered tumor cells to mice, the authors observed a significant antitumor and antimetastatic effect in mice inoculated with the MCA2005IL-28 in comparison with those injected with the parental tumor cells.

	IFN-λ production	Cell proliferation	MHC I antigen expression
B16 cells	-	++++	+
B16. IFN-λ cells	+ + + + + ++ +	+++	+ + + + + ++ +
B16. IFN-λ Res. cells	+ + + + + ++ +	+++	+

	Tumor necrosis	Inflammation	Tumor vascularization	Tumor mitotic rate
B16 cells	+ +	+/-	+ + + + + +	**>14/HPF**
B16. IFN-λ cells	+ + + + + +	-	+ +	**5-10/HPF**
B16. IFN-λ Res. cells	+ + + +	-	+ +	**15/HPF**
B16/B16. IFN-λ cells	+ + + + + +	-	+ +	**3-5/HPF**
B16/ B16. IFN-λ Res. cells	+ + + + + +	-	+ +	**6-10/HPF**

Table 1. Constitutive production of IFN-λ-induced tumor alteration. *In vitro* (Top) and *in vivo* (Bottom) analysis of the engineered B16 cells constitutively producing IFN-λ (B16.IFN-λ cells and B16.IFN-λ Res. cells). In contrast to the parental B16 and B16.IFN-λ cells, B16.IFN-λ Res. cells are completely resistant to IFN-λ, as indicated by MHC class I antigen expression unaffected by the presence of IFN-λ. HPF (High-Powered Field)

5.2 Investigation of the antitumor activities of IFN-λ in comparison with those of IFN-α in a BNL mouse model of hepatocellular carcinoma (HCC)

HCC is the most prevalent type of liver cancer. It is the fifth most common solid tumor and the third leading cause of cancer-related death worldwide. It is also the second most lethal cancer with the five-year survival rate below 9% (Farazi and DePinho, 2006; Lau and Lai, 2008; Sherman, 2005). Treatment options for HCC are limited mainly because of the inefficiency of existing anticancer chemotherapeutic drugs against HCC. Unfortunately, due to a lack of biomarkers and screening for HCC, most patients are diagnosed at advanced stages of the disease and do not meet strict selection criteria for potentially curative surgical tumor resection or orthotopic liver transplantation (OLT) (Mazzaferro et al., 2008, 2009; Taketomi et al., 2008) In patients with unresectable HCC and preserved liver function, transarterial chemoembolization (TACE) has been shown to prolong survival. However TACE is rarely curative, and progression-free survival beyond 24 months is not frequent (Georgiades et al., 2008; Lau and Lai, 2008). For patients with advanced disease, systemic chemotherapy is of limited benefit because of the resistance of HCC to existing anticancer drugs and the fact that about 50% of patients with HCC die secondary to liver failure from cirrhosis (Di Bisceglie et al., 1998; Nagai and Sumino, 2008). HCC occurs most frequently in patients with cirrhosis as a result of chronic HBV and HCV infections, and alcohol abuse (El-Serag, 2002; Sherman, 2005). Although the link between the cancer and the viral infection is not fully understood yet, there is some suggestion that viral infection interferes with signal transduction and consequently, disrupts the normal, controlled growth of cells.

Since IFN-α is used in the clinic for the treatment of chronic HCV and HBV infections, several studies evaluated the effect of IFN treatment on the incidence of HCC (Sherman, 2005). It was previously shown that the systemic administration of high doses and long-term IFN-α into nude mice bearing human HCC with high metastatic potential, following curative resection, inhibited tumor metastasis and recurrence (Wang et al., 2003). The majority of clinical studies also concluded that IFN therapy, alone or in combination with ribavirin, decreased the incidence of HCC, particularly in patients with sustained virological response (Fattovich et al., 1998; Lin et al., 2007; Omata et al., 2005; Yu et al., 2006). Therefore, IFN alone or, perhaps, in combination with other drugs can be used as a preventive therapy against the development of HCC in HCV and HBV-infected patients. However, numerous side effects limit the overall tolerability of IFN-α, particularly in patients with cirrhosis (Llovet et al., 2000; Lo et al., 2007; Ueshima et al., 2008).

In the following part of this section, we describe our findings on the antitumor properties of IFN-λ on the BNL mouse model of HCC. To evaluate the antitumor activities of both IFN-λ and IFN-α, we used a gene therapy approach as previously described (Lasfar et al., 2006). We expressed IFN-λ and IFN-α genes under a strong constitutive promoter in BNL cells and selected stable cell lines, BNL-IFN-λ and BNL-IFN-α, constitutively expressing IFN-λ and IFN-α (Abushahba et al., 2010). Since the constitutive expression of IFN-λ at the tumor site was found to affect the tumorigenicity of B16 melanoma cells *in vivo* (Lasfar et al., 2006), we examined whether similar effects of IFN-λ would be displayed in the case of BNL hepatoma. Mice injected with BNL.vector or parental BNL cells developed tumors in 4 to 6 weeks, whereas the tumor appearance for BNL.IFN-λ cells was significantly delayed. Similar effects were obtained in mice inoculated with BNL.IFN-α cells. These experiments demonstrated that constitutive expression of IFNs at the tumor site resulted in the delay of tumor growth *in vivo*. Interestingly, we found that IFN-α and IFN-λ exhibited similar antitumor activities (Abushahba et al., 2010).

6. Antitumor mechanisms of IFN-α and IFN-λ

6.1 Antitumor mechanisms of IFN-α

Despite the antiproliferative effects of IFN-α on cells, it seems that the direct effects on tumor cells may not be the major mechanism by which IFN-α displays its antitumor activity. IFN-α can act indirectly on the tumor by inhibiting angiogenesis which is induced by the tumors and is required to promote their growth and metastasis (Sidky and Borden, 1987). In mice bearing human tumors, it was clearly demonstrated that the antitumor activity of IFN-α is associated with the inhibition of tumor angiogenesis in bladder carcinoma (Dinney et al., 1998) and prostate cancer (Dong et al., 1999). The involvement of the immune system in the antitumor mechanism of IFN-α was strongly suggested by Gresser and coll. Early studies in tumor models have shown that an intact immune system was essential in IFN-α-induced antitumor activities. The inhibition of FLC (Friend Leukemia Cells) by IFN-α in mice was shown to depend on the activation of host cells, such as NK cells and macrophages (Gresser et al., 1994). Both host humoral and cellular immune mechanisms were involved in the continued suppression of Friend erythroleukemia metastases after IFN-α treatment in mice (Gresser, 1991). In addition, effective adaptive immunotherapy was observed in a T-cell lymphoma model, after the injection of tumor-sensitized spleen cells and IFN-α. By using antibodies against different immune cell populations, it has been shown that CD4+ T lymphocytes and CD8+ T lymphocytes were the major effectors in the antitumor activities induced by IFN-α (Kaido et al., 1994; 1995).

6.2 Antitumor mechanism of IFN-λ

Although IFN-α and IFN-λ signal quite similarly (Figure 1), the mechanisms underlying the antitumor activity of IFN-λ may be qualitatively different from IFN-α. As previously described, we initially investigated whether type III IFNs also possessed antitumor activities utilizing a gene therapy approach in the B16 melanoma model. B16 melanoma cells that were engineered to constitutively secrete IFN-λ and were either sensitive or resistant to IFN-λ, were transplanted into two groups of mice. Potent antitumoral activity was observed for both groups of mice. Since secreted IFN-λ did not affect the proliferation rate of B16 melanoma cells *in vitro*, studies in the B16 melanoma model suggested that IFN-λ acted through host mechanisms to elicit its antitumor activity (Lasfar et al., 2006). However, we did not observe a significant long-lasting immunity, implying that there may be a lack of effective adaptive immunity in the mice which rejected the tumor. On the other hand, we noticed a reduction in tumor vascularity in the presence of IFN-λ, suggesting a potential role of IFN-λ in the tumor microenvironment (Lasfar et al., 2006). Since we found that keratinocytes are highly sensitive to IFN-λ and they are known to interact with melanocytes, the cells from which the melanoma originates, we suggested that IFN-λ delivery to the tumor microenvironment may affect the function of the keratinocytes as well as other stroma cells thereby promoting inhibition of tumor growth (Lasfar et al., 2006) (Figure 5).

Natural Killer (NK) cells, the major effectors of innate immunity, could also be recruited to the tumor microenvironment and help destroy the tumor cells. Two groups have reported that NK cells played a role in the antitumor mechanisms of IFN-λ. Sato and coll. (Sato et al., 2006) have described the involvement of NK cells in melanoma and colon cancer antitumor responses. They have shown that transient transduction of B16 cells with mouse IFN-λ cDNA, enhanced MHC class I and Fas expression, suppressed cell proliferation by inducing increased caspase-3/7 activity and increased $p21^{Waf1/Cip1}$ levels and dephosphorylated Rb (Ser^{780}) *in vitro* (Sato et al., 2006). This meant that IFN-λ was able to induce cell cycle arrest and apoptotic cell death *in vitro*. In addition, they have demonstrated that overexpression of IFN-λ inhibited local and pulmonary metastatic tumor formation *in vivo*. Depletion of NK cells, by injecting an anti-asialo GM1 antibody before tumor cells injection, revealed that NK cells are important in this IFN-λ-mediated tumor growth inhibition *in vivo*, suggesting that IFN-λ activated the innate immune response (Sato et al., 2006). Numasaki and coll. (Numasaki et al., 2007) have also implicated NK cells, polymorphonuclear neutrophils and $CD8^+$ T cells in the antitumoral activity induced by IFN-λ in the MCA205 murine fibrosarcoma mouse model. Inoculation of MCA205-IFN-λMCA205-IFN-λ cells, into mice enhanced IFN-γ production and cytotoxic T cell activity in the spleen. The antitumor activity of IFN-λ was partially dependent on IFN-γ. In addition, IFN-λ increased the total number of splenic NK cells in severe combined immunodeficiency (SCID) mice, enhanced IL-12-induced IFN-γ production *in vivo,* and expanded spleen cells in C57BL/6 mice. Furthermore, they reported that IL-12 augmented the IFN-λ-mediated antitumor activity in the presence or absence of IFN-γ. Based on their findings, they suggested that IFN-λ is able to induce both innate and adaptive immune responses to suppress *in vivo* tumor growth (Numasaki et al., 2007).

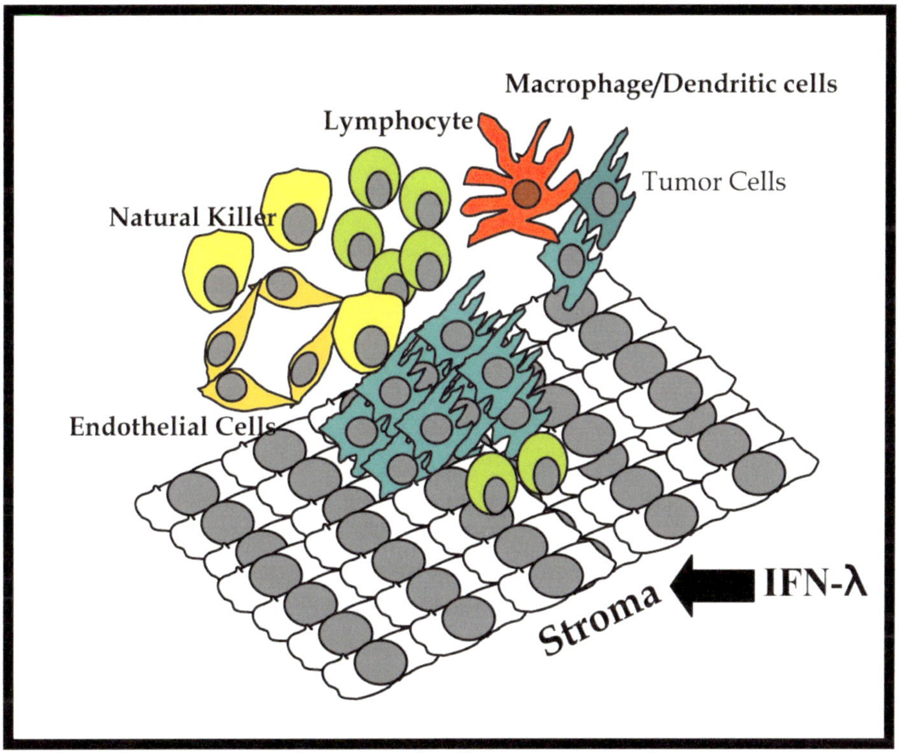

Fig. 5. Potential role of IFN-λ in the tumor, microenvironment. The IFN-λ delivered to the tumor microenvironment may induce its potent antitumor activity by modulating the interaction between the tumor cells and the normal cells, including the recruited immune cells.

Our recent study in the BNL hepatoma model also revealed that NK cells are implicated in the antitumor activity induced by IFN-λ and probably more potently than in the antitumor activity induced by IFN-α. However, in contrast to IFN-α, we did not detect any response after *in vitro* treatment of NK cells by IFN-λ, suggesting that IFN-λ may activate other cells, which then mediate NK cell activation (Abushahba et al., 2010). There was also a marked NK cell infiltration in IFN-λ producing tumors. In addition, IFN-λ and, to a lesser extent, IFN-α enhanced immunocytotoxicity of splenocytes primed with irradiated BNL cells. Splenocyte cytotoxicity against BNL cells was dependent on IL-12 and IFN-γ, and mediated by dendritic cells. In contrast to NK cells, isolated from spleen, CD11c+ and mPDCA+ dendritic cells responded directly to IFN-λ, suggesting that the effects of IFN-λ on NK cells are mediated by other IFN-λ-responsive cells, such as DCs (Abushahba et al., 2010). On the other hand, a significant decrease in CD4+CD25+Foxp3+ Tregs was observed in mice inoculated with BNL cells secreting IFN-α, whereas the moderate decrease in Tregs observed in mice receiving BNL cells secreting IFN-λ was not statistically significant (Abushahba et al., 2010). Therefore, antitumor mechanisms activated by IFN-α and IFN-λ may differ; IFN-λ increased the number of NK cells at the tumor site whereas IFN-α had a stronger effect on Tregs in the BNL model.

These studies altogether suggest that although IFN-α and IFN-λ signal quite similarly (Figure 1), differences exist in their biological potency, kinetics and the sets of target cells sensitive to IFN-λ and IFN-α. Therefore, these two types of IFNs may have distinct physiological functions.

7. IFN-λ as a potential ally rather than alternative to IFN-α

Unlike IFN-α, only a small subset of cells are sensitive to IFN-λ, implying that its potential clinical use may be associated with limited side effects. This presumption raises the question whether IFN-λ could be an alternative to IFN-α in cancer therapy. However, despite the severe and numerous side effects inherent to IFN-α treatment (Moschos et al., 2005), we believe that alternative treatment to IFN-α should be weighed first against the real benefits to patients in terms of overall survival and their tumor clearance. We have, demonstrated in the BNL hepatoma model that the combination of IFN-λ and IFN-α could achieve a stronger antitumor activity in comparison with the use of each IFN alone (Lasfar et al., 2008). The benefits of the combination therapy of IFN-λ and IFN-α have been demonstrated by both a gene therapy approach and direct administration of IFNs to the mice bearing the tumors. The mice injected with BNL cells secreting both IFN-λ and IFN-α can completely reject the tumor, in contrast to the mice that only received the BNL.IFN-λ cells or the BNL.IFN-α cells. Furthermore, mice bearing established tumors and treated with exogenous IFN-λ and IFN-α, showed a drastic tumor repression. This effect was observed when the IFNs were delivered locally and even at low doses. Therefore, we believe that IFN-λ is not simply acting like IFN-α, with reduced side effects, but can be combined with IFN-α to achieve efficient antitumor activity. Combination of IFN-λ with low doses of IFN-α, which are sub-therapeutic but less toxic (Kleeberg et al., 2004), may improve IFN therapy and benefit cancer patients. Combinational therapy of IFN-λ and IFN-α may achieve ultimate antitumor activity by inducing complementary mechanisms directly on the tumor cells or by indirectly modulating the tumor microenvironment, thereby leading to the stimulation of the immune response against the tumor and the inhibition of tumor angiogenesis. By acting with different intensities on the same targets, IFN-λ and IFN-α may generate a high level of synergy, leading to a potent antitumor activity.

8. Conclusion

Similarly to IFN-α, IFN-λ has been shown to play an important role in cancer and viral disease treatment. Although the two IFNs act through an identical signaling pathway in the cell, the pattern of their activity seems to be different *in vivo*, implying that IFN-λ and IFN-α are not redundant cytokines. By acting on some targets with different intensity, we believe that IFN-λ and IFN-α act in concert to better control tumor development *in vivo*. Therefore, to achieve better treatments for viral diseases or cancers, we believe that the development of a combination therapy rather than the use of each IFN alone will be more beneficial for the patients. The combination of IFNs with other cytokines, growth factors, or their antagonists could also be a viable strategy for the improvement of the IFN therapy. Transforming Growth Factor-beta (TGFβ) which plays a dual role in cancer, mediating tumor suppresive activities at early stages and prooncogenic activities at later stages of tumor progression (Javelaud et al., 2008), could represent one potentially important modulator or mediator of the IFN response. In different cancers, inculding melanoma, several cellular pathways modulate the activity of TGFβ (Lasfar and Cohen-Solal, 2010). Understanding the potential crosstalks between IFN-α, IFN-λ and other cytokines or growth factors, such as TGFβ, could be rewarding and lead to new preclinical studies in animal models and new clinicals trials resulting in better cancer treatments.

9. Acknowledgment

We thank Dr. Sergei Kotenko for his valuable support and useful discussions. We also thank Dr. Andrew de la Torre and Dr. Walid Abushahba for their input in the hepatoma antitumor studies. We are grateful for the direct or indirect help of Dr. Ion Gresser, Dr. Jeanne Wietzerbin, Dr. Christian Billard, Dr. Jean-Pierre Kolb, Dr. Michael Tovey and Dr. Sidney Pestka.

10. References

Abushahba, W., Balan, M., Castaneda, I., Yuan, Y., Reuhl, K., Raveche, E., De La Torre, A., Lasfar, A., and Kotenko, S. V. (2010). Antitumor activity of type I and type III interferons in BNL hepatoma model. Cancer Immunol Immunother *59*, 1059-1071.

Ank, N., Iversen, M. B., Bartholdy, C., et al. (2008). An important role for type III interferon (IFN-lambda/IL-28) in TLR-induced antiviral activity. J Immunol *180*, 2474-2485.

Ank, N., West, H., Bartholdy, C., Eriksson, K., Thomsen, A. R., and Paludan, S. R. (2006). Lambda interferon (IFN-lambda), a type III IFN, is induced by viruses and IFNs and displays potent antiviral activity against select virus infections in vivo. J Virol *80*, 4501-4509.

Biron, C. A. (2001). Interferons alpha and beta as immune regulators--a new look. Immunity *14*, 661-664.

Brand, S., Beigel, F., Olszak, T., et al. (2005). IL-28A and IL-29 mediate antiproliferative and antiviral signals in intestinal epithelial cells and murine CMV infection increases colonic IL-28A expression. Am J Physiol Gastrointest Liver Physiol *289*, G960-968.

Bullens, D. M., Decraene, A., Dilissen, E., Meyts, I., De Boeck, K., Dupont, L. J., and Ceuppens, J. L. (2008). Type III IFN-lambda mRNA expression in sputum of adult and school-aged asthmatics. Clin Exp Allergy *38*, 1459-1467.

Cascinelli, N., Belli, F., Mackie, R. M., Santinami, M., Bufalino, R., and Morabito, A. (2001). Effect of long-term adjuvant therapy with interferon alpha-2a in patients with regional node metastases from cutaneous melanoma: a randomised trial. Lancet *358*, 866-869.

Clemens, M. J. (2003). Interferons and apoptosis. J Interferon Cytokine Res *23*, 277-292.

Coccia, E. M., Severa, M., Giacomini, E., Monneron, D., Remoli, M. E., Julkunen, I., Cella, M., Lande, R., and Uze, G. (2004). Viral infection and Toll-like receptor agonists induce a differential expression of type I and lambda interferons in human plasmacytoid and monocyte-derived dendritic cells. Eur J Immunol *34*, 796-805.

Dai, J., Megjugorac, N. J., Gallagher, G. E., Yu, R. Y., and Gallagher, G. (2009). IFN-{lambda}1 (IL-29) inhibits GATA3 expression and suppresses Th2 responses in human naive and memory T cells. Blood.

Dellgren, C., Gad, H. H., Hamming, O. J., Melchjorsen, J., and Hartmann, R. (2009). Human interferon-lambda3 is a potent member of the type III interferon family. Genes Immun *10*, 125-131.

Der, S. D., Zhou, A., Williams, B. R., and Silverman, R. H. (1998). Identification of genes differentially regulated by interferon alpha, beta, or gamma using oligonucleotide arrays. Proc Natl Acad Sci U S A *95*, 15623-15628.

Di Bisceglie, A. M., Carithers, R. L., Jr., and Gores, G. J. (1998). Hepatocellular carcinoma. Hepatology *28*, 1161-1165.

Ding, L., Linsley, P. S., Huang, L. Y., Germain, R. N., and Shevach, E. M. (1993). IL-10 inhibits macrophage costimulatory activity by selectively inhibiting the up-regulation of B7 expression. J Immunol *151*, 1224-1234.

Dinney, C. P., Bielenberg, D. R., Perrotte, P., Reich, R., Eve, B. Y., Bucana, C. D., and Fidler, I. J. (1998). Inhibition of basic fibroblast growth factor expression, angiogenesis, and growth of human bladder carcinoma in mice by systemic interferon-alpha administration. Cancer Res *58*, 808-814.

Dong, Y., Rohn, W. M., and Benveniste, E. N. (1999). IFN-gamma regulation of the type IV class II transactivator promoter in astrocytes. J Immunol *162*, 4731-4739.

Doyle, S. E., Schreckhise, H., Khuu-Duong, K., et al. (2006). Interleukin-29 uses a type 1 interferon-like program to promote antiviral responses in human hepatocytes. Hepatology *44*, 896-906.

Dumoutier, L., Tounsi, A., Michiels, T., Sommereyns, C., Kotenko, S. V., and Renauld, J. C. (2004). Role of the interleukin (IL)-28 receptor tyrosine residues for antiviral and antiproliferative activity of IL-29/interferon-lambda 1: similarities with type I interferon signaling. J Biol Chem *279*, 32269-32274.

El-Serag, H. B. (2002). Hepatocellular carcinoma: an epidemiologic view. J Clin Gastroenterol *35*, S72-78.

Farazi, P. A., and Depinho, R. A. (2006). Hepatocellular carcinoma pathogenesis: from genes to environment. Nat Rev Cancer *6*, 674-687.

Fattovich, G., Giustina, G., Sanchez-Tapias, J., et al. (1998). Delayed clearance of serum HBsAg in compensated cirrhosis B: relation to interferon alpha therapy and disease prognosis. European Concerted Action on Viral Hepatitis (EUROHEP). Am J Gastroenterol *93*, 896-900.

Ge, D., Fellay, J., Thompson, A. J., et al. (2009). Genetic variation in IL28B predicts hepatitis C treatment-induced viral clearance. Nature *461*, 399-401.

Georgiades, C. S., Hong, K., and Geschwind, J. F. (2008). Radiofrequency ablation and chemoembolization for hepatocellular carcinoma. Cancer J *14*, 117-122.

Gresser, I. (1991). Antitumour effects of interferons: past, present and future. Br J Haematol *79 Suppl 1*, 1-5.

Gresser, I., Kaido, T., Maury, C., Woodrow, D., Moss, J., and Belardelli, F. (1994). Interaction of IFN alpha/beta with host cells essential to the early inhibition of Friend erythroleukemia visceral metastases in mice. Int J Cancer *57*, 604-611.

Havell, E. A., Berman, B., Ogburn, C. A., Berg, K., Paucker, K., and Vilcek, J. (1975). Two antigenically distinct species of human interferon. Proc Natl Acad Sci U S A *72*, 2185-2187.

Hong, S. H., Cho, O., Kim, K., Shin, H. J., Kotenko, S. V., and Park, S. (2007). Effect of interferon-lambda on replication of hepatitis B virus in human hepatoma cells. Virus Res *126*, 245-249.

Hou, W., Wang, X., Ye, L., Zhou, L., Yang, Z. Q., Riedel, E., and Ho, W. Z. (2009). Lambda interferon inhibits human immunodeficiency virus type 1 infection of macrophages. J Virol *83*, 3834-3842.

Isaacs, A., and Lindenmann, J. (1957). Virus interference. I. The interferon. Proc R Soc Lond B Biol Sci *147*, 258-267.

Jankowski, W. J., Davey, M. W., O'malley, J. A., Sulkowski, E., and Carter, W. A. (1975). Molecular structure of human fibroblast and leukocyte interferons: probe by lectin and hydrophobic chromatography. J Virol *16*, 1124-1130.

Javelaud, D., Alexaki, V. I., and Mauviel, A. (2008). Transforming growth factor-beta in cutaneous melanoma. Pigment Cell Melanoma Res *21*, 123-132.

Johnston, S. L. (2007). Innate immunity in the pathogenesis of virus-induced asthma exacerbations. Proc Am Thorac Soc *4*, 267-270.

Jordan, W. J., Eskdale, J., Boniotto, M., Rodia, M., Kellner, D., and Gallagher, G. (2007a). Modulation of the human cytokine response by interferon lambda-1 (IFN-lambda1/IL-29). Genes Immun *8*, 13-20.

Jordan, W. J., Eskdale, J., Srinivas, S., Pekarek, V., Kelner, D., Rodia, M., and Gallagher, G. (2007b). Human interferon lambda-1 (IFN-lambda1/IL-29) modulates the Th1/Th2 response. Genes Immun *8*, 254-261.

Kaido, T., Maury, C., Schirrmacher, V., and Gresser, I. (1994). Successful immunotherapy of the highly metastatic murine ESb lymphoma with sensitized CD8+ T cells and IFN-alpha/beta. Int J Cancer *57*, 538-543.

Kaido, T. J., Maury, C., and Gresser, I. (1995). Host CD4+ T lymphocytes are required for the synergistic action of interferon-alpha/beta and adoptively transferred immune cells in the inhibition of visceral ESb metastases. Cancer Res *55*, 6133-6139.

Kalvakolanu, D. V. (2004). The GRIMs: a new interface between cell death regulation and interferon/retinoid induced growth suppression. Cytokine Growth Factor Rev *15*, 169-194.

Kelly, C., Klenerman, P., and Barnes, E. (2011). Interferon lambdas: the next cytokine storm. Gut.

Kirkwood, J. M., Ibrahim, J., Lawson, D. H., Atkins, M. B., Agarwala, S. S., Collins, K., Mascari, R., Morrissey, D. M., and Chapman, P. B. (2001). High-dose interferon alfa-2b does not diminish antibody response to GM2 vaccination in patients with resected melanoma: results of the Multicenter Eastern Cooperative Oncology Group Phase II Trial E2696. J Clin Oncol *19*, 1430-1436.

Kirkwood, J. M., Strawderman, M. H., Ernstoff, M. S., Smith, T. J., Borden, E. C., and Blum, R. H. (1996). Interferon alfa-2b adjuvant therapy of high-risk resected cutaneous melanoma: the Eastern Cooperative Oncology Group Trial EST 1684. J Clin Oncol *14*, 7-17.

Kleeberg, U. R., Suciu, S., Brocker, E. B., Ruiter, D. J., Chartier, C., Lienard, D., Marsden, J., Schadendorf, D., and Eggermont, A. M. (2004). Final results of the EORTC 18871/DKG 80-1 randomised phase III trial. rIFN-alpha2b versus rIFN-gamma versus ISCADOR M versus observation after surgery in melanoma patients with either high-risk primary (thickness >3 mm) or regional lymph node metastasis. Eur J Cancer *40*, 390-402.

Kotenko, S. V., Gallagher, G., Baurin, V. V., Lewis-Antes, A., Shen, M., Shah, N. K., Langer, J. A., Sheikh, F., Dickensheets, H., and Donnelly, R. P. (2003). IFN-lambdas mediate antiviral protection through a distinct class II cytokine receptor complex. Nat Immunol *4*, 69-77.

Kugel, D., Kochs, G., Obojes, K., Roth, J., Kobinger, G. P., Kobasa, D., Haller, O., Staeheli, P., and Von Messling, V. (2009). Intranasal administration of alpha interferon reduces seasonal influenza A virus morbidity in ferrets. J Virol *83*, 3843-3851.

Labie, D., and Gilgenkrantz, H. (2010). [IL28 (interferon lambda3) gene polymorphisms and response to IFN-alpha treatment in patients infected with hepatitis virus C]. Med Sci (Paris) *26*, 225-226.

Langer, J. A., Cutrone, E. C., and Kotenko, S. (2004). The Class II cytokine receptor (CRF2) family: overview and patterns of receptor-ligand interactions. Cytokine Growth Factor Rev *15*, 33-48.

Lasfar, A., Abushahba, W., De La Torre, A., Castaneda, I., Kotenko, S. V., and Reuhl, K. (2008). IFN Therapy in TIB75 HCC Model: Combination of IFN-lambda and IFN-alpha induces complete remission. Hepathology *48, 4(suppl), #191.*

Lasfar, A., and Cohen-Solal, K. A. (2010). Resistance to transforming growth factor beta-mediated tumor suppression in melanoma: are multiple mechanisms in place? Carcinogenesis *31*, 1710-1717.

Lasfar, A., Lewis-Antes, A., Smirnov, S. V., et al. (2006). Characterization of the mouse IFN-lambda ligand-receptor system: IFN-lambdas exhibit antitumor activity against B16 melanoma. Cancer Res *66*, 4468-4477.

Lau, W. Y., and Lai, E. C. (2008). Hepatocellular carcinoma: current management and recent advances. Hepatobiliary Pancreat Dis Int *7*, 237-257.

Lazaro, C. A., Chang, M., Tang, W., Campbell, J., Sullivan, D. G., Gretch, D. R., Corey, L., Coombs, R. W., and Fausto, N. (2007). Hepatitis C virus replication in transfected and serum-infected cultured human fetal hepatocytes. Am J Pathol *170*, 478-489.

Le Bon, A., and Tough, D. F. (2002). Links between innate and adaptive immunity via type I interferon. Curr Opin Immunol *14*, 432-436.

Li, M., Liu, X., Zhou, Y., and Su, S. B. (2009). Interferon-{lambda}s: the modulators of antivirus, antitumor, and immune responses. J Leukoc Biol.

Li, W., Lewis-Antes, A., Huang, J., Balan, M., and Kotenko, S. V. (2008). Regulation of apoptosis by type III interferons. Cell Prolif *41*, 960-979.

Lin, S. M., Yu, M. L., Lee, C. M., Chien, R. N., Sheen, I. S., Chu, C. M., and Liaw, Y. F. (2007). Interferon therapy in HBeAg positive chronic hepatitis reduces progression to cirrhosis and hepatocellular carcinoma. J Hepatol *46*, 45-52.

Littman, S. J., Faltynek, C. R., and Baglioni, C. (1985). Binding of human recombinant 125I-interferon gamma to receptors on human cells. J Biol Chem *260*, 1191-1195.

Llovet, J. M., Sala, M., Castells, L., Suarez, Y., Vilana, R., Bianchi, L., Ayuso, C., Vargas, V., Rodes, J., and Bruix, J. (2000). Randomized controlled trial of interferon treatment for advanced hepatocellular carcinoma. Hepatology *31*, 54-58.

Lo, C. M., Liu, C. L., Chan, S. C., Lam, C. M., Poon, R. T., Ng, I. O., Fan, S. T., and Wong, J. (2007). A randomized, controlled trial of postoperative adjuvant interferon therapy after resection of hepatocellular carcinoma. Ann Surg *245*, 831-842.

Maher, S. G., Sheikh, F., Scarzello, A. J., Romero-Weaver, A. L., Baker, D. P., Donnelly, R. P., and Gamero, A. M. (2008). IFNalpha and IFNlambda differ in their antiproliferative effects and duration of JAK/STAT signaling activity. Cancer Biol Ther *7*, 1109-1115.

Mangia, A., Thompson, A. J., Santoro, R., et al. (2010). An IL28B polymorphism determines treatment response of hepatitis C virus genotype 2 or 3 patients who do not achieve a rapid virologic response. Gastroenterology *139*, 821-827, 827 e821.

Marcello, T., Grakoui, A., Barba-Spaeth, G., Machlin, E. S., Kotenko, S. V., Macdonald, M. R., and Rice, C. M. (2006). Interferons alpha and lambda inhibit hepatitis C virus replication with distinct signal transduction and gene regulation kinetics. Gastroenterology *131*, 1887-1898.

Mazzaferro, V., Chun, Y. S., Poon, R. T., Schwartz, M. E., Yao, F. Y., Marsh, J. W., Bhoori, S., and Lee, S. G. (2008). Liver transplantation for hepatocellular carcinoma. Ann Surg Oncol *15*, 1001-1007.

Mazzaferro, V., Llovet, J. M., Miceli, R., et al. (2009). Predicting survival after liver transplantation in patients with hepatocellular carcinoma beyond the Milan criteria: a retrospective, exploratory analysis. Lancet Oncol *10*, 35-43.

Mccarthy, J. J., Li, J. H., Thompson, A., Suchindran, S., Lao, X. Q., Patel, K., Tillmann, H. L., Muir, A. J., and Mchutchison, J. G. (2010). Replicated association between an IL28B gene variant and a sustained response to pegylated interferon and ribavirin. Gastroenterology *138*, 2307-2314.

Meager, A., Visvalingam, K., Dilger, P., Bryan, D., and Wadhwa, M. (2005). Biological activity of interleukins-28 and -29: comparison with type I interferons. Cytokine *31*, 109-118.

Mennechet, F. J., and Uze, G. (2006). Interferon-lambda-treated dendritic cells specifically induce proliferation of FOXP3-expressing suppressor T cells. Blood *107*, 4417-4423.

Merlin, G., Falcoff, E., and Aguet, M. (1985). 125I-labelled human interferons alpha, beta and gamma: comparative receptor-binding data. J Gen Virol *66 (Pt 5)*, 1149-1152.

Montes-Cano, M. A., Garcia-Lozano, J. R., Abad-Molina, C., Romero-Gomez, M., Barroso, N., Aguilar-Reina, J., Nunez-Roldan, A., and Gonzalez-Escribano, M. F. (2010). Interleukin-28B genetic variants and hepatitis virus infection by different viral genotypes. Hepatology *52*, 33-37.

Mordstein, M., Kochs, G., Dumoutier, L., Renauld, J. C., Paludan, S. R., Klucher, K., and Staeheli, P. (2008). Interferon-lambda contributes to innate immunity of mice against influenza A virus but not against hepatotropic viruses. PLoS Pathog *4*, e1000151.

Mordstein, M., Neugebauer, E., Ditt, V., et al. (2010). Lambda interferon renders epithelial cells of the respiratory and gastrointestinal tracts resistant to viral infections. J Virol *84*, 5670-5677.

Morrow, M. P., Pankhong, P., Laddy, D. J., Schoenly, K. A., Yan, J., Cisper, N., and Weiner, D. B. (2009). Comparative ability of IL-12 and IL-28B to regulate Treg cell populations and enhance adaptive cellular immunity. Blood.

Mosbruger, T. L., Duggal, P., Goedert, J. J., et al. (2010). Large-scale candidate gene analysis of spontaneous clearance of hepatitis C virus. J Infect Dis *201*, 1371-1380.

Moschos, S., Varanasi, S., and Kirkwood, J. M. (2005). Interferons in the treatment of solid tumors. Cancer Treat Res *126*, 207-241.

Muir, A. J., Shiffman, M. L., Zaman, A., et al. (2010). Phase 1b study of pegylated interferon lambda 1 with or without ribavirin in patients with chronic genotype 1 hepatitis C virus infection. Hepatology *52*, 822-832.

Muller, U., Steinhoff, U., Reis, L. F., Hemmi, S., Pavlovic, J., Zinkernagel, R. M., and Aguet, M. (1994). Functional role of type I and type II interferons in antiviral defense. Science *264*, 1918-1921.

Nagai, H., and Sumino, Y. (2008). Therapeutic strategy of advanced hepatocellular carcinoma by using combined intra-arterial chemotherapy. Recent Pat Anticancer Drug Discov *3*, 220-226.

Novak, A. J., Grote, D. M., Ziesmer, S. C., Rajkumar, V., Doyle, S. E., and Ansell, S. M. (2008). A role for IFN-lambda1 in multiple myeloma B cell growth. Leukemia *22*, 2240-2246.

Numasaki, M., Tagawa, M., Iwata, F., Suzuki, T., Nakamura, A., Okada, M., Iwakura, Y., Aiba, S., and Yamaya, M. (2007). IL-28 elicits antitumor responses against murine fibrosarcoma. J Immunol *178*, 5086-5098.

Omata, M., Yoshida, H., and Shiratori, Y. (2005). Prevention of hepatocellular carcinoma and its recurrence in chronic hepatitis C patients by interferon therapy. Clin Gastroenterol Hepatol *3*, S141-143.

Pestka, S. (2007). The interferons: 50 years after their discovery, there is much more to learn. J Biol Chem *282*, 20047-20051.

Pestka, S., Krause, C. D., and Walter, M. R. (2004). Interferons, interferon-like cytokines, and their receptors. Immunol Rev *202*, 8-32.

Rauch, A., Kutalik, Z., Descombes, P., et al. (2010). Genetic variation in IL28B is associated with chronic hepatitis C and treatment failure: a genome-wide association study. Gastroenterology *138*, 1338-1345, 1345 e1331-1337.

Robek, M. D., Boyd, B. S., and Chisari, F. V. (2005). Lambda interferon inhibits hepatitis B and C virus replication. J Virol *79*, 3851-3854.

Sato, A., Ohtsuki, M., Hata, M., Kobayashi, E., and Murakami, T. (2006). Antitumor activity of IFN-lambda in murine tumor models. J Immunol *176*, 7686-7694.

Sheppard, P., Kindsvogel, W., Xu, W., et al. (2003). IL-28, IL-29 and their class II cytokine receptor IL-28R. Nat Immunol *4*, 63-68.

Sherman, M. (2005). Hepatocellular carcinoma: epidemiology, risk factors, and screening. Semin Liver Dis *25*, 143-154.

Sidky, Y. A., and Borden, E. C. (1987). Inhibition of angiogenesis by interferons: effects on tumor- and lymphocyte-induced vascular responses. Cancer Res *47*, 5155-5161.

Srinivas, S., Dai, J., Eskdale, J., Gallagher, G. E., Megjugorac, N. J., and Gallagher, G. (2008). Interferon-lambda1 (interleukin-29) preferentially down-regulates interleukin-13 over other T helper type 2 cytokine responses in vitro. Immunology *125*, 492-502.

Stewart, W. E., 2nd, Declercq, E., De Somer, P., Berg, K., Ogburn, C. A., and Paucker, K. (1973). Antiviral and non-antiviral activity of highly purified interferon. Nat New Biol *246*, 141-143.

Suppiah, V., Moldovan, M., Ahlenstiel, G., et al. (2009). IL28B is associated with response to chronic hepatitis C interferon-alpha and ribavirin therapy. Nat Genet *41*, 1100-1104.

Taketomi, A., Soejima, Y., Yoshizumi, T., Uchiyama, H., Yamashita, Y., and Maehara, Y. (2008). Liver transplantation for hepatocellular carcinoma. J Hepatobiliary Pancreat Surg *15*, 124-130.

Tanaka, Y., Nishida, N., Sugiyama, M., et al. (2009). Genome-wide association of IL28B with response to pegylated interferon-alpha and ribavirin therapy for chronic hepatitis C. Nat Genet *41*, 1105-1109.

Ueshima, K., Kudo, M., Nagai, T., et al. (2008). Combination therapy with S-1 and pegylated interferon alpha for advanced hepatocellular carcinoma. Oncology *75 Suppl 1*, 106-113.

Uze, G., and Monneron, D. (2007). IL-28 and IL-29: newcomers to the interferon family. Biochimie *89*, 729-734.

Valle, M. J., Jordan, G. W., Haahr, S., and Merigan, T. C. (1975). Characteristics of immune interferon produced by human lymphocyte cultures compared to other human interferons. J Immunol *115*, 230-233.

Wang, L., Wu, W. Z., Sun, H. C., Wu, X. F., Qin, L. X., Liu, Y. K., Liu, K. D., and Tang, Z. Y. (2003). Mechanism of interferon alpha on inhibition of metastasis and angiogenesis of hepatocellular carcinoma after curative resection in nude mice. J Gastrointest Surg *7*, 587-594.

Witte, K., Gruetz, G., Volk, H. D., Looman, A. C., Asadullah, K., Sterry, W., Sabat, R., and Wolk, K. (2009). Despite IFN-lambda receptor expression, blood immune cells, but not keratinocytes or melanocytes, have an impaired response to type III interferons: implications for therapeutic applications of these cytokines. Genes Immun.

Wolk, K., Witte, K., Witte, E., et al. (2008). Maturing dendritic cells are an important source of IL-29 and IL-20 that may cooperatively increase the innate immunity of keratinocytes. J Leukoc Biol *83*, 1181-1193.

Yu, M. L., Lin, S. M., Chuang, W. L., Dai, C. Y., Wang, J. H., Lu, S. N., Sheen, I. S., Chang, W. Y., Lee, C. M., and Liaw, Y. F. (2006). A sustained virological response to interferon or interferon/ribavirin reduces hepatocellular carcinoma and improves survival in chronic hepatitis C: a nationwide, multicentre study in Taiwan. Antivir Ther *11*, 985-994.

Zitzmann, K., Brand, S., Baehs, S., Goke, B., Meinecke, J., Spottl, G., Meyer, H., and Auernhammer, C. J. (2006). Novel interferon-lambdas induce antiproliferative effects in neuroendocrine tumor cells. Biochem Biophys Res Commun *344*, 1334-1341.

16

Intramuscular *IL-12* Electrogene Therapy for Treatment of Spontaneous Canine Tumors

Maja Cemazar[1], Gregor Sersa[1], Darja Pavlin[2] and Natasa Tozon[2]
[1]*Institute of Oncology Ljubljana, Department of Experimental Oncology*
[2]*University of Ljubljana, Veterinary Faculty Ljubljana, Clinic for Small Animal Medicine and Surgery*
Slovenia

1. Introduction

In the last two decades an enormous progress has been made in research of gene therapy, translating this new therapeutic approach from preclinical level to a large number of clinical trials, which presented encouraging results in treatment of a number of different diseases, from a single gene disorders to a more complex diseases, such as cancer. According to the Journal of Gene Medicine, at present more than 1400 human clinical trials investigating effects of gene therapy have been conducted, over 2/3 for therapy of cancer (www.wiley.com/genmed/clinical). With the advances in the field of gene therapy, this new therapeutic tool is steadily gaining its acceptance also in clinical veterinary medicine. In the last decade, a number of gene therapy clinical trials have been conducted on companion animals, employing both viral and nonviral vectors and evaluating its effects primarily in oncologic, haematologic, musculoskeletal and cardiovascular diseases (Bergmann et al., 2003; Bodles-Brakhop et al., 2008; Dow et al., 2005; Draghia-Akli et al. 2002; Herzog et al., 2001; Huttinger et al., 2008; Jahnke et al., 2007; Kamstock et al., 2006; Kornegay et al., 2010; Ohshima et al., 2009; Pavlin et al., 2011; Siddiqui et al., 2007; Sleeper et al., 2010; Z. Wang et al., 2007). Such clinical trials on companion animals not only play an essential role for progress of veterinary medicine, but also provide invaluable data for human clinical research, which cannot be gained from strictly preclinical research on experimental animals.
With gene therapy having versatile applications, different approaches have been developed, utilizing delivery of therapeutic genes into a variety of target tissues. The first reports on using skeletal muscle as a target for gene delivery have been published in the 1990's and since then, extensive evidence has been presented that skeletal muscle is a suitable target tissue for gene therapy (Wolff et al., 1990). The main advantages of skeletal muscle are high capacity of protein synthesis and post-mitotic status of muscle fibers which enable long-lasting transgene expression. Muscle targeted transgene delivery can lead to either local intramuscular secretion or systemic delivery of transgene products, thus having potential for treatment of both muscular and non-muscular disorders. The clinical applications of muscle targeted gene therapy are mainly correction of gene deficits in the muscle tissue (e.g. muscle dystrophies), intravascular release of therapeutic proteins resulting in expansion of this therapy on systemic level (e.g.immunomodulation) and DNA vaccination against tumor antigens or infectious agents. Intramuscular gene therapy in veterinary medicine has already been successfully applied for a variety of indications in a number of different animal

species, for example in cattle and sheep (Howell et al., 2008; Mena et al., 2001; Tollefsen et al., 2003), horses (Brown et al., 2008), pigs (Brown et al., 2004; Gravier et al., 2007) as well as cats (Brown et al., 2009; Ross et al., 2006; Walker et al, 2005) and dogs. In dogs mainly *ex vivo* delivery approach and viral vectors have been used in different disease models, primarily for treatment of hemophilia B, muscle dystrophies and in therapy of ischemic heart disease (Arruda et al. 2010; Banks & Chamberlain, 2008; Dixon & Spinale, 2009; Hasbrouck & High, 2008; Haurigot et al., 2010; Herzog et al., 2001; Katz et al., 2010; Ohshima et al., 2009; L. Wang & Herzog, 2005; Z. Wang et al., 2007, 2009).

The most straightforward introduction of foreign transgenes into skeletal muscle is simple intramuscular injection of naked plasmid DNA, which can result in a sustained transgene expression (Budker et al., 2000; Lu et al., 2003; Wolff et al., 1990). The main disadvantage of this method, which severely limits its therapeutic potential, is low transfection efficiency and pronounced variability of inter-individual levels of gene expression (Mir et al., 1999). Both described limitations of this gene delivery technique can be ameliorated by different methods, one of them being electroporation.

Electroporation is a physical method for delivery of various molecules into the cells by transiently increasing permeability of cell membrane with application of controlled external electrical field to the target cells (Neumann et al., 1982). It displays effectiveness for a broad spectrum of applications, in both *in vitro* and *in vivo* settings. *In vitro* it is already routinely used as a method for intracellular delivery of a variety of molecules, e. g. RNA, DNA, dyes, ions, chemotherapeutic drugs, etc. *In vivo* it has shown a great potential for two prospective therapeutic approaches in oncology, electrochemotherapy and electrogene therapy (EGT), both already used in clinical practice in both human and veterinary medicine (Cemazar et al., 2008; Daud et al. 2008; Kodre et al., 2005; Mir et al., 1998; Pavlin et al., 2011; Reed et al., 2010; Sersa et al., 2000; Tozon et al., 2001, 2005). This method of transgene delivery can be applied to almost any tissue in a living organism, with research focused primarily on tumor tissue, skin and skeletal muscle (Cemazar & Sersa, 2007). Electroporation based transfection of skeletal muscle or muscle targeted EGT has been proven to be one of the most efficient and simple methods among different nonviral delivery methods currently under investigation (Cemazar & Sersa, 2007; Gehl et al., 1999). It combines injection of therapeutic plasmid DNA into the muscle with subsequent electroporation of the target tissue, resulting in dramatically, up to 2000-times, increased long-term local gene expression lasting more than one year (Aihara & Miyaziki et al., 1998; Mir et al., 1999; Tevz et al., 2008).

In the last few years, the number of reports on successful intramuscular EGT in dogs is steadily increasing. Therapeutic genes, delivered into canine skeletal muscle with this technique are genes encoding growth hormone releasing hormone (GHRH) (Bodles-Brakhop et al., 2008; Brown et al., 2009; Draghia-Akli et al., 2002), human coagulation factor IX (hF.IX) (Fewell et al., 2001) and interleukin-12 (IL-12) (Pavlin et al., 2008). These studies showed a considerable clinical effect of intramuscular EGT in canine patients. *GHRH* EGT resulted in dramatically improved clinical condition of dogs with cancer, resulting in prolonged life span and improved quality of life (Bodles-Brakhop et al., 2008; Draghia-Akli et al., 2002). In dogs with chronic renal failure the same therapy improved kidney function and anemia associated with kidney disease, leading to overall improved health and survival rate (Brown et al., 2009). Intramuscular *hF.IX* EGT led to significant increase in levels of hF.IX in dogs, which can be predicted to have therapeutic effect in animal models of hemophilia B (Fewell et al., 2001). An important aspect of these studies is the fact that the procedure was successfully performed on both healthy and diseased dogs, demonstrating that even debilitated, cachectic and immunocompromised animals are capable of systemic shedding of transgenes resulting in clinical effect of intramuscularly delivered therapeutic genes.

IL-12 is a heterodimeric protein composed of two covalently linked subunits, a 35 kDa light chain (also known as p35 or IL-12α) and a 40 kDa heavy chain (known as p40 or IL-12β). The discovery of IL-12 in 1989 revealed its strong effect on both innate immune system through induction of IFN-γ production from natural killer (NK) cells as well as on adaptive immune system through generation of cytotoxic T Lymphocytes (Kobayashi et al., 1989; Trinchieri et al., 1992). Based on these biological actions it was predicted that this cytokine is required for resistance to bacterial and intracellular parasites, as well as for the establishment of organ-specific autoimmunity (Trinchieri, 2003) and was considered that it shows possible therapeutic potential for treatment of diseases, which would favorably respond to its immunomodulating actions. With the additional discovery of its antiangiogenic effects (Voest et al., 1995), IL-12 became one of the most promising cytokines for treatment of malignant diseases.

A model of mechanisms involved in the antitumor effects of IL-12 predict that IL-12 directly activates cells of the adaptive (CD4+ and CD8+ T cells) and innate arm of immunity by helping to prime T cells increasing their survival, enhancing T cell, and NK cell effector functions as well as promoting induction of IFN-γ secretion. IFN-γ in turn acts directly on tumor cells and other cell components within the tumor, by enhancing recognition of tumor cells by T cells through MHC class I processing and presentation and by modifications of extracellular matrix, which result in reduced antiangiogenesis and tumor invasion. The end result of these actions is impediment of tumor growth and ultimately eradication of the tumor. The first preclinical studies in the early 1990s with recombinant IL-12 protein in cancer treatment indeed showed its antitumor and antimetastatic activity (Brunda et al., 1993; Nastala et al., 1994). Unfortunately, potent antitumor effect established on preclinical level did not translate to clinical setting, demonstrating only limited therapeutic effect with serious toxic side-effects in the first clinical studies (Atkins et al., 1997). Therefore new therapeutic approaches for *in vivo* delivery of IL-12 have been investigated, with gene transfer of *IL-12* introducing safer and more effective treatment method compared to systemic application of recombinant protein.

As one of therapeutic gene delivery methods, *IL-12* EGT has been utilized in a number of different tumor models both on preclinical level and in clinical trials (Cemazar et al., 2010). Using electroporation, the therapeutic gene has been delivered into tumor tissue or skeletal muscle and EGT has been used either as a single therapy or in combination with other therapeutic genes and agents (e.g. *IL-18, IL-27,* herpes virus thymidine kinase, tetanus toxin fragment C) or different treatment methods, e.g. electrochemotherapy or radiotherapy (Cemazar et al., 2010; Kamensek & Sersa, 2008). These studies established that *IL-12* EGT shows remarkable local and systemic antitumor effects, including significant growth delay and even achieving complete long-term regression of treated tumors, induction of long-term antitumor immunity, antimetastatic activity and prolongation of survival in treated animals. Direct antitumor effect in established tumors is generally better achieved with local intratumoral delivery of therapeutic gene, whereas intramuscular delivery results especially in good antimetastatic activity (Hanna et al., 2001; Lee et al., 2003; Li et al., 2005; Lucas et al., 2002; Tevz et al., 2009).

In preclinical studies the murine tumor models, which favorably responded to *IL-12* EGT, were melanoma (L.C. Heller & R. Heller, 2010), lymphoma (Lee et al., 2003), soft tissue sarcoma (Pavlin et al., 2009; Tevz et al., 2009) and a variety of different carcinomas (Cemazar et al., 2010; L.C. Heller et al., 2005). In clinical settings, intratumoral *IL-12* EGT has been successfully used both in humans (Daud et al., 2008), as well as dogs (Cutrera et al., 2008; Pavlin et al., 2011; Reed et al., 2010). In all of presently published studies in tumor-bearing dogs, EGT has been performed with intratumoral delivery of *IL-12* either alone (Chuang et al., 2009; Pavlin et al., 2011), or in combination with electrochemotherapy with bleomycin (Cutrera et al, 2008; Reed et al., 2010). The only published intramuscular *IL-12* EGT in dogs was performed on healthy experimental beagles (Pavlin et al., 2008), showing feasibility, efficacy and safety of this approach. However, similar approach to *IL-12* gene therapy in tumor-bearing companion animals has not yet been described.

The aim of our study was to evaluate effects of intramuscular EGT with plasmid encoding human IL-12 in dogs with spontaneously occurring tumors. For this purpose, 1 mg of plasmid encoding human IL-12 was injected into *m. semitendinosus* of 6 patients with 4 different tumor types. Systemic transgene release and induction of IFN-γ response was determined by repeated measurements of hIL-12 and canine IFN-γ (cIFN-γ) in patients' sera. Possible side effects of the procedure were monitored with regular clinical examinations and determination of selected hematology and biochemistry parameters.

2. Materials and methods

2.1 Animals

All animals participating in this study were referred to the Clinic for small animal medicine and surgery, Veterinary faculty of Ljubljana, University of Ljubljana, Slovenia, for evaluation of different types of spontaneously occurring tumors. Prior to inclusion, written consent for participation in the study was obtained from the owners and the study was approved by the Ethical Committee at the Ministry of Agriculture, Forestry and Food of the Republic of Slovenia (approval No. 323-451/2004-9). Six dogs of five different breeds corresponded to the inclusion criteria, their age ranging from 3 - 13 years (Table 1). Inclusion criteria for the study comprised at least one cytologically or histologically confirmed tumor nodule, good general health status of the animal with the basic hematology and biochemistry profile within reference limits and normal renal and cardiovascular function. In these animals intramuscular EGT was performed either as an adjuvant therapy to conventional therapeutical procedures, specific for each tumor type or as single therapy in a patient, where other therapies were not possible or acceptable by the owner.

The study cohort comprised of three dogs with intermediately (*i.e.* grade II) (Figure 1) and poorly differentiated (*i.e.* grade III) (Figure 2) mast cell tumors (MCT) in different clinical stages, and one dog with each: pulmonary histiocytic sarcoma (PHS) (Figure 3), osteosarcoma (OSA) (Figure 4) and mammary adenocarcinoma (MAC) (Table 1).

One patient with MCT had metastatic disease involving local lymph nodes, and neither of patients had clinically detectable distant metastases. Two of the patients, one with MCT and one with mammary adenocarcinoma, had recurrent disease after marginal surgery. Histological or cytological diagnosis was established with examination of tumor biopsies and local lymph node fine needle aspiration in all tumors except OSA. Superficial tumors were measured in three perpendicular directions and their volume was calculated using the formula: $V = a \times b \times c \times \pi/6$.

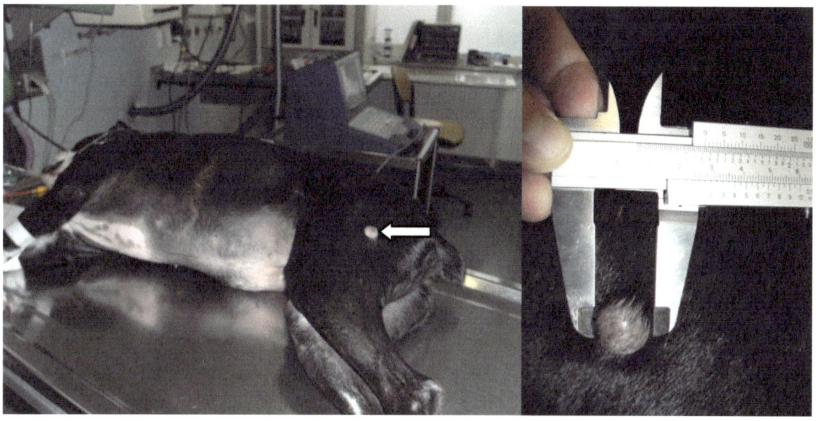

Fig. 1. Patient no. 2, German boxer with grade II MCT in the gluteal region, which was surgically removed and at the same time intramuscular EGT performed in the contralateral leg. Arrow indicats the position of the tumor.

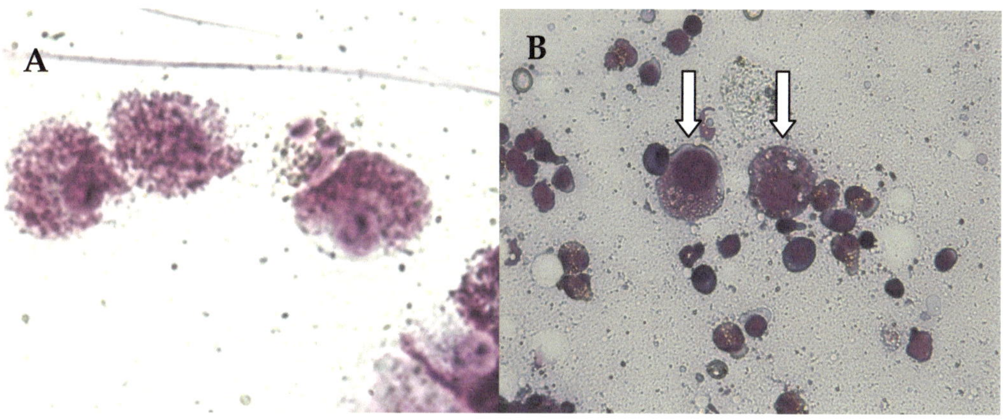

Fig. 2. Fine needle aspirate of poorly differentiated MCT (gradus III) in patient no. 3 (Giemsa stain). A: Tumor aspirate; B: Aspirate of prescapular lymph node with mast cell infiltrations (metastases of primary tumor in local lymph nodes) (arrows).

Before the treatment, staging of the disease according to modified WHO criteria in each patient was performed with clinical examinations, abdominal ultrasonography, thoracic radiography and basic bloodwork with biochemistry profile. Bloodwork included complete blood count with differential white blood cell count, performed with an automated laser hematology analyzer (Technicon H*1, Bayer, Germany) with species-specific software (H*1 Multi-Species V30 Software). Determination of selected biochemistry parameters (serum concentrations of urea and creatinine and activity of serum alkaline phosphatase and alanine aminotransferase) was performed using automated chemistry analyzer Technicon RA-XT (Bayer, Germany). Basal determinations of serum concentrations of human IL-12 and canine IFN-γ using ELISA kits (Human IL-12 Quantikine ELISA kit and Canine IFN-γ Quantikine ELISA kit, respectively, both R&D System, Minneapolis, MN, USA) were also performed.

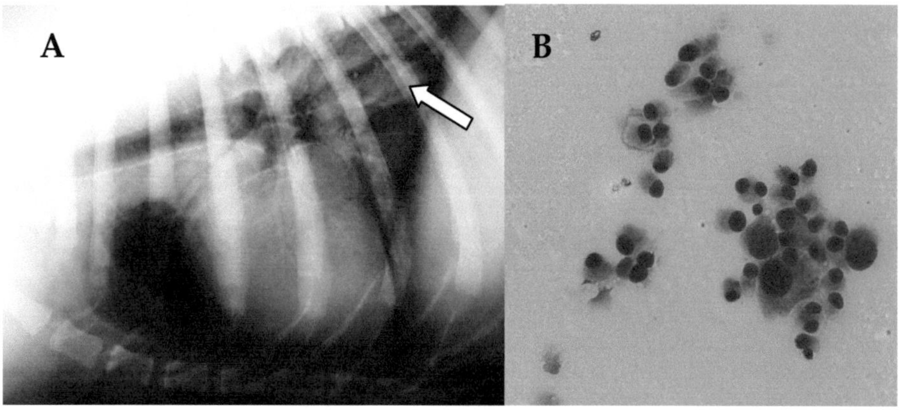

Fig. 3. Patient no. 4 with pulmonary histiocytic sarcoma. A: Thoracic radiograph of the patient depicting a solid mass in caudal lobe of the lungs (arrow); B: Fine needle aspirate of the tumor showing large round typically vacuolated histiocytic cells with high degree of anisokariosis (Giemsa stain; 400 times magnification).

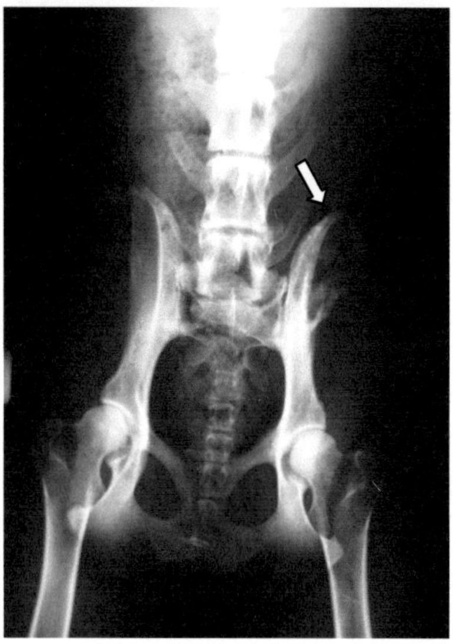

Fig. 4. Radiograph of pelvis in patient no. 5 showing predominantly osteolytic lesions on the iliac bone involving pars compacta (arrow), consistent with radiological presentation of osteosarcoma.

Each patient received one EGT treatment. In five of six treated animals, EGT was performed as an adjuvant therapy to conventional treatment procedures (Table 1). In all three dogs with MCT, tumor nodules were marginally surgically removed prior to or concomitantly with EGT and two of these patients also received systemic chemotherapy, which consisted of either vincristine and methyprednisolone protocol (0.5 - 0.7 mg/m^2 and 1 mg/kg, respectively) or CCNU (lomustine, 60 - 90 mg/m^2). In the patient with mammary adenocarcinoma, the tumor was surgically removed with marginal excision before performing EGT. The patient with pulmonary histiocytic sarcoma received one cycle of CCNU chemotherapy (60 mg/m^2), applied two weeks after EGT. The only exception, in which EGT was performed as a single therapy was the dog with OSA in which location of the tumor (pelvis) precluded surgical treatment and the owner refused palliative radiotherapy.

Pt. No.	Breed	Age (yrs)/ Gender	Tumor type	Tumor location	Clinical stage	Therapy (listed chronologically)
1	German boxer	7/M	Mast cell tumor Gradus III	Front leg	II[a]	• Marginal surgery • Systemic chemotherapy (V+M 4 cycles) • EGT
2	German boxer	3/FS	Mast cell tumor Gradus II	Hind leg	I[a]	• Surgery with clear surgical margins concomitantly with EGT
3	Lhasa-apso	13/FS	Mast cell tumor Gradus III	Neck Metastases in local lymph nodes Recurrence after surgery	III[a]	• Marginal surgery • EGT • Systemic chemotherapy (V+M 2 cycle; CCNU 1 cycles)
4	Bernese mountain dog	6/M	Pulmonary histiocytic sarcoma	Lungs	N/A	• EGT • CCNU 1 cycle
5	Doberman Pinscher	8/FS	Osteosarcoma	Pelvis (ilium)	N/D	• EGT
6	Crossbreed	11/FS	Mammary adenocarcinoma	Mammary gland (D2-4) Recurrence after surgery	III[b]	• Surgery (partial mastectomy) • EGT

a - clinical stage according to modified WHO clinical staging system for mast cell tumors (Thamm & Vail, 2007)

b - clinical stage according to Owen LN, Classification of tumors in domestic animals, Geneva, 1980, WHO

M: male, FS: spayed female, V+M: vincristine/methylprednisolone chemotherapy protocol, N/A: not applicable, N/D: not determined

Table 1. Summary of dogs' characteristics and histories

2.2 Plasmid preparation

The pORF-hIL-12 plasmid (InvivoGen, Toulouse, France), encoding human IL-12, was selected based on published data indicating that canine and human IL-12 share approximately 90% genetic identity based on amino acid sequence analysis (Buettner et al., 1998). Furthermore, it has already been shown that in *in vitro* settings, human IL-12 activates proliferation of canine peripheral blood mononuclear cells (PBMC), consequently triggering a number of immune responses in canine PBMCs (Phillips et al., 1999). The plasmid was prepared using the Qiagen Maxi Endo-Free kit (Qiagen, Hilden, Germany), according to manufacturer's instructions and diluted to concentration of 1 mg/ml. Purified plasmid DNA was subjected to quality control and quantity determinations, performed by agarose gel electrophoresis and by means of spectrophotometry.

2.3 Electrogene therapy procedure

EGT was performed in the patients under general anesthesia, which was induced with propofol (Propoven 10 mg/ml, Fresenius Kabi Austria GmbH, Graz, Austria) and maintained with isoflurane (Forane, Abbott Laboratories LTD, Queensborough, UK). During the anesthesia the animals were receiving Hartmann's solution (B. Braun Melsungen AG, Melsunen, Germany) at the rate of 10 ml/kg of bodyweight/h. Hair on the right femoral region was clipped and the area surgically prepared, followed by intramuscular injection of 1 mg of sterile solution of therapeutic plasmid into *m. semitendinosus* using 1 ml syringe with 22 G needle (Figure 5). The position of the needle was slightly changed during the emptying of syringe, allowing the content of syringe to infiltrate the target tissue more uniformly. Ten minutes later, electric pulses were applied to plasmid infiltrated muscle with electric pulses generator Cliniporator™ (IGEA s.r.l., Carpi, Italy), using intramuscularly placed needle electrodes N-18-4B (IGEA s.r.l., Carpi, Italy), which consist of 2 arrays, each composed of 4 electrodes with 4 mm distance between them. One HV pulse (600 V/cm, 100 µs) was delivered, followed by 4 LV pulses (80 V/cm, 100 ms, 1 Hz), with 1 second lag between the HV and LV pulses. Postsurgically, analgesia was provided to all dogs with single intravenous application of carprofen (Rimadyl, Pfizer Animal Health, Dundee, United Kingdom; 4mg/kg of bodyweight). When they fully recovered from anesthesia, they were released from the hospital. The treated femoral area was protected with suitable dressing in order to prevent licking and any possible contact of humans or animals with the electroporated region.

2.4 Evaluation of response to the therapy

Animals were examined 7, 14 and 28 days after EGT and monthly thereafter until any cytokine was detected in three consecutive samples. Each follow-up included the same diagnostic procedures as pre-therapy examination. At each examination, response to the therapy was evaluated with determination of serum concentrations of both previously mentioned cytokines, as described above, measurements of tumor nodules, where applicable and notification of possible side effects. For evaluation of local effects, measurements of tumor nodules, where applicable, were performed.

2.5 Evaluation of possible side effects of the procedure

The possible occurrence of local and systemic side effects was evaluated at each follow-up with clinical examination of the patients, assessment of electroporated area for appearance of any adverse effects to either plasmid solution or electroporation of the tissue (e.g. swelling, erythema, pain, secretions, tissue necrosis etc). Blood samples were collected at each follow-up for the same bloodwork as during the staging of the disease prior to EGT in order to evaluate possible systemic toxicity of the procedure.

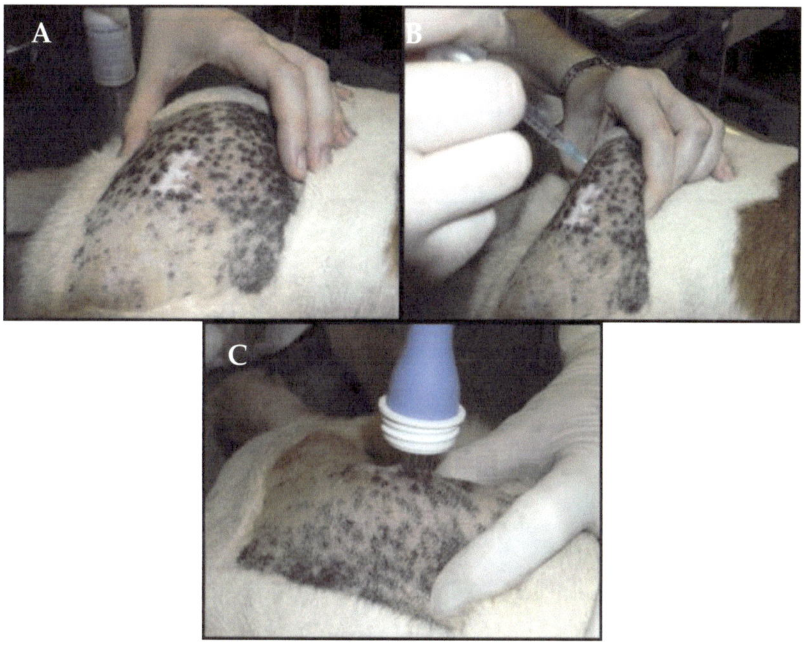

Fig. 5. Intramuscular EGT procedure. A: Surgically prepared femoral region; B: Intramuscular application of plasmid solution; C: Transcutaneous intramuscular placement of needle electrodes.

3. Results

3.1 Response to the therapy

In four out of six treated patients, serum concentrations of human IL-12 and/or canine IFN-γ were detected, among these responders were all three patients with MCT and the patient with PHS (Figure 6). Human IL-12 was detected in serum of a MCT patient 7 days after the procedure in concentration 17 pg/ml. IFN-γ was detected in single or multiple samples of all four mentioned patients, in concentrations ranging from 6.5 to 246.8 pg/ml, 4 to 28 days after the EGT procedure (Table 2). None of the patients had any detectable hIL-12 or IFN-γ in samples taken before the EGT procedures.

In these four patients, surprisingly long survival times after EGT were achieved (Table 2), even though intramuscular *IL-12* EGT did not have any effect on volumes of measurable tumor nodules. The dog with recurrent grade III MCT and lymph node metastases (clinical stage III) and the dog with PHS received additional chemotherapy 2 weeks after EGT; however the chemotherapeutic protocols were shortly discontinued due to severe side effects both patients developed. Even though the delivered chemotherapy in these two patients was inadequate to be effective and result in potential systemic antitumor effect, the dog with MCT survived 6 and the dog with PHS 8 months after the EGT procedure. The other two patients with detected IL-12 and/or IFN-γ had grade II and grade III MCTs. In the dog with grade II MCT (clinical stage I), the tumor nodule was marginally surgically removed and at the same time intramuscular *IL-12* EGT performed, without any additional therapy. In the last dog, grade III MCT (clinical stage II) was treated with marginal excision and full chemotherapy with vincristine and methylprednisolone, followed by intramuscular

IL-12 EGT. These two patients had complete response to the therapy without local recurrence or metastatic disease, surviving for over 4 and 3 years, respectively.

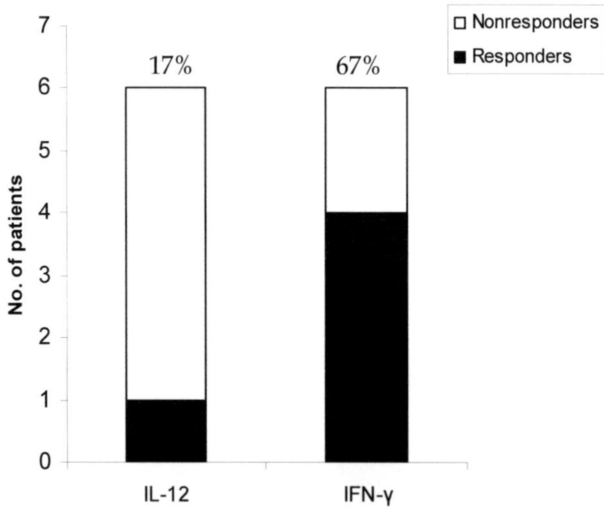

Fig. 6. Graph representing percentage of treated animals, which responded to intramuscular EGT with systemic release of either cytokine (i.e. responders) versus animals without systemically detectable cytokine (i.e. nonresponders).

Pt. No.	Tumor type	IL-12 (pg/ml)	IFN-γ (pg/ml)	Timing of sample collection after EGT	Follow-up after EGT	Response to the therapy
1	Mast cell tumor Gradus III	17.0 -	- 246.8	7 days 28 days	> 3 years	CR
2	Mast cell tumor Gradus II	-	6.5	7 days	> 4 years	CR
3	Mast cell tumor Gradus III	-	80	7 days	6 months	PD
4	Pulmonary histiocytic sarcoma	- -	37.1 104.2	7 days 14 days	8 months	SD
5	Osteosarcoma	-	-		5.5 months	SD
6	Mammary adenocarcinoma	-	-		2 months	PD

Table 2. Response to the therapy in the treated patients. CR: complete response, PD: progressive disease, SD: stable disease

In the other two patients (OSA and recurrent extensive MAC), neither cytokine was detected in serum at any time point after surgery. The dog with OSA survived for 165 days without any additional treatment, except pharmacological pain management and was euthanized due to progression of pain, unresponsive to analgesic therapy, without any radiologically evident distant metastases. The patient with MAC was euthanized 2 months after EGT due to progression of the disease (growth of tumor).

	Before EGT	Week 1	Week 4	Week 5	Week 6	Week 8	Week 11	Week 14	Ref. values
Therapy:		V+M: Cycle 1	V+M: Cycle 2	V+M: Stop		CCNU: Cycle 1	CCNU: Stop		
WBC	13.64	21.41	15.84	3.29	16.25	19.78	13.51	12.96	6.0-18.0
RBC	8.45	6.85	6.12	6.55	7.10	6.35	6.89	6.59	5.1-8.5
HCT	0.57	0.47	0.44	0.47	0.52	0.47	0.51	0.48	0.35-0.55
Neutro	8.43	16.48	12.27	1.29	12.31	17.25	10.48	12.2	3.0-11.8
Urea	10.2	N/D	9.2	12.1	11.9	13.2	8.03	10.5	3.0-12.5
Crea	107.4	N/D	90.6	111.3	114.9	109.5	96.9	118.1	44.2-132.6
SAP	92.6	77.0	113.3	N/D	107.5	112.9	671.1	287.9	25-117
ALT	65.4	64.6	50.7	N/D	62.1	78.1	312.5	84.1	23-90

Table 3. Hematological and biochemistry results in the patient No. 3 with high grade MCT, receiving *IL-12* EGT, followed by two different systemic chemotherapy protocols, applied only partially due to induction of marked side effects. Clinically relevant abnormalities in the bloodwork subsided after discontinuation of chemotherapy, demonstrating that the toxicity was caused by chemotherapy and not *IL-12* EGT WBC: white blood cells, RBC: red blood cell, HCT: hematocrit, Neutro: neutrophils, Crea: creatinine, SAP: serum alkaline phosphatase, ALT: alanine aminotransferase, V+M: vincristine/methylprednosolone chemotherapy protocol, N/D: not detected

3.2 Side effects of the procedure

In order to evaluate possible side effects at each follow-up, clinical examination as well as bloodwork with emphasis on kidney and liver function of patients was performed, due to known hepato- and nephrotoxicity of systemic recombinant IL-12 based therapy. We did not detect any side effects, which could be attributed to IL-12 toxicity, with hematological and biochemistry parameters staying within reference limits immediately after the procedure. In two of the patients marked hematological abnormalities were detected after induction of chemotherapy after EGT, which were attributed to the used chemotherapeutic agents, rather than EGT, since they were typical and well documented side effects of selected chemotherapy (i.e. leucopenia due to immunosuppression with vincristine and activation of serum alkaline phosphatase and alanin aminotrasferase due to hepatotoxicity of CCNU) (Table 3). In these two patients the abnormal values returned within the reference limits shortly after discontinuation of chemotherapy.

EGT procedure also did not cause any local side effects, for example swelling or inflammation of the electroporated area despite local invasiveness of the procedure, which was performed with intramuscularly placed needle electrodes (Figure 7).

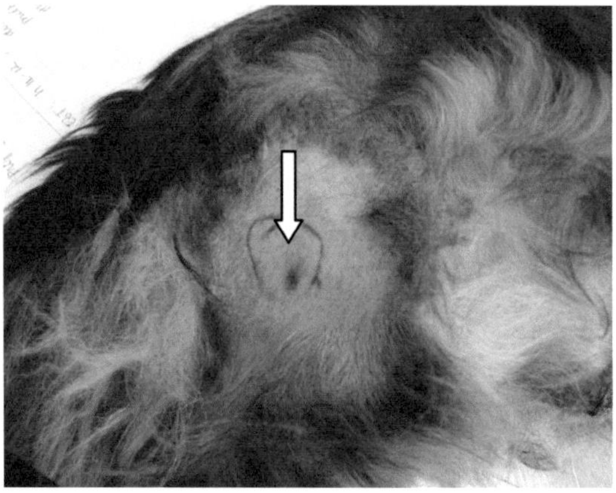

Fig. 7. The site of intramuscular EGT (arrow) in patient with mammary adenocarcinoma 2 days after the procedure without any signs of local side effects following invasive procedure

4. Discussion

Results of our study indicate that in canine cancer patients, intramuscular *IL-12* EGT is a safe procedure, which can result in systemic shedding of human IL-12 and possibly trigger IFN-γ response in treated patients, leading to prolonged disease free period and survival of treated animals.

In all of our patients, EGT was performed with a single intramuscular application of 1 mg of therapeutic plasmid encoding human IL-12, followed by delivery of one high voltage pulse and four low voltage pulses. Four out of six patients responded to the therapy with systemically detectable human IL-12 and/or IFN-γ concentrations. Systemic release of encoded transgene products in sufficient concentrations to elicit biological effect was already demonstrated after intramuscular EGT with different therapeutic genes in dogs (Brown et al., 2009; Draghia-Akli et al., 2002; Fewell et al., 2001; Pavlin et al., 2008; Tone et al., 2004). In preclinical studies, intramuscular *IL-12* EGT displayed systemic antitumor effect due to systemic release of IL-12 and IFN-γ in several tumor models (Hanna et al., 2001; Lee et al., 2003; Lucas et al., 2002, 2003; Tevz et al., 2009; Zhu & Li, 2008). Compared to these studies, we achieved relatively low systemic concentrations of IL-12, whereas the serum concentrations of IFN-γ were comparable to concentrations achieved in experimental animals (Lucas et al., 2002; Tevz et al., 2009).

It is possible that more pronounced response to the therapy with higher systemic cytokine concentrations in treated patients could be achieved with application of either higher plasmid dose or with more repetitions of EGT procedure. Even though Fewell and colleagues achieved systemic release of therapeutic concentration of human coagulation factor IX with a single intramuscular EGT of therapeutic plasmid, extremely high dose of therapeutic plasmid had to be delivered, even up to 3 mg of plasmid/kg of bodyweight (Fewell et al., 2001). Similarly, different experiments showed that in large animals the level of systemically secreted transgene product is dose and volume dependent with increased transgene expression correlating with increase in plasmid dose and volume until a certain saturating dose (Khan et al., 2003). On the other hand, in studies where therapeutic plasmid encoding GHRH was used, biological effects were achieved after single EGT with plasmid doses as low as 10 - 100 µg of plasmid per kg of bodyweight (Brown et al., 2009; Draghia-

Akli et al., 2002; Tone et al., 2004). As established in preclinical research, size and construction of plasmid plays an important role in effectiveness of electroporation-based delivery of DNA *in vivo* (Cemazar & Sersa, 2007). This fact could in part explain such striking differences in plasmid doses, which were needed in different studies on dogs to exert systemically detectable transgene product release. Therefore in the future, optimization of dose with dose escalation studies should be attempted for each therapeutic plasmid.

Another possible improvement of systemic transgene release could be in multiple consecutive repetitions of EGT procedure. Several previous studies on different animal tumor models demonstrated, that more than one either intratumoral or intramuscular application of plasmid encoding IL-12 is necessary to achieve adequate therapeutic response in treated animals, even without systemically detectable IL-12 concentrations (Heinzerling et al., 2001; L.C. Heller et al., 2006; Lucas & R. Heller, 2003; Tevz et al., 2009). For example in melanoma tumor model significantly better therapeutic response was achieved with increasing the number of intratumoral applications or with addition of intramuscular gene delivery (Lucas & R. Heller, 2003). Similarly, four consecutive intramuscular *IL-12* EGTs resulted in a significantly better systemic release of IL-12, compared to a single EGT procedure (Tevz et al., 2009).

Another possible explanation for nonresponders is that the timing of the samples collections was not optimal, since the samples were collected every 1 to 2 weeks in the first month and monthly thereafter. According to published literature, the time of the highest systemic release of IL-12 and IFN-γ achieved after intramuscular *IL-12* EGT is greatly variable. In different studies, the highest serum concentration of IL-12 was achieved between 4 and 17 days after EGT procedure, followed by the elevation of IFN-γ serum level with approximately 4-5 days delay (Lucas et al., 2002; Tevz et al., 2009). Kinetics of systemic IL-12 release varies even within the same species. In mice intramuscular EGT with the same plasmid dose results in significantly different systemic transgene release depending on strain of treated animals (Tevz et al., 2009). For example, in C57Bl/6 strain, serum concentration of IL-12 reached peak on day 6 (Tevz et al., 2009) or day 10 (Lucas et al., 2002) after EGT and abruptly declined to approximately half of peak concentration in the next few days. On the other hand, in A/J mice strain, serum concentration of IL-12 reached plateau by day 6, which lasted until approximately day 14, followed by a slow decline. Even more surprising is the fact, that in C57Bl/6 strain approximately three-times higher serum concentrations of IL-12 were achieved compared to A/J strain. The underlying mechanisms responsible for these discrepancies in transgene expression are not yet explained. Therefore even in a relatively homogenous group of experimental animals, determination of optimal serum collection timing is not as straightforward. Based on these findings, in such a heterogenic group as dogs, greatly varying in size and other physical attributes, a more thorough examination of cytokine release after intramuscular EGT should be attempted. Data on kinetics of transgene release in dogs after intramuscular *IL-12* EGT would be helpful for clinical application to determine the best time intervals for treatment repetitions in each individual patient in order to achieve the maximum therapeutic effect.

In our study, intramuscular EGT did not exert such pronounced local antitumor effect on treated tumors compared to direct intratumoral *IL-12* EGT (Chuang et al. 2009; Pavlin et al., 2011). In four of our patients, where tumors were not surgically removed and the size of intact tumors could be repeatedly measured, there was no regression in tumor size after performed EGT. In comparison, with intratumoral *IL-12* EGT volumes of treated canine mast cell tumors reduced significantly by over 50% (Pavlin et al., 2011) and even complete remissions were achieved in experimentally induced transmissible veneral tumors in dogs (Chuang et al., 2009). This discrepancy in antitumor effectiveness of intratumoral versus intramuscular *IL-12* EGT has already been shown in experimentally induced tumors in preclinical studies. Usually, intratumoral *IL-12* EGT results in better direct antitumor effect, demonstrated as growth delay and reduction of treated tumors' size, compared to intramuscular route of gene delivery (Lucas et al., 2002, 2003). On the other hand, intramuscular *IL-12* EGT exhibits pronounced antimetastatic effect with high systemic concentrations of IL-12 and stable induction of IFN-γ response (Hanna et al., 2001; Tevz et al., 2009). With intramuscular route of therapeutic gene delivery, relatively low proportion of complete regressions is achieved, typically around 15-40%, depending on model of treated tumor (Lee et al., 2003; Lucas et al., 2003; Tevz et al., 2009), whereas in some of the reported studies, complete response with intramuscular *IL-12* EGT was not achieved (Hanna et al., 2001). In comparison, intratumoral *IL-12* EGT generally results in approximately 60-80% complete response rate in treated tumors (L.C. Heller et al., 2006; Lucas et al., 2003), even reaching 100% curability (Pavlin et al., 2009). Based on results of preclinical work it can be concluded that the main advantage of intramuscular *IL-12* EGT lies in its systemic effects, namely antimetastatic activity and consequently prolongation of treated animals survival time (Lee et al., 2003; Lucas et al., 2002; Tevz et al., 2009; Zhu & Li, 2008).

Even though we treated a relatively small number of animals, their survival times after EGT were longer compared to survival times associated with specific tumor types from literature review. For example, the patient with PHS was euthanized over 8 months after EGT and a single application of CCNU due to progression of clinical signs, namely dispnoa and exercise intolerance. According to the literature, median survival time for dogs with PHS, treated with full CCNU chemotherapy (four consecutive applications every 3 weeks), is 96-106 days (Fulmer & Maudlin, 2007; Rassnick et al., 2010; Skropuski et al., 2007). In this patient, CCNU therapy was discontinued after one application due to pronounced hepatotoxicity, therefore probably exerting only negligible therapeutic effect. The patient with OSA survived 5.5 months, whereas reported median survival time for dog with OSA without any treatment is 1 - 3 months (Selvarajah et al., 2009). In three patients with higher grade MCTs, relatively long survival times were achieved. In canine MCT, survival strongly correlates with histological grade of the tumor and clinical stage of the disease (Patnaik et al., 1984), with very high recurrence rate after surgical therapy in more aggressive higher grade tumors (Fox, 2002; Thamm & Vail, 2007). The patient with grade III MCT in clinical stage III of the disease with recurrent growth of tumor tissue immediately after marginal resection of MCT and metastases in local lymph nodes survived for 6 months after EGT before being euthanized due to progression of the disease. Two weeks after EGT, consecutively two different systemic chemotherapies were started, each discontinued shortly after induction due to severe side-effects, therefore none of the chemotherapy protocol was administered long enough to reach any therapeutic potential. In comparison to these three patients, veterinary literature reports approximately 30% local recurrence of incompletely excised grade II MCT (Thamm & Vail, 2007) and only 7% partial response rate, without any complete responses, to full chemotherapy protocol utilizing vincristine (McCaw et al., 1997). For patients with grade III MCT, median survival time of 3 months after surgery without any additional therapy is reported (Thamm & Vail, 2007).

In preclinical studies intramuscular *IL-12* EGT conveyed in successful transgene expression and systemic release of significant concentrations of IL-12, therefore raising concerns regarding safety of this therapeutic approach, based on described toxicity of systemic application of recombinant IL-12. It has been established that systemic recombinant IL-12 therapy can exhibit serious adverse effects, including elevated body temperature, headaches, nausea and vomiting, nephro- and hepatotoxicity (Leonard et al., 1997) and application of high dose of rIL-12 was linked with temporary immunosuppression (neutropenia, lymphopenia, thrombocytopenia and anemia) (Motzer et al., 1998), which would not be favorable for effective immunotherapy. Therefore monitoring of renal and hepatic function in patients receiving any IL-12 based therapy is strongly recommended. These adverse effects are presumably due to toxicity of IFN-γ response induced by circulating IL-12 (Car et al., 1999; Leonard et al., 1997; Ryffel, 1996). Toxic side effects in human patients appeared when serum concentration of IFN-γ exceeded 6.0 ng/ml (Leonard et al., 1997), whereas experimental animals tolerated serum concentrations as high as 300 ng/ml without any severe adverse reactions (Leonard et al., 1997). A comprehensive study of intratumoral *IL-12* EGT toxicity has been conducted, with evaluation of changes in weight and blood biochemistry and haematology parameters, as well as histopatological examination of several different tissues of treated animals (L.C. Heller et al., 2006). Even though a pronounced antitumor effect was achieved on melanoma tumor model, no significant side effects of the procedure were observed (L.C. Heller et al., 2006). Although sporadically, significant abnormalities in bloodwork were detected, they were clinically irrelevant for the treated animals. The only histopathologic abnormality was late-onset inflammation associated with the kidney without any biochemical markers of decreased kidney function. Nevertheless, these findings did not reflect in any impairment of general health of treated animals. Nevertheless, in this study no systemically detectable concentrations of either IL-12 or IFN-γ were achieved. Therefore its conclusions can not directly demonstrate safety of intramuscular *IL-12* EGT as well, since intramuscular route of therapeutic gene administration can result in significant systemic concentrations of both IL-12 and IFN-γ. In preclinical studies, side-effects of the procedure were not so thoroughly investigated, however, available data show that intramuscular *IL-12* EGT, compared to intratumoral, can exhibit more pronounced, but still tolerable side effects, mainly transient significant reduction of bodyweight at the highest serum concentrations of IL-12 and IFN-γ (Tevz et al., 2009).

Clinical status of all animals enrolled in our study remained unaltered for the first 8 weeks after the EGT procedure. In the two patients with progressive disease (one patient with MCT and a patient with MAC), deterioration of general health was observed after 6 and 2 months, respectively, which reflected the increased tumor burden and was not a consequence of any toxic effects of the procedure. Hematology as well as biochemistry parameters of collected blood samples remained mostly within reference limits throughout the observation period. Few clinically significant alterations were observed in two patients receiving systemic chemotherapy. In the patient with PHS elevation of serum activities of enzymes ALT and SAP, which are biomarkers of liver function, was observed. However, this change occurred a week after induction of chemotherapy with CCNU, which exhibits known hepatotoxicity (Kristal et al., 2004). In the first two weeks after EGT, before the chemotherapy was started, no abnormalities in bloodwork were observed in this patient, despite detecting elevated serum levels of IFN-γ in blood samples collected 7 and 14 days after EGT. Furthermore, the increase in activities of both enzymes was only transient and their values normalized immediately after cessation of systemic chemotherapy. Similarly, transient haematological abnormalities were detected in the patient with MCT, receiving first immunosuppressive chemotherapy consisting of vincristine and methylprednisolone and later CCNU. Bloodwork alterations were related to toxicity of these chemotherapy protocols, since they were displayed only after induction of chemotherapy and not around the time, when elevated levels of IFN-γ in patient's serum was detected. Other patients with systemically detectable IFN-γ, even as high as 246.8 pg/ml, did not display any abnormalities in their bloodwork assays. Therefore we can conclude, that the observed hepatotoxicity and immunosuppression were due to pharmacological agents rather than a side effect of *IL-12* gene therapy.

5. Conclusion

In conclusion, the results of this study indicate, that intramuscular *IL-12* EGT in dogs with spontaneously occurring tumors, is a feasible, simple and safe procedure, which exerts systemic transgene release of IL-12 and induction of IFN-γ response in treated animals, making it promising treatment modality in veterinary medicine. In the future, refinement of treatment protocols in different canine tumors should be performed, with respect to investigating kinetics of cytokine release, defining optimal plasmid dose, number of treatment repetitions and effect of combination with other treatment protocols (e.g. local intratumoral plasmid delivery or electrochemotherapy) in order to achieve effective long-term antitumor effect in canine cancer patients.

6. Acknowledgement

The authors acknowledge the financial support of the state budget by Slovenian Research Agency (Projects No. P3-0003, P4-0053 and J3-2277). We would also like to thank dr. Tanja Plavec, dr. Tanja Svara and Estera Pogorevc for their help with cytology samples and radiographs of the patients.

7. References

Aihara, H. & Miyaziki, J. (1998). Gene transfer into muscle by electroporation in vivo, *Nat Biotechnol*, Vol.16, No.9, (September 1998), pp. 867-870

Arruda,V.R., Stedman, H.H., Haurigot, V., Buchlis, G., Baila, S., Favaro, P., Chen, Y., Franck, H.G., Zhou, S., Wright, J.F., Couto, L.B., Jiang, H., Pierce, G.F., Bellinger, D.A., Mingozzi, F., Nichols, T.C., High, K.A. (2010). Peripheral transvenular delivery of deno-associated viral vectors to skeletal muscle as a novel therapy for hemophilia B, *Blood*, Vol.115, No.23, (June 2010), pp. 4678-4688

Atkins, M.B., Robertson, M.J., Gordon, M., Lotze, M.T., DeCoste, M., DuBois, J.S., Ritz, J., Sandler, A.B., Edington, H.D., Garzone, P.D., Mier, J.W., Canning, C.M., Battiato, L., Tahara, H., Sherman, M.L. (1997). Phase I evaluation of intravenous recombinant human interleukin 12 in patients with advanced malignancies, *Clin Cancer Res.*, Vol.3, No.3, (March 1997), pp.409-417

Banks, G.B. & Chamberlain, J.S. (2008). The value of mammalian models for duchenne muscular dystrophy in developing therapeutic strategies, *Curr Top Dev Biol*, Vol.84, pp. 431-453

Bergman, P.J., McKnight, J., Novosad, A., Charney, S., Farrelly, J., Craft, D., Wulderk, M., Jeffers, Y., Sadelain, M., Hohenhaus, A.E., Segal, N., Gregor, P., Engelhorn, M., Riviere, I., Houghton, A.N., Wolchok, J.D. (2003). Long-term survival of dogs with advanced malignant melanoma after DNA vaccination with xenogeneic human tyrosinase: a phase I trial, *Clin Cancer Res*, Vol.9, No.4, (April 2003), pp.1284-1290

Bodles-Brakhop, A.M., Brown, P.A., Pope, M.A., Draghia-Akli, R. (2008). Double-blinded, Placebo-controlled plasmid GHRH trial for cancer-associated anemia in dogs, *Mol Ther*, Vol.16, No.5, (May 2008), pp.862-870

Brown, P.A., Bodles-Brakhop, A., Draghia-Akli, R. (2008). Plasmid growth hormone releasing hormone therapy in healthy and laminitis-afflicted horses-evaluation and pilot study, *J Gene Med*, Vol.10, No.5, (May 2008), pp.564-574

Brown, P.A., Bodles-Brakhop, A.M., Pope, M.A., Draghia-Akli, R. (2009). Gene therapy by electroporation for the treatment of chronic renal failure in companion animals, *BMC Biotechnol*, (January 2009), 9:4

Brunda, M.J., Luistro, L., Warrier, R.R. et al. (1993). Antitumor and antimetastatic activity of interleukin 12 against murine tumors, *J Exp Med*, Vol.178, No.4, (October 1993), pp.1223-1230

Budker, V., Budker, T., Zhang, G., Subbotin, V., Loomis, A., Wolff, J.A. (2000). Hypothesis: naked plasmid DNA is taken up by cells in vivo by a receptor-mediated process, *J Gene Med*, Vol.2, No.2, (March 2000), pp. 76-88

Buettner, M., Belke-Louis, G., Rziha, H.J., McInnes, C., Kaaden, O.R. (1998). Detection, cDNA cloning and sequencing of canine interleukin 12, *Cytokine*, Vol.10, No.4, (April 1998), pp.241-248

Car, B.D., Eng, V.M., Lipman, J.M., Anderson, T.D. (1999). The toxicology of interleukin-12: a review. *Toxicol Pathol*, Vol.27, No.1, (January 1999), pp.58-63.

Cemazar, M. & Sersa, G. (2007). Electrotransfer of therapeutic molecules into tissues. *Curr Opin Mol Ther*, Vol.9, No.6, (December 2007), pp.554–562

Cemazar, M., Tamzali, Y., Sersa, G., Tozon, N., Mir, L.M., Miklavcic, D., Lowe, R., Teissie, J. (2008). Electrochemotherapy in veterinary oncology, *J Vet Intern Med*, Vol.22, No.4, (July 2008), pp.826-831

Cemazar M, Jarm T, Sersa G. Cancer electrogene therapy with interleukin-12, *Curr Gene Ther*, Vol.10, No.4, pp.300-311

Cutrera, J., Torrero, M., Shiomitsu, K., Mauldin, N., Li, S. (2008). Intratumoral bleomycin and IL-12 electrochemogenetherapy for treating head and neck tumors in dogs, *Methods Mol Biol*, Vol.423, pp.319-325

Daud, A.I., DeConti, R.C., Andrews, S., Urbas, P., Riker, A.I., Sondak, V.K., Munster, P.N., Sullivan, D.M., Ugen, K.E., Messina, J.L., Heller, R. (2008). Phase I trial of interleukin-12 plasmid electroporation in patients with metastatic melanoma *J Clin Oncol*, Vol.26, No.36, (December 2008), pp.5896-5903

Dixon, J.A. & Spinale, F.G. (2009). Large animal models of heart failure: a critical link in he translation of basic science to clinical practice, *Circ Heart Fail*, Vol.2, No.3, (May 2009), pp. 262-271

Dow, S., Elmslie, R., Kurzman, I., MacEwen, G., Pericle, F., Liggitt, D. (2005). Phase I study of liposome-DNA complexes encoding the interleukin-2 gene in dogs with osteosarcoma lung metastases, *Hum Gene Ther*, Vol.16, No.8, (August 2005), pp.937-946

Draghia-Akli, R., Hahn, K.A., King, G.K., Cummings, K.K., Carpenter, R.H. (2002). Effects of plasmid-mediated growth hormone-releasing hormone in severely debilitated dogs with cancer, *Mol Ther*, Vol.6, No.6, (December 2002), pp.830-836

Fewell, J.G., MacLaughlin, F., Mehta, V., Gondo, M., Nicol, F., Wilson, E., Smith, L.C. (2001). Gene therapy for the treatment of hemophilia B using PINC-formulated plasmid delivered to muscle with electroporation, *Mol Ther*, Vol.3, No.4, (April 2001), pp.574-583

Fox, L.E. (2002). Mast Cell Tumors. In: *Cancer in dogs and cats: medical and surgical management, 2nd ed.*, Morrison, W.B., ed., pp.451-460, Teton NewMedia, Jackson Hole, ISBN: 1-893441-47-4

Fulmer, A.K. & Mauldin, G.E. (2007). Canine histiocytic neoplasia: An overview, *Can Vet J*, Vol.48, No.10, (October 2007), pp.1046-1050

Gehl, J., Sorensen, T.H., Nielsen, K., Raskmark, P., Nielsen, S.L., Skovsgaard, T., Mir, L.M. (1999). In vivo electroporation of skeletal muscle: threshold, efficacy and relation to electric field distribution, *Biochim Biophys Acta*, Vol.1428, No.2-3, (August 1999), pp.233-240

Gravier, R., Dory, D., Laurentie, M., Bougeard, S., Cariolet, R., Jestin, A. (2007). In vivo tissue distribution and kinetics of a pseudorabies virus plasmid DNA vaccine after intramuscular injection in swine, *Vaccine*, Vol.25, No.39-40, (September 2007), pp.6930-6938

Hanna, E., Zhang, X., Woodlis, J., Breau, R., Suen, J., Li, S. (2001). Intramuscular electroporation delivery of IL-12 gene for treatment of squamous cell carcinoma located at distant site, *Cancer Gene Ther*, Vol.8, No.3, (March 2001), pp.151-157

Hasbrouck, N.C. & High, K.A. (2008). AAV-mediated gene transfer for the treatment of hemophilia B: problems and prospects, *Gene Ther*, Vol.15, No.11, (June 2008), pp.870-875

Haurigot, V., Mingozzi, F., Buchlis, G., Hui, D.J., Chen, Y., Basner-Tschakarjan, E., Arruda, V.R., Radu, A., Franck, H.G., Wright, J.F., Zhou, S., Stedman, H.H., Bellinger, D.A., Nichols, T.C., High, K.A. (2010). Safety of AAV factor IX peripheral transvenular gene elivery to muscle in hemophilia B dogs, *Mol Ther*, Vol.18, No.7, (July 2010), pp.1318-1329

Heinzerling, L.M., Feige, K., Rieder, S., Akens, M.K., Dummer, R., Stranzinger, G., Moelling, K. (2001). Tumor regression induced by intratumoral injection of DNA coding for human interleukin 12 into melanoma metastases in gray horses, *J Mol Med*, Vol.78, No.12, pp.692-702

Heller, L.C., Merkler, K., Westover, J., Cruz, Y., Coppola, D., Benson, K., Daud, A., Heller, R. (2006). Evaluation of toxicity following electrically mediated interleukin-12 gene delivery in a B16 mouse melanoma model, *Clin Cancer Res*, Vol.12, No.10, (May 2006), pp.3177-3183

Heller, L.C. & Heller, R. (2010). Electroporation gene therapy preclinical and clinical trials for melanoma, *Curr Gene Ther*, Vol.10, No.4, (August 2010), pp.312-317

Herzog, R.W., Mount, J.D., Arruda, V.R., High, K.A., Lothrop, C.D. Jr. (2001). Muscle-directed gene transfer and transient immune suppression result in sustained partial correction of canine hemophilia B caused by a null mutation, *Mol Ther*, Vol. 4, No.3., (September 2001), pp.192-200

Howell, J.M., Walker, K.R., Davies, L., Dunton, E., Everaardt, A., Laing, N., Karpati, G. (2008). Adenovirus and adeno-associated virus-mediated delivery of human myophosphorylase cDNA and LacZ cDNA to muscle in the ovine model of

McArdle's disease: expression and re-expression of glycogen phosphorylase, *Neuromuscul Disord*, Vol.18, No.3, (March 2008), pp.248-258

Hüttinger, C., Hirschberger, J., Jahnke, A., Köstlin, R., Brill, T., Plank, C., Küchenhoff, H., Krieger, S., Schillinger, U. (2008). Neoadjuvant gene delivery of feline granulocyte-macrophage colony-stimulating factor using magnetofection for the treatment of feline fibrosarcomas: a phase I trial, *J Gene Med*, Vol.10, No.6, (June 2008), pp.655-667

Jahnke, A., Hirschberger, J., Fischer, C., Brill, T., Köstlin, R., Plank, C., Küchenhoff, H., Krieger, S., Kamenica, K., Schillinger, U. (2007). Intra-tumoral gene delivery of feIL-2, feIFN-gamma and feGM-CSF using magnetofection as a neoadjuvant treatment option for feline fibrosarcomas: a phase-I study, *J Vet Med A Physiol Pathol Clin Med*, Vol.54, No.10, (December 2007), pp.599-606

Kamensek, U. & Sersa, G. (2008). Targeted gene therapy in radiotherapy, *Radiol Oncol*, Vol.42, No.3, pp.115-135

Kamstock, D., Guth, A., Elmslie, R., Kurzman, I., Liggitt, D., Coro, L., Fairman, J., Dow, S. (2006). Liposome-DNA complexes infused intravenously inhibit tumor angiogenesis and elicit antitumor activity in dogs with soft tissue sarcoma, *Cancer Gene Ther*, Vol.13, No.3, (March 2006), pp.306-317

Katz, M.G., Swain, J.D., White, J.D., Low, D., Stedman, H., Bridges, C.R. (2010). Cardiac gene therapy: optimization of gene delivery techniques in vivo, *Hum Gene Ther*, Vol.21, No.4, (April 2010), pp.371-380

Khan, A.S., Smith, L.C., Abruzzese, R.V., Cummings, K.K., Pope, M.A., Brown, P.A., Draghia-Akli, R. (2003). Optimization of of electroporation parameters for the intramuscular delivery of plasmids in pigs. DNA Cell Biol, Vol.22, No.12, (December 2003), pp.807-814

Kobayashi, M., Fitz, L., Ryan, M., Hewick, R.M., Clark, S.C., Chan, S., Loudon, R., Sherman, F., Perussia, B., Trinchieri, G. (1989). Identification and purification of natural-killer cell stimulatory factor (NKSF), a cytokine with multiple biologic effects on human-lymphocytes, *J Exp Med*, Vol.170, No.3, (September 1989), pp.827-845

Kodre, V., Cemazar, M., Pecar, J., Sersa, G., Cor, A., Tozon, N. (2009). Electrochemotherapy compared to surgery for treatment of canine mast cell tumours, *In Vivo*, Vol.23, No.1, (January 2009), pp.55-62

Kornegay, J.N., Li, J., Bogan, J.R., Bogan, D.J., Chen, C., Zheng, H., Wang, B., Qiao, C., Howard, J.F. Jr., Xiao, X. (2010). Widespread muscle expression of an AAV9 human mini-dystrophin vector after intravenous injection in neonatal dystrophin-deficient dogs, *Mol Ther*, Vol.18, No.8, (August 2010), pp.1501-1508

Kristal, O., Rassnick, K.M., Gliatto, J.M., Northrup, N.C., Chretin, J.D., Morrison-Collister, K., Cotter, S.M., Moore, A.S. (2004). Hepatotoxicity associated with CCNU (lomustine) chemotherapy in dogs, *J Vet Intern Med*, Vol.18, No.1, (January 2004), pp.75-80

Lee, S.C., Wu, C.J., Wu, P.Y., Huang, Y.L., Wu, C.W., Tao, M.H. (2003). Inhibition of established subcutaneous and metastatic murine tumors by intramuscular electroporation of the interleukin-12 gene, *J Biomed Sci*, Vol.10, No.1, (January 2003), pp.73-86

Leonard, J.P., Sherman, M.L., Fisher, G.L., Buchanan, L.J., Larsen, G., Atkins, M.B., Sosman, J.A., Dutcher, J.P., Vogelzang, N.J., Ryan, J.L. (1997). Effects of single-dose interleukin-12 exposure on interleukin-12-associated toxicity and interferon-gamma production, *Blood*, Vol.90, No.7, (October 1997), pp.2541-2548

Li, S., Zhang, L., Torrero, M., Cannon, M., Barret, R. (2005). Administration route- and immune cell activation-dependant tumor eradication by IL-12 electrotransfer, *Mol Ther*, Vol.12, No.5, (November 2005), pp.942-949

Lu, Q., Bou-Gharion, G., Partridge, T.A. (2003). Non-viral gene delivery in skeletal muscle: a protein factory, *Gene Ther*, Vol.10, No.2, (January 2003), pp.131-142

Lucas, M.L., Heller, L., Coppola, D., Heller, R. (2002). IL-12 plasmid delivery by in vivo electroporation for the successful treatment of established subcutaneous B16.F10 melanoma, *Mol Ther*, Vol.5, No.6, (June 2002), pp.668-675

Lucas, M.L. & Heller, R. (2003). IL-12 gene therapy using an electrically mediated nonviral approach reduces metastatic growth of melanoma, *DNA and Cell Biol*, Vol.22, No.12, (December 2003), pp.755-763

McCaw, D.L., Miller, M.A., Bergman, P.J., Withrow, S.J., Moore, A.S., Knapp, D.W., Fowler, D., Johnson, J.C. (1997). Vincristine therapy for mast cell tumors in dogs, *J Vet Intern Med*, Vol.11, No.6, (November 1997), pp. 375-378

Mena, A., Andrew, M.E., Coupar, B.E. (2001). Rapid dissemination of intramuscularly inoculated DNA vaccines, *Immunol Cell Biol*, Vol.79, No.1, (February 2001), pp.87-89

Mir, L.M., Glass, L.F., Sersa, G., Teissié, J., Domenge, C., Miklavcic, D., Jaroszeski, M.J., Orlowski, S., Reintgen, D.S., Rudolf, Z., Belehradek, M., Gilbert, R., Rols, M.P., Belehradek, J. Jr., Bachaud, J.M., DeConti, R., Stabuc, B., Cemazar, M., Coninx, P., Heller, R. (1998). Effective treatment of cutaneous and subcutaneous malignant tumours by electrochemotherapy, *Br J Cancer*, Vol.77, No.12, (June 1998), pp.2336-2342

Mir, L.M., Bureau, M.F., Gehl, J., Rangara, R., Rouy, D., Caillaud, J.M., Delaere, P., Branellec, D., Schwartz, B., Scherman, D. (1999). High-efficiency gene transfer into skeletal muscle mediated by electric pulses, *Proc Natl Acad Sci U S A*, Vol.96, No.8, (April 1999), pp.4262-4267

Motzer, R.J., Rakhit, A., Schwartz, L.H., Olencki, T., Malone, T.M., Sandstrom, K., Nadeau, R., Parmar, H., Bukowski, R. (1998). Phase I trial of subcutaneous recombinant human interleukin-12 in patients with advanced renal cell carcinoma, *Clin Cancer Res*, Vol.4, No.5, (May 1998), pp.1183-1191

Nastala, C.L., Edington, H.D., McKinney, T.G., Tahara, H., Nalesnik, M.A., Brunda, M.J., Gately, M.K., Wolf, S.F., Schreiber, R.D., Storkus, W.J. (1994). Recombinant IL-12 administration induces tumor regression in association with IFN-gamma production, *J Immunol*, Vol.153, No.4, (August 1994), pp.1697-1706

Neumann, E., Schaefer-Ridder, M., Wang, Y., Hofschneider, P.H. (1982). Gene transfer into mouse lyoma cells by electroporation in high electric fields, *EMBO*, Vol.1, No.7, pp.841-845

Ohshima, S., Shin, J.H., Yuasa, K., Nishiyama, A., Kira, J., Okada, T., Takeda, S. (2009). Transduction efficiency and immune response associated with the administration of AAV8 vector into dog skeletal muscle, *Mol Ther*, Vol.17, No.1, (Jauary 2009), pp.73-80

Patnaik, A.K., Ehler, W.Y., MacEwen, E.G. (1984). Canine cutaneous mast cell tumors: morphological grading and survival in 83 dogs, *Vet Pathol*, Vol.21, No.5, (september 1984), pp.469-474

Pavlin, D., Tozon, N., Sersa, G., Pogacnik, A., Cemazar, M. (2008). Efficient electrotransfection into canine muscle, *Technol Cancer Res Treat*, Vol.7, No.1, (February 2008), pp. 45-54

Pavlin, D., Cemazar, M., Kamensek, U., Tozon, N., Pogacnik, A., Sersa, G. (2009). Local and systemic antitumor effect of intratumoral and peritumoral IL-12 electrogene therapy on murine sarcoma, *Cancer Biol Ther*, Vol.8, No.22, (November 2009), pp.2114-2122

Pavlin, D., Cemazar, M., Cor, A., Sersa, G., Pogacnik, A., Tozon, N. (2011). Electrogene therapy with interleukin-12 in canine mast cell tumors, *Radiol Oncol*, Vol.45, No.1, (March 2011), pp.31-39

Phillips, B.S., Padilla, M.L., Dickerson, E.B., Lindstrom, M.J., Helfand, S.C. (1999). Immunostimulatory effects of human recombinant interleukin-12 on peripheral blood mononuclear cells from normal dogs, *Vet Immunol Immunopathol*, Vol.70, No.3-4, (September 1999), pp.189-201

Ross, C.J., Twisk, J., Bakker, A.C., Miao, F., Verbart, D., Rip, J., Godbey, T., Dijkhuizen, P., Hermens, W.T., Kastelein, J.J., Kuivenhoven, J.A., Meulenberg, J.M., Hayden, M.R. (2006). Correction of feline lipoprotein lipase deficiency with adeno-associated virus serotype 1-mediated gene transfer of the lipoprotein lipase S447X beneficial mutation, *Hum Gene Ther*, Vol.17, No.5, (May 2006), pp.487-499

Rassnick KM, Moore AS, Russell DS, Northrup NC, Kristal O, Bailey DB, Flory AB, Kiselow MA, Intile JL. Phase II, open-label trial of single-agent CCNU in dogs with previously untreated histiocytic sarcoma, *J Vet Intern Med*, Vol.24, No.6, (November 2010), pp.1528-1531

Ryffel, B. (1996). Unanticipated human toxicology of recombinant proteins, *Arch Toxicol Suppl*, Vol.18, pp.333-341

Selvarajah, G.T., Kirpensteijn, J., van Wolferen, M.E., Rao, N.A., Fieten, H., Mol, J.A. (2009). Gene expression profiling of canine osteosarcoma reveals genes associated with short and long survival times, *Molecular Cancer*, No. 8, (September 2009), pp.72

Sersa, G., Stabuc, B., Cemazar, M., Miklavcic, D., Rudolf, Z. (2000). Electrochemotherapy with cisplatin: clinical experience in malignant melanoma patients, *Clin Canc Res*, Vol.6, No.3, (March 2000), pp.863-867

Siddiqui, F., Li, C.Y., Larue, S.M., Poulson, J.M., Avery, P.R., Pruitt, A.F., Zhang, X., Ullrich, R.L., Thrall, D.E., Dewhirst, M.W., Hauck, M.L. (2007). A phase I trial of hyperthermia-induced interleukin-12 gene therapy in spontaneously arising feline soft tissue sarcomas, *Mol Cancer Ther*, Vol.6, No.1, (January 2007), pp.380-389

Skorupski, K.A., Clifford, C.C., Paoloni, M.C, Lara-Garcia, A., Barber, L., Kent, M.S., LeBlanc, A.K., Sabhlok, A., Mauldin, E.A., Shofer, F.S., Couto, C.G., Sørenmo, K.U. (2007). CCNU for the treatment of dogs with histiocytic sarcoma, *J Vet Intern Med*, Vol21, No.1, (January 2007), pp. 121–126

Sleeper, M.M., Bish, L.T., Sweeney, H.L. (2010). Status of therapeutic gene transfer to treat canine dilated cardiomyopathy in dogs, *Vet Clin North Am Small Anim Pract*, Vol.40, No.4, (July 2010), pp.717-724

Tevz, G., Kranjc, S., Cemazar, M., Kamensek, U., Coer, A., Krzan, M., Vidic, S., Pavlin, D., Sersa, G. (2009). Controlled systemic release of interleukin-12 after gene electrotransfer to muscle for cancer gene therapy alone or in combination with ionizing radiation in murine sarcomas, *J Gene Med*, Vol.11, No.12, (December 2009), pp.1125-1137

Thamm, D.H. & Vail, D.M. (2007). Mast Cell Tumors, In: *Withrow and MacEwen's small animal clinical oncology*, Withrow, S.J. & Wail, D.M., eds., pp.402-416, Saunders, St. Louis, ISBN: 9780-7216-0558-6

Tollefsen, S., Vordermeier, M., Olsen, I., Storset, A.K., Reitan, L.J., Clifford, D., Lowrie, D.B., Wiker, H.G., Huygen, K., Hewinson, G., Mathiesen, I., Tjelle, T.E. (2003). DNA injection in combination with electroporation: a novel method for vaccination of farmed ruminants, *Scand J Immunol*, Vol.57, No.3, (March 2003), pp.229-238

Tone, C.M., Cardoza, D.M., Carpenter, R.H., Draghia-Akli, R. (2004). Long-term effects of plasmid-mediated growth hormone releasing hormone in dogs, *Cancer Gene Ther*, Vol.11, No.5, (May 2004), pp.389-396

Tozon, N., Sersa, G., Cemazar, M. (2001). Electrochemotherapy: potentiation of local antitumour effectiveness of cisplatin in dogs and cats, *Anticancer Res*, Vol.21, No.4A, (July 2001), pp.2483-2488

Tozon, N., Kodre, V., Sersa, G., Cemazar, M. (2005). Effective treatment of perianal tumors in dogs with electrochemotherapy, *Anticancer Res*, Vol.25, No.2A, (March 2005), pp.839-845

Trinchieri, G., Wysocka, M., D'Andrea, A., Rengaraju, M., Aste-Amezaga, M., Kubin, M., Valiante, N.M., Chehimi, J. (1992). Natural killer cell stimulatory factor (NKSF) or interleukin-12 is a key regulator of immune response and inflammation, *Prog Growth Factor Res*, Vol.4, No.4, pp.355-368

Trinchieri G. Interleukin-12 and the regulation of innate resistance and adaptive immunity, *Nat Rev Immunol*, Vol.3, No.2, (February 2003), pp.133-146

Voest, E.E., Kenyon, B.M., O'Reilly, M.S., Truitt, G., D'Amato, R.J., Folkman, J. (1995). Inhibition of angiogenesis in vivo by interleukin 12, *J Natl Cancer Inst*, Vol.87, No.8, (April 1995), pp. 581-586

Walker, M.C., Mandell, T.C., Crawford, P.C., Simon, G.G., Cahill, K.S., Fernandes, P.J., MacLeod, J.N., Byrne, B.J., Levy, J.K. (2005). Expression of erythropoietin in cats treated with a recombinant adeno-associated viral vector, *Am J Vet Res*, Vol.66, No.3, (March 2005), pp.450-456

Wang, L. & Herzog, R.W. (2005). AAV-mediated gene transfer for treatment of hemophilia, *Curr Gene Ther*, Vol.5, No.3, (June 2005), pp.349-360

Wang, Z., Kuhr, C.S., Allen, J.M., Blankinship, M., Gregorevic, P., Chamberlain, J.S., Tapscott, S.J., Storb, R. (2007). Sustained AAV-mediated dystrophin expression in a canine model of Duchenne muscular dystrophy with a brief course of immunosuppression, *Mol Ther*, Vol.15, No.6, (June 2007), pp.1160-1166

Wang, Z., Chamberlain, J.S., Tapscott, S.J., Storb, R. (2009). Gene therapy in large animal models of muscular dystrophy, *ILAR J*, Vol.50, No.2, pp.187-198

Wolff, J.A., Malone, R.W., Williams, P., Chong, W., Acsadi, G., Jani, A., Felgner, P.L. (1990). Direct gene transfer into mouse muscle in vivo, *Science*, Vol.247, (March 1990), pp.1465-1468

Zhu, S. & Li, S. (2008). Systemic IL-12 gene therapy for treating malignancy via intramuscular electroporation, *Methods Mol Biol*, No.423, pp.327-337

Part 3

Gene Therapy of Other Diseases

17

Gene Therapy Targets and the Role of Pharmacogenomics in Heart Failure

Dimosthenis Lykouras[1], Christodoulos Flordellis[2] and Dimitrios Dougenis[1]
[1]Department of Cardiothoracic Surgery, University Hospital of Patras
[2]Department of Pharmacology, School of Medicine, University of Patras
Greece

1. Introduction

Heart failure is supposed to be one of the most important causes of morbidity and mortality in the developed countries (McMurray JJ, 2000) (Cowie MR, 2000). It is not a disease by itself but it is a consequent condition of a number of co-existing factors including arterial hypertension, coronary artery heart disease and myocardiopathies. The quality of life of the patient is affected in heart failure more than in other diseases (Stewart AL, 1989) and the cost for the care providing system is estimated to be 22 billion $ each year in the United States (American Heart Association, 2000). Thus, investigating into heart failure causal factors and into management possibilities is of high importance in order to provide the essential help to the patients. It should be marked that the most important causal factor of heart failure is ischemic heart disease, thus we are dealing with heart failure developed after an ischemic episode if not mentioned else.

The currently used drugs can manage effectively the main symptoms of heart failure and may control the symptoms of this condition. Nevertheless, judging by the numbers of morbidity and especially mortality, which remain high, we can assume that new research fields have to be developed in order to provide new effective therapies for heart failure.

The progress in the technology and in biologic science allows the development of new optimized and individualized drugs with the aid of pharmacogenomics. Moreover, novel effective therapies emerge from the use of gene therapy and stem cell transplantation in the therapeutic strategies against heart failure after an ischemic episode.

2. Currently available therapy for heart failure

The main strategy for the currently available therapies used in the management of heart failure is to: a) reduce the preload, b) reduce the after load and c) improve the myocardial contraction.

Depending on the New York Heart Association (NYHA) classification for heart failure there are four categories based upon the patient's quality of life due to the symptoms. In NYHA Stage I the patient faces no symptoms when performing normal everyday work. In NYHA Stage II the patient has mild symptoms in everyday life, which are relieved at rest. In NYHA Stage III the patient has moderate symptoms that may affect the physical activity, which are only relieved at rest. Finally, in NYHA Stage IV the patients faces severe symptoms which are present even at rest. Table 1 and Fig.1 demonstrate the main pharmaceutical categories used taking into consideration the NYHA Stage.

NYHA Stage	**Stage I**	**Stage II**	**Stage III**	**Stage IV**
Symptoms	**None**	**Mild**	**Moderate**	**Severe**
ACE inhibitors	**Yes**	**Yes**	**Yes**	**Yes**
AT1R blockers	Alternatively to ACE inhibitors, when adverse reactions present (cough)			
beta-blockers	After ACS, hypertension	Yes	Yes	Yes
Diuretics	Hypertension, edema	Yes	Yes	Yes
Aldosterone antagonists	Not needed	In hypokalemia	Yes	Yes
Digoxin	In atrial fibrosis	In atrial fibrosis	Yes	Yes

Table 1. Main pharmaceutical categories used depending on NYHA Stage. (NYHA: New York Heart Association, ACE: Angiotensin Converting Enzyme, ACS: Acute Coronary Syndrome)

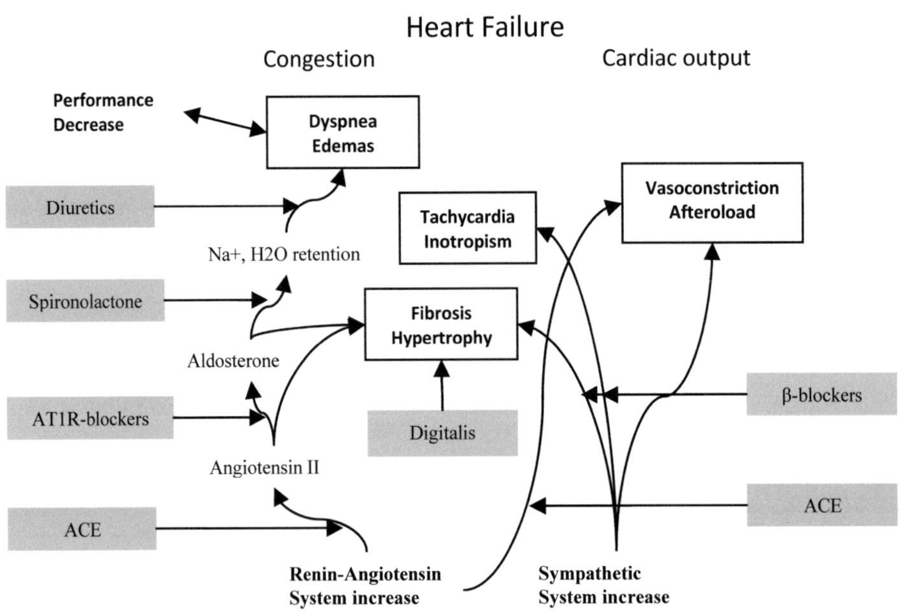

Fig. 1. Drugs used in the management of heart failure and their mechanism of action.

The great and increasing number of patients suffering from heart failure after ischemic episodes worldwide provide with the need to improve and individualize existing therapies and to develop novel treatments based on the promising tools of the biology and computer science.

3. Pharmacogenomics in heart failure

3.1 Introduction to pharmacogenomics

In distinction to rare mutations that cause a disease, genetic polymorphisms, which are frequently occurring mutations, do not cause disease. Instead, they may affect the disease onset and outcome, the clinical cause of a disease or even response to a drug treatment. Genetic polymorphisms act either through alteration of the biochemic phenotype of the gene products as a mask for other directly involved polymorphisms (linkage disequilibrium).
The extensive use of drugs in various populations has shown that the efficacy and toxicity amongst the users may differ a lot. In the USA it is estimated that 100.000 of patients die and 2.200.000 suffer from adverse reactions attributed to drugs. The incidence in patients in a hospital environment is up to 6-7% and the adverse reaction to drugs is 4th amongst death causes (Lazarou J, 1998).
The adverse reactions and the pharmaceutical targets are the main investigational fields with the aid of genetic analysis and computer science. In many cases the efficacy of a drug can be attributed to gene polymorphisms that encode enzymes that metabolize the drug itself, drug carriers or its targets. The study of genetic diversity the adverse reaction could be predicted and the safety and efficacy of the drug could be improved. The most effective therapy could be prescribed based on the special genetic alterations that the patient carries (March R, 2001) (Veenstra D, 2000). In the future, each patient could have an "individualized drug" that would be suitable to the genetic profile.

3.2 Discovery of new targets

The discovery of genomic regions of interest requires the DNA of the cell, which contains all the essential genetic information. Therefore, we can use the following techniques:
1. Development of a cDNA library that derives from the mRNA of the studied cellular type. This library contains only the expressed gene of the specific tissue.
2. Extraction of the whole DNA from the chromosomes of the studied cells. In this case the derivative DNA contains both introns and exons. Thus, computational tools and biologic techniques, such as "western blot" are required in order to define the areas of interest.

3.2.1 DGE profiling (Differential Gene Expression)

DGE is a technique which is used to measure the difference of the mRNA that is the product of a specific gene or a number of gene between two tissues. Therefore, we can find the specific genes expressed in a pathologic tissue, for example an ischemic tissue, and connect the gene to the phenotype. Thus, we can define genes responsible for the pathogenesis of a certain condition. The most important types of DGE is GeneCalling (Shimkets RA, 1999) and SAGE (de Waard V, 1999). GeneCalling has been used in a number of studies in murine models involving the Atrial Natriuretic Peptide and the TGF-β (Shimkets RA, 1999) (Geng YJ, 1999). The SAGE method has been used in the identification of genes participating in atherogenesis in the myocardial tissue (de Waard V, 1999).

3.2.2 Database of expressed genes

The database of expressed genes contains information from cDNA sequences that derive from total mRNA of the studied tissue. Therefore, if we know a specific gene that is expressed, then we are aware of the proteins that are produced. Special softwares are used in the analyses such as PHRED and PHRAP (Ewing B, 1998). In the case of heart failure genes that are involved in the coagulation and the formation of the vasculature in the endothelium have already been scanned.

3.2.3 ExPg (Expression Pharmacogenomics)

The ExPg is a tool that can be used to improve the safety and efficacy of the drugs. The most time consuming part of a drug development is the toxicity and efficacy tests. The ExPg could reduce time in the pharmaceutic development and also predict the possible adverse reaction of a novel drug (Gould Rothberg BE, 2001). Moreover, the ExPg could be used for the evaluation of known metabolic and signaling pathways of the cell.

3.2.4 SNPs (Single Nucleotide Polymorphisms)

The SNPs are changes of a single base that may cause alterations in the protein product and having an impact on the functionality of the protein. Genetic polymorphisms may be the reason why patients may have a different response to a certain drug therapy, because a polymorphism may affect the metabolism of the drug or its receptors. Therefore, a better knowledge of possible polymorphisms may give a better prediction of the efficacy of a therapy. A map including the main polymorphisms involved in heart failure, atheromatosis, thrombosis and dyslipidemia could be produced.

4. Gene therapy in heart failure

The biologic progress has provided us with new knowledge regarding the mechanisms involved in the restoration of the heart after an ischemic episode. The novel view of the disease allows the use of gene therapy in order to a) facilitate revascularization in the ischemic myocardium, b) protect from free radicals and oxidative stress and c) improve myocardial contraction.

4.1 Introduction to gene therapy

The techniques used in gene therapy involve the introduction of a normal allele of a gene either because the cell does not express the gene or because the gene is under-expressed in that kind of cell. Before performing gene therapy a lot of work is needed to prepare the induction of the new gene. More specifically the following steps are followed:

1. Isolation of the target gene
2. Development of a specific gene vector
3. Specification of the target cells
4. Definition of route of administration
5. Identification of other potential uses of the gene

One might wonder what the importance of gene therapy is and why it is not effective to produce the protein that is missing and administer it to the patient afterwards. This would be available in large scale production schemes by the means of genetically altered bacteria. Nevertheless, the infusion of the protein is not curative, because of the half-life of the growth factors and the factors helping in angiogenesis that are used in the case of heart failure.

4.1.1 Isolation of the target gene

The isolation of a gene can be achieved after the production of a cDNA library that contains the total unique genes expressed in a specific tissue. The DNA contained in a cDNA library is not genomic, therefore it contains only the encoding sequences of the DNA.

The procedure of the construction of a cDNA library consists of the following steps:
1. Isolation of the total amount of mRNA that is produced in the target cells,
2. Hybridization using a multi-T promoter,
3. Synthesis of complementary DNA (cDNA) to the mRNA prototype using the enzyme reverse transcriptase,
4. Degradation of the mRNA by the means of an alkali,
5. Synthesis of the second DNA strand using nucleotides and the enzyme DNA polymerase.

The cDNA library contains only the exons of the genes that are expressed in the specific tissue; therefore the cDNA can show the activity of the studied tissue.

4.1.2 Development of a specific gene vector

As soon as the isolation of the gene that is to be administered to the patient is achieved, an appropriate vector is needed in order to deliver the gene to the target cells. The methods of genetic engineering are utilized and the gene is induced into a special agent (usually a virus or a chemical substance) that is used to perform transfection of the targeted cellular population. Therefore, the genome of the virus is inserted in the genome of the cell together with the gene that was previously inserted in the viral genome.
A number of chemical agents as well as viruses are used to deliver genes to target cells and these are presented in the following table (Table 2).

	Advantages	Disadvantages
Plasmids	Well-tolerated Safe (Kastrupa J, 2001)	Transfer towards the nucleus is not so easy (Laham RJ, 2001)
Adeno-virus	It may transfect differentiating as well as stale cells Very good percentage of transfection	It is not inserted in the nucleus Possibility of reaction against the adeno-virus (Lehrman S, 1999)
Retro-virus	Inserted in the genome Stable during transport	It can only used in transfection of multiplying cells (Flugelman MY, 1992)
Lenti-virus	Subtype of retro-virus that may be inserted in stable cells This type of virus is quite stable during the procedure (Sakoda T, 1999)	
AAV (adeno-associated-based vector)	Inserted in the genome This vector is quite stable during the procedure Stable cells can be transfected as well	Only 4,7 kb can be inserted Possibility of mutations (Shimpo M, 2002)
Liposomes - Oligonucleotides (ODN-based)	Very easy to use Selective for the endothelium Special alterations can improve the availability and reduce toxicity (Felgner PL, 1995)	

Table 2. Chemical compounds and virus used in gene therapy.

4.1.3 Specification of the target cells

The target cell has to be defined carefully in order to achieve the best curative result. In the case of heart failure, the smooth muscle cells of the heart are targeted, because in most cases of heart failure ischemia has already occurred. Soon after ischemia is induced, a number of genes alter their expression as a result of changes that take place. Therefore, it is important to targeting proteins as these described in the following table (Table 3) in the specified cells of the myocardium.

Gene	Function
Heat shock proteins	Protection of cellular integrity, metabolism and homeostasis after serious injury
Growth factors: Brain-Derived Neurotrophiv factor Vascular Endothelial Growth Factor	Protection and regeneration of neural and vascular networks
Modulators of apoptosis: Plasminogen activator inhibitor 1	Anti-apoptotic factor
Transcription factors: Liver regenerating factor - Atf3	Regulation of augmentation, anti-apoptotic factor
Cell survival promoters: B-cell translocation gene-2 Growth arrest and DNA-damage inducible gene 45a)	Promote cellular survival, neural protection, DNA protection

Table 3. Genes altering their expression in case of ischemia of the myocardium.

4.1.4 Definition of route of administration

The route of administration has to be defined so as the target gene is transported to the target cells in order to perform the transfection of the target tissue cells. In the case of heart failure after ischemia, the gene can be transported to: a) the epicardium (injection), b) the endocardium (catheter), c) the coronary arteries (catheter), d) pericardium (injection).

4.1.5 Identification of other potential uses of the gene

The use of a target gene in the therapy of a certain condition such as heart failure does not exclude a possible use of the gene in another therapeutic strategy, where there is a similar pathophysiology or malfunction of the studied gene or group of genes. Therefore, the identification of other potential uses of the target gene is always important.

4.2 Targets of gene therapy in heart failure

The most important cause that leads to heart failure is the ischemia of the myocardium, thus the post-ischemic myocardium is going to be discussed more extensively. The heart muscle fails to keep up to the body needs, because of the ischemia, therefore heart failure symptoms present.

Soon after the crucial period of the ischemia onset in the myocardial tissue, a large number of genes alter their expression, as a result to the new environment that lacks oxygen. Consequently, only 20 minutes after the induction of ischemia an up-regulation of the expression of Heat Shock Protein (HSP) genes is reported, especially HSP 27, 40, 70, 86 and 105 kDa. These proteins mainly help the ischemic tissue to maintain its integrity and homeostasis (Currie RW, 1987).

Furthermore, an increase in the expression of growth factors is measured, especially of the Vascular Endothelial Growth Factor (VEGF), the Brain-Derived Growth Factor (BDNF), which play an important role in the continuation of the stability of the myocardial and neural infrastructure of the myocardium (Das DK, 1995).
The Activating Transcription Factor (Atf-3), that is also known as a factor protecting the liver, plays a major role in the activation and the regulation of the growth by controlling the expression of genes involved in late response (such as the genes that control the synthesis of the DNA) (Nobori K, 2002). Moreover, the Atf-3 can stop the procedure of apoptosis that may have been initiated as a response to ischemia (Kwaan HC, 2000).
Finally, other genes that promote cellular survival are the Btg2 (B-cell translocation gene 2) and the Gadd45a (Growth arrest and DNA damage-inducible gene 45 alpha), which can also promote the stability of the genome and its resistance in stress conditions (Hollander MC, 1999).

4.2.1 Angiogenesis and revascularization in the myocardium

VEGF (Vascular Endothelial Growth factor)

The VEGF is an angiogenetic glucoprotein that binds to the heparin and plays a major role in the development of new vasculature in the ischemic myocardium (Symes JF, 2001). A large number of studies have investigated into the procedure of revascularization and the regeneration of the vascular infrastructure of the myocardium that takes place soon after the onset of the ischemia, and it is known that the VEGF is facilitated by a transcriptional factor that is promoted by hypoxia (hypoxia-inducible factor-1). Six different structural genes of the VEGF have already been found, but their efficacy in angiogenesis is comparable. The VEGF gene was the first gene to be used in experiments of gene therapy for heart failure.
Clinical trials has shown so far that the transport of the gene in the target cell is possible by the means of plasmid DNA through an direct injection in the ischemic myocardium (Losordo DW, 1998) (or with the aid of mini-thoracotomy) (Fortuin Jr FD, 2003). In other studies an adeno-virus was used in order to achieve tranfection of the target cellular population after the injection of the gene-adeno-viral agent (Rosengart TK, 1999).
All the studies performed in order to evaluate the use of VEGF gene in gene therapy have demonstrated an increase in the level of VEGF in the myocardium without substantial side-effects that were initially supposed to emerge (such as hemangiomas or reticulopathy) (Symes JF, 1999) (Vale PR, 2000). Moreover, the effect of the therapy on the symptoms of heart failure was remarkable as angina was significantly reduced and the nitrate-free periods were longer (Vale PR, 2001).

FGF (Fibroblast Growth Factor)

Apart from the VEGF, the activation of angiogenesis can also be initiated by the Fibroblast Growth Factor. Clinical trials so far demonstrate that the administration of FGF-2 gene into the coronary artery vasculature can be well tolerated except for episodic hypotension that may be present for 1 up to 3 days (Fortuin Jr FD, 2003) (Simons M, 2002). In the patients that received the Fibroblast Growth Factor gene, 6 months after the therapy, their score in stress test was improved, the angina symptoms were significantly reduced, the ischemic part of the heart was smaller and the wall of the myocardium was thickened (Unger EF, 2000).
The transport of the FGF gene can be achieved using an adeno-virus. The administration can be done through intra-coronary artery injection (Grines CL, 2002) (Grines CL, 2003). The

effect of the therapy on heart failure was remarkable as angina was significantly reduced and the nitrate-free periods were longer than before gene therapy.

4.2.2 Protection from reperfusion injury

The revascularization after the episode of ischemia is crucial for the myocardium. However, the formation of new vasculature towards the right direction is very important, otherwise further ischemia may develop either because of oxidative stress products or because of clot formation. Possible genes which are involved in the reduction of free radicals and lower the oxidative stress impact have already been discovered and investigated. The Superoxide Dismutase gene (SOD) and the Heme Oxygenase-1 gene (HO-1) have been used in trials involving animal models. Nevertheless, there are no clinical trials in humans showing the possibility of using these target genes for avoiding reperfusion gene in post-ischemic myocardium.

SOD (Superoxide Dismutase)

It is known that the administration of the superoxide dismutase gene in rabbits soon after ischemia of the myocardium can reduce the development of stunning myocardium (Li Q, 1998). The target gene of SOD, which was acquired from a cDNA library, was inserted in the genome of an adenovirus (Ad5/CMV/Ec-SOD) and was injected through a catheter. This special vector was selected, because of its selectivity to extracellular binding positions of the liver (Karlsson K, 1998), where the gene can be securely "stored" in order to act only when it is needed, without causing inflammation to the myocardium. As a result the revascularization of the myocardial tissue was improved, without any loss in the functionality of the tissue.

HO-1 (Heme Oxygenase 1)

The Heme Oxygenase gene 1 (HO-1) has been investigated as a potential target for gene therapy in experimental murine models, where reperfusion injury was present due to revascularization after an ischemic episode (Melo LG, 2002). A human gene was inserted in an adeno-viral vector and then was injected on the epicardium on the wall of the left ventricle (Platt JL, 1998). The transportation of the gene resulted in the reduction by 75% of the ischemic myocardium and in a reduction of pro-inflammatory and pro-apoptotic factors. When planning gene therapy in order to eliminate the oxidative stress it is essential to take into consideration the fact that in patients with an ischemic episode there is an increased probability of recurrent episodes of ischemia of the myocardium. Therefore, the gene that is to be used should be highly expressed in ischemic periods in order to be more effective. The HO-1 gene therapy does not seem to have lasting effect on the myocardial tissue, while the administration together with the SOD gene may lead to adverse reactions (mitochondrial function disruption, CO overproduction) (Tang YL, 2004).

A special type of vectors called "vigilant vectors" was developed so as to be activated only in an ischemic environment (Phillips MI, 2002). The trials were performed in a murine model, where a vigilant plasmid containing the HO-1 gene was administrated after an acute ischemic episode. This experiment demonstrated less fibrotic regions in the newly developed vasculature, an increased expression of the HO-1 gene and improved myocardial contraction (Tang YL, 2004).

Parstatin: a cryptic peptide involved in cardioprotection

Thrombin activates protease-activated receptor 1 by proteolytic cleavage of the N-terminus. Although much research has focused on the activated receptor, little is known about the 41-

amino acid N-terminal peptide (parstatin). It has been shown that parstatin would protect the heart against ischaemia-reperfusion injury (Routhu KV, 2010).

A single treatment of parstatin administered prior to ischaemia may cause immediate cardioprotection by recruiting the Gi-protein activation pathway including p38 MAPK, ERK1/2, NOS, and K(ATP) channels. Parstatin acts on both the cardiomyocytes and the coronary circulation to induce cardioprotection. This suggests a potential therapeutic role of parstatin in the treatment of cardiac injury resulting from ischaemia and reperfusion (Strande JL, 2009).

4.2.3 Improvement of myocardial contraction

The role of Ca++ and phospholamban

The intracellular bank of Ca++ in the ischemic myocardium that fails to keep up with the heart needs has been another target in gene therapy studies and experiments. It is known that the activity of the SERCA2a channel (Sarcoplasmic Reticulum Ca++ adenosine trophosphatase 2a channel) is reduced, resulting in decreased myocardial contraction. In murine models the gene of SERCA2a channel was inserted in an adeno-viral vector (Ad.SERCA2a) and was administered through an injection on the aorta, leading to improved myocardial contraction (Miyamoto MI, 2000) (del Monte F, 2001).

The signaling with the Ca++ levels in myocardial cells also depends on the activity of an calcium-binding protein (called S100A1) that shares a positive inotrope action and is found to be at low levels in the ischemic tissue (Remppis A, 1996) (Most P, 2004). However, trials have shown that the administration of the respective gene can improve the myocardial contraction, may increase the levels of Ca++ and facilitate the activity of the SERCA2a channel. Thus, the use of this gene may be effective.

The antagonism of the activity of phospholamban by the means of gene techniques has been investigated as well. Phospholamban has an action against SERCA2a channel; therefore its blockade can be beneficial for the myocardial tissue. A number of trials both in murine models and in humans have been accomplished (Ziolo MT, 2005) (del Monte F, 2002). An adenoviral vector was used in the trials. The results demonstrated improved contraction as the levels of phospholamban decreased 48 h after the administration of the vector.

The β-ARs (β-adrenergic receptors)

The most important actions of the beta-adrenergic receptor are the regulation of the cardiac rhythm and the myocardial contraction as a response to catecholamines. The myocardial β-ARs are equally distributed in the atria and the ventricles (Ahlquist RP, 1948) (Brodde OE, 1993). There are subtypes β1, β2, β3 and the ratio is β1AR:β2AR=4:1.

The β-ARs belong to the family of the G protein-coupled receptors (GPCRs), also known as seven-transmembrane domain receptors 7TM. Once a catecholamine is recognized, the receptor shifts conformation and, thus, mechanically activates the G protein, which detaches from the receptor. The receptor can now either activate another G protein or switch back to its inactive state. The resulting G_{α} and $G_{\beta\gamma}$ subunits become active. The G_{α} activates adenyl cyclase towards the formation of cAMP, that controls the ion channels and has a positive action on myocardial contraction (Dohlman HG, 1991) (Hartzell HC, 1988).

The receptor is not active eternally as it is de-activated by the means of GPCR kinase (GRK), which are serine/threonine kinases. These are very selective molecules that bind and phosphorylate only previously activated receptors. The myocardial sup-types are GRK1 and

GRK2 also named as βARK1 and βARK2 respectively (Hausdorff WP, 1990) (Benovic JL, 1989).
It is known that in heart failure the density and the sensitivity of the β-adrenergic receptors are reduced. Moreover, the levels of the βARK1 are increased which suggests a crucial role of the βARK1 in the de-activation of the β-receptor.
When the myocardial failure commences, the β-adrenergic agonists (epinephrine or nor-epinephrine) can be effectively used as they can increase the preload. Nevertheless, in the chronic condition of heart failure the myocardial load cannot benefit from the use of β-agonists due to the decrease in the density and sensitivity of their receptors (Bristow MR, 1982) (Ungerer M, 1996).
The blockade of the βARK1 by the means of gene therapy could be effective as in this case the de-activating role of the βARK1 would be stopped, thus permitting the β-agonists to remain effective even in chronic administration.
Another view of the matter shows the need to discover the role of β-arrestin. The muscles that act under the continuous action of the sympathetic system, β1-adrenergic receptors mediate a β-arrestin activation of the EGFR, thus initiating cardioprotective pathways that compensate the toxic action of increased catecholes (Noma T, 2007). Therefore, it is suggested that there are two signaling pathways, one that is G-protein dependent and another one that is b-arrestin dependent. The meaning of these findings is obvious as the design of special drugs that selectively activate or block adrenergic action can be achieved.

5. Stem cell transplantation in heart failure

The potential use of stem cells for regenerative medicine and for the treatment of genetic disease has rarely been out of the news. Discussion has focused mainly on the use of human embryonic stem cells, which in culture have the capacity to generate all cell types. However, initial hopes for stem-cell therapy have been somewhat dampened by both technical and ethical problems. Recent studies have therefore created a great deal of excitement. They show that fully differentiated somatic cells (such as skin fibroblasts) can be reprogrammed to make cells similar to embryonic stem cells (Douglas R, 2008).
Experimental studies and clinical trials have revealed that Mesenchymal Stem Cells (MSCs) not only differentiate into cardiomyocytes and vascular cells, but also secrete amounts of growth factors and cytokines which may mediate endogenous regeneration via activation of resident cardiac stem cells and other stem cells, as well as induce neovascularization, anti-inflammation, anti-apoptosis, anti-remodeling and cardiac contractility in a paracrine manner. It has also been postulated that the anti-arrhythmic and cardiac nerve sprouting potential of MSCs may contribute to their beneficial effects in cardiac repair. Most molecular and cellular mechanisms involved in the MSC-based therapy after myocardial infarction is still unclear at present (Wen Z, 2010).

6. Conclusion

To sum up, it is clear that the careful study of human genome can lead to new innovative views of the pathogenesis of heart failure after an ischemic episode. Therefore, the clarification of the genetic mechanisms which are involved in heart failure will give a boost to novel genetic therapies and improvement of the existing pharmaceutical therapies.

7. References

Ahlquist RP. 1948. A study of the adrenergic receptors. *Am J Physiol.* 1948, 153:586–600.

American Heart Association. 2000. *Heart and stroke statistical update.* s.l. : American Heart Association, 2000.

Benovic JL, DeBlasi A, Stone WC, Caron MG, Lefkowitz RJ. 1989. b-adrenergic receptor kinase: primary structure delineates a multigene family. *Science.* 1989, 246(4927):235–40.

Bristow MR, Ginsburg R, Minobe W, Cubicciotti RS, Sageman WS, Lurie K. 1982. Decreased catecholamine sensitivity and b-adrenergicreceptor density in failing human hearts. *New Engl J Med.* 1982, 307(4):205–11.

Brodde OE. 1993. b-adrenoceptors in cardiac disease. *Pharmacol Ther.* 1993, 60(3):405–30.

Corrente G, Guardavaccaro D, Tirone F. 2002. PC3 potentiates NGF-induced differentiation and protects neurons from apoptosis. *Neuroreport.* 2002, 13:417–422.

Cowie MR, Wood DA, Coats AJ, Thompson SG, Suresh V, Poole- Wilson PA. 2000. Survival of patients with a new diagnosis of heart failure: a population based study. *Heart.* 2000, 83(5):505–10.

Currie RW. 1987. Effect of ischemia and perfusion temperature on the synthesis of stress-induced (heat-shock) proteins in isolated and perfused rat hearts. *J Mol Cell Cardiol.* 1987, 19:795–808.

Das DK, Maulik N, Moratu II. 1995. Gene expression in acute myocardial stress. Induction by hypoxia, ischemia, reperfusion, hyperthermia and oxidative stress. *J Mol Cell Cardiol.* 1995, 27:181–193.

de Waard V, van den Berg BM, Veken J, Schultz-Heienbrok R, Pannekoek H, van Zonneveld AJ. 1999. Serial analysis of gene expression to assess the endothelial cell response to an atherogenic stimulus. *Gene.* 1999, 226:1-8.

del Monte F, Harding SE, Dec GW. 2002. Targeting phospholamban by gene transfer in human heart failure. *Circulation.* 2002, 105:904–907.

del Monte F, Williams E, Lebeche D. 2001. Improvement in survival and cardiac metabolism after gene transfer of sarcoplasmic reticulum Ca2+-ATPase in a rat model of heart failure. *Circulation.* 2001, 104:1424–1429.

Dohlman HG, Thorner J, Caron MG, Lefkowitz RJ. 1991. Model systems for the study of seven-transmembrane-segment receptors. *Annu Rev Biochem.* 1991, 60:653–88.

Douglas R. 2008. A New Dawn for Stem-Cell Therapy. *N Engl J Med.* 2008, 358:964-966.

Ewing B, Hillier L, Wendl MC, Green P. 1998. Base-calling of automated sequencer traces using phred. I. Accuracy assessment. *Genome Res.* 1998, 8:175-85.

Felgner PL, Tsai YJ, Sukhu L, Wheeler CJ, Manthorpe M, Marshall J, Cheng SH. 1995. Improved cationic lipid formulations for in. vivo gene therapy. *Ann NY Acad Sci.* 1995, 772, 126-39.

Fitzgerald LW, Burn TC, Brown BS. 2000. Possible role of valvular serotonin 5-HT(2B) receptors in th cardiopathy associated with fenfluramine. *Mol Pharmacol.* 2000, 57:75-81.

Flugelman MY, Jaklitsch MT, Newman KD, Casscells W, Bratthauer GL, Dichek DA. 1992. Low level in vivo gene transfer into the arterial wall through a perforated balloon catheter. *Circulation.* 1992, 85, 1110-7.

Fortuin Jr FD, Vale P, Losordo DW. 2003. One-year followup of direct myocardial gene transfer of vascular endothelial growth factor-2 using naked plasmid DNA by way of thoracotomy in no-option patients. *Am J Cardiol.* 2003, 92:436–439.

Geng YJ, Ishikawa Y, Vatner DE. 1999. Apoptosis of cardiac myocytes in Gs alpha transgenic mice. *Circ Res.* 1999, 84:34-42.

Gould Rothberg BE. 2001. The use of animal models in expression pharmacogenomic analysis. *Pharmacogenomics J.* 2001, 1:48-58.

—. 2001. The use of animal models in expression pharmacogenomic analysis. *Pharmacogenomics J.* 2001, 1:48-58.

Grines CL, Watkins MW, Helmer G. 2002. Angiogenic gene therapy (AGENT) trial in patients with stable angina. *Circulation.* 2002, 105:1291–1297.

Grines CL, Watkins MW, Mahmarian JJ. 2003. A randomized, double-blind, placebo-controlled trial of Ad5FGF-4 gene therapy and its effect on myocardial perfusion in patients with stable angina. *J Am Coll Cardiol.* 2003, 42:1339–1347.

Hartzell HC. 1988. Regulation of cardiac ion channels by catecholamines, acetylcholine and second messenger systems. *Prog Biophys Mol Biol.* 1988, 52(3):165–247.

Hausdorff WP, Caron MG, Lefkowitz RJ. 1990. Turning off the signal: desensitization of b-adrenergic receptor function. *FASEB J.* 1990, 4(11):2881-9.

Hollander MC, Sheikh MS, Bulavin DV. 1999. Genomic instability in Gadd45a-deficient mice. *Nat Genet.* 1999, 23:176–184.

Hsu JC, Bravo R, Taub R. 1992. Interaction among LRF-1, JunB, c-Jun, and c-Fos define a regulatory program in the G1 phase of liver regeneration. *Mol Cell Biol.* 1992, 12:4654–4665.

Karlsson K, Marklund SL. 1998. Heparin-, dextran sulfate-, and protamine-induced release of extracellular-superoxide dismutase to plasma in pigs. *Biochim Biophys Acta.* 1998, 967:110–114.

Kastrupa J, Jørgensena E, Drvotab V, Thuesend L, Bøtkerd HE, Gyöngyösie M, Glogare D, Rückb A, Bin Islamc K, Sylvénb C. 2001. Intramyocardial Injection of Genes with a Novel Percutaneous Technique: Initial Safety Data of the Euroinject One Study. *Heart Drug.* 2001, 1:299-304.

Kirshenbaum LA, de Moissac D. 1997. The bcl-2 gene product prevents programmed cell death of ventricular myocytes. *Circulation.* 1997, 96:1580–1585.

Kwaan HC, Wang J, Svoboda K. 2000. Plasminogen activator inhibitor 1 may promote tumour growth through inhibition of apoptosis. *Br J Cancer.* 2000, 82:1702–1709.

Laham RJ, Simons M, Sellke F. 2001. Gene transfer for angiogenesis in coronary artery disease. *Annu Rev Med.* 2001, 2, 485-502.

Lazarou J, Pomeranz BH. 1998. Incidence of adverse reactions on hospitalized patients. A meta-analysis of prospective studies. *JAMA.* 1998, 279, 1200–1205.

Lehrman S. 1999. Virus treatment questioned after gene therapy death. *Nature.* 1999, 401, 517-8.

Li Q, Bolli R, Qiu Y. 1998. Gene therapy with extracellular superoxide dismutase attenuates myocardial stunning in conscious rabbits. *Circulation.* 1998, 98:1438–1448.

Losordo DW, Vale PR, Symes JF. 1998. Gene therapy for myocardial angiogenesis: Initial clinical results with direct myocardial injection of phVEGF165 as sole therapy for myocardial ischemia. *Circulation.* 1998, 98:2800–2804.

March R. 2001. Pharmacogenomics - legal, ethical and regulatory considerations. *Pharmacogenomics.* 2001, 2, 317–327.

Matsui T, Li L, del Monte F. 1999. Adenoviral gene transfer of activated phosphatidylinositol 3′-kinase and Akt inhibits apoptosis of hypoxic cardiomyocytes in vitro. *Circulation.* 1999, 100:2373–2379.

McMurray JJ, Stewart S. 2000. Epidemiology, aetiology, and prognosis of heart failure. *Heart.* 2000, 83(5): 596–602.

Melo LG, Agrawal R, Zhang L. 2002. Gene therapy strategy for long-term myocardial protection using adeno-associated virus-mediated delivery of heme oxygenase gene. *Circulation.* 2002, 105:602–607.

Miyamoto MI, del Monte F, Schmidt U. 2000. Adenoviral gene transfer of SERCA2a improves left-ventricular function in aortic-banded rats in transition to heart failure. *Proc Natl Acad Sci USA.* 2000, 97:793–798.

Most P, Pleger ST, Völkers M. 2004. Cardiac adenoviral S100A1 gene delivery rescues failing myocardium. *J Clin Invest.* 2004, 114:1550–1563.

Nobori K, Ito H, Tamamori-Adachi M. 2002. ATF3 inhibits doxorubicin-induced apoptosis in cardiac myocytes: A novel cardioprotective role of ATF3. *J Mol Cell Cardiol.* 2002, 34:1387–1397.

Noma T, Lemaire A, Naga Prasad SV. 2007. Beta-arrestin mediated beta-1 adrenergic receptor transactivation of the EGFR confers cardioprotection. *J Clin Invest.* 2007, 117: 2445-58.

Okubo S, Wildner O, Shah MR. 2001. Gene transfer of heat-shock protein 70 reduces infarct size in vivo after ischemia/reperfusion in rabbit heart. *Circulation.* 2001, 103:877–881.

Phillips MI, Tang Y, Schmidt-Ott K. 2002. Vigilant vector: Heart-specific promoter in an adeno-associated virus vector for cardioprotection. *Hypertension.* 2002, 39:651–655.

Platt JL, Nath KA. 1998. Heme oxygenase: Protective gene or Trojan horse. *Nat Med.* 1998, 4:1364–1365.

Remppis A, Greten T, Schafer BW. 1996. Altered expression of the Ca2+-binding protein S100A1 in human cardiomyopathy. *Biochim Biophys Acta.* 1996, 1313:253–257.

Rosengart TK, Lee LY, Patel SR. 1999. Angiogenesis gene therapy: Phase I assessment of direct intramyocardial administration of an adenovirus vector expressing VEGF121 cDNA to individuals with clinically significant severe coronary artery disease. *Circulation.* 1999, 100:468–474.

Routhu KV, Tsopanoglou NE, Strande JL. 2010. Parstatin(1-26): the putative signal peptide of protease-activated receptor 1 confers potent protection from myocardial ischemia-reperfusion injury. *J Pharmacol Exp Ther.* 2010, 332(3):898-905.

Sakoda T, Kasahara N, Hamamori Y, Kedes L. 1999. A high-titer lentiviral production system mediates efficient transduction of differentiated cells including beating cardiac myocytes. *J Mol Cell Cardiol.* 1999, 31, 2037-47.

Shimkets RA, Lowe DG, Tai JT. 1999. Gene expression analysis by transcript profiling coupled to a gene database query. *Nat Biotechnol.* 1999, 17:798-803.

Shimpo M, Ikeda U, Maeda Y, Takahashi M, Miyashita H, Mizukami H, Urabe M, Kume A, Takizawa T, Shibuya M, Ozawa K, Shimada K. 2002. AAV-mediated VEGF gene transfer into skeletal muscle stimulates angiogenesis and improves blood flow in a rat hindlimb ischemia model. *Cardiovasc Res.* 2002, 53, 993-1001.

Simons M, Annex BH, Laham RJ. 2002. Pharmacological treatment of coronary artery disease with recombinant fibroblast growth factor-2: Double-blind, randomized, controlled clinical trial. *Circulation.* 2002, 105:788–793.

Soeda S, Oda M, Ochiai T. 2001. Deficient release of plasminogen activator inhibitor-1 from astrocytes triggers apoptosis in neuronal cells. *Brain Res.* 2001, 91:96–103.

Stewart AL, Greenfield S, Hays RD, Wells K, Rogers WH, Berry SD. 1989. Functional status and well-being of patients with chronic conditions. Results from the medical outcomes study. *JAMA.* 1989, 262(7):907–13.

Strande JL, Widlansky ME, Tsopanoglou NE, Su J, Wang J, Hsu A, Routhu KV, Baker JE. 2009. Parstatin: a cryptic peptide involved in cardioprotection after ischaemia and reperfusion injury. *Cardiovasc Res.* 2009, 15;83(2):325-34.

Symes JF. 2001. Gene therapy for ischemic heart disease: Therapeutic potential. *Am J Cardiovasc Drugs.* 2001, 1:159–166.

Symes JF, Losordo DW, Vale PR. 1999. Gene therapy with vascular endothelial growth factor for inoperable coronary artery disease. *Ann Thor Surg.* 1999, 68:830–837.

Tang YL, Tang Y, Zhang YC. 2004. Protection from ischemic heart injury by a vigilant heme oxygenase-1 plasmid system. *Hypertension.* 2004, 43:746–751.

Ulrich P, Cerami A. 2001. Protein glycation, diabetes, and aging. *Recent Prog Horm Res.* 2001, 56:1–21.

Unger EF, Goncalves L, Epstein SE. 2000. Effects of a single intracoronary injection of basic fibroblast growth factor in stable angina pectoris. *Am J Cardiol.* 2000, 85:1414–1419.

Ungerer M, Kessebohm K, Kronsbein K, Lohse MJ, Richardt G. 1996. Activation of b-adrenergic receptor kinase during myocardial ischemia. *Circ Res.* 1996, 79(3):455–60.

Vale PR, Losordo DW, Milliken CE. 2000. Left ventricular electromechanical mapping to assess efficacy of phVEGF165 gene transfer for therapeutic angiogenesis in chronic myocardial ischemia. *Circulation.* 2000, 102:965–974.

–. 2001. Randomized, single-blind, placebo-controlled pilot study of catheterbased myocardial gene transfer for therapeutic angiogenesis using left ventricular electromechanical mapping in patients with chronic myocardial ischemia. *Circulation.* 2001, 103:2138–2143.

Vasan S, Zhang X, Zhang X, Kapurniotu A, Bernhagen J, Teichberg S. 1996. An agent cleaving glucose-derived protein crosslinks in vitro and in vivo. *Nature.* 1996, 382:275–8.

Veenstra D. 2000. Assessing the cost-effectiveness of pharmacogenomics. *AAPS PharmSci.* 2000, 2, 29.

Velculescu VE, Zhang L, Vogelstein B, Kinzler KW. 1995. Serial analysis of gene expression. *Science.* 1995, 270:484-7.

Wen Z, Zheng S, Zhou C, Wang J, Wang T. 2010. Repair mechanisms of bone marrow mesenchymal stem cells in myocardial infarction. *J Cell Mol Med.* 2010, Dec 28.

Zile M, Gaasch W, Little W, Francis G, Tavazzi L, Cleland J. 2004. A phase II, double-blind, randomized, placebo-controlled, dose comparative study of the efficacy, tolerability, and safety of MCC-135 in subjects with chronic heart failure, NYHA class II/III (MCC-135-GO1 study): rationale and design. *J Card Fail.* 2004, 10:193–199.

Ziolo MT, Martin JL, Bossuyt J. 2005. Adenoviral gene transfer of mutant phospholamban rescues contractile dysfunction in failing rabbit myocytes with relatively preserved SERCA function. *Circ Res.* 2005, 96:815–817.

18

Gene Therapy of the Heart through Targeting Non-Cardiac Cells

Guro Valen
University of OsloDepartment of Physiology/Center for Heart Failure Research
Norway

1. Introduction

To combat ischemic heart disease in the clinical scenarios of open heart surgery, unstable coronary syndromes, percutaneous coronary interventions, or thrombolysis, different research approaches are used to improve clinical treatments. The most dreaded long term consequence of ischemic heart disease - heart failure - is another clinical diagnosis where the treatment we have to offer is less than optimal. Some researchers are attempting to omit the reason for cardiovascular disease through targeting the process of atherosclerosis. Others adress the pathophysiology of restenosis, which may occurr after balloon dilatation of atherosclerotic lesions. Yet others adress improved treatment of the myocardium which has undergone an infarction, where the building of new blood vessels, strengthening of the contractile apparatus, and recruitment of new cells to areas of necrosis may be therapeutical end-points. Arrthythmias may occur due to reperfusion injury, after long-term morphological changes in the heart, or due to endogenous causes related to changes of the conduction system; new therapies are required for improved treatment. Novel treatments for dysfunctional, calsified heart valves are subject to other lines of investigations. Gene therapy and cell therapy using genetic engineering of stem cells will be the focus of this chapter, in particular the current status of treatments directed towards the myocardium itself in ischemic heart disease will be discussed. Gene therapy and to a lesser extend cell therapy have been used both clinically and experimentally to combat acute ischemia, remodeling and heart failure. However, the protected location of the heart of the heart inside the thoracic cavity, the nature of cardiac cells with minimal ability of entering cell cycle, and the electrophysiological properties of the heart render this organ with some particular challenges for gene therapy.

2. Gene therapy for myocardial protection

Delivery of DNA to hearts as well as other organs has been performed in animal experiments, and clinical studies in "no-option" patients have been conducted. Many clinical trials with gene therapy in cardiovascular patients have recently been reviewed (Lavu at al., 2010, Lyon et al., 2011). A general challenge with gene delivery to the heart is low transfection efficacy (the cardiomyocyte does not enter cell cycle), cell injury/inflammation, and unwanted sideeffects. There are several options on routes of DNA

delivery to the heart. One alternative is intravascular delivery, which can be directed through coronary arteries or retrogradely into the coronary sinus. An arterial approach which requires open coronary arteries may not be suitable for patients with coronary artery disease if the target is treating cardiomyocytes rather than vascular cells. Pericardial gene delivery has been attempted, but there are rather few publications with that particular route of delivery. Another option is direct intracardiac delivery, which has been tried clinically and experimentally (Isner, 2002, Semenza, 2004, Vinge et al., 2008). In general it is difficult to achieve a lasting transfection through this invasive approach, which may be delivery of naked DNA or DNA ligated to a vector. Viral vectors used for cardiovascular therapy are most commonly adenovirus, adenoasscociated virus, and to a lesser extent lentivirus. A third possibility is systemic delivery with "something" that directs the DNA/RNA to a specific cell. The "something" in question may be adenovirus or adenoassociated virus, which have been most extensively used for genetic correction of cardiovascular disorders. Adenovirus have the advantage of being easy to manipulate, can be produced in high titers, and have a large transgene cloning capacity (Vinge et al., 2008). However, adenovirus elicit an inflammatory response. Development of so-called "gutted or gutless" adenovirus, where the immunogenic viral epitopes are removed, may become an option in the future (Vinge et al., 2008). Adenoassociated virus are not associated with any human disease, produce a stable and long-lasting gene expression, and easily transfect cardiac muscle cells. The latter is especially the case with some of the newer serotypes, of which serotype 9 is most cardiotropic (Bush et al., 2008, Zancarelli et al., 2008). A disadvantage is that only small constructs (less than 5 kb) can be packed into adenoassociated virus (AAV). Non-viral vectors are also in use and will be briefly discussed.
Further considerations in cardiac gene therapy are which cells are to be treated and what do we want to overexpress or silence (Vinge et al., 2008). The possibilities range from targeting the vasculature to stabilize atherosclerotic plaques, prevent neointima formation, reduce atherosclerosis, induce angiogenesis, to improve survival of cardiomyocytes, improve function of cardiomyocytes, to reduce pathologic remodelling, and to prevent arrhythmia generation. Choice of gene construct and delivery route will depend on this. Genes encoding for factors which have intracellular effects should be delivered to a large population of cells to correct the underlying pathology, while genes encoding for secretory factors require fewer successfully transfected cells provided gene expression lasts (Isner, 2002). RNA interference or silencing, a possibility for gene knockdown, is predominantly at an animal experimental level. Experimentally, RNA interference though short hairpin RNA silencing the RNA polymerase of Coxsackie B3 virus packed into AAV2 successfully treated cardiac dysfunction in mice with coxsackieB cardiomyopathy (Fechner et al., 2008). In that study, the AAV2-construct was given intravenously. The same group have also used phospholamban silencing in short hairpin RNA delivered systemically through a AAV9 vector to normalize left ventricular remodelling after phenylephrine-induced hypertrophy (Suckau et al., 2009). RNA silencing will not be discussed further in this chapter.

2.1 Viral vectors

The first experimental studies on cardiac gene therapy used intramyocardial delivery with plasmid DNA, demonstrating the feasibilty of envisioning cardiac gene transfer (Acsadi et al., 1991, Lin et al., 1990, Burrick et al., 1992). Although those studies were successful in the terms of being able to cause transgene expression up to six months later in cardiomyocytes, the number of transfected myocytes was estimated to be as low as 60-100 cells (Ascadi et al., 1991). This lead to the search for vectors to enhance nuclear uptake, where viral vectors have been most extensively studied. Adenovirus was first attempted. Guzman and coworkers injected an adenoviral vector containing β-galactosidase (1993) into the myocardium, and was able to see a stronger signal than that evoked by plasmid containing the same molecular marker. However, the expression lasted only one week, and was accompanied by an inflammatory response (Guzman et al. 1993). Subsequently viral titers and protein production have been extensively studied and optimized, as have anatomic location and duration of adenoviral based gene expression in the heart (French et al., 1994, Magovern et al., 1996, Barr et al., 1994). Delivery of therapeutic genes with adenoviral vectors has been performed with success. For instance, adenoviral based delivery of DNA encoding for β2-adrenoceptors enhanced cardiac function in hamsters with cardiomyopathy (Tomiyasu et al., 2000). However, although adenovirus was the first vector to be used for cardiac gene therapy and has been useful for "proof of concept" as well as some initial clinical trials (Lavu et al., 2010), it may not be of large scale therapeutic use for the future. Adenovirus are double-stranded DNA viruses, with a high effeciency of delivery and expression of their genome in nuclei of dividing and non-dividing cells (Voplers & Kochanek, 2004). They are relatively large viral structures, with the capacity to carry constructs of up to 30 kB (Lyon et al., 2011). However, despite the fact that they are relatively cheap to produce in high titers and with a reasonably high purity, a major issue is that they evoke an immune response. As naturally occurring pathogens, patients are likely to have encountered them previously. Thus immune responses leading to destruction of cells containing adenovirus in the heart is a likely outcome. The latter factor also limits the time frame of therapeutic gene expression (Lyon et al., 2011). However, since work on gene therapy of the heart started with adenoviral vectors, the experience in use of this vector is high, and it is an excellent tool for basic science studies to evaluate the therapuetic potential of novel genes.

Attempts are being made to reduce the immunogenicity of adenoviruses, removing the viral genome and viral proteins. The third generation of "gutless" adenovirus have low immunogenicity, and longer transgene expression (Chen et al., 1997). Direct myocardial delivery of gutless adenovirus resulted in less inflammation than the first generation virus, but the gene expression was not high and it was short-lasting (Fleury et al., 2004). Another still remaining problem with adenovirus in the heart is the affinity for other organs such as gastrointestinal tract, liver, respiratory tract, and muscle, causing side effects in clinical trials (Lavu et al., 20120, Lyon et al., 2011).

Adenoassociated viruses (AAV) are currently without comparison the most suitable vectors for cardiovascular gene transfer. AAVs are not associated with any human pathology although 20-40% of all humans may have antibodies to them, making them attractive and safe for clinical treatment. AAVs exist in different seroforms, which have different affinity for the heart. The most recent serotyope, AAV9, is more cardiotropic than any other known virus and will transfect nearly 100% of all heart cells (Vandendriessche et al., 2007). AAV9 causes a sustained cardiac expression of the delivered gene, with little leakage to other organs (Bish et al., 2008, Inagaki et al., 2006, Zincarelli et al., 2008, Pacak et al., 2006). AAV1, 6, and 8 also have relatively high tropism to the heart, and since they have been around for a longer time, they have come further into clinical studies. AAV have been used for intracardiac, intravascular, and systemic gene delivery. Hitherto more than 20 clinical trials using AAV vectors have delivered the vectors to hundreds of patients without observing any adverse effects (Lyon et al. 2011, Leon et al. 2010). A major advantage of AAV9 is that a systemic approach to gene delivery can be used, thus avoiding some of the challenges of the other viral vectors.

Retroviruses are RNA viruses which integrate into the host cell chromosome after enzymatic conversion to DNA. Retroviral vectors are modified to retain the part of the genome which is neccessary to initiate reverse transcription into the target cell, while the rest of the viral genome is removed (Lyon et al., 2011). Integration of virus into the cell requires cell division, which is why this vector can be suitable for therapies against endothelial or smooth muscle cells such as in avoiding atherosclerosis or restenosis, but less suitable for cardiomyocytes which have a low division rate. However, the insertion of retrovirus into the host genome may cause mutations, potentially leading to malignancies which can be passed on into the germline to offspring.

Lentiviruses belong to the retroviridae family, and include vectors derived from the human immunodeficiency virus type I (HIV-1). Wild-type HIV-1 have an affinity for T-cell subpopulations, limiting their usability for cardiovascular purposes. Hybrid "pseudotyped" lentivirus have been produced to expand their tropism for other cell types. In the context of transfecting cardiomyocytes, lentiviral-based vectors are as effecient as adenoviruses, with transgene expression lasting longer (Yoshimitsu 2006). They can incorporate constructs up to 8 kB in size (Yoshimitsu). Lentivirurses are especially favoured in studies targeting transfection of endothelial cells or smooth muscle cells (Sakoda et al., 2007). The major obstacle towards a large-scale employment of lentivirus is currently uncertainties regarding safety. Modifications of the virus to avoid any risk of human disease are being performed, and may in the future lead to a larger therapeutic potential (Lyon et al. 2011).

2.2 Intrapericardial gene delivery

In theory, injection of DNA into the intrapericardial space may offer an environment which is relatively constant (no blood flow), and would be a relatively non-invasive approach for getting DNA to the heart. However, an intrapericardial injection can not lead to directed gene delivery, in the sense that there is no control over uptake in a specific type of cell or a specific area of the heart such as into the border zone of myocardial infarction. It is noteworthy that few publications exist using this option. Zhang and coworkers delivered adenoviral based LacZ into the pericardium of neonatal mice through a percutaneous puncture, and three days later found LacZ activity in the endocardium, epicardium, and myocardium (Zhang et al., 1999). However, the same regimen did not lead to wide-spread expression in adult hearts, in which hepatic transduction was found in high levels (Zhang et al., 1999). Using a transdiagfragmatic approach, Fromes et al. (1999) delivered adenoviral based β-galactodase intrapericardially in rats. Positive staining was found exclusively in pericardial cells. Mixing the virus with proteolytic enzymes increased transgene expression intramyocardially within a short time later, but the expression did not last, and there was leakage to other organs (Fromes et al., 1999). In the canine myocardium, March and coworkers (1999) delivered adenovirus based LacZ through a penetrating catheter. This lead to a pericardial-located activity of LacZ. The abscence of publications using this delivery approach for the last decade suggests that this is not a delivery route for the future.

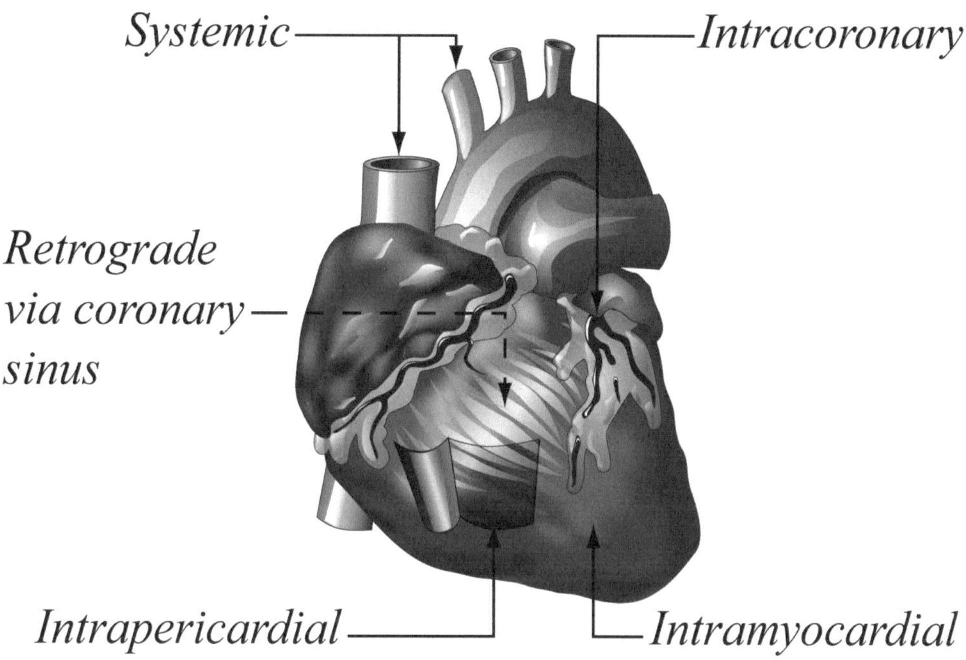

Fig. 1. The cartoon depicts possible routes of delivery of either stem cells or DNA with or without a vector to the heart. Systemic delivery is suitable only when DNA is ligated to a cardiotropic vector.

2.3 Intramyocardial gene delivery

Gene delivery to the heart of either plasmid DNA or DNA ligated to a vector has been performed for decades both in experimental and in clinical trials (Lavu et al., 2010, Katz et al., 2010). Regardless of whether the injection is of plasmid DNA or DNA ligated to a vector, intramyocardial injections are invasive and do not have a clinical appeal. One can envision injection of DNA during open heart surgery when the heart is exposed anyway, or catheter-based delivery when a patient is undergoing invasive arterial procedures. However, except for open heart surgery with direct visualization the accuracy of such an approach is not high - if the intention is delivery of genes i.e. into an ischemic border zone to induce angiogenesis, it will be very difficult to control where exactly the injection site is in relation to where it would be wished to be. The approach has, however, given us invaluable research information on the therapeutic potential and limitations of genes thought to correct underlying pathologies. Many studies have used intramyocardial injections of DNA to induce angiogenesis. Delivery of the transcription factor GATA-4 ligated to an adenoviral vector before coronary artery ligation resulted in improved left ventricular function and reduced infarct size (Rysä et al., 2010). This was due to increased angiogenesis, decreased apoptosis, and mobilization of cardiac stem cells in GATA-4 treated hearts. AAV-based transfection with angiogenin in an *in vivo* infarction model reduced remodelling, induced angiogenesis, and attenuated cardiac dysfunction four weeks later (Zhao et al., 2006). Therapeutic use of AAV9-vascular endothelial growth factor-B is cardioprotective in canine pacing-induced dilated cardiomyopathy, but not due to formation of new vessels (Pepe et al., 2010). Delivery of adenoviral vector-ligated vascular endothelial growth factor B to rats with angiotensin II-induced hypertrophy leads to reduction of diastolic dysfunction, increasing capillary area but not density (Serpi et al., 2011). In a chronic ischemia model in rats, AAV2-based delivery of both vascular endothelial growth factor A and - B were protective (Zentilin et al., 2010). Vascular endothelial growth factor B was more protective than A, reducing apoptosis and remodelling and preserving heart function in the absence of angiogenesis. Hepatocyte growth factor delivered by adenovirus into the myocardium following myocardial infarction preserved cardiac function, reduced remodelling and apoptosis, and induced angiogenesis (Jayasankar et al., 2003). Other studies have used antiinflammatory agents injected into the myocardium to combat ischemic heart disease and its consequences. Adenoviral-based expression of inhibitory kappa B-alpha in a rat infarction model improved heart function six weeks later (Trescher et al., 2004). AAV9 based delivery of heme oxygenase-1 into the myocardium before myocardial infarction had infarct reducing, anti-inflammatory, and antiapoptotic effects (Melo et al., 2002). Intramyocardial injection with inducible nitric oxide synthase ligated to adenovirus had an infarct-reducing effect both short-term and long-term (Li et al., 2006). This effect was mediated by inducible cyclooxygenase and nuclear factor kappa B (Liet al., 2007). Other cardioprotective genes in various models of heart disease are the inhibitor of matrix metalloproteinase TIMP-1 (Jayasankar 2004), the cell cycle regulator cyclin A2 (Woo et al., 2006), the regulator of organ development sonic hedgehog (Kusano et al., 2005); Notch1, regulator of cell proliferation and differentiation (Kratsios et al., 2010), the beta adrenoceptor receptor betaARKct (Rengo et al., 2009), and sphingosine kinase 1, a protective protein kinase (Duan et al., 2007). Thus, a major insight into possible therapeutic genes has been provided by this gene delivery route. Intramyocardial gene delivery is likely to remain a powerful research tool for testing the therapeutic potiential of genes in experimental models in the future. However, the future clinical gene therapies are unlikely to involve intramyocardial delivery at a large scale.

2.4 Intravascular delivery

Cardiac intravascular gene delivery has been performed through antegrade coronary artery delivery, non-selective intracoronary delivery (i.e. left ventricular injection), and retrogradely through the coronary sinus (Katz et al., 2010). Common for these approaches is the need to occlude the coronary circulation temporarily to allow virus to migrate into cells. The attractive aspect of this approach is the possibility of a minimally invasive delivery procedure through a catheter well within established clinical procedures (at least the antegrade technique) and the possibility to deliver into all four heart chambers. The first studies using coronary artery delivery resulted in very few transfected cells (Longeart et al., 2001, Hayase et al., 2005, Kaplitt et al., 1996). Later studies have refined delivery methods to some degree. With a recombinant AAV2 vector ligated to deliver enhanced green fluorescent protein, Kaspar and collegues (2005) used rats for indirect intracoronary delivery. Rats had transgene expression lasting up to 12 months, with a gradient of expression across the left ventricular wall, the epicardium expressing much more than the endocardium. There was evidence of AAV2 vector genome in liver and lungs of injected animals (Kaspar et al., 2005). Lai and coworkers (2004) delivered DNA encoding for adenylyl cyclase 6 ligated to an adenoviral vector into all three major coronary arteries of pigs with heart failure, using a vasodilator at the time of delivery, and compared with delivery of saline. Three weeks later left ventricular function was improved in the pigs recieving adenylyl cyclase 6. Gene expression in left ventricular biopsies evaluated with PCR was increased, although in which cells was not adressed (Lai et al., 2004). The success of intravascular gene delivery may depend on the target cell; if it is vascular, the chance of success may increase compared with a cardiac cell target. However, anything that enters the coronary circulation must enter the general circulation, reducing the clinical appeal of this approach. A special situation where this mode of delivery may be attractive is during open heart surgery with cardioplegic arrest.

2.5 Gene therapy using non-viral vectors

Although improvements are made in modifying viral vectors, reducing immunogenicity and increasing duration and amount of gene expression and narrowing the expression to target cells, researchers are travelling on alternative routes to deliver genes to the heart. Several non-viral techniques are used to improve the transfection efficacy of plasmids such as liposomes, polymers, electroporation, and nanotechnology (Holladay et al. 2010, Lukyanenko 2007). The status of these approaches are recently reviewed elsewhere (Holladay et al. 2010, Lukyanenko 2007).

3. Cardioprotection by cell therapy

Stem cell therapy for protecting hearts is a large topic. For readers particularly interested in the field, the recent reviews by Novotny et al. (2008), Beeres at al. (2008), and Atoui et al. (2008) are excellent. Stem cells are divided into committed and uncommitted cells, where the latter are the true stem cells in the sense that they are undifferenciated, capable of self-renewal, and multipotent (Novotny et al., 2008, Beeres et al., 2008, Atoui et al., 2008). These types of cells include multipotent bone marrow or adipose tissue derived mesenchymal stem cells and embryonic stem cells. Commited progenitor cells are more differentiated, and include endothelial progenitor cells, fetal cardiomyocytes, and autologous skeletal myoblasts. Experimental studies have successfully been able to induce neovascularization, increase cardiomyocyte survival, and improve postinfarct function through using cell transplantation. However, why it works is not completely clarified. Some investigators believe that stem cells dedifferentiate into cardiomyocytes, but not all studies confirm this finding (Silva et al., 2005, Cinnaird et al., 2004, Cocher et al., 2001, Murry et al., 2004). Possibly there is a fusion between the transplanted cells and the endogenous cardiomyocytes (Beeres et al., 2008). Possibly also the transplanted cells lead to recruitment of resident cardiac progenitor cells (Novotny et al., 2008, Beeres et al., 2008). Paracrine effects may be of importance. As transplanted cells have a short life span in their new environment, these effects will be transitory. Some suggested mechanisms of action are autocrine or paracrine release of cytokines and growth factors that will stimulate new vessel formation, inhibit apoptosis, rescue injured cardiomyocytes, and reduce pathologic remodelling. Recently, endogenous cardiac stem cells are reported to have even more promising potential for correcting cardiac pathologies. These cells are a large topic beyond the scope of this chapter (Bolli & Chaudrey, 2010).

Therapeutic use of stem cells is now a clinical reality, but there is need for more laboratory work before this field can become useful in patients at a large scale. At the moment we do not know the optimal cell for delivery, the optimal amount of cells, or which route of delivery (as for gene therapy, intramyocardial, intravascular through artery or vein, pericardial and other approaches have all been performed) that will give the best outcome.

Genetically modifed cells may act as transgene carriers and be used to deliver therapeutic targets to cardiac tissue. Transfected cells of different origins have been used in animal experiments to induce angiogenesis, increase contractility, decrease fibrosis, improve remodelling, and improve graft cell survival.

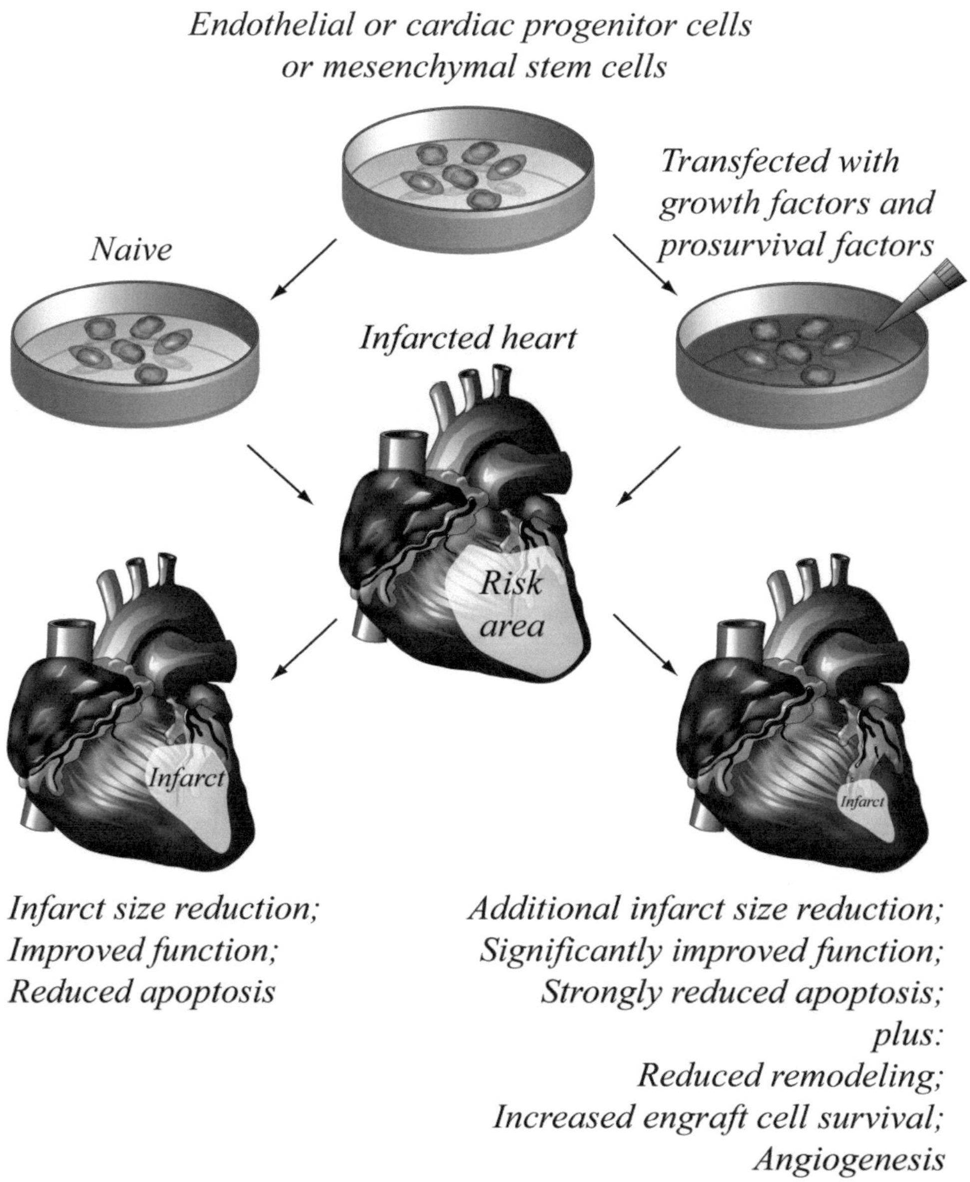

Fig. 2. The advantages of using genetically engineered stem cells versus naive stem cells are illustrated. Naive stem cells do rescue myocardium, but the effects are much more pronounced when stem cells are genetically engineered.

3.1 Genetically engineered stem cells as cardioprotective agents

Based on the assumption that the major effect of stem cells is through their paracrine effects, quite a few works have focused on genetically engineered stem cells to produce angiogenic factors, with the perspective to both increase survival of the transplanted cell and to enhance the formation of new blood vessels in the infarcted heart. For instance, bone-marrow derived endothelial progenitor cells were expanded and transduced with AAV to overexpress insulin-like growth factor 1. Then the autologous cells were transplanted into the infarct area of rats (Sen et al., 2010). Three months later rats receiving insulin-like growth factor 1 transduced cells as opposed to LacZ-transduced cells had improved myocardial function, reduced apoptosis, increased number of capillaries, and increased cardiomyocyte proliferation in the infarct area. There was no dissemination of transduced cells into other organs (Sen et al., 2010). In a model of neointima formation in hypercholesterolemic rats, endothelial progenitor cells transduced to overexpress hepatocyte growth factor were delivered. The transduced cells homed to the vascular site of injury more than untreated cells, and this caused a decreased neointima formation and increased endothelialization (Song et al., 2009). Colony stimulating factor-1 was used to transfect primary autologous rat myoblasts, which were transplanted into the myocardium of rats with postinfarction heart failure (Aharinejad et al., 2008). Left ventricular function evaluated by echocardiography was improved in hearts of rats treated with with autologous colony stimulating factor myoblasts. This protection was not found after delivery of untransduced myoblasts or plasmid DNA encoding for colony stimulating factor. In a similar model myoblasts transduced with human growth factor were able to improve heart function, increase capillary density, and reduced apoptosis (Rong et al., 2008). Mesenchymal stem cells engineered to overexpress adrenomedullin transplanted after myocardial infarction improved cardiac function more than naive mesenchymal stem cells (Jo et al., 2007). The growth factor angiopoietin-1 in modified mesenchymal stem cells has reduced ischemic damage when injected shortly after ischemia in rat hearts (Sun et al., 2007). In pigs, mononuclear cells were extracted from peripheral blood and induced to overexpress vascular endothelial growth factor retrogradely delivered through the coronary sinus. The transduced cells induced angiogenesis and reduced postischemic ventricular dysfunction four weeks later (Hagikura et al., 2010). Vascular endothelial growth factor ligated to mesenchymal stem cells under the control of a hypoxia response element induced ischemia-responsive production of vascular endothelial growth factor when transplanted into the ischemic myocardium (Kim et al., 2010). This caused an increased retainment of genetically altered mesenchymal stem cells in the infarcted heart compared with naive cells, reduction of apoptosis, and reduced remodelling. Also hypoxia-regulated heme oxygenase-1 overexpressing mesenchymal stem cells transplanted into the infarcted ventricular wall improved survival of transplanted cells, improved heart function, and reduced cell death (Tang et al., 2005).

Genetic modification of stem cells also improves cell survival and outcome of ischemia models when the gene in question is not considered to be a secretory molecule. Treatment of mesenchymal stem cells to overexpress connexin 43 followed by injection into infarcted myocardium improves left ventricular function and reduces cell death (Wang et al., 2010). Mesenchymal stem cells overexpressing heat shock protein of the 20 kDa family has similar beneficial effects (Wang et al., 2009). In the latter study, the authors provide evidence that the protective effect could be through increased secretion of proteins, where vascular endothelial growth factor, insulin-like growth factor, and fibroblast growth factor were released from transfected cells. The authors speculate that the relased growth factors were due to a detected activation of the protein kinase Akt (Wang et al., 2009). Indeed, mesenchymal stem cells overexpressing Akt itself transplanted into the ischemic myocardium improved left ventricular function, reduced infarct size, reduced apoptosis, increased mobilization of cardiac progenitor cells (c-kit+), and reduced collagen deposition (Mangi et al., 2003). The beneficial effects were dependent on the amount of transplanted cells. In a follow up study, the authors found that the mechanism for cardioprotection was not through stem cell fusion with cardiomyocytes, which occurred infrequently, and not due to differentiation of stem cells into cardiomyocytes (Noiseux et al. 2006). Another protein kinase associated with myocardial protection, Pim-1 kinase, was transfected into cardiac progenitor cells before injection into ischemic myocardium (Fischer et al., 2009). When animals were observed up to 32 weeks later, improved function and reduced infarct size was accompanied by increased survival of engrafted cells, increased vascularization, and increased number of c-kit+ cells (Fischer et al., 2009). Consequently, secondary secretory effects of genetic manipulation with a factor acting intracellularly is indicated. The antiapoptotic molecule Bcl2 has been used to transfect cardiomyoblasts (Kutcha et al., 2006) and mesenchymal stem cells (Li et al, 2007) before transplantation into infarcted myocardium, leading to improved function and survival of both engrafted cells and infarcted myocardium. Mesenchymal stem cells transfected with Bcl2 had an increased secretion of vascular endothelial growth factor in vitro, and an increased capillary density in vivo (Li et al., 2007). Finally, a few studies have used genes coding for antiinflammatory factors as enrichment of stem cells to improve survival of engrafted stem cells and the heart. Mesenchymal stem cells overexpressing the interleukin-18 binding protein, the naturally occurring inhibitor of the proinflammatory cytokine interleukin 18, improved cardioprotection more than that observed with unmodified stem cells (Wang et al., 2009). The beneficial effects observed on heart function, remodelling, and infarct size could have been due to increased secretion of vascular endothelial growth factor and decreased interleukin 6 levels in hearts of animals treated with genetically modified cells. Mesenchymal stem cells have also been used to overexpress the chemokine receptors CCR1 and CXCR2 before intramyocardial injection into infarcted heart (Huang et al., 2010). Stem cells with overexpression of CCR1 had increased survival intramyocardially, which was accompanied by less cardiac remodelling, increased capillarization, and improved cardiac function in both acute and chronic (4 weeks) observation times. The effect was not found when cells were overexpressing CXCR2, which lead to similar findings as with naive mesenchymal stem cells (Huang et al., 20010).

To conclude, we still have a long way to go to fully understand the mechanisms by which stem cells may protect hearts and which cell type and number that should be used for future therapies. However, it is well documented that genetic engineering of stem cells with both secretory factors and primarily intracellularly acting factors improve engrafted cell survival as well as survival of the myocardium. Many of the studies mentioned above using a primary intracellularly acting factor have documented secondary secretory effects.

4. Cardiac gene therapy using a peripheral approach

A downside with intracardiac delivery of either genes or genetically modified cells is the relative invasiveness of the method. It is possible to envision effects in the heart through a

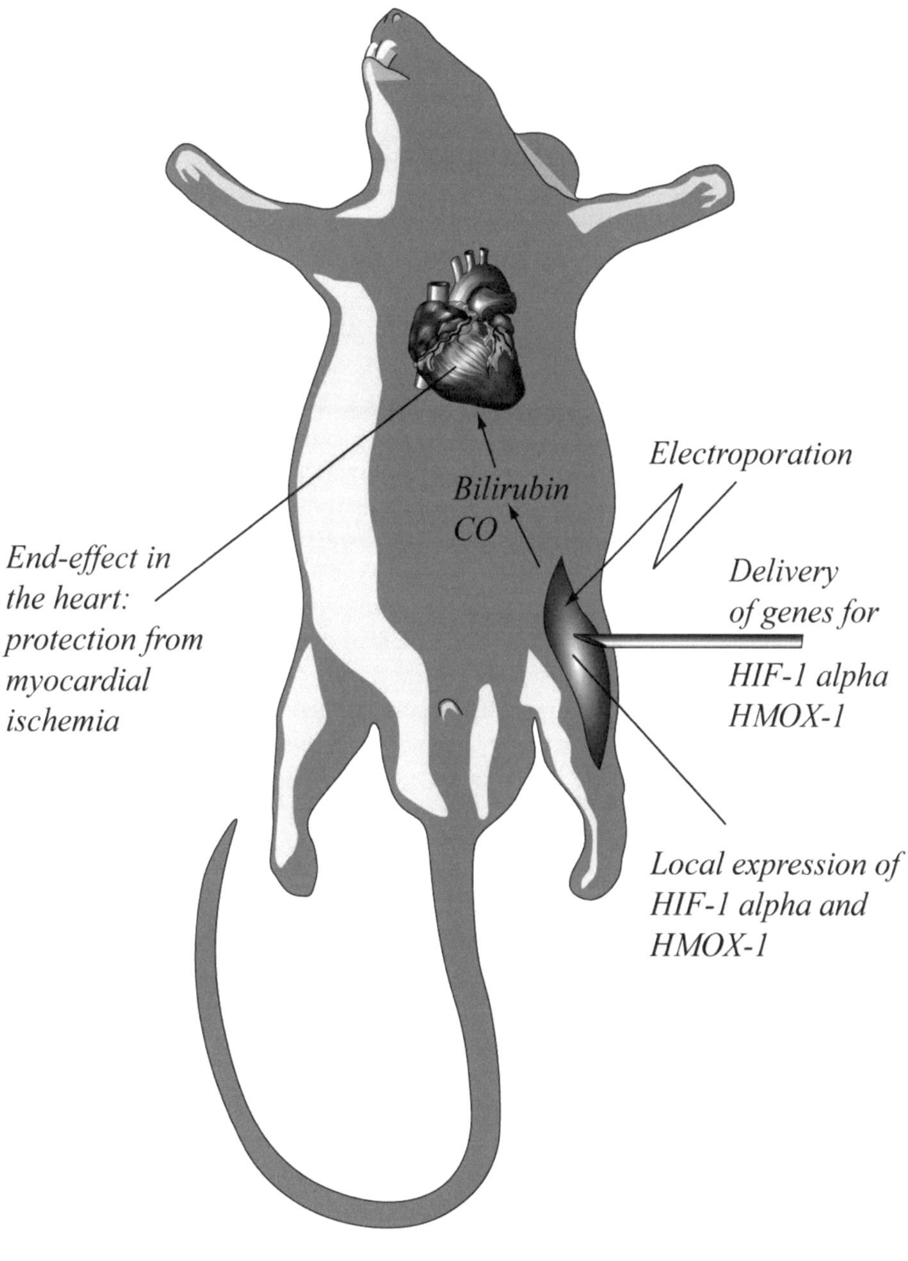

Fig. 3. The cartoon depicts the principle of remote gene therapy delivering plasmid DNA into the skeletal muscle, increasing nuclear uptake by electroporation, and achieving myocardial protection.

peripheral approach, building upon the principle of general organ protection evoked by pre- or postconditioning (Przyklenk et al., 1993). Preconditioning is the observation that brief episodes of ischemia and reperfusion to an organ will protect the organ against a later ischemic event (Murry et al., 1986), while postconditioning is the observation that brief episodes of ischemia and reperfusion at the start of reperfusion will reduce organ damage (Zhao et al., 2003). It is shown that the protection afforded by these brief episodes of ischemia and reperfusion provide an universal organ protection termed remote preconditioning (Przyklenk et al., 1993). In a series of experiments we have delivered plasmid DNA encoding for hypoxia-inducible factor 1alpha (HIF-1α) into an easily accessible peripheral organ, the quadriceps skeletal muscle. Others have shown that the skeletal muscle may serve as an endocrine organ, stably secreting endocrine factors into the blood stream after delivery of plasmid DNA and enhancing nuclear uptake by electroporation (Mathisen et al., 1999). This gives a very local increase of gene expression, transfecting a few skeletal muscle fibers in the treated muscle and with no leakage to other organs (Czibik et al 2009a, 2009b). The skeletal muscle expression of HIF-1α lasted for 8 weeks (not investigated longer) (Czibik et al., 2009a). When hearts were isolated and Langendorff-perfused with global ischemia and reperfusion, they had improved function and reduced infarct size compared with hearts of mice which were not pretreated with HIF-1α (Czibik et al., 2009a). To attempt to unravel mechanisms underlying the beneficial effects of HIF-1α, a Taqman low density array of some 47 HIF-regulated genes was performed on samples of the transfected skeletal muscle one week later. Several genes encoding for growth factors were increased in the transfected muscle, among them insulin-like growth factor 2, heme oxygenase-1, adrenomedullin, and platelet derived growth factor B (Czibik et al. 2009a). When these factors were used to protect the cardiomyocyte cell line HL-1 cells against injury evoked by hydrogen peroxide, heme oxygenase-1 (HMOX-1) was beyond comparison most protective, with effects similar to that of HIF-1α (Czibik et al. 2009b).

HMOX-1 is an inducible member of the heme oxygenase family of proteins, also consisting of the constitutive heme oxygenase-2 and the less well characterized heme oxygenase-3 (Durante et al., 2010, Wu et al., 2010). HMOX-1 expression is induced by its substrates: heme, oxidants, heavy metals, cytokines, growth factors, hemodynamic forces, gases, hypoxia, and hormones (Wu et al., 2011). Many transcription factors may be involved in its regulation. Some of them are HIF-1α, nuclear factor kappa B, activator protein 1, and nuclear factor E2-related factor (Wu et al., 2011). HMOX-1 catalyzes the degradation of heme into biliverdin, free iron, and carbon monoxide (Maines et al., 1986). Biliverdin is subsequently rapidly reduced to bilirubin by the enzyme biliverdin reductase. HMOX-1 is expressed in a plethora of cell types, including cardiac and vascular cells. Carbon monoxide, most known as a toxic gas, is recognized as an intracellular signalling molecule (Maines et al., 1986, Verma et al., 1993). Carbon monoxide has many cellular effects which have recently been reviewed elsewhere (Abraham & Kappas, 2008); in this context, it can be summarized that it may have antiinflammatory and antiapoptotic effects, lead to vasorelaxation, reduce lipid peroxidation and proliferation of vascular smooth muscle cells, and possibly induce angiogenesis. Bilirubin was shown to have antioxidant effects already in 1987 (Stocker et al.). Since then evidence supports that bilirubin regulates cellular redox states, reduces the formation of reactive oxygen species, and has antiinflammatory effects through decreasing the expression leukocyte adhesion molecules and neutrophil adhesion. Free iron may induce ferritin expression leading to iron sequestration. Thus, HMOX-1 through its downstream products is potentially very suitable for protection of cardiomyocytes.

When the HIF-1α gene was delivered in vivo into skeletal muscle of rats, the expression of HMOX-1 was increased, accompanied by increased serum bilirubin (Czibik et al., 2009b, Czibik et al., 2011). When a HMOX-1 blocker was given together with plasmid DNA encoding for HIF-1α and the hearts isolated and perfused with induced global ischemia, the beneficial effect of gene therapy was abolished (Czibik et al., 2009b). Delivery of plasmid DNA endocing for HMOX-1 before isolated heart perfusion mimicked the beneficial effects of HIF-1α (Czibik et al.,2009b). Gene delivery of HIF-1α into the skeletal muscle protected the heart ex vivo, and in vitro, and was also evaluated to be highly cardioprotective in an in vivo model of cardiac ischemia-reperfusion with remodelling six weeks later (Czibik et al., 2009a, 2009b, 2011). Unfortunately, systemic delivery of HIF-1α induced a general angiogenesis evident as increased CD31 positive staining in the electroporated muscle with gene delivery, the contralateral muscle, and in the heart (Czibik et al., 2009a, 2009b, 2011). Downstream factors to hypoxia inducible factor may turn out to be cardioprotective without the unwanted side-effects. Delivery of plasmid DNA encoding for HMOX-1 into the skeletal muscle before in vivo infarction protects against postinfarct remodelling without causing angiogenesis (manuscript in progress). Thus, these promising results from mice experimental studies should now be tested in larger animals as a bridge to human therapy.

5. Conclusion

For the treatment of cardiovascular disease, gene therapy may become an alternative in the near future. Gene delivery through intravascular approaches, intramyocardial injection, and pericardial route have been tried using plasmid DNA, adeno-, retro-, lenti-, and adenoassociated viral vectors. Of the viral vectors, adenoassociated virus serotype 9 is the most promising, as it is cardiotropic and can be delivered systemically. Stem cells are another approach to novel therapies against ischemic heart disease. Stem cells can be delivered through the same routes as genes. At the moment the mechanism of stem cell-induced protection of the heart is not well understood - the cells tend to stay shortly in the myocardium, and to a low degree fuse with cardiomyocytes or differentiate into cardiomyocytes. Possibly paracrine effects of stem cells are the reason for cardioprotection. Genetic engineering of stem cells improves the therapeutic effect of transplanted cells, both when the engineering is for a secretory factor and when it is overexpressing a factor primarily working intracellularly, and secondarily secretory. Gene therapy of the heart can also be evoked through using the skeletal muscle as a site of gene transfer, where delivery of plasmid DNA encoding for both hypoxia-inducible factor 1 alpha and its downstream target heme oxygenase-1 protects cardiomyocytes in vivo, ex vivo, and in vitro.

6. Acknowledgement

Arkady Rutkovskiy, MD, is gratefully acknowledged for making illustrations. Jarle Vaage, MD, PhD, read and commented on the manuscript. Financial support was recieved by the Norwegian Health Association, The Norwegian Women's Public Health Association, and the University of Oslo.

7. References

Abraham, N. G.; Kappas, A. (2008). Pharmacological and clinical aspects of heme oxygenase. *Pharmacological Reviews* 60: 79-127.

Ascadi, G., Jiao, S., Jani, A., Duke, D., Williams, P., Chong, W., Wolff, J.A. (1991) Direct gene transfer and expression into rat heart in vivo. *New Biol* 3:71-81.

Aharinejad ,S., Abraham, D,, Paulus, P., Zins, K., Hofman, M., Michilits, W., Gyöngyösi, M., Macfelda, K., Lucas, T., Treschner, K., Grimm, M., Stanley, E.R. (2008). Colony-stimulating factor-1 transfection of myoblasts improves the repair of failing myocardium following autologous myoblast transplantation. *Cardiovasc Res* 79:395-404.

Atoui, R., Shum-Tim, D., Chiu, R.C.J. (2008). Myocardial regenerative therapy: immunologic basis for the potential universal donor cells. *Ann Thorac Surg* 86:327-334.

Barr, E., Carroll, J., Kalynych, A.M., Tripathy, S.K., Kozarsky, K., Wilson, J.M., Leiden, J.M. (1994). Efficient catheter-mediated gene transfer into the heart using replication-deficient adenovirus. *Gene Ther* 1:51-58.

Beeres, S.L.M.A., Atsma, D., van Ramshorst, J., Schalij, M.J., Bax, J.J. (2008). Cell therapy for ischemic heart disease. *Heart* 94:1214-1226.

Bish, L.T., Morine, K., Sleeper, M.M., Sanmiguel, J., Wu, D., Gao, G., Wilson, J.M., Sweeney, L. (2008). AAV9 provides global cardiac gene transfer superior to AAV1, AAV6, AAV7, and AAV8 in the mouse and rat. *Hum Gene Ther* 19:1359-1368.

Bolli, P., Chaudhry, H.W. (2010). Molecular physiology of cardiac regeneration. *Ann NY Acad Sci* 1211:113-126.

Buttrick, P.M., Kass, A., Kitsis, R.N., Kaplan, M.L., Leinwand, L.A. (1992). Behaviour of genes directly injected into the rat heart in vivo. *Circ Res* 3:193-198.,

Chen, H.H., Mack, L.M., Kelly, R., Ontell, M., Kochanek, S., Clemens, P.R. (1997). Persistance in muscle of an adenoviral vector that lacks all viral genes. *Proc Nat Acad Sci USA* 94: 1654-1650.

Czibik, G., Martinov, V., Ruusalepp, A., Sagave, J., Skare, Ø., Valen, G. (2009). In vivo remote delivery of DNA encoding for hypoxia-inducible factor 1 alpha reduces myocardial infarct size. *Clinical and Translational Science* 1:33-40.

Czibik, G., Sagave, J., Martinov, V., Ishaq, B., Sohl, M., Sefland, I., Carlsen, H., Blomhoff, R., Farnebo, F., Valen, G. (2009). Cardioprotection by hypoxia-inducible factor 1 alpha transfection in skeletal muscle is critically dependent on heme oxygenase activity in mice. *Cardiovasc Res* 82:107-114.

Czibik, G., Gravning, J., Martinov, V., Ishaq, B., Attramadal, H., Valen, G. (2011). Remote delivery of DNA encoding for hypoxia-inducible factor 1 alpha is protective against in vivo myocardial ischemia-reperfusion injury. *Life Sciences* 16:71-78.

Duan, H.F., Wang, H., Yi, J., Liu, H.J., Zhang, T., Lu, Y., Wu, C.T., Wang, L.S. (2007). Adenoviral gene transfer of sphingosine kinase 1 protects heart against ischemia/reperfusion-induced injury and attenuates its postischemic failure. *Hum Gene Ther* 18:1119-1128.

Durante, W. (2010). Targeting heme oxygenase-1 in vascular disease. *Current Drug Targets* 11: 1504-1516.

Fechner, H., Sipo, I., Westernmann, D., Pinkert, S., Wang, X., Suckau, L., Kurreck, J., Zeichhardt, H., Müller, O., Vetter, R., Erdmann, V., Tschope, C., Poller, W. (2008). Cardiac—targeted RNA interference mediated by an AAV9 vector improves cardiac function in coxackievirus B3 cardiomyopathy. *J Mol Med* 86:987-997.

Fischer, K.M., Cottage, C.T., Wu, W., Din, S., Gude, N.A., Avitabile, D., Quijada, P., Collins, B.L., Fransioli, J., Sussman, M.A. (2009). Enhancement of myocardial regeneration through genetic engineering of cardiac progenitor cells expressing Pim-1 kinase. *Circulation* 120:2077-2087.

Fleury, S., Driscoli, R., Simeoni, E., Dudler, J., von Segesser, L.K., Kappenberger, L., Vassalli, G. (2004). Helper-dependent adenovirus vectors devoid of all viral genes cause less myocardial inflammation compared with first-generation adenovirus vectors. *Basic Res Cardiol* 99:247-258.

French, B.A., Mazur, W., Geske, R.S., Bolli, R. (1994). Direct in vivo transfer to porcine myocardium using replication-deficient adenoviral vectors. *Circulation* 90:2412-2424.

Fromes, Y., Salmon, A., Wang, X., Collin, H., Rouche, A., Hagege, A., Schwartz, K., Fiszman, M.Y. (1999). Gene delivery to the myocardium by intraperitoneal injection. *Gene Ther* 6:683-688.

Guzman, R.J., Lemarchand, P., Crystal, R.G., Epstein, S.E., Finkel, T. (1993). Efficient gene transfer into myocardium by dierct injection of adenovirus vectors. *Circ Res* 73:1202-1207.

Hagikura, K., Fukuda, N., Yokoyama, S., Yuxin, L., Kusumi, Y., Matsumoto, T., Ikeda, Y., Kunimoto, S., Takayama, T., Jumabay, M., Mitsumata, M., Saito, S., Hirayama, A., Mugishima, H. (2010). Low invasive angiogenic therapy for myocardial infarction by retrograde transplantation of mononuclear cells expressing the VEGF gene. *Int J Cardiol* 142:56-64.

Hayase, M., del Monte, F., Kawase, Y., MacNeill, B.D., McGregor, J., Yoneyama, R., Hoshino, K., Tsuji, T., De Grand, A.M., Gwathmey, J.K., Frangioni, J.V., Hajjar, R.J. (2005). Catheter-based antegrade intracoronary viral gene delivery with coronary Venous blockade. *Am J Physiol* 288:H2995-H3000.

Huang, J., Zhang, Z., Guo, J., Ni, A., Deb, A., Zghang, L., Mirotsou, M., Pratt, R.E., Dzau, V.J. (2010). Genetic modification of mesenchymal stem cells overexpressing CCR1 increases cell viability, migration, engratfment, and capillary density in the injured myocardium. *Circ Res* 106:1753-1762.

Inagaki, K., Fuess, S., Storm, T.A., Gibson, G.A., Mctiernen, C.F., Kay, M.A., Nakai, H. (2006). Robust systemic transduction with AAV9 vectors in mice; Efficient global cardiac gene transfer superior to that of AAV8. *Molecular Therapy* 14:45-53.

Isner, J.M. (2002). Myocardial gene therapy. *Nature* 415:234-239.

Jayasankar, V., Woo, Y.J., Bish, L.T., Pirolli, T.J., Chatterjee, S., Berry, M.F., Burdick, J., Gardner, T.J., Sweeney, H.L. (2003). Gene transfer of hepatocyte growth factor attenuates postinfarction heart failure. *Circulation* 108 Supl1:I1230-1236.

Jayasankar, V., Woo, Y.J., Bish, L.T., Pirolli, T.J., Berry, M.F., Burdick, J., Bhalla, R.C., Sharma, R.V., Gardner, T.J., Sweeney, H.L. (2004). Inhibition of matrix metalloproteinase activity by TIMP-1 gene transfer effectively treats ischemic cardiomyopathy. *Circulation* 110 Supl1:I1180-1186.

Jo, J., Nagaya, N., Miyhara, Y., Kataoka, M., Harada-Shiba, M., Kangawa, K., Tabata, Y. (2007). Transplantation of genetically engineered mesenchymal stem cells improves cardiac function in rats with myocardial infarction: benefit of a nonviral vector, cationized dextran. *Tissue Eng* 13:313-322.

Kaplitt, M.G., Xiao, X., Samulski, R.J., Li, J., Ojamaa, K., Klein, I.L., Makimura, H., Kaplitt, M.J., Strumpf, R.K., Diethrich, E.B. (1996). Long-term gene transfer in porcine myocardium after coronary infusion of an adeno-associated virus vector. *Ann Thorac Surg* 62-1669-1676.

Kaspar, B.K., Roth, D.M., Lai, N.C., Drumm, J.D., Erickson, D.A., McKirnan, M.D., Hammond, H.K. (2005). Myocardial gene transfer and long-term expression following intracoronary delivery of adeno-associated virus. *J Gene Medicine* 7:316-324.

Katz, M.G., Swain, J.D., Tomasulo, C.E., Sumaroka, M., Fargnoli, A., Bridges, C.R. (2011). Current strategies for myocardial gene delivery. *J Mol Cell Cardiol* epub ahead of print

Kim, H.K., Moon, H.H., Kim, H.A., Hwang, K.C., Lee, M., Choi, D. (2011). Hypoxia-inducible vascular endothelial growth factor –engineered mesenchymal stem cells prevent myocardial ischemic injury. *Molecular Therapy* 19:741-750.

Kinnaird, T., Stabile, E., Burnett, M.S., Shou, M., Lee, C.W., Barr, S., Fuchs, S., Epstein, S.E. (2004). Local delivery of marrow-derived stromal cells augments collateral perfusion through paracrine mechanisms. *Circulation* 109:1543-1549.

Kochner, A.A., Schuster, M.D., Szaboics, M.J. (2001). Neovascularization of ischemic myocardium by human bone-marrow-derived angioblasts prevents cardiomyocyte apoptosis, reduces remodeling and improves cardiac function. *Nat Med* 7:430-436.

Kratsios, P., Catela, C., Salimova, E., Huth, M., Berno, V., Rosenthal, N., Mourkioti, F.(2010). Distinct roles for cell-autonomous Notch signalling in cardiomyocytes of the embryonic and adult heart. *Circ Res* 106:559-572.

Kusano, K.F., Pola, R., Murayama, T., Curry, C., Kawamoto, A., Iwakura, A., Shintani, S., Li, M., Asai, J., Tkebuchava, T., Thorne, T., Takenaka, H., Aikawa, R., Goukassian, D., von Samson, P., Hamada, H., Yoon, Y.S., Silver, M., Eaton, E., Ma, H., Heyd, L., Kearney, M., Munger, W., Porter, J.A., Kishore, R., Losordo, D.W. (2005). Sonic hedgehog myocardial gene therapy; tissue repair through transient reconstitution of embryonic signalling. *Nat Med* 11:1197-1204.

Kutschka, I., Kofidis, T., Chen, I.Y., von Degenfeld, G., Zwierzchoniewska, M., Hoyt, G., Lebl, D.R., Hendry, S.L., Sheikh, A.Y., Cooke, D.T., Connolly, A., Blau, H.M., Gambhir, S.S., Robbins, R.C. (2006). Adenoviral human BCL-2 transgene expression attenuates early donorcell death after cardiomyoblast transplantation into ischemic rat hearts. *Circulation* 114:174-178.

Lai, N.C., Roth, D.M., Gao, M.H., Tang, T., Dalton, N., Lai, Y.Y., Spellman, M., Clopton, P., Hammond, H.K. (2004). Intracoronary adenovirus encoding adenylyl cyclase VI increases left ventricular function in heart failure. *Circulation* 110:330-336.

Lavu, M., Gundewar, S., Lefer, D.J. (2011). Gene therapy for ischemic heart disease. *J Mol Cell Cardiol* 50:742-750.

Li, Q., Guo, Y., Tan, W., Stein, A.B., Dawn, B., Wu, W.J., Zhu, X., Lu, X., Xu, X., Siddiqui, T., Tiwari, S., Bolli, R. (2006). Gene therapy with iNOS provides long-term protection against myocardial infarction without adverse functional consequences. *Am J Physiol* 290:H584-589.

Li, Q., Guo, Y., Tan, W., Ou, G., Wu, W.J., Sturza, D., Dawn, B., Hunt, G., Cui, C., Bolli, R. (2007). Cardioprotection afforded by inducible nitric oxide synthase gene therapy is mediated by cyclooxygenase-2 via a nuclear factor-kappaB dependent pathway. *Circulation* 116:1577-1584.

Li, W., Ma, N., Ong, L.L., Nesselmann, C., Klopsch, C., Ladilov, Y., Furlani, D., Piechaczek, C., Moebius, J.M., Lützow, K., Lendlein, A., Stamm, C., Li, R.K., Steinhoff, G. (2007). Bcl-2 engineered MSCs inhibited apoptosis and improved heart function. *Stem Cells* 8:2118-2127.

Lin, H., Parmacek, M.S., Morle, G., Bolling, S., Leiden, J.M. (1990). Expression of recombinant genes in myocardium in vivo after direct injection of DNA. *Circulation* 82:2217-2221.

Logeart, D., Hatem, S.N., Heimburger, M., Roux, A.L., Michel, J.B., Mercadier, J.J. (2001). How to optimize in vivo gene transfer to cardiac myocytes: mechanical or pharmacological procedures? *Hum Gene Ther* 12:1601-1610.

Lyon, A.R., Sato, M., Hajjar, R.J., Samulski, R.J., Harding, S.E. (2008). Gene therapy: Targeting the myocardium. *Heart* 94:89-99.

Maines, M.D., Trakshel, G.M., Kutty, R.K. (1986). Characterization of two constitutive forms of rat liver microsomal heme oxygenase; only one molecular species of the enzyme is inducible. *J Biol Chem* 261: 411-419.

Magovern, C.J., Mack, C.A., Zhang, J., Hahn, R.T., Ko, W., Isom, O.W., Crystal, R.G., Rosengart, T.K. (1996). Direct in vivo gene transfer to canine myocardioum using a replication-deficient adenoviral vector. *Ann Thorac Surg* 62:425-433.

Mangi, A.A., Noiseux, N., Kong, D., He, H., Rezvani, M., Ingwall, J.S., Dzau, V.J. (2003). Mesenchymal stem cells modified with Akt prevent remodeling and restore performance of infarcted hearts. *Nat Med* 9:1195-1201.

March, K.L., Woody, M., Mehdi, K., Zipes, D.P., Bradtly, M., Trapnell, B.C. (1999). Efficient in vivo catheter-based pericardial gene transfer mediated by adenoviral vectors. *Clin Cardiol* 22:123-129.

Mathiesen, I., Lømo, T. (1999). Electropermeabilization of skeletal muscle enhances gene transfer in vivo. *Gene Ther* 6:508-14.

Melo, L.G., Agrawal, R., Zhang, L., Rezvani, M., Mangi, A.A., Ehsan, A., Griese, D.P., Dell'Acqua, G., Mann, M.J., Oyama, J., Yet, S.F., Layne, M.D., Perrella, M.A., Dzau, V.J. (2002). Gene therapy strategy for long-term myocardial protection using adeno-associated virus-mediated delivery of heme oxygenase gene. *Circulation* 105:602-607.

Murry, C.E., Jennings, R.B., Reimer, K.A. (1986). Preconditioning with ischemia: a delay in lethal injury in ischemic myocardium. *Circulation* 74: 1124-1136.

Murry, C.E., Soonpaa, M.H., Reinecke, H., Nakajima, H., Rubart, M., Pasumarthi, K.B., Virag, J.I., Bertelmez, S.H., Poppa, V., Bradford, G., Dowell, J.D., Williams, D.A., Field, L.J. (2004). Haematopoietic stem cells do not transdifferentiate into cardiac myoblasts in myocardial infarcts. *Nature* 428:664-668.

Noiseux, N., Gnecchi, M., Lopez-Ilasaca, M., Zhang, L., Solomon, S.D., Deb, A., Dzau, V.J., Pratt, R.E. (2006). Mesenchymal stem cells overexpressing Akt dramatically repair infarcted myocardium and improve cardiac function despite infrequent cellular fusion or differentiation. *Mol Ther* 14:840-850.

Novotny, N.M., Ray, R., Markel, T.A., Crisostomo, P.R., Wang, M., Meldrum, D.R. (2008). Stem cell therapy in myocardial repair and remodelling. *J Am Coll Surg* 207:423-434.

Pacak, C.A., Mah, C.S., Thattaliyath, B.D., Conlon, T.J., Lewis, M.A., Cloutier, D.E., Zolotukhin, I., Tarantal, A.F., Byrne, B.J. (2006). Recombinant adeno-associated virus serotype 9 leads to preferential cardiac transduction in vivo. *Circ Res* 99:e3-e9.

Pepe, M., Mamdani, M., Zentilin, L., Csiszar, A., Qanud, K., Zacchigna, S., Ungvari, Z., Puliqadda, U., Moimas, S., Edwards, J.G., Hintze, T.H., Giacca, M., Recchia, F.A. (2010). Intramyocardial VEGF-B167 gene delivery delays the progression towards congestive failure in dogs with pacing-induced dilated cardiomyopathy. *Circ Res* 106:1893-1903.

Przyklenk, K., Bauer, B., Ovize, M., Kloner, R.A., Whittaker, P. (1993). Regional ischemic 'preconditioning' protects remote virgin myocardium from subsequent sustained coronary occlusion. *Circulation* 87:893-899.

Rengo, G., Lymperopoulus, A., Zincarelli, C., Donniacuo, M., Soltys, S., Rabinowitz, J.E., Koch, W.J. (2009). Myocardial adeno-associated virus serotype 6-betaARKct gene therapy improves cardiac function and normalizes the neurohormonal axis in chronic heart failure. *Circulation* 119:89-98.

Rong, S.L., Lu, Y.X., Wang, X.L., Wang, Y.J., Chang, C., Wang, Y.Q., Liu, Q.Y., Gao, Y.Z., Mi, S.H. (2008). Effects of transplanted myoblasts transfected with human growth hormone gene on improvement of ventricular function of rats. *Chin Med J* 121:347-354.

Rysä, J., Tenhunen, O., Serpi, R., Soini, Y., Nemer, M., Leskinen, H., Ruskoaho, H. (2010). GATA-4 is an angigenic survival factor of the infarcted heart. *Circ Heart Fail* 3:440-450.

Sakoda, T., Kasahara, N., Kedes, L., Ohyanagi, M.. (2007). Lentiviral vector-mediated gene transfer to endothelial cells compared with adenoviral and retroviral vectors. *Prep Biochem Biotechnol* 37:1-11.

Semenza, G. (2004). O2-regulated gene expression: transcriptional control of cardio-respiratory physiology by HIF-1. *J Appl Physiol* 96:1173-1177.

Sen, S., Merchan, J., Dean, J., Li, M., Gavin, M., Silver, M., Tkebuchava, T., Yoon, Y.S., Rasko, J.E.J., Aikawa, R. (2010). Autologous transplantation of endothelial progenitor cells genetically modified by adeno-associated viral vector delivering insulin-like growth factor-1 gene after myocardial infarction. *Human Gene Therapy* 21;1327-1334.

Serpi, R., Tolonen, A.M., Huusko, J., Rysä, J., Tenhunen, O., Ylä-Herttuala, S., Ruskoaho, H. (2011). Vascular endothelial growth factor-B gene transfer prevents angiotensin II-induced diastolic dysfunction via proliferation and capillary dilatation in rats. *Cardiovasc Res* 89:204-213.

Silva, G.V., Livotsky, S., Assad, J.A., Sousa, A.L., Martin, B.J., Vela, D., Coulter, S.C., Lin, J., Ober, J., Vaughn, W.K., Branco, R.V., Oliveira, E.M., He, R., Geng, Y.J., Willerson, J.T., Perin, E.C. (2005). Mesenchymal stem cells differentiate into an endothelial phenotype, enhance vascular density, and improve heart function in a canine chronic ischemia model. *Circulation* 111:150-156.

Song, M.B., Yu, X.J., Zhu, G.X., Chen, J.F., Zhao, G., Huang, L. (2009). Transfection of HGF gene enhances endothelial progenitor cell (EPC) function and improves EPC transplant efficiency for balloon-induced arterial injury in hypercholesterolemic rats. *Vascul Pharmacol* 51:205-213.

Suckau, L., Fechner, H., Chemaly, E., Krohn, S., Hadri, L., Kockskämper, J., Westerman, D., Bisping, E., Ly, H., Wang, X., Kawase, Y., Chen, J., Liang, L., Sipo, I., Vetter, R., Weger, S., Kurreck, J., Erdmann, V., Tschope, C., Pieske, B., Lebeche, D., Schultheiss, H.-P., Hajjar, R.J., Poller, W.C. (2009). Long-term cardiac-targeted RNA interference for the teratment of heart failure restores cardiac function and reduces pathological hypertrophy. *Circulation* 119:1241-1252.

Stocker, R., Yamamoto, Y., McDonagh, A.F., Glazer, A.N., Ames, B.N. (1987). Bilirubin is an antioxidant of possible physiological importance. *Science* 235: 1043-1046.

Sun, L., Cui, M., Wang, Z., Feng, X., Mao, J., Chen, P., Kangtao, M., Chen, F., Zhou, C. (2007). Mesenchymal stem cells modified with angiopoietin-1 improve remodelling in a rat model of acute myocardial infarction. *Biochem Biophys Res Commun* 357:779-784.

Svensson, E.C., Marshall, D.J., Woodard, K., Lin, H., Jiang, F., Chu, L., Leiden, J.M. (1999). Efficient and stable transduction of cardiomyocytes after intramyocardial injection or intracoronary perfusion with recombinant adeno-associated virus vectors. *Circulation* 99:201-205.

Tang, Y.L., Tang, Y., Zhang, Y.C., Qian, K., Shen, L., Phillips, M.I. (2005). Improved graft mesenchymal stem cell survival in ischemic heart with a hypoxia-regulated heme oxygenase-1 vector. *J Am Coll Cardiol* 46:1339-1350.

Tomiyasu. K., Oda, Y., Nomura, M., Satoh, E., Fushiki, S., Imanishi, J., Kondo, M., Mazda, O. (2000). Direct intracardiomuscular transfer of b2-adrenergic receptor gene augments cardiac output in cardiomyopathic hamsters. *Gene Ther* 7:2087-2093.

Treschner, K., Bernecker, O., Fellner, B., Gyöngösi, M., Krieger, S., Demartin, R., Wolner, E., Podesser, B.K. (2004). Adenovirus-mediated overexpression of inhibitor kappa B-alpha attenuates postinfarct remdoeling in the rat heart. *Eur J Cardiothorac Surg* 26:960-967.

Verma ,A., Hirsch, D.J., Glatt, C.E., Ronnett, G.V., Snyder, S.H. (1993). Carbon monoxide: a putitative neural messenger. *Science* 259: 381-384.

Vinge, L.E., Raake, P.W., Koch, W. (2008). Gene therapy in heart failure. *Circ Res* 102:1458-1470.

Volpers, C., Kochanek, S. (2004). Adenoviral vectors for gene transfer and therapy. *J Gen Med* 6(suppl 1):S164-S171).

Wand, D., Shen, W., Zhang, F., Chen, M., Chen, H., Cao, K. (2010). Connexin-43 promotes survival of mesenchymal stem cells in ischaemic heart. *Cell Biol Int* 34:415-423.

Wang, M., Tan, J., Meldrum, K.K., Dinarello, C.A., Meldrum, D.R. (2009). IL-18 binding protein-expressing mesenchymal stem cells improve myocardial protection after ischemia or infarction. *Proc Natl Acad Sci* 106:17499-17504.

Wang, X., Zhao, T., Huang, W., Wang, T., Qian, J., Xu, M., Kranias, E.G., Wang, Y., Fan, G.C. (2009). Hsp20-engineered mesenchymal stem cells are resistant to oxidative stress via enhanced activation of Akt and increased secretion of growth factors. *Stem Cells* 12:3021-3031.

Woo, Y.J., Panlilio, C.M., Cheng, R.K., Liao, G.P., Atluri, P., Hsu, V.M., Cohen, J.E., Chaudry, H.W. (2006). Therapeutic delivery of cyclin A2 induces myocardial regeneration and enhances cardiac function in ischemic heart failure. *Circulation* 114(Supl.1):I206-213.

Wu, M.-L., Ho, Y.-C., Yet, S.-F. (2011). A central role of heme oxygenase-1 in cardiovascular protection. *Antioxidants & Redox signalling* ;epub ahead of print.

Yoshimitsu, M., Higuchi, K., Dawood, F., Rasaiah, V.I., Ayach, B., Chen, M., Liu, P., Medin, J.A. (2006). Correction of cardiac abnormalities in fabry mice by direct intraventricular injection of a recombinant lentiviral vector that engineers expression of alpha-galactosidase A. *Circ J* 70:1503-1508.

Zancarelli, C., Soltys, S., Rengo, G., Rabinowitz, J.E. (2008). Analysis of AAV serotypes 1-9 mediated expression and tropism in mice after systemic injection. *Mol Ther* 16:1073-1080.

Zentilin, L., Puligadda, U., Lionetti, V., Zacchigna, S., Collesi, C., Pattarini, L., Ruozi, G., Camporesi, S., Sinagra, G., Pepe, M., Recchia, F.A., Giacca, M. (2010). Cardiomyocyte VEGFR-1 activation by VEGF-B induces compensatory hypertrophy and preserves cardiac function after myocardial infarction. *FASEB J* 24:1467-1478.

Zhang, J.C.L., Woo, Y.J., Swain, J.L., Sweeney, H.L. (1999). Efficient transmural cardiac gene transfer by intrapericardial injection in neonatal mice. *J Mol Cell Cardiol* 31:721-732.

Zincarelli, C., Soltys, S., Rengo, G., Rabinowitz, J.E. (2008). Analysis of AAV seroptypes 1-9 mediated gene expression and tropism in mice after systemic injection. *Molecular Therapy* 16:1073-1080.

Zhao, Z.Q., Corvera, J.S., Halkos, M.E., Kerendi, F., Wang, N.P., Guyton, R.A., Vinten-Jonasen, J. (2003). Inhibition of myocardial injury by ischemic postconditioning during reperfusion: comparison with ischemic preconditioning. *Am J Physiol Heart Circ Physiol* 285:H579-88.

Zhao, X.Y., Hu, S.J., li, J., Mou, Y., Chan, C.F., Jin, J., Sun, J., Zhu, Z.H. (2006). rAAV-mediated angiogenin gene transfer induces angiogenesis and modifies left ventricular remodeling in rats with myocardial infarction. *J Mol Med* 84:1033-1046.

19

Transplantation of Sendai Viral Angiopoietin-1-Modified Mesenchymal Stem Cells for Ischemic Heart Disease

Jianhua Huang[1,4], Huishan Wang[2] and Hirofumi Hamada[3]
[1]Department of Cardiothoracic Surgery, Ningxia People's Hospital, YinChuan,
[2]Department of Cardiac Surgery, Shenyang Northern Hospital, ShenYang,
[3]Department of Molecular Medicine, Sapporo Medical University, Sapporo,
[4]Department of Tissue Engineering, LiaoNing Medical University, Jinzhou,
[1,2,4]China
[3]Japan

1. Introduction

Ischemic heart disease is one of the major threatens to human heath. Despite great advances in the treatment of it, the cardiac infarction caused by heart ischemia still represents a significant cause of morbidity and mortality. Recently, MSCs therapy has been emerged as one of the potential treatments for ischemic heart disease [1-4]. Although MSCs can differentiate into endothelial [5], cardiac cell [6], and secret a range of cytokines [7], there are mounting evidences which showed paracrine effect is the major mechanism for the therapeutic effect of MSCs in the ischemic heart [8-10]. Thus, the supplement of genes that can enhance angiogenesis or cell survival is one of the attractive strategies for MSCs therapy [11].

The Ang-1 has been reported to improve angiogenesis in ischemic heart [12,13]. Ang-1 has also been found as an apoptotic survival factor [14-16]. Therefore, the combination of Ang-1 gene and MSCs would be an alternative method to enhance the effects of MSCs. However, when performing the combination of Ang-1 gene and MSCs therapy, a vector that has high transductive efficiency to MSCs is needed.

Sendai virus is a murine parainfluenza virus type I, and is a single-stranded RNA virus. Sendai virus is considered to be non-pathogenic to humans [17]. Efficient gene transduction into various primary cultured cells and tissues by recombinant virus vector has been reported [18-22]. Furthermore, it replicates in the cytoplasma and poses no risk of integration into the genomic DNA. These characteristics of the Sendai virus make it a potential vector for combined gene and cell therapy.

In our previously study, we found Sendai viral vector (SeV) has high transductive efficiency to MSCs even at low MOI [23]. To further investigate its clinical practicality, we infected SeV to the MSCs in vitro at low MOI with short time exposure. We also injected MSCs modified with SeVhAng-1 into the ischemic heart of rats to investigate its effect on angiogenesis and engraftment of MSCs in the ischemic heart.

2. Materials and methods

2.1 Animals

Lewis rats were obtained from the Animal Research Centre of the Fourth Military Medical University, Xi'an (China) and maintained on a 12-hour light: 12-hour dark in a 20–25°C environment. The Ethics Committee for Animal Experiments of the Fourth Military Medical University approved all animal work (Permit number: 20531) and the experimental protocols strictly complied with the institutional guidelines and the criteria outlined in the "Guide for Care and Use of Laboratory Animals".

2.2 Sendai virus vectors

Sendai virus vectors containing the E.coli β-galactosidase gene (SeVLacZ) or the human angiopoietin-1 gene (SeVhAng-1) were used [24]. For the construction of genomic cDNA of SeVhAng1, the human Ang-1 open reading frame was cloned from a human cDNA library and amplified using the polymerase chain reaction with primers containing SeV-specific transcriptional regulation signal sequences: 5'-TTGCGGCCGCCAAAGTTCAATGACAGTTTTCCTTTCCTTTCCTCTCTG-3'a nd5'ATTGCGGCCGCGATGAACTTTCACCCTAAGTTTTTCTTACTACGGTCAAAAATCT AAAGTTCGAATCATCATAGTTGTGGAACG-3', and was subsequently inserted into the NotI site of pSeV18+b(+) [25] to generate pSeVhAng-1. The pSeVhAng-1 was transfected into LLC-MK2 cells previously infected with vaccinia virus vTF7-3 [26], which expresses T7 polymerase. The T7-drived full-length recombinant SeVhAng-1 RNA genomes were encapsulated with N, P and L proteins, which were derived from the respective cotransfected plasmids. Forty hours later, the transfected cells were injected into 10 day-old embryonated chicken eggs to amplify the recovered virus [27]. The Sendai virus titer was determined by a hemagglutination assay using chicken red blood cells, and the virus was stored at -70 °C until use.

2.3 MSCs source

MSCs cultures were prepared according to the protocol reported previously. Briefly, under sterile conditions, the femur and tibia of 2 month-old male Lewis rats were excised, with special attention given to remove all connective tissue attached to bones. Bone marrow plugs were extracted from the bones by flushing the bone marrow cavity with Dulbecco's modified Eagle's medium (DMEM). Marrow plug suspension was dispersed by passing it through subsequent pipettes of decreasing sizes. After a homogenous cell suspension was achieved, the cells were plated, cultured in DMEM containing 10% fetal bovine serum, and incubated at 37°C humidified atmosphere with 5% CO_2 for 3 days before the first medium change.

2.4 In vitro SeV transduction

After 70% confluence of cultured MSCs in the dish, SeVLacZ at 10 MOI were infected to the MSCs with different time exposure (1 minute to 60 minutes). After 48 hr, both chmiluminescent assay of MSCs infected with SeVLacZ at 10 MOI with different time exposure and X-gal staining of MSCs infected with SeVLacZ at 10 MOI with 1 minute exposure were performed as previous described [28].

2.5 Expression of hAng-1 in MSCs by SeVhAng-1 transduction

Human Ang-1 expression in MSCs was detected after 2 days of transduction with SeVhAng-1 by Western blot. MSCs were washed twice with cold PBS and suspended in a cold lysis buffer (20 mmol/L HEPES, pH 7.5, 150 mmol/L NaCl, 1 mmol/L EDTA, 0.5% Triton X-100, protease inhibitors [complete, Roche]). Similar quantities of the soluble fractions (20μg) were separated by SDS-PAGE, transferred onto nitrocellulose membranes, and blocked overnight in blocking solution at 4°C. The membranes were incubated for 1 hr with mouse anti-human monoclonal antibodies to Ang-1 (Santa Cruz Biotechnology), followed by anti-mouse secondary antibody conjugated to horseradish peroxidase (Zymed, Inc., South San Francisco, CA) for 1 hr at room temperature. An enhanced chemiluminescence substrate system ECL Plus (Amersham Biosciences UK, Little Chalfont, UK) was used to visualize HRP. The ß-actin protein levels were assayed as the internal control.

2.6 Animal model

Lewis rats (female, weight 200-250 g) were used in the experiment. The rat was anesthetized with IP injection of ketamine(100mg/kg) and xylizine (10mg/kg), and intubated with a 17-gague needle sheath. After intubation, the rat was supported with a rodent respirator. A left lateral thoractomy was made, the heart was exposed and LAD was ligated with 6-0 suture [12]. Immediately after LAD ligation, $5x10^{6}$ MSCs were injected into the heart at 2 sites of peri-infarct area of the heart.

2.7 Evaluation of heart function

After 4 weeks of LAD ligation, the heart function was evaluated by echocardiography as previously described [29]. FS was used as a main index for the evaluation of heart function.

2.8 Evaluation of infarct size

We evaluated the infarct size of the heart as previously described [12]. Four weeks after myocardial infarction, rats were deeply anesthetized with inhalation of diethyl ether, injected with a mixture of ketamine hydrochloride (50 mg/kg) and xylazine (4 mg/kg), and killed by rapid exision of the heart. The excised hearts were immediately soaked in cold saline for 10s to remove excess blood from the ventricles and fixed in neutral-buffered 4% formalin for 48 h. Paraffin-embedded samples were sectioned at 10 μm, and Masson's trichrome staining was performed to delineate scar tissue from viable myocardium. Masson's trichrome-stained sections were captured as digital images and analyzed by NIH Image software.

2.9 Capillary density measurement

After 28 days of LAD ligation, the heart was harvest and snap-frozen in liquid nitrogen. Cryosections of 10 μm were made. The endothelial cells were stained with anti-CD31 monoclonal antibody (Pharmingen) as first antibody, followed by a biotinylated anti-mouse IgG as second antibody, and an avidin-HRP conjugate for color reaction (DAB paraffin IHC staining module, Ventana Medical Systems, Inc., Tucson, AZ). The sections were observed under microscope, 5 fields were randomly selected in the peri-infarct area of each section, and CD31-positive cells were counted in a blinded manner. The number of CD 31-positive cells in each field was used as an index of capillary density.

2.10 Analysis of Ang-1 expression and its effect on p-Akt in the ischemic heart

We injected MSCs modified with or without SeVhAng-1 into the ischemic heart of the rats and determined the effect of Ang-1 overexpression on p-Akt as previously described. In brief, after 2 days injection of MSCs modified with or without SeVhAng-1 into the ischemic heart, the heart was harvested and put into 4 ml lysis buffer, and incubated for 5 min on ice. The cardiac muscle was homogenized with a mixing homogenizer (Kinematica AG, Littau switzerland). The homogenates were heated at 95 °C for 10 min and centrifuged at 12,000g for 10 min. After determination of protein concentration in supernatants by BCA methods, total protein (40 μg) was subjected to SDS page in 5-20% Tris-glycine gels, subsequently transferred to nitrocellulose membranes and blocked overnight in blocking solution at 4°C. The membranes were incubated for 1 hr with mouse anti-human monoclonal antibodies to Ang-1 (Santa Cruz Biotechnology), p-Akt (ser473) and t-Akt (Signaling Technology, Beverly, MA) followed by anti-mouse secondary antibody conjugated to horseradish peroxidase (Zymed, Inc., South San Francisco, CA) or anti-rabbit secondary antibody conjugated to horseradish peroxidase (Amersham Biosciences UK, Buckinghamshire, England) for 1 hr at room temperature. An enhanced chemiluminescence substrate system ECL Plus (Amersham Biosciences UK, Little Chalfont, UK) was used to visualize HRP.

2.11 TUNEL staining

After 2 days injection of MSCs modified with or without SeVhAng-1, the heart was harvested, and cryosections were cut and randomly selected for TUNEL staining as described by manufacture (Roche).

2.12 Real-time polymerase chain reaction for MSCs survival in the ischemic heart

Real-time PCR was performed to detect Y-chromosomal DNA in the ischemic heart of female rat injected with male MSCs as previously reported [30]. In brief, after 2 days of MSCs injection, the heart was harvested, the DNA of the tissue was extracted with the Qiagen Kit (Qiagen, Mississauga, Ontario, Canada). Real-time PCR was performed with SYBR-Green (Applied Biosystems, Foster City, Calif). The SYBR-Green I dye binds to the double-stranded product, resulting in an increase in fluorescence detected by the ABI 7900HT Sequence Detection System (Applied Biosystems). A specific sequence of rat Sry3 gene in the Y chromosome was targeted. The genomic DNA taken from male MSCs was used to obtain a standard curve. The primer pairs were 5'-GCA TTT ATG GTG TGG TCC CGC GG-3' and 5'-GGC ACT TTA ACC CTT CGA TGA GGC-3'. The cycling conditions were 5 minutes at 50°C, 10 minutes at 95°C for activation of polymerase, and then 30 seconds at 95°C for denaturation, 60 seconds at 62°C inducing annealing, and 30 seconds at 72°C for extension. Forty-five cycles were used. After amplification, dissociation curves were obtained to discriminate between specific and nonspecific products.

2.13 Statistical analysis

Data were expressed as means ± standard deviations (SD). Statistical comparisons were performed using ANOVA followed by Bonferroni/Dunn testing. A p value less than 0.05 was considered to be statistically significant.

3. Results

3.1 Transductive efficiency of SeV to the MSCs

To determine the transductive efficiency of SeV to MSCs, we infected SeVLacZ to MSCs at 10 MOI with 1 minute exposure, and performed X-Gal staining after 48 h of infection. The results showed that Sendai viral vector almost had 100% transductive efficiency to MSCs even at 10 MOI with 1 mintue exposure. We also performed time course effect of the Sendai viral vector on the transductive efficiency to the MSC by chemiluminescent assay. Interestingly, we found that Sendai viral vector almost had the same protein expression at every time point checked (1 minute to 60 minutes). This indicates Sendai viral vector is ideal candidate for combined gene and cell therapy in clinical practice for its high transductive efficiency at low MOI with short time exposure.

3.2 SeVhAng-1 transduction to MSCs mediated efficient Ang-1 expression

To determine the expression of hAng-1 by SeVhAng-1-modified MSCs, Western blot were performed. We used a human Ang-1 antibody which has cross reaction with rat Ang-1 for Western blot. The result showed an obviously increased expression of Ang-1 in MSCs modified with SeVhAng-1.

3.3 SeVhAng-1-modified MSCs injection decreased heart infarction and improved cardiac function after LAD ligation

After 4 weeks of LAD ligation, the cardiac function was evaluated by echo. The FS was 39.0 ± 3.5, 32.0 ± 2.8 and 21.1 ± 3.3 in the SeVhAng-1-modified MSCs-, MSCs- and medium-treated groups, respectively, and there was a significant difference between the SeVhAng-1-modified MSCs and the medium ($p<0.01$), there was also a significant difference between SeVhAng-1-modified MSCs and sole MSCs ($p<0.05$). We then sacrificed rats after 4 weeks, the hearts were harvested, and Masson's trichrome staining was performed. The infarct size was 24.5 ± 4.8%, 32.5 ± 4.4% and 42.5 ± 5.1% in the SeVhAng-1-modified MSCs-, MSCs- and medium-treated groups, respectively, and there was a significant difference between the SeVhAng-1-modified MSCs and the medium ($p<0.01$), there was also a significant difference between SeVhAng-1-modified MSCs and sole MSCs ($p<0.05$).

3.4 SeVhAng-1-modified MSCs injection increased capillary density in ischemic heart

After 28 days of SeVhAng-1-modified MSCs injection, the immunostaining of CD31 on the cryosections of the cardiac muscle was carried out. The capillary density was 204.8 ± 18.3, 150.2 ±1 6.2 and 77.4 ± 13.8 per field in the SeVhAng-1-modified MSCs-, MSCs- and medium-treated groups, respectively, and there was a significant difference between the SeVhAng-1-modified MSCs and the medium($p<0.01$), there was also a significant difference between SeVhAng-1-modified MSCs and sole MSCs ($p<0.05$).

3.5 Overexpression of Ang-1 increased p-Akt and decreased apoptosis in the ischemic heart

MSCs secrete numerous cytokines and growth factors in hypoxic condition. However, the Ang-1 secretion is not obvious elevated [10,31]. Thus, we inferred that Ang-1, which is secreted by SeVhAng-1-modified MSCs, would play some role during early period of cardiac infarction. To prove this, we injected MSCs modified with or without SeVhAng-1 into the ischemic heart of rats. First, we determined by Western blot whether the overexpression of Ang-1 by MSCs had an effect on the expression of p-Akt in the ischemic heart. The result showed that p-Akt expression obviously increased in ischemic heart treated by SeVhAng-1-modified MSCs, compared with that by sole MSCs. Because activated Akt has the effect of anti-apoptosis, we further determined whether increased p-Akt decreases apoptosis in the ischemic heart. We found that overexpression of Ang-1 by SeVhAng-1-modified MSCs decreased the apoptosis which may include endothelial cells, cardiac myocytes or MSCs in the ischemic heart, compared with that by sole MSCs. We further determined whether increased p-Akt improves survival of MSCs injected into the ischemic heart. By real time detection of *sry* gene in the female heart tissue samples at 2 days after sex-mismatched cell transplantation, We found that overexpression of Ang-1 by SeVhAng-1-modified MSCs significantly improved survival of MSCs per se in the ischemic heart ($p<0.01$), compared with that by sole MSCs.

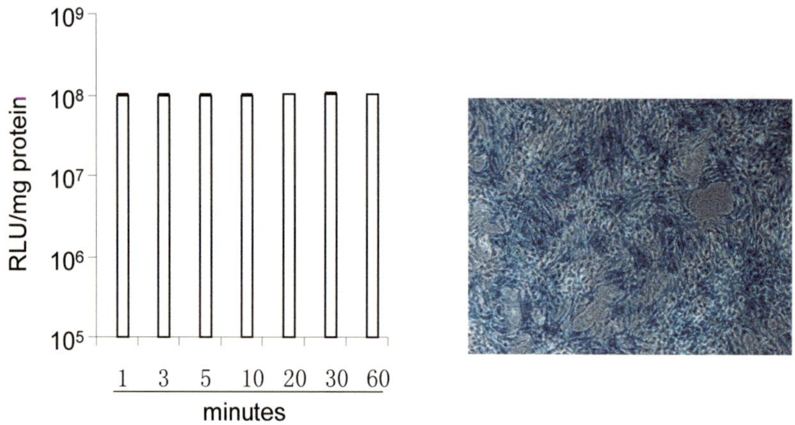

Fig. 1. Transductive efficiency of Sendai viral vector to MSCs. A, MSCs were infected with 10 MOI SeVLacZ with different time exposure, the chemiluminescent assay showed Sendai viral vector had high transductive efficiency to MSCs even with short time exposure, and 1 minute exposure by SeVLacZ almost had the same transductive efficiency to the MSCs as 60 minutes exposure did. B, X-gal staining of MSCs infected with 10 MOI Sendai viral vector.

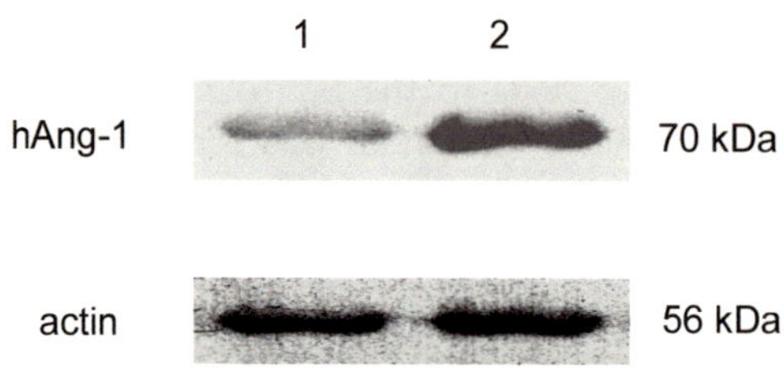

Fig. 2. SeVhAng-1 mediated efficient hAng-1 expression in MSCs. Representative Western blot detection of hAng-1 expression after 10 MOI SeVhAng-1 infected to the MSCs with 1 minute exposure. Lane 1, MSCs without transduction of SeVhAng-1; lane 2, MSCs with transduction of SeVhAng-1. The experiments were repeated 3 times.

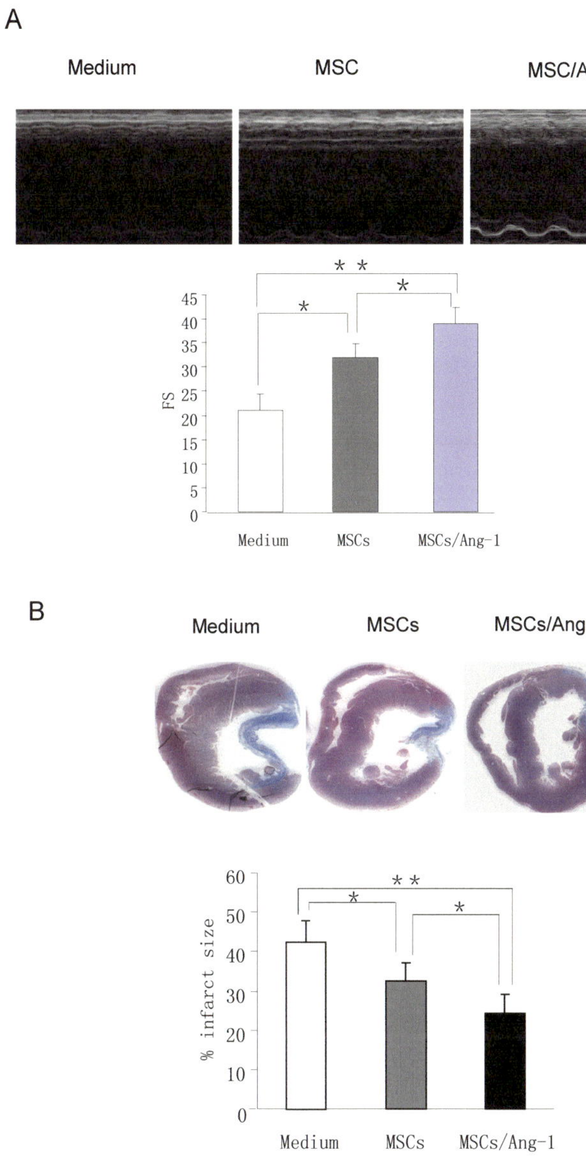

Fig. 3. Effect of SeVhAng-1 modified MSCs on heart with LAD liagation. A, representive echo measurement of cardiac function at 28 days after LAD ligation. left, ischemic heart injected with medium; middle, ischemic heart injected with MSCs; right, ischemic heart injected with SeVhAng-1 modified MSCs. SeVhAng-1 modified MSCs significantly improved cardiac function, *$p < 0.05$ versus sole MSCs and **$p < 0.01$ versus medium, n=5 in each group. B, Masson's trichrome staining of the heart at 28 days after LAD ligation. left, ischemic heart injected with medium; middle, ischemic heart injected with MSCs; right, ischemic heart injected with SeVhAng-1 modified MSCs. SeVhAng-1 modified MSCs significantly decreased infarct size, *$p < 0.05$ versus sole MSCs and **$p < 0.01$ versus medium, n=5 in each group.

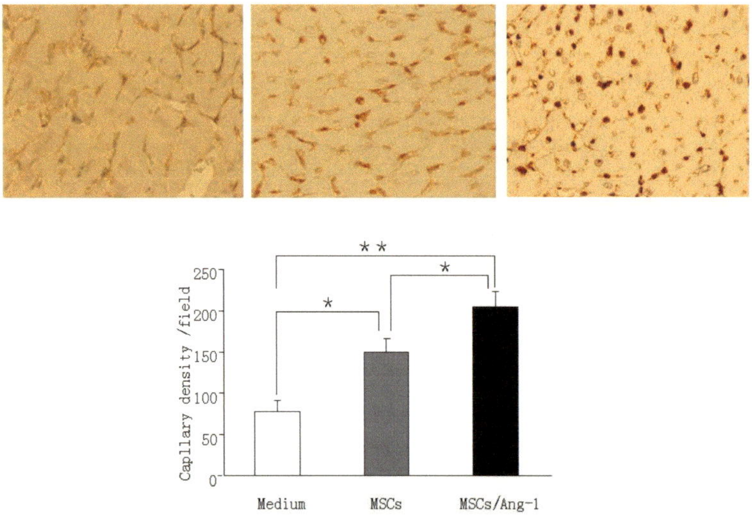

Fig. 4. A, capillary density at 28 days after injection of SeVhAng-1 modified MSCs into the ischemic heart. Left, heart injected with medium; middle, heart injected with sole MSCs; right, heart injected with SeVhAng-1-modified MSCs, magnification, ×400. B, SeVhAng-1 significantly increased the capillary density compared with controls. *$p < 0.01$ versus medium and *$p < 0.05$ versus MSCs, n=5 in each group.

4. Discussion

In the present study, we found that Sendai viral vector had high transductive efficiency to MSCs even at low MOI with short time exposure. Both MSCs modified with SeVhAng-1 and MSCs improved the cardiac function in rats after heart infarction. However, MSCs modified with SeVhAng-1 had better improvement of cardiac function, compared with sole MSCs. This indicated that SeVhAng-1-modified MSCs could serve as a more effective therapy for ischemic heart disease.

Among various vectors, adenoviral vector is widely used for combination of gene and cell therapy in recent years. However, because of lower expression of the CAR receptor for the binding of adenovirus in MSCs, the transductive efficiency of adenoviral vector to the MSCs is not so satisfactory, especially at low MOI [23, 31]. SeV has been proved to have high transductive efficiency in a broad range of tissues, including the airway epithelial cells, vasculature tissues, skeletal muscles, activated T cells, stem cells and neural tissues. In our previously study, we found Sendai viral vector (SeV) has high transductive efficiency to MSCs even at low MOI [23]. In present study, we further found that SeV had high transductive efficiency to MSCs at low MOI with short time exposure. This characteristic of SeV overcomes the shortcoming of needing relatively long time exposure to the MSCs by current available vectors such as adenoviral vector, and makes it an ideal vector for combined stem cell and gene therapy in clinical practice.

Although MSCs can differentiate into cardiomyocytes and endothelial cells, the magnitude of incorporation of MSCs into vascular structures or regenerating cardiomycytes is too low to explain the functional recovery of ischemic heart by MSCs. Kinnaird et al found that MSCs can secret a range of cytokines such as VEGF and bFGF in hypoxic condition and suggested the paracrine mechanism of MSCs is one of the major causes of angiogenetic effect by MSCs [9,10]. Nevertheless, hypoxic condition does not increase Ang-1 expression in MSCs [10, 32]. Because Ang-1 plays an important role in angiogenesis, the supplement of Ang-1 seems to have significant importance for MSCs in treating ischemic heart disease. In the present study, we got a high expression of Ang-1 by transduction of SeVhAng-1 to the MSCs, which had an enhanced angiogenesis effect in the ischemic heart compared with sole MSCs.

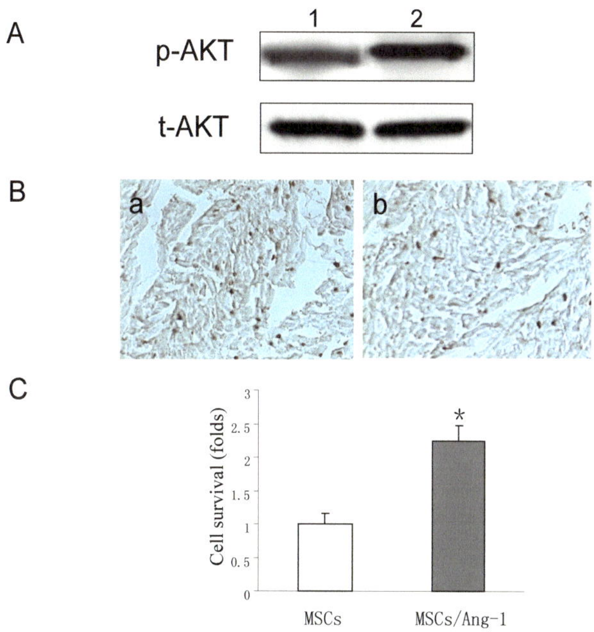

Fig. 5. Effect of overexpression of Ang-1 on p-Akt and MSCs survival in the ischemic heart. A, lane 1, heart injected with MSCs; lane 2, heart injected with SeVhAng-1- modified MSCs. SeVhAng-1- modified MSCs obviously increased expression of Ang-1 and p-Akt in the ischemic heart. The experiments were repeated 3 times. B, a, heart injected with MSCs; b, heart injected with MSCs modified with SeVhAng-1. Apoptotic cell were stained brown, magnification, ×400. SeVhAng-1-modified MSCs obviously decreased apoptosis, compared with the sole MSCs. C , Real-time polymerase chain reaction for *sry* gene in the female heart muscle samples at 2 days after sex-mismatched cell transplantation. The fold change in *sry* gene expression in different animal groups was calculated. The results showed SeVhAng-1-modified MSCs significantly improved MSCs survival, compared with the sole MSCs. *$p<0.01$ versus sloe MSCs.

The high rate of death occurs after MSCs transplantation because of inflammation, loss of survival signal from matrix attachments [33] and cytotoxic factors in the ischemic heart [34]. For these reasons, the enhancement of MSCs engraftment in hostile circumstance is becoming one of attractive strategies to improve its therapeutic effects [35-38]. Ang-1 prevents endothelial cell apoptosis [16] and promotes cardiac muscle survival [39] via activation of Akt pathways. Accordingly, overexpression of Ang-1 by SeVhAng-1-modified MSCs may also have protective effect to MSCs per se which is beneficial to the engraftment of MSCs in the ischemic heart. Indeed, we found SeVhAng-1-modified MSCs significantly increased p-AKT expression, which improved survival of MSCs injected into the ischemic heart. This protective effect by SeVhAng-1-modified MSCs would be beneficial to the enhancement of angiogenesis during the period of heart ischemia.

Our study indicated that Sendai viral vector has high transductive efficiency to the MSCs even at low MOI with short time exposure, and MSCs modified with SeVhAng-1 enhances the angiogenetic effect of MSCs. In addition, the SeVhAng-1 modification increases survival of MSCs in the ischemic heart. SeVhAng-1-modified MSCs may serve as a more effective and practical tool in dealing with ischemic heart disease.

5. Acknowledgements

We thank Takeo Yamamoto for his technical assistance in vector construction.

6. Footnotes

Competing Interests: The authors have declared that no competing interests exist.

Funding: This work was partly supported by a grant to HJ from National Natural Science foundation of China (30960379). The funders had no role in study design, data collection and analysis, decision to publish, or preparation of the manuscript. No current external funding sources for this study.

7. References

[1] Nagaya N, Fujii T, Iwase T, Ohgushi H, Itoh T, et al. Intravenous administration of mesenchymal stem cells improves cardiac function in rats with acute myocardial infarction through angiogenesis and myogenesis.Am J Physiol Heart Circ Physiol. 2004; 287(6):H2670-2676.

[2] Pittenger MF, Martin BJ. Mesenchymal stem cells and their potential as cardiac therapeutics.Circ Res. 2004; 95(1):9-20.

[3] Dick AJ, Guttman MA, Raman VK, Peters DC, Pessanha BS, et al. Magnetic resonance fluoroscopy allows targeted delivery of mesenchymal stem cells to infarct borders in Swine. Circulation. 2003; 108(23):2899-2904.

[4] Dai W, Hale SL, Martin BJ, Kuang JQ, Dow JS, et al. Allogeneic mesenchymal stem cell transplantation in postinfarcted rat myocardium: short- and long-term effects. Circulation. 2005; 112(2):214-223.

[5] Silva GV, Litovsky S, Assad JA, Sousa AL, Martin BJ, et al. Mesenchymal stem cells differentiate into an endothelial phenotype, enhance vascular density, and improve heart function in a canine chronic ischemia model. Circulation. 2005; 111:150-156.

[6] Toma C, Pittenger MF, Cahill KS, Byrne BJ, Kessler PD. Human mesenchymal stem cells differentiate to a cardiomyocyte phenotype in the adult murine heart. Circulation. 2002; 105:93-98.

[7] Iwase T, Nagaya N, Fujii T, Itoh T, Murakami S, et al. Comparison of angiogenic potency between mesenchymal stem cells and mononuclear cells in a rat model of hindlimb ischemia. Cardiovasc Res. 2005; 66:543-551.

[8] Gnecchi M, Zhang Z, Ni A, Dzau VJ. Paracrine mechanisms in adult stem cell signaling and therapy. Circ Res. 2008; 103(11):1204-1219.

[9] Kinnaird T, Stabile E, Burnett MS, Shou M, Lee CW, et al. Local delivery of marrow-derived stromal cells augments collateral perfusion through paracrine mechanisms. Circulation. 2004; 109:1543-1549.
[10] Kinnaird T, Stabile E, Burnett MS, Saji M, Lee CW, et al. Marrow-derived stromal cells express genes encoding a broad spectrum of arteriogenic cytokines and promote in vitro and in vivo arteriogenesis through paracrine mechanisms. Circ Res. 2004; 94:678-685.
[11] Penn MS, Mangi AA. Genetic enhancement of stem cell engraftment, survival, and efficacy. Circ Res. 2008; 102(12):1471-1482.
[12] Takahashi K, Ito Y, Morikawa M, Kobune M, Huang J, et al. Adenoviral-delivered angiopoietin-1 reduces the infarction and attenuates the progression of cardiac dysfunction in the rat model of acute myocardial infarction. Mol Ther. 2003; 8(4):584-592.
[13] Zhou L, Ma W, Yang Z, Zhang F, Lu L, et al. VEGF165 and angiopoietin-1 decreased myocardium infarct size through phosphatidylinositol-3 kinase and Bcl-2 pathways. Gene Ther. 2005; 12:196-202.
[14] Papapetropoulos A, Garcia-Cardena G, Dengler TJ, Maisonpierre PC, Yancopoulos GD, et al. Direct actions of angiopoietin-1 on human endothelium: evidence for network stabilization, cell survival, and interaction with other angiogenic growth factors. Lab Invest. 1999; 79:213-223.
[15] Holash J, Maisonpierre PC, Compton D, Boland P, Alexander CR, et al. Vessel cooption, regression, and growth in tumors mediated by angiopoietins and VEGF. Science.1999; 284:1994-1998.
[16] Kim I, Kim HG, So JN, Kim JH, Kwak HJ, et al. Angiopoietin-1 regulates endothelial cell survival through the phosphatidylinositol 3'-Kinase/Akt signal transduction pathway.Circ Res. 2000; 86(1):24-29.
[17] Bitzer M, Armeanu S, Lauer UM, Neubert WJ. Sendai virus vectors as an emerging negative-strand RNA viral vector system. J Gene Med. 2003; 5:543-553.
[18] Yonemitsu Y, Kitson C, Ferrari S, Farley R, Griesenbach U, et al. Efficient gene transfer to airway epithelium using recombinant Sendai virus. Nat Biotechnol. 2000; 18:970-973.
[19] Masaki I, Yonemitsu Y, Komori K, Ueno H, Nakashima Y, et al. Recombinant Sendai virus-mediated gene transfer to vasculature: a new class of efficient gene transfer vector to the vascular system. Faseb J. 2001; 15:1294-1296.
[20] Li HO, Zhu YF, Asakawa M, Kuma H, Hirata T, et al. A cytoplasmic RNA vector derived from nontransmissible Sendai virus with efficient gene transfer and expression. J Virol. 2000; 74:6564-6569.
[21] Okano S, Yonemitsu Y, Nagata S, Sata S, Onimaru M, et al. Recombinant Sendai virus vectors for activated T lymphocytes. Gene Ther. 2003; 10:1381-1391.
[22] Jin CH, Kusuhara K, Yonemitsu Y, Nomura A, Okano S, et al. Recombinant Sendai virus provides a highly efficient gene transfer into human cord blood-derived hematopoietic stem cells. Gene Ther. 2003; 10:272-277.
[23] Piao W, Wang H, Inoue M, Hasegawa M, Hamada H, et al. Transplantation of mesenchymal cells modified with SeVhAng1 for ischemic limb disease. Angiogenesis 2010；13:203-210
[24] Huang J, Inoue M, Hasegawa M, Tomihara K, Tanaka T, et al. Sendai viral vector mediated angiopoietin-1 gene transfer for experimental ischemic limb disease. Angiogenesis. 2009; 12:243-249.

[25] Hasan MK, Kato A, Muranaka M, Yamaguchi R, Sakai Y, et al. Versatility of the accessory C proteins of Sendai virus: contribution to virus assembly as an additional role. J Virol. 2000; 74:5619-5628.
[26] Fuerst TR, Niles EG, Studier FW,Moss B. Eukaryotic transient-expression system based on recombinant vaccinia virus that synthesizes bacteriophage T7 RNA polymerase. Proc Natl Acad Sci U S A. 1986; 83:8122-8126.
[27] Kato A, Sakai Y, Shioda T, Kondo T, Nakanishi M, et al. Initiation of Sendai virus multiplication from transfected cDNA or RNA with negative or positive sense. Genes Cells. 1996; 1:569-579.
[28] Huang J, Ito Y, Kobune M, Sasaki K, Nakamura K, et al. Myocardial injection of CA promoter-based plasmid mediates efficient transgene expression in rat heart. J Gene Med. 2003; 5:900-908.
[29] Jiang S, Haider HKh, Idris NM, Salim A, Ashraf M. Supportive interaction between cell survival signaling and angiocompetent factors enhances donor cell survival and promotes angiomyogenesis for cardiac repair. Circ Res. 2006; 99(7):776-784.
[30] Shujia J, Haider HK, Idris NM, Lu G, Ashraf M. Stable therapeutic effects of mesenchymal stem cell-based multiple gene delivery for cardiac repair.Cardiovasc Res. 2008;77(3):525-533.
[31] Tsuda H, Wada T, Ito Y, Uchida H, Dehari H, et al. Efficient BMP2 gene transfer and bone formation of mesenchymal stem cells by a fiber-mutant adenoviral vector. Mol Ther. 2003; 7:354-365.
[32] Ohnishi S, Yasuda T, Kitamura S, Nagaya N. Effect of hypoxia on gene expression of bone marrow-derived mesenchymal stem cells and mononuclear cells. Stem Cells. 2007; 25:1166-1177.
[33] Zhang M, Methot D, Poppa V, Fujio Y, Walsh K, et al. Cardiomyocyte grafting for cardiac repair: Graft cell death and anti-death strategies. J Mol Cell Cardiol. 2001; 33: 907-921
[34] Geng YJ. Molecular mechanisms for cardiovascular stem cell apoptosis and growth in the hearts with atherosclerotic coronary disease and ischemic heart failure. Ann N Y Acad Sci. 2003; 1010: 687-697.
[35] Duan HF, Wu CT, Wu DL, Lu Y, Liu HJ, et al. Treatment of myocardial ischemia with bone marrow-derived mesenchymal stem cells overexpressing hepatocyte growth factor. Mol Ther. 2003; 8: 467–474.
[36] Song H, Kwon K, Lim S, Kang SM, Ko YG, et al. Transfection of mesenchymal stem cells with the FGF-2 gene improves their survival under hypoxic conditions. Mol Cells. 2005;19: 402–407.
[37] Jo J, Nagaya N, Miyahara Y, Kataoka M, Harada-Shiba M, et al. Transplantation of genetically engineered mesenchymal stem cells improves cardiac function in rats with myocardial infarction: benefit of a novel nonviral vector, cationized dextran. Tissue Eng. 2007; 13: 313–322.
[38] Matsumoto R, Omura T, Yoshiyama M, Hayashi T, Inamoto S, et al. Vascular endothelial growth factor-expressing mesenchymal stem cell transplantation for the treatment of acute myocardial infarction. Arterioscler Thromb Vasc Biol. 2005; 25: 1168–1173.
[39] Dallabrida SM, Ismail N, Oberle JR, Himes BE, Rupnick MA. Angiopoietin-1 promotes cardiac and skeletal myocyte survival through integrins. Circ Res. 2005; 96:e8-24.

20

Using Factor VII in Hemophilia Gene Therapy

Bahram Kazemi
Shahid Beheshti University of Medical Sciences
Iran

1. Introduction

Human blood at physiological conditions is kept as fluid through precise system called homeostasis, if damage to the vessel, causing the system will be restored by vessel wall. Cases no regulation or homeostasis disorders, thrombosis (intravascular coagulation) or bleeding occur. In normal conditions, the secretion of vascular endothelial heparin-like and trmbomodulin molecules prevent blood coagulation and secretion of nitric oxide and prostacyclin prevent platelet aggregation and blood brings the liquid keeps. Homeostasis has three stages: vasoconstriction, platelet plug formation and blood coagulation, blood coagulation are reactions in which plasma zymogens become active enzymes that create the clotting reaction. Coagulation reactions will be set with inhibitory and stimulatory mechanisms. Coagulation is a regulatory process that keeps the blood flowing. Blood coagulation has two external and internal pathways (Figure 1), tissue factor and FVII form the external pathway, internal pathway is formed of FVIII, FIX and FXI (Ramanarayana et al., 2011; Ellison, 1977).

2. Hemophilia

Hemophilia had recognized in the fifth century BC, first the Jews law passed that when a woman has two dead boys doing the circumcision her third son should not be circumcised, they showed the mother will transmit the disease to her sons (History of hemophilia, 2011). Genetic and hereditary pattern of hemophilia was carefully described in 1803 by the American physician John Conrad Otto. He supposed that the bleeding was occurring due to lack of blood anti hemophilic factor (Cahill & Colvin, 1997). Glossary of hemophilia was developed for this disease in 1828 at the University of Zurich. Anti-hemophilia globin was discovered in 1937 by Patek and Tylor at Harvard University (History of Hemophilia Disease, 2011). The two forms of hemophilia A and B were distinguished in 1952 by Pavlosky, the Brazilian physician. Both diseases are sex-dependent and occur in males (Cahill & Colvin, 1977).

3. Causes hemophilia

Hemophilia is a genetic disorder happens in coagulation FVIII (hemophilia A) or FIX (hemophilia B) and are related to the X chromosome. Hemophilia A is a disease due to genetic defects in coagulation FVIII (Furie et al., 1994; White & Shoemaker, 1989) It is identified by Hoyer and Breckenridge (Hoyer & Breckenridge, 1968) and then by Denson for the first time (Denson et al., 1969). They showed that there was not FVIIIa in the plasma of the most people with hemophilia. Hemophilia B caused by genetic defects occur in the coagulation FIX; the FIX deficiency will inhibit the activation of FX by FVIIa through external coagulation pathway (Furie et al., 1994; Thompson, 1986). About half The patients who suffer from severe hemophilia A there is a large inversion in intron 22 of their FVIII mRNA (Figure 2) which it is repeated (Arruda et al., 1995; Deutz-Terlouw et al., 1995; Okamoto et al., 1995; Pieneman et al., 1995; Van de Water et al., 1995; Goodeve et al., Jenkins et al., 1994; 1994; Naylor et al., 1993; Naylor et al., 1992). Different alleles of the VNTR (di nucleotides) have observed in intron 13 of FVIII in people with hemophilia A (Kochhan et al., 1994).

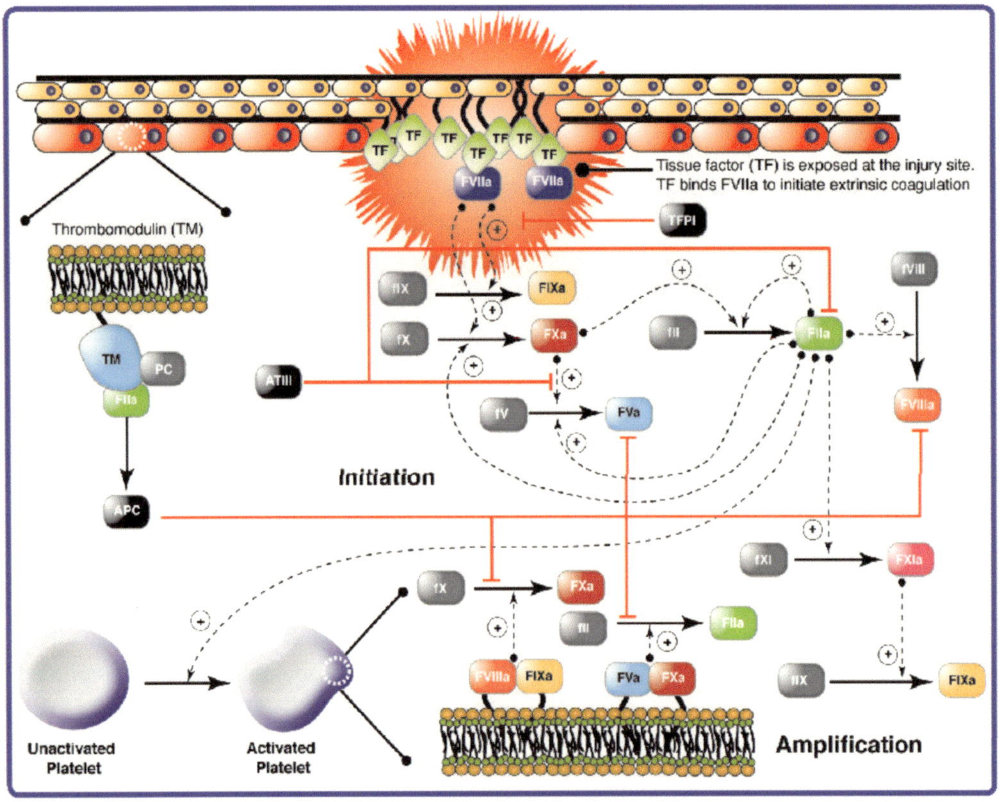

Fig. 1. External and internal pathways of blood coagulation process. (Reference http://www.varnerlab.org/coagulation)Read phonetically

Hemophilia A is occurring one for 5000-10000 birthday boys and hemophilia B one for 20,000 to 34,000 birthday boys (Dimitrios et al., 2009). The bleeding in joints of hemophilia patients the wound bleeding is longer continued (Petkova et al., 2004). The position of FVIII gene is Xq28 and of FIX is Xq27.1 location on distal long arm of chromosome X (Figure 3). The FVIII gene has 186 kb organized in 26 exons (about 9 kb) (Figure 4). There are detected some gene mutations on FVIII as insertion, deletions or point mutations which involved in the reduced or cut up in FVIII activation (Ramanarayana et al., 2011; Salviato et al., 2002; Cahill & Colvin, 1997; Arruda et al., 1995; Naylor et al., 1991; Higuchi et al., 1989; Youssoufian et al., 1987; Gitschier et al., 1985;). The FVIII organized in A, B and C domains

(Figure 5), which B domain is highly glycosylated and do not involve in FVIII activities (Eaton et al., 1986).

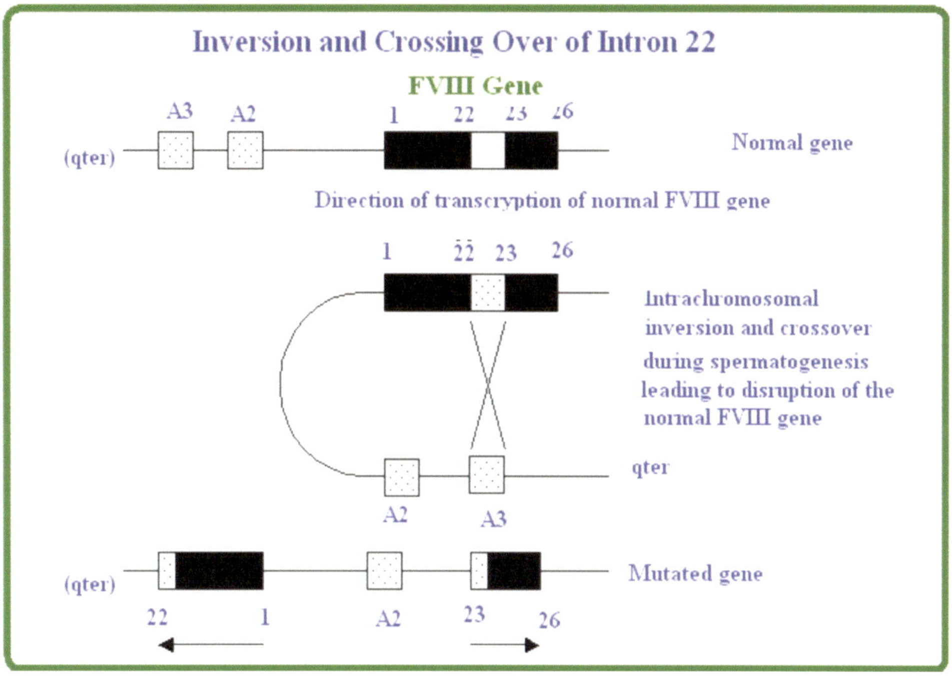

Fig. 2. Genetic mutation in intron 22 of FVIII (Schwartz et al., 2011)

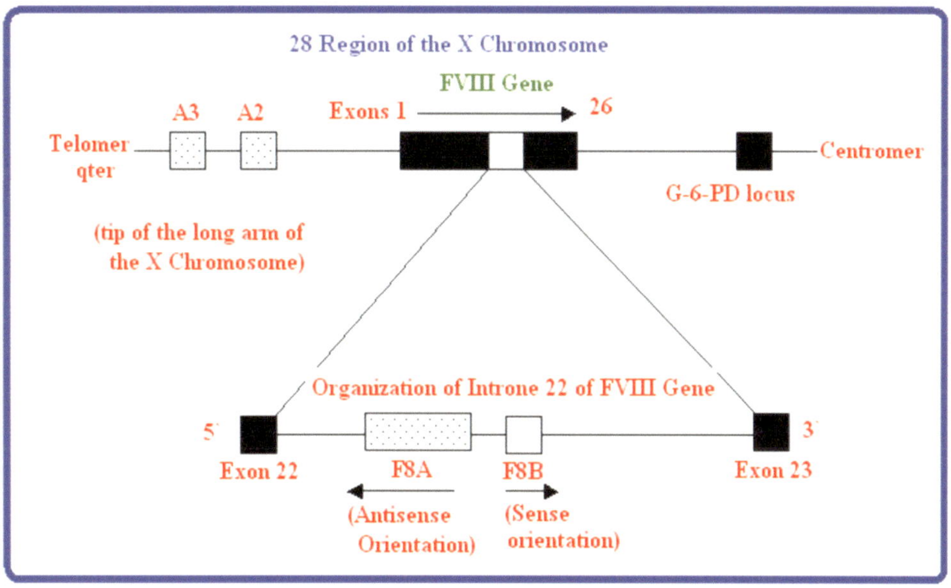

Fig. 3. The Map of FVIII on the long arm of chromosome X (Schwartz et al., 2011)

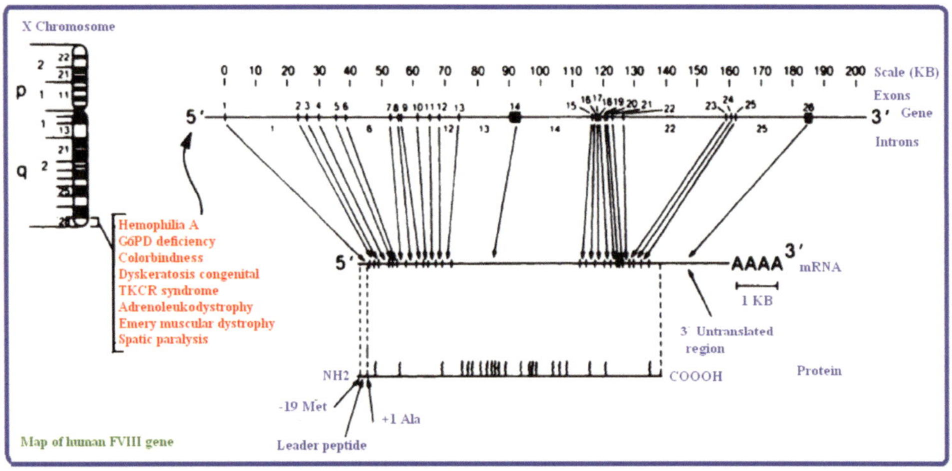

Fig. 4. Genetic map of FVIII (White & Shoemaker, 1989)

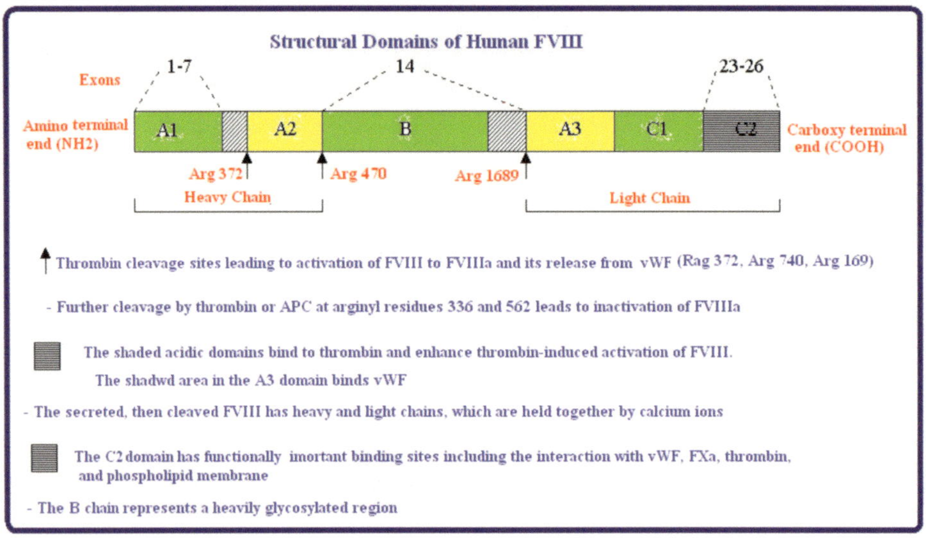

Fig. 5. The domains organization of FVIII (Schwartz et al., 2011)

4. Diagnosis of hemophilia

Laboratory diagnosis of hemophilia is done based on activated partial thromboplastin time (aPTT), prothrombin time (PT), platelet count and bleeding time. There is an abnormally in the initial section of internal coagulation pathway at the prolonged aPTT and normal PT. The normal aPTT should not be reject the FVIII deficiencies (hemophilia A), the aPTT is not enough sensitive too reduced amount of FVIII C. Prolonged PT alone, or PT and aPTT do not specify of hemophilia A, the liver diseases, overdose of warfarin or heparin and the distribution intravascular coagulation (DIC) can cause this coagulophaty. Thrombocytopenia alone cannot cause of hemophilia A. The nature and severity of bleeding is performed with cell blood counts (CBC) and differentiation also check for blood in the stool and urine (Schwartz et al., 2011). Knights and Ingram in 1967 were used thromboplastin time assay for hemophilia A and B differentiation. Based on their test when alumina is added to normal plasma do not see the harm of FVIII, but FIX is deleted, remove the alumina from plasma FIX will re- back up. If thromboplastin time is increased in males with a history of prolonged bleeding, test is repeated after adding or removing alumina from the plasma. If thromboplastin time is shorter than the control, the patient is suffering from hemophilia A, but if thromboplastin time is shortened after the removal of the alumina, patient is suffering from hemophilia B (Knights & Ingram, 1967). Stites et al (1971) and Essien and Ingram (1967) were distinguished hemophilia A and B by FVIII inhibitory antibodies.

The test results in children and adults are different. Clotting Index and coagulability in hemophilia patients significantly lower than non-hemophilia one. In this test, coagulability of FVIII treated blood varies by the replaced FVIII type. rFVIII clotting index is lower than of derived plasma one (Goldenberg et al., 2006). Firshein and colleagues were diagnosed prenatal hemophilia A using radioimmunometric by fetal plasma and fetoscope by amniotic fluid at second trimester in pregnancy women (Firshein et al., 1979), other researchers were developed radoimmunometric method for measurements of FVIII antibody (Hoyer et al., 1985; Hellings et al., 1982; Ljung R, Holmberg, 1982). Antonarakis et al were analyzed FVIII gene for possibility detection of prenatal and hemophilia carrier through gene cloning method (Antonarakis et al., 1985), the problems and limitations of these methods were evaluated by other researchers (Graham et al., 1985). The PCR RFLP method was used for prenatal diagnosis and hemophilia A carrier for the first time in 1990s (Rudzki et al., 1996; Herrmann et al., 1988; Kogan et al., 1987;). Missense and nonsense point mutations in FVIII gene of hemophilia A patient, prenatal and carrier hemophilia A were detected using DGGE method (Gitschier, 1989). Ball and colleagues were used oral cells, urine and hair follicles samples to identify prenatal and carrier hemophilia A (Ball et al., 1990). Various polymorphism and mutations have been detected in FVIII gene of hemophilia A patients (Wacey et al., 1996' Antonarakis et al, 1995; Naylor et al., 1991; Baranov et al., 1990; Gécz et al., 1990; Jedlicka et al., 1990; Sadler et al., 1990; Surin et al., 1990; Wehnert et al., 1990a; Wehnert et al., 1990b). Establishment the PCR technique in diagnostic laboratories was a large change in DNA analysis of FVIII gene for detecting carriers and individuals with hemophilia A (Song et al., 1993; Feng, 1991; Wadelius et al., 1991; Wu, 1991). Detection of unknown mutations is performed by universal mutation detection system methods such as SSCP (Arruda et al., 1995; Pieneman et al., 1995; David et al., 1994). Hemophilia diagnosis with PGD method was used by Michaelides (2006) and colleagues For the first time in 2006; they were diagnosed two point mutations in FVIII gene of donor (IVF) blastomere. Acquired hemophilia due to FVIII autoantibody is a rare disease and occurs one in a million, yearly; its mortality is 20 percent (Shetty et al., 2010).

5.1 Treatment of hemophilia A

Hemophilia treatment doing by replacing the natural (Brackmann & Gormsen, 1977) or recombinant FVIII (Kaufman, 1991) via intravenous injection. The half life of transfused FVIII in normal individuals or patients with hemophilia is 8 to 12 hours (White & Shoemaker, 1989). Using recombinant serum proteins in the treatment of hemophilia began in 1990 (Liras, 2008), but Homate P / humate-P is a derived pasteurized human plasma which was approved in Germany in 1981 and used administered intravenous injection for

25 years to control bleeding in patients with hemophilia A and von Willebrand disease (Berntorp, 2009; Carter & Scott, 2007; Czapek et al, 1988). The main presentation following hemophilia treatment is creating inhibitory antibodies against the FVIII which observed 5% in patients with hemophilia B and 40 -20 percent in patients with severe hemophilia A (Hong & Stachnik, 2010; Kempton et al., 2010; Eckhardt et al., 2009; Ghosh & Shetty, 2009; von Auer et al., 2005; Sharathkumar wt al., 2003; Scharrer, 1999; de Biasi et al., 1994). Complication inhibitory antibodies seem to produce with plasma-derived FVII severe than with recombinant one (Lusher, 2002; Lusher, 2000), also with FVIII (Qadura et al., 2009; Delignat et al., 2007; Goudemand et al., 2006; Yoshioka et al., 2003; Fijnvandraat et al, 1997). The B cell epitopes mutated, produced FVIII inhibitory antibody is reduced, and some one proposed that this phenomenon is safe vaccine for people with hemophilia (Parker et al, 2004). Antibody production against FVIII has been studied in hemophilia patients and indicates that most nonsense mutations and large deletions in FVIII gene and chromosomal recombination lead to produce FVIII inhibitory antibody (Schwaab et al., 1995). Treatment of hemophilia by FVIII overdose administration is effective for producer antibodies hemophilia patients (Scandella et al., 2000).

The OBI (BDD- rpFVIII) was introduced by Ipsen and Inspiration Biopharmaceuticals Inc Company and passed clinical trial phases 1 and 2. It shows porcine FVIII biochemical properties and procoagulant activity and less immunogenicity than plasma derived pFVIII (Toschi, 2010).

In 1960 Los Angeles Red Cross Blood Center was treated hemophilia patients using anti hemophilic globin (Rapaport et al., 1960). 1-Deamino-8-d-arginine vasopressin (DDAVP) (a FVII autologous) have been used instead of plasma derived factors for treatment of hemophilia A and B (Mannucci et al., 1977). Hultin and colleagues were used cyclophosphamide as immunosuppression drug for antibody producer hemophilia patients (Hultin et al., 1976). Lian et al. were treated hemophilia using cyclophosphamide, vincristine and prednisone (CVP) (Lian et al., 1989). Blatt et al were removed FVIII inhibitory antibody with prothrombin complex concentrates (PCC) (Blatt et al., 1977). Paleyanda and colleagues were transferred FVIII cDNA into pig lactate system; the pig was produced FVIII more than 10 times as normal plasma (**Paleyanda** et al., 1997). Specific thrombin anticoagulant Bivalirudin (Krolick, 2005) and monoclonal antibody Retoximab (Franchini, 2007; Wiestner et al., 2002) are also used for hemophilia treatment and patients with FVIII autoantibody, respectively. Idiotype vaccines will neutralize anti human FVIII antibody in hemophilia A patients (Lacroix-Desmazes et al., 2002).

Production and characterization of recombinant FVIII for the treatment of hemophilia was conducted in 1984 for the first time (Toole et al., 1984; Wood et al., 1984). Use of recombinant proteins to replace clotting factors and treatment of hemophilia opened a new arena in treatment of disease. Circulating blood factors are the first generation recombinant proteins and second generation drugs made by recombinant DNA and protein engineering technology cause changes in proteins for specific applications, like FVIIa (Levy & Levi, 2009; Pipe, 2008). FVII alone or in combination with its analogues have been used to reduce bleeding (Lauritzen el al., 2008a; Lauritzen et al., 2008b; Allen et al., 2007). Use of recombinant FVIIa for hemophilia patients with FVIII antibody (Obergfell et al., 2010; Margaritis, 2010; Margaritis et al., 2010), also people who have bleeding into the joint or prevent bleeding in surgery is economically efficient (Stephens et al., 2007).

5.2 Gene therapy of hemophilia A

For the first time in 1996, Connelly et al were administrated intravenous hemophilia dog by adenovirus containing hFVIII gene in which related protein was detectable in plasma for two weeks (Connelly et al., 1996a). Connelly and colleagues were injected adenovirus containing BDD- hFVIII gene through the tail artery into mice; hFVIII was detected in plasma by ELISA method (Connelly et al., 1999; Connelly et al. 1995). Dwarki and colleagues were transfected fibroblast by retrovirus containing BDD- FVIII gene, transfected fibroblasts were transferred into mice, human FVIII was observed in plasma after one week (Dwarki et al., 1995). Connelly et al were transferred adenovirus containing hFVIII gene into mice, hFVIII was stable in mouse for five months. (Connelly et al., 1996b). Ill et al were prepared suitable plasmid with necessary elements for FVIII expression in liver cells (Ill et al., 1997). Zhang et al were prepared a mini-adenovirus containing FVIII -equipped human albumin gene promoter for hemophilia A gene therapy. This structure was transferred to cell line; the hFVIII was consistently produced in mouse transferred ell line (Zhang et al., 1999). Gene therapy of hemophilia were done by liver cell transfected by adeno associated viruses or lentiviral viruses containing FVIII and FIX. Also use non-viral vector is also considered. Antibody production in gene therapy of hemophilia with FVIII and FIX can be depended on vector serotype (viral), expression rate (a long time, especially in the liver), the promoter used, method of gene delivery and transduced cell types (Margaritis et al., 2009; Ohmori et al., 2008; VandenDriessche et al., 2003; Chuah et al., 2001).

To overcome adenovirus toxicity phenomena, Andrews and colleagues were used adenovirus defected early genes E1, E2a, E3, E4 (four-generation defected vector), and transferred albumin promoter –controlled FVIII gene into mice, but was not suitable for use in vivo (Andrews et al., 2001). Chuah et al were inhibited bleeding in hemophilia A SCID mice using intravenous injection of adenovirus carrying BDD -FVIII gene (Chuah et al., 2003). Shi et al believed that platelet/ megakaryocyte is a target for hemophilia A gene therapy, they were transferred equipted specific platelet glycoprotein IIb promoter BDD-hFVIII to Domi cells, hFVIII was biosynthesised (Shi et al., 2003). Sarkar and colleagues were transferred AAV carrying hFVIII to deficient FVIII mice through portal, intravenous and spleen injections, they observed secreted hFVIII in transgenic animals but no in neonatal animal (Sarkar et al., 2003). Scallan et al were transferred FVIII gene into mice by AAV2 vector. The construct was equipped with liver cell specific promoter (Scallan et al., 2003). Kang and colleagues were used liver specific promoter equipted FIV retrovirus containing BDD- hFVIII gen for intravenous injection in hemophilia mice, hFVIII was secreted in mice for months without anti FVIII antibody production (Kang et al., 2005). Kumaran et al were treated hemophilia mice by cell therapy, a mixture of hepatocytes, liver endothelial sinusoids and liver kupffer cells was injected into mice peritoneum, FVIII was observed in mouse blood (Kumaran et al., 2005). Jiang et al were transferred FVIII in to hemophilia dog by AAV types 2, 5, 6 and 8, their report indicated that the performance of virus types 2 and 5 for gene therapy is more than viruses type 6 and 8 (Jiang et al., 2006). Sarkar et al believed that gene therapy duration in the dog with AAV8 containing FVIII have prolonged up to two years (Sarkar et al., 2006). Durable gene therapy based on AAV containing FVIII have also been reported by McCormack and colleagues (McCormack et al., 2006). Shi and colleagues findings suggest that targeted FVIII gene expression by platelets specific promoter is effective in the treatment of hemophilia A (Shi et al., 2006). Shi and colleagues were suggested that ectopic expression of FVIII in platelets with lentiviral virus via bone marrow gene therapy is effective for human hemophilia treatment They were transferred lentiviral vector containing FVIII - Induced glycoprotein IIb platelet specific promoter into null mice bone marrow, the permanent secretion of FVIII in platelets lysates mice was observed. (Shi et al., 2007). Liu and colleagues were targeted rDNA of HL7702 hepatocytes by non-viral vector pHrneo containing FVIII gene for treatment of hemophilia (Liu et al., 2007). Doering has been transferred swine FVIII gene into mouse bone marrow mesenchymal cells for hemophilia treatment (Doering, 2008). Ishiwata and colleagues have been treated hemophilia mice using AAV8 vector containing canine BDD -FVIII gene (Ishiwata et al., 2009). Sabatino and colleagues report indicated that canine BDD- FVIII dogs is stable than human BDD- FVIII, it can be considered in the hemophilia treatment (Sabatino et al., 2009). Doering et al were transferred hFVIII - sFVIII hybrid in to hematopoietic stem cells with lentiviral vector; cells expressed FVIII more than 100-8 times of cells transfected with hFVIII only (Doering et al., 2009). Zatloukal and colleagues report suggested that expressed FVIII would be observed if the adenovirus containing FVIII -transfected fibroblasts or mayoblasts move into liver or spleen cells, but do not observe in the transfected muscle cells (Zatloukal et al., 1995). Because there are no acceptable phenotypic correction of hemophilia mice, Liars was used induced pluri potent stem cell therapy technology, these cells suggested converting into all cells and can be transfected by recombinant AAV or lentiviral vectors (Liars, 2011). Studies conducted so far suggest that blood factors gene therapy with AAV in animal muscle (dogs and mice) was healthy for FIX, but did not sufficiently much success for FVIII (Haurigot et al., 2010; Wang & Herzog, 2005). It is believed that the clinical correction of hemophilia B depends on the dose of vector transfer into muscular hosts (mice and dogs) (Hagstrom et al., 2000; Kay et al., 2000).

5.3 Hemophilia gene therapy with factor VII

Activated FVII is used as recombinant factor VII (rFVII) can go around process dependent coagulation FVIII and FIX (Mackman et al., 2007), it helps blood coagulation through extrinsic pathway. It is an ideal choice in the treatment of patients with FVIII producing antibodies and hemophilia patients to be considered (Johannessen etal., 2000; Lauritzen et al., 2008a). FVII is used in patient`s surgery with hemophilia A (Lauritzen et al., 2008a) also effective in term of homostatic process (Hedner et al., 2000; Kenet et al., 1999). The VIIa (Novoseven; rhFVIIa) has been achieved great success in treating patients with hemophilia. On the FVIII or FIX defects or presence of inhibitory antibodies, FVIIa – tissue factor complex will activate coagulation FX. FVIIa can activate coagulation cascade which cause clot formation and bleeding is inhibited (Hong & Stachnik, 2010; Levy & Levi, 2009). The main drug problems are short half-life (3-6 hours) and highly price (Ramanarayana et al., 2011; Puetz, 2010; Agersø et al., 2011;), more than one full dose of medication, especially for homeostasis regulation during surgeries are required. Hence, research groups around the world are trying different methods of gene transfer to express stable FVIIa in cells without the need to drug re administration (Ramanarayana et al., 2011). After biosynthesis of rhFVII as zymogen, it will be cut by proteases and biologically active through purification process (Huntington, 2009). The produced protein will breaks down at Arg152 and Ile153 to FVIIa. It is proposed that FVII gene transfer eliminates short half-life of rFVII and FVIII inhibitory antibody production (Ramanarayana et al., 2011). Emamgholipour et al (2009) and Margaritis (2010) established furin enzyme digestion site between Arg152 and Ile153 to generate FVIIa from FVII zymogene break down inside the targeted cell during FVII gene therapy strategy (Figure 6). Margaritis and colleagues were successfully corrected canine hemophilia B with this method

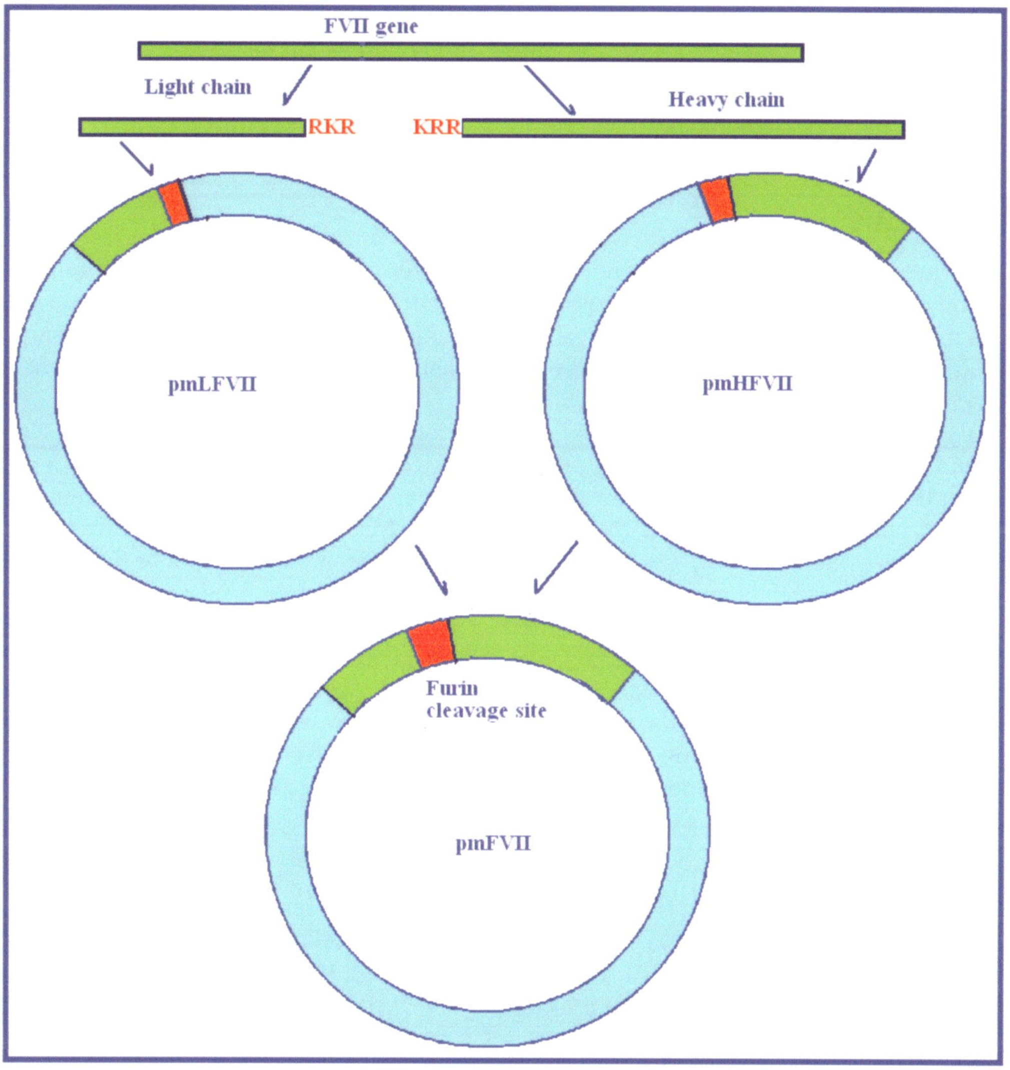

Fig. 6. Mutagenesis method to create furin digestion site on the FVII protein (Proposed based on Emamgholipour et al., 2009; Margaritis, 2010)

(Margaritis et al., 2004). Margaritis and colleagues were injected the mice through gene therapy by AAV contained FVII gene, FVII was produced in host cells (Margaritis et al., 2004). Miller et al were injected mice muscle myoblasts with plasmids coding FVIII and FVII cDNA (muscle specific elements and poly A were placed on both sides of genes); they were observed FVII and related antibody after 4-5 days. They believed that post translation modification process was occurred in the muscle cells (Miller et al., 1995). Tomokiyo and colleagues showed that the composition of plasma FVIIa and FXa in the treatment of monkeys hemophilia B more effective than FVIIa alone (Tomokiyo et al., 2003). Ohmori et al have been used ectopic expression FVIIa in platelets to hemophilia A treatment, they were transferred SIV containing platelet glycoprotein Ib alpha specific promoter into bone marrow cells, was lead to FVII expression on the platelets surface. This construct was corrected mouse hemophilia A phenotype (Ohmori et al., 2008). Margaritis have been treated canine hemophilia by AAV containing FVII through the portal vein (Margaritis et al., 2009). To overcome the repeated injection problem, Obergfell and colleagues were studied hemophilia treatment and suggested permanent expression of FVII in canine hemophilia model through gene therapy method (Obergfell et al., 2010).

6. Conclusion

There are some reported of FVIII and FIX gene transfer by viral vectors in animal models, but no evidence so far reported successful treatment of human hemophilia gene therapy by this method. Researchers have used FVII to overcome antibody production in treatment of FVIII deficiency. Despite several reports of curing hemophilia A with FVII in animals, there is no yet successful reported in human.

Methods proposed for the future: reviewing the history of hemophilia gene therapy by viral vectors, identified several reasons that cannot be sure of the viruses used for gene transfer: 1) Application of viruses is associated with inappropriate chromosomal insertion and makes the undesirable point mutations (Nakai et al., 2003; Miller et al., 2002). 2) Viruses are carcinogens (Check, 2003). 3) The viruses will cause the host immune response (Lefesvre et al., 2003) which is temporarily being transgene. 4) Because viruses genome are great than non-viral vectors the sequences of the viruses cannot be controlled by reseaechers. 5) Preparation of this vector requires a lot of time and money. Although non-viral gene transfer is less efficient than virus vector but have been told no above disadvantages and their use for gene transfer in human can be safer than viruses. Vectors are suggested to be prepared as non-viral vector for targeting the rDNA locus of human genome by homologous recombination method, and as ex vivo gene transfer in humans to be done with them.

7. Acknowledgment

This work was supported by Iran National Science Foundation (project no.843083) and was done in Cellular and Molecular Biology Research Center of Shahid Beheshti University of Medical Sciences, the author's thanks directors.

8. References

Agersø H, Brophy DF, Pelzer H, Martin J, Carr M, Hedner U, Ezban M (2011). Recombinant human factor VIIa (rFVIIa) cleared principally by antithrombin following intravenous administration in hemophilia patients. *J Thromb Haemost*; 9(2): 333-338. ISSN: 1538-7933

Allen GA, Persson E, Campbell RA, Ezban M, Hedner U, Wolberg AS (2007). A variant of recombinant factor VIIa with enhanced procoagulant and antifibrinolytic activities in an in vitro model of hemophilia. *Arterioscler Thromb Vasc Biol* ;27(3):683-689. ISSN 1049-8834

Andrews JL, Kadan MJ, Gorziglia MI, Kaleko M, Connelly S (2001). Generation and characterization of E1/E2a/E3/E4-deficient adenoviral vectors encoding human factor VIII. *Mol Ther*; 3 (3):329- 336. ISSN: 1525-0016

Antonarakis SE, Waber PG, Kittur SD, Patel AS, Kazazian HH Jr, Mellis MA, Counts RB, Stamatoyannopoulos G, Bowie EJ, Fass DN, et al. (1985). Hemophilia A. Detection of molecular defects and of carriers by DNA analysis. *N Engl J Med*; 313(14): 842-848. ISSN 0028-4793

Antonarakis SE, Kazazian HH, Tuddenham EG (1995). Molecular etiology of factor VIII deficiency in hemophilia A. *Hum Mutat*; 5(1): 1-22. ISSN: 1059-7794

Arruda VR, Pieneman WC, Reitsma PH, Deutz-Terlouw PP, Annichino-Bizzacchi JM, Briët E, Costa FF (1995). Eleven novel mutations in the factor VIII gene from Brazilian hemophilia A patients. *Blood*; 86(8): 3015-3020. ISSN 0006-4971

Ball J, Warnock LJ, Preston FE (1990). Rapid assessment of haemophilia A carrier state by non-invasive techniques using the polymerase chain reaction. *J Clin Pathol*; 43(6): 505-507. ISSN:0021-9746

Baranov VS, Aseev MV, Gorbunova VN, Ivashchenko TE, Mikhaĭlov AV, Gornostaeva NI, Surin VL (1990). Use of molecular and genetic approaches in prenatal diagnosis and prevention of hemophilia A and Duchenne muscular dystrophy. *Akush Ginekol* (Mosk) ;(11): 26-28. ISSN: 0002-3906

Bartlett A, Dormandy KM, Hawkey CM, Stableforth P, Voller A (1976). Factor-VIII-related antigen: measurement by enzyme immunoassay. *Br Med J*; 1(6016): 994-996. ISSN: 09598138

Berntorp E.(2009). Haemate P/Humate-P: a systematic review. *Thromb Res*;124 Suppl 1: S11-4. ISSN:0049-3848

Blatt PM, White GC 2nd, McMillan CW, Roberts HR (1977). Treatment of anti-factor VIII antibodies. *Thromb Haemost*; 38(2): 514-523. ISSN:0340-6245

Brackmann HH, Gormsen J (1977): Massive factor-VIll infusion in haemophiliac with factor-VIll inhibitor, high responder. Lancet; 2: 933. ISSN: 0140-6736

Cahill MR, Colvin BT (1997). Haemophilia. *Postgrad Med J*; 73: 201-206. ISSN: 0022-3859

Carter NJ, Scott LJ (2007). Human Plasma von Willebrand Factor/Factor VIII Complex (Haemate(R) P/Humate-P(R)): In von Willebrand Disease and Haemophilia A. *Drugs*: 67 (10): 1513-1519. ISSN 0012-6667

Check E (2003). Cancer risk prompts US to curb gene therapy. *Nature*. Mar 6;422(6927):7. ISSN : 0028-0836

Chuah MK, Collen D, VandenDriessche T (2001). Gene therapy for hemophilia. *J Gene Med*; 3(1): 3-20. ISSN: 1099-498X

Chuah MK, Schiedner G, Thorrez L, Brown B, Johnston M, Gillijns V, Hertel S, Van Rooijen N, Lillicrap D, Collen D, VandenDriessche T, Kochanek S (2003). Therapeutic factor VIII levels and negligible toxicity in mouse and dog models of hemophilia A following gene therapy with high-capacity adenoviral vectors. *Blood*;101(5):1734-1743. ISSN: 0006-4971

Connelly S, Mount J, Mauser A, Gardner JM, Kaleko M, McClelland A, Lothrop CD Jr (1996a). Complete short-term correction of canine hemophilia A by in vivo gene therapy. *Blood*; 88(10): 3846-3853. ISSN: 0006-4971

Connelly S, Smith TA, Dhir G, Gardner JM, Mehaffey MG, Zaret KS, McClelland A, Kaleko M (1995). In vivo gene delivery and expression of physiological levels of functional human factor VIII in mice. *Hum Gene Ther*; 6(2): 185-193. ISSN: 1043-0342 ISSN: 1043-0342

Connelly S, Gardner JM, Lyons RM, McClelland A, Kaleko M (1996b). Sustained expression of therapeutic levels of human factor VIII in mice. *Blood* ; 87(11): 4671-4677. ISSN: 0006-4971

Connelly S, Andrews JL, Gallo-Penn AM, Tagliavacca L, Kaufman RJ, Kaleko M (1999). Evaluation of an adenoviral vector encoding full-length human factor VIII in hemophiliac mice. *Thromb Haemost*; 81(2): 234-239. ISSN:0340-6245

Czapek EE, Gadarowski JJ Jr, Ontiveros JD, Pedraza JL (1988). Humate-P for treatment of von Willebrand disease [letter]. *Blood*; 72: 1100. ISSN: 0006-4971

David D, Moreira I, Lalloz MR, Rosa HA, Schwaab R, Morais S, Diniz MJ, de Deus G, Campos M, Lavinha J, et al (1994). Analysis of the essential sequences of the factor VIII gene in twelve haemophilia A patients by single-stranded conformation polymorphism. *Blood Coagul Fibrinolysis*; 5(2): 257-264. ISSN: 1473-5733

de Biasi R, Rocino A, Papa ML, Salerno E, Mastrullo L, De Blasi D (1994). Incidence of factor VIII inhibitor development in hemophilia A patients treated with less pure plasma derived concentrates. *Thromb Haemost*; 71(5): 544-7. ISSN:0340-6245

Delignat S, Dasgupta S, André S, Navarrete AM, Kaveri SV, Bayry J, André MH, Chtourou S, Tellier Z, Lacroix-Desmazes S (2007). Comparison of the immunogenicity of different therapeutic preparations of human factor VIII in the murine model of hemophilia A. *Haematologica* ;92(10): 1423-1426. ISSN is 0390-6078

Denson KW, Biggs R, Haddon ME, Borrett R, Cobb K (1969). Two types of haemophilia (A+ and A-): a study of 48 cases. *Br J Haematol*; 17(2): 163-171. ISSN 0007-1048

Deutz-Terlouw PP, Losekoot M, Olmer R, Pieneman WC, de Vries-v d Weerd S, Briët E, Bakker E (1995). Inversion in the factor VIII gene: improvement of carrier detection and prenatal diagnosis in Dutch haemophilia A families. *J Med Genet*; 32(4): 296-300. ISSN: 0148-7299

Dimitrios P Agaliotis, Robert A Zaiden, Saduman Ozturk (2009). Hemophilia, Overview. http://emedicine.medscape.com/article/210104-overview

Doering CB, Denning G, Dooriss K, Gangadharan B, Johnston JM, Kerstann KW, McCarty DA, Spencer HT (2009). Directed engineering of a high-expression chimeric transgene as a strategy for gene therapy of hemophilia A. *Mol Ther*; 17(7): 1145-1154. ISSN: 1525-0016

Doering CB (2008). Retroviral modification of mesenchymal stem cells for gene therapy of hemophilia. *Methods Mol Biol*; 433: 203-212. ISSN: 1064-3745

Dwarki VJ, Belloni P, Nijjar T, Smith J, Couto L, Rabier M, Clift S, Berns A, Cohen LK. (1995). Gene therapy for hemophilia A: production of therapeutic levels of human factor VIII in vivo in mice. *Proc Natl Acad Sci U S A*; 92(4): 1023-1027. 0027-8424. ISSN

Eaton DL, Wood WI, Eaton D, Hass PE, Hollingshead P, Wion K, Mather J, Lawn RM, Vehar GA & Gorman C (1986). Construction and characterization of an active factor VIII variant lacking the central one-third of the molecule. *Biochemistry*; 25(26): 8343-8327. ISSN:1742-464X

Eckhardt CL, Menke LA, van Ommen CH, van der Lee JH, Geskus RB, Kamphuisen PW, Peters M, Fijnvandraat K (2009). Intensive peri-operative use of factor VIII and the Arg593-->Cys mutation are risk factors for inhibitor development in mild/moderate hemophilia A. *J Thromb Haemost*; 7(6): 930-937. ISSN: 1538-7933

Ellison N (1977). Diagnostic and management of Bleeding disorders. *Anesthesiology*; 47(2): 171-180. ISSN: 0003-3022

Emamgholipour S, Bandehpour M, Shabani P, Maghen L, Yaghmaee B, Kazemi B (2009). Mutagenesis in sequence encoding of human factor VII for gene therapy of hemophilia. DARU; 17(4): 294-298. ISSN : 1560-8115

Essien EM, Ingram GI (1967). Diagnosis of haemophilia: use of an artificial factor-VIII-deficient human plasma system. *J Clin Pathol*; 20(4): 620-623. ISSN:0021-9746

Feng J (1991). Gene diagnosis of hemophilia A by PCR. *Zhongguo Yi Xue Ke Xue Yuan Xue Bao*; 13(5): 384-388. ISSN: 0376-2491

Franchini M (2007). Rituximab in the treatment of adult acquired hemophilia A: a systematic review. *Crit Rev Oncol Hematol*; 63(1):47-52. ISSN: 1040-8428

Fijnvandraat K, Turenhout EA, van den Brink EN, ten Cate JW, van Mourik JA, Peters M, Voorberg J (1997). The missense mutation Arg593 --> Cys is related to antibody formation in a patient with mild hemophilia A. *Blood*; 89(12): 4371-2377. ISSN: 0006-4971

Firshein SI, Hoyer LW, Lazarchick J, Forget BG, Hobbins JC, Clyne LP, Pitlick FA, Muir WA, Merkatz IR, Mahoney MJ (1979). Prenatal diagnosis of classic hemophilia. *N Engl J Med*; 300(17): 937-941. ISSN: 0028-4793

Forbes CD, King J, Prentice CR, McNicol GP (1972). Serum enzyme changes after intramuscular bleeding in patients with haemophilia and Christmas disease. *J Clin Patho*; 25(12): 1034-1037. ISSN:0021-9746

Furie B, Limentani SA, Rosenfield CG (1994). A Practical Guide to the Evaluation and Treatment of Hemophilia. *Blood;* 84 (1): 3-9. ISSN: 0006-4971

Gécz J, Kádasi L, Poláková H, Ferák V (1990). Use of DNA analysis in the diagnosis and prevention of hemophilia A. *Bratisl Lek Listy*; 91(3): 219-224. ISSN: 0006-9248

Ghosh K, Shetty S (2009). Immune response to FVIII in hemophilia A: an overview of risk factors. *Clin Rev Allergy Immunol*; 37(2): 58-66. ISSN: 1080-0549

Gitschier J (1989). Molecular genetics of hemophilia A. *Schweiz Med Wochenschr*; 119(39): 1329-1331. ISSN, 0036-7672

Gitschier J, Wood WI, Tuddenham EG, Shuman MA, Goralka TM, Chen EY, Lawn RM (1985). Detection and sequence of mutations in the factor VIII gene of haemophiliacs. *Nature*; 315(6018):427-430. ISSN : 0028-0836

Goldenberg, NA, Hathaway WE, Jacobson L, et al. (2006). "Influence of Factor VIII on Overall Coagulability and Fibrinolytic Potential of Haemophilic Plasma as Measured by Global Assay: Monitoring in Hemophilia A." *Haemophilia.*; 12: 605-614. ISSN 1351-8216

Goodeve A, Preston FE, Peake IR (1994). Factor VIII gene rearrangements in patients with severe haemophilia A. *Lancet*; 343: 329-330. ISSN: 0140-6736

Goudemand J, Rothschild C, Demiguel V, Vinciguerrat C, Lambert T, Chambost H, Borel-Derlon A, Claeyssens S, Laurian Y, Calvez T (2006). Influence of the type of factor VIII concentrate on the incidence of factor VIII inhibitors in previously untreated patients with severe hemophilia A. *Blood*; 107(1): 46-51. ISSN: 0006-4971

Graham JB, Green PP, McGraw RA, Davis LM (1985). Application of molecular genetics to prenatal diagnosis and carrier detection in the hemophilias: some limitations. *Blood*; 66(4): 759-764. ISSN: 0006-4971

Hagstrom JN, Couto LB, Scallan C, Burton M, McCleland ML, Fields PA, Arruda VR, Herzog RW, High KA (2000). Improved muscle-derived expression of human coagulation factor IX from a skeletal actin/CMV hybrid enhancer/promoter. Blood; 95(8): 2536-42. ISSN: 0006-4971

Haurigot V , Mingozzi F, Buchlis G, Hui D , Chen Y, Tschakarjan EB, Arruda V, Radu A, Franck HG, Wright JF, Zhou S, Stedman HH, Bellinger DA, Nichols5 TC & High KA (2010). Safety of AAV Factor IX Peripheral TransvenularGene Delivery to Muscle in Hemophilia B Dogs. *Mol Ther*; 18 (7): 1318–1329. ISSN: 1525-0016

Hedner U (2000). NovoSeven as a universal haemostatic agent. *Blood Coagul Fibrinolysis;* 11 Suppl 1: S107-111. ISSN: 0957-5235

Hellings JA, van Leeuwen FR, Over J, van Mourik JA (1982). 1712. Immunoradiometric assay of VIII:CAg, a potential tool to detect human anti-VIII:C antibodies. *Thromb Res* 15; 26(4):297-302. ISSN:0049-3848

Herrmann FH, Kruse T, Wehnert M, Vogel G, Wulff K (1988). First experiences in application of RFLP analysis for carrier detection in preparation of prenatal diagnosis of hemophilia A in the GDR. *Folia Haematol Int Mag Klin Morphol Blutforsch;* 115(4): 489-93. ISSN : 1087-0156

Higuchi M, Kochhan L, Schwaab R, Egli H, Brackmann HH, Horst J, Olek K (1989). Molecular defects in hemophilia A: identification and characterization of mutations in the factor VIII gene and family analysis. *Blood;* 74(3): 1045-1051. ISSN: 0006-4971

History of hemophilia. http://www.hemophilia-information.com/history-of-hemophilia.html

History of Hemophilia Disease. http://www.buzzle.com/articles/history-of-hemophilia-disease.html

Hong I, Stachnik J (2010). Unlabeled uses of factor VIIa (recombinant) in pediatric patients. *Am J Health Syst Pharm;* 67(22):1909-19. ISSN: 0815-9319

Hoyer LW, Breckenridge RT (1968). Immunologic studies of antihemophilic factor (AHF, factor VIII): cross-reacting material in a genetic variant of hemophilia A. *Blood;* 32(6): 962-971. ISSN: 0006-4971

Hoyer LW, Carta CA, Golbus MS, Hobbins JC, Mahoney MJ (1985). Prenatal diagnosis of classic hemophilia (hemophilia A) by immunoradiometric assays. *Blood;* 65(6):1312-1317. ISSN: 0006-4971

Hultin MB, Shapiro SS, Bowman HS, Gill FM, Andrews AT, Martinez J, Eyster EM, Sherwood WC (1976). Immunosuppressive therapy of Factor VIII inhibitors. *Blood;* 48(1): 95-108. ISSN: 0006-4971

Huntington JA. (2009). Slow thrombin is zymogen-like. *J Thromb Haemost;* Suppl 1: 159-64. ISSN: 1538-7933

Ill CR, Yang CQ, Bidlingmaier SM, Gonzales JN, Burns DS, Bartholomew RM, Scuderi P (1997). tion of the human factor VIII complementary DNA expression plasmid for gene therapy of hemophilia A. *Blood Coagul Fibrinolysis;* Suppl 2:S23-30. ISSN: 0957-5235

Ishiwata A, Mimuro J, Mizukami H, Kashiwakura Y, Takano K, Ohmori T, Madoiwa S, Ozawa K, Sakata Y (2009). Liver-restricted expression of the canine factor VIII gene facilitates prevention of inhibitor formation in factor VIII-deficient mice. *J Gene Med* ; 11(11): 1020-1029. ISSN: 1099-498X

Jedlicka P, Greer S, Millar DS, Grundy CB, Jenkins E, Mitchell M, Mibashan RS, Kakkar VV, Cooper DN (1990). Improved carrier detection of haemophilia A using novel RFLPs at the DXS115 (767) locus. *Hum Gene;* 85(3): 315-318. ISSN: 0340-6717

Jenkins PV, Collins PW, Goldman E, McCraw A, Riddell A, Lee CA, Pasi KJ (1994). Analysis of intron 22 inversions of the factor VIII gene in severe hemophilia A: implications for genetic counseling. *Blood;* 84(7): 2197-2201. ISSN: 0006-4971

Jiang H, Lillicrap D, Patarroyo-White S, Liu T, Qian X, Scallan CD, Powell S, Keller T, McMurray M, Labelle A, Nagy D, Vargas JA, Zhou S, Couto LB, Pierce GF (2006). Multiyear therapeutic benefit of AAV serotypes 2, 6, and 8 delivering factor VIII to hemophilia A mice and dogs. *Blood;* 108(1): 107-115. ISSN: 0006-4971

Johannessen M, Andreasen RB, Nordfang O (2000). Decline of factor VIII and factor IX inhibitors during long-term treatment with NovoSeven. *Blood Coagul Fibrinolysis;* 11(3): 239-242. ISSN: 0957-5235

Kang Y, Xie L, Tran DT, Stein CS, Hickey M, Davidson BL, McCray PB Jr (2005). Persistent expression of factor VIII in vivo following nonprimate lentiviral gene transfer. *Blood;* 106(5): 1552-1558. ISSN: 0006-4971

Kaufman RJ (1991). Developing rDNA products for treatment of hemophilia A. *Trends Biotechnol;* 9(10): 353-359. ISSN: 0167-7799

Kay MA, Manno CS, Ragni MV, Larson PJ, Couto LB, McClelland A, Glader B, Chew AJ, Tai SJ, Herzog RW, Arruda V, Johnson F, Scallan C, Skarsgard E, Flake AW, High KA (2000). Evidence for gene transfer and expression of factor IX in haemophilia B patients treated with an AAV vector. *Nat Genet;* 24(3): 257-261. ISSN:1061-4036

Kempton CL, Soucie JM, Miller CH, Hooper C, Escobar MA, Cohen AJ, Key NS, Thompson AR, Abshire TC (2010). Non-severe hemophilia A the risk of inhibitor after intensive factor treatment is greater in older patients: a case-control study. *J Thromb Haemost;* 8(10): 2224-2231. ISSSN: 1538-7933

Kenet G, Walden R, Eldad A, Martinowitz U (1999). Treatment of traumatic bleeding with recombinant factor VIIa. *Lancet;* 354(9193): 1879. ISSN: 0140-6736

Knights SF, Ingram GIC (1967). Partial thromboplastin time test with kaolin: diagnosis of haemophilia and Christmas disease without natural reference plasmas. *J clin. Path;* 20: 616-619. ISSN:0021-9746

Kochhan L, Lalloz MR, Oldenburg J, McVey JH, Olek K, Brackmann HH, Tuddenham EG, Schwaab R (1994). Haemophilia A diagnosis by automated fluorescent DNA detection of ten factor VIII intron 13 dinucleotide repeat alleles. *Blood Coagul Fibrinolysis;* 5(4): 497-501. ISSN: 0957-5235

Kogan SC, Doherty M, Gitschier J (1987). An improved method for prenatal diagnosis of genetic diseases by analysis of amplified DNA sequences. Application to hemophilia A. *N Engl J Med;* 317(16):985-990. ISSN: 0028-4793

Krolick MA (2005). Successful percutaneous coronary intervention in a patient with severe haemophilia A using bivalirudin as the sole procedural anticoagulant. *Haemophilia;* 11(4): 415-417. ISSN 1351-8216

Kumaran V, Benten D, Follenzi A, Joseph B, Sarkar R, Gupta S (2005). Transplantation of endothelial cells corrects the phenotype in hemophilia A mice. *J Thromb Haemost;* 3(9): 2022-2031. ISSN: 1538-7933

Lacroix-Desmazes S, Bayry J, Misra N, Kaveri SV, Kazatchkine MD (2002). The concept of idiotypic vaccination against factor VIII inhibitors in haemophilia A. *Haemophilia;*8 Suppl 2:55-59. ISSN 1351-8216

Lauritzen B, Tranholm M, Ezban M (2008a). rFVIIa and a new enhanced rFVIIa-analogue, NN1731, reduce bleeding in clopidogrel-treated and in thrombocytopenic rats. *J Thromb Haems;* 7(4): 651- 657. ISSN: 1538-7933

Lauritzen B, Hedner U, Johansen PB, Tranholm M, Ezban M (2008b). Recombinant human factor VIIa and a factor VIIa-analogue reduces heparin and low molecular weight heparin (LMWH)-induced bleeding in rats. *J Thromb Haemost*; 6(5): 804-811. ISSN: 1538-7933

Lefesvre P, Attema J, Lemckert A, Havenga M, van Bekkum D (2003). Genetic heterogeneity in response to adenovirus gene therapy. *BMC Mol Biol*. 5; 4: 4. ISSN 1471-2199

Levy JH, Levi M (2009). A modified recombinant factor VIIa: can we make it work Harder, Better, Faster, Stronger?. *J Thromb Haemo*st; 7(9): 1514- 1516. ISSN: 1538-7933

Lian EC, Larcada AF, Chiu AY (1989). Combination immunosuppressive therapy after factor VIII infusion for acquired factor VIII inhibitor. *Ann Intern Med*; 110(10): 774-778. ISSN: 0003-4819

Liars A (2011). Induced human pluripotent stem cells and advanced therapies Future perspectives for the treatment of haemophilia?*Thromb Res*; 2011 Mar 9. [Epub ahead of print] ISSN:0049-3848

Liras A (2008). Recombinant proteins in therapeutics: haemophilia treatment as an example. *Int Arch Med*, 1:4 ISSN 1755-7682

Liu X, Liu M, Xue Z, Pan Q, Wu L, Long Z, Xia K, Liang D, Xia J (2007). Non-viral ex vivo transduction of human hepatocyte cells to express factor VIII using a human ribosomal DNA-targeting vector. *J Thromb Haemost*; 5(2): 347-351. ISSN: 1538-7933

Ljung R, Holmberg L (1982). Immunoradiometric assay of inhibitors of antihaemophilic factor A. *Acta Paediatr Scand*; 71(6): 1019-1023. ISSN: 0001-656X

Lusher JM (2000). Hemophilia treatment. Factor VIII inhibitors with recombinant products: prospective clinical trials. *Haematologica*; 85(10 Suppl): 2-5; discussion 5-6. ISSN: 0390-6078

Lusher JM (2002). First and second generation recombinant factor VIII concentrates in previously untreated patients: recovery, safety, efficacy, and inhibitor development. *Semin Thromb Hemost*; 28(3): 273-276. ISSN: 0094-6176

Mackman N, Tilley RE, Key NS (2007). Role of the extrinsic pathway of blood coagulation in hemostasis and thrombosis. *Arterioscler Thromb Vasc Biol*; 27(8): 1687-1693. ISSN 1049-8834

Mannucci PM, Ruggeri ZM, Pareti FI, Capitanio A (1977).1-Deamino-8-d-arginine vasopressin: a new pharmacological approach to the management of haemophilia and von Willebrands' diseases. *Lancet*; 1(8017): 869-872. ISSN: 0140-6736

Margaritis P, Arruda VR, Aljamali M, Camire RM, Schlachterman A, High KA (2004). Novel therapeutic approach for hemophilia using gene delivery of an engineered secreted activated Factor VII. *Clin Invest*; 113(7): 1025-1031. ISSN: 0021-9738

Margaritis P (2010). Long-term expression of canine FVIIa in hemophilic dogs. *Thromb Res;* 125 Suppl 1:S60-62. ISSN:0049-3848

Margaritis P, Roy E, Aljamali MN, Downey HD, Giger U, Zhou S, Merricks E, Dillow A, Ezban M, Nichols TC, High KA (2009). Successful treatment of canine hemophilia by continuous expression of canine FVIIa. *Blood*; 113(16): 3682-3689. ISSN 0006-4971

McCormack WM Jr, Seiler MP, Bertin TK, Ubhayakar K, Palmer DJ, Ng P, Nichols TC, Lee B (2006). Helper-dependent adenoviral gene therapy mediates long-term correction of the clotting defect in the canine hemophilia A model. *J Thromb Haemost*; 4(6): 1218-1225. ISSN: 1538-7933

Michaelides K, Tuddenham EG, Turner C, Lavender B, Lavery SA (2006). Live birth following the first mutation specific pre-implantation genetic diagnosis for haemophilia A. *Thromb Haemost*; 95(2): 373-379. ISSN: 1538-7933

Miller G, Steinbrecher RA, Murdock PJ, Tuddenham EG, Lee CA, Pasi KJ, Goldspink G (1995). Expression of factor VII by muscle cells in vitro and in vivo following direct gene transfer: modelling gene therapy for haemophilia. *Gene Ther;* 2(10): 736-742. ISSN : 0969-7128

Miller DG, Rutledge EA, Russell DW (2002). Chromosomal effects of adeno-associated virus vector integration. *Nat Genet;* 30(2): 147-8. ISSN: 1061-4036

Nakai H, Montini E, Fuess S, Storm TA, Grompe M, Kay MA (2003). AAV serotype 2 vectors preferentially integrate into active genes in mice. *Nat Genet;* 34(3): 297-302. ISSN: 1061-4036

Naylor J, Brlnke A, Hassock S, M.Green P, Giannelll F (1993). Characteristic mRNA abnormality found in half the patients with severe haemophilia A is due to large DNA inversions. *Human Molecular Genetics;* 2(11): 1773-1778. ISSN: 0964-6906

Naylor JA, Green PM, Montandon AJ, Rizza CR, Giannelli F (1991). Detection of three novel mutations in two haemophilia A patients by rapid screening of whole essential region of factor VIII gene. *Lancet;* 337(8742): 635-639. ISSN: 0140-6736

Naylor JA, Green PM, Rizza CR, Giannelli F (1992). Factor VIII gene explains all cases of haemophilia A. *Lancet;* 340(8827):1066-1067. ISSN: 0140-6736

Nowotny C, Niessner H, Thaler E, Lechner K (1976). Sonography: a method for localization of hematomas in hemophiliacs. *Haemostasis;* 5(3): 129-135. ISSN:0301-0147

Obergfell A, Nichols T, Ezban M (2010). Animal models of FVIIa gene expression: their role in the future development of haemophilia treatment. *Haemophilia;* 16 Suppl 2: 24-27. ISSN 1351-8216

Ohmori T, Ishiwata A, Kashiwakura Y, Madoiwa S, Mitomo K, Suzuki H, Hasegawa M, Mimuro J, Sakata Y (2008). Phenotypic correction of hemophilia A by ectopic expression of activated factor VII in platelets. *Mol Ther;* 16(8): 1359-1365. ISSN: 1525-0016

Okamoto Y, Kojima T, Katsumi A, Yamazaki T, Hamaguchi M, Nishida M, Suzumori K, Saito H (1995). Carrier detection and prenatal diagnosis for hemophilia A using the inversion analysis of the factor VIII gene. *Rinsho Ketsueki;* 36(11): 1252-1256. ISSN: 0485-1439

Paleyanda RK, Velander WH, Lee TK, Scandella DH, Gwazdauskas FC, Knight JW, Hoyer LW, Drohan WN, Lubon H (1997). Transgenic pigs produce functional human factor VIII in milk. *Nat Biotechnol;*15(10):971-997. ISSN : 1087-0156

Parker ET, Healey JF, Barrow RT, Craddock HN, Lollar P (2004). Reduction of the inhibitory antibody response to human factor VIII in hemophilia A mice by mutagenesis of the A2 domain B-cell epitope. *Blood;* 104(3):704-710. ISSN 0006-4971

Petkova R, Chakarov S, Kremensky I (2004). Genetic analysis of haemophilia A in Bulgaria. *BMC Blood Disord;* 4(1): 2. ISSN 1471-2326

Puetz J (2010). Optimal use of recombinant factor VIIa in the control of bleeding episodes in hemophilic patients. *Drug Des Devel Ther;* 4: 127-337. ISSN: 1177-8881

Pieneman WC, Deutz-Terlouw PP, Reitsma PH, Briët E (1995). Screening for mutations in haemophilia A patients by multiplex PCR-SSCP, Southern blotting and RNA analysis: the detection of a genetic abnormality in the factor VIII gene in 30 out of 35 patients. *Br J Haematol;* 90(2): 442-449. ISSN: 0007-1048

Pipe SW (2008). Recombinant clotting factors. Thromb Haemost ; 99: 840–850.

Ramanarayana J, Krishnan GS, Hernandez-Ilizaliturri. Factor VII. http://emedicine.medscape.com/article/209585-overview

Qadura M, Waters B, Burnett E, Chegeni R, Bradshaw S, Hough C, Othman M, Lillicrap D (2009). Recombinant and plasma-derived factor VIII products induce distinct splenic cytokine microenvironments in hemophilia A mice. *Blood* ; 114(4): 871-880. ISSN 0006-4971

Rapaport SI, Patch MJ, Casey JE (1960). The antihemophilic globulin in plasma; content of freshly frozen single-donor plasma units prepared by the Los Angeles Red Cross Blood Center. *Calif Med*; 93:208-210.. ISSN:0008-1264

Rudzki Z, Rodgers SE, Sheffield LJ, Lloyd JV (1996). Detection of carriers of haemophilia A: use of bioassays and restriction fragment length polymorphisms (RFLP). *Aust N Z J Med*; 26(2): 195-205. ISSN: 0004-8291

Sabatino DE, Freguia CF, Toso R, Santos A, Merricks EP, Kazazian HH Jr, Nichols TC, Camire RM, Arruda VR (2009). Recombinant canine B-domain-deleted FVIII exhibits high specific activity and is safe in the canine hemophilia A model. *Blood*; 114(20): 4562-4565. ISSN 0006-4971

Sadler JE (1990). Recombinant DNA methods in hemophilia A: carrier detection and prenatal diagnosis. *Semin Thromb Hemost* ; 16(4): 341-347. ISSN:0094-6176

Salviato R, Belvini D, Are A, Radossi P, Tagariello G (2002). Large FVIII gene deletion confers very high risk of inhibitor development in three related severe haemophiliacs. *Haemophilia*; 8(1): 17-21. ISSN 1351-8216

Sarkar R, Mucci M, Addya S, Tetreault R, Bellinger DA, Nichols TC, Kazazian HH Jr (2006). Long-term efficacy of adeno-associated virus serotypes 8 and 9 in hemophilia a dogs and mice. *Hum Gene Ther*; 17(4): 427-439. ISSN: 1043-0342

Sarkar R, Xiao W, Kazazian HH Jr (2003). A single adeno-associated virus (AAV)-murine factor VIII vector partially corrects the hemophilia A phenotype. *J Thromb Haemost*; 1(2): 220-226. ISSN:1538-7933

Scallan CD, Liu T, Parker AE, Patarroyo-White SL, Chen H, Jiang H, Vargas J, Nagy D, Powell SK, Wright JF, Sarkar R, Kazazian HH, McClelland A, Couto LB (2003). Phenotypic correction of a mouse model of hemophilia A using AAV2 vectors encoding the heavy and light chains of FVIII. *Blood*; 102(12):3919- 3926. ISSN 0006-4971

Scandella D, Reyes H, Felch M, Sakurai Y (2000). Characterization of antibodies to factor VIII in hemophilia A patients treated by immune tolerance therapy. *Haematologica*; 85(10 Suppl): 86-88. ISSN: 0390-6078

Scharrer I (1999). Recombinant factor VIIa for patients with inhibitors to factor VIII or IX or factor VII deficiency. *Haemophilia*; 5(4): 253-259. ISSN 1351-8216

Schwaab R, Brackmann HH, Meyer C, Seehafer J, Kirchgesser M, Haack A, Olek K, Tuddenham EG, Oldenburg J (1995). Haemophilia A: mutation type determines risk of inhibitor formation. *Thromb Haemost* ; 74(6): 1402-1406. ISSN:0340-6245

Schwartz RA, Klujszo E, McKenna Ri. FVIII. http://emedicine.medscape.com/article/201319-overview

Sharathkumar A, Lillicrap D, Blanchette VS, Kern M, Leggo J, Stain AM, Brooker L, Carcao MD (2003). Intensive exposure to factor VIII is a risk factor for inhibitor development in mild hemophilia A. *J Thromb Haemost*; 1(6): 1228-1236. ISSN: 1538-7933

Shetty S, Bhave M, Ghosh K (2010). Acquired hemophilia A: Diagnosis, aetiology, clinical spectrum and treatment options. *Autoimmun Rev*. 2010 Nov 27. [Epub ahead of print]. ISSN: 1568-9972

Shi Q, Wilcox DA, Fahs SA, Weiler H, Wells CW, Cooley BC, Desai D, Morateck PA, Gorski J, Montgomery RR (2006). Factor VIII ectopically targeted to platelets is therapeutic in hemophilia A with high-titer inhibitory antibodies. *J Clin Invest*; 116(7): 1974-1982. ISSN: 0021-9738

Shi Q, Wilcox DA, Fahs SA, Fang J, Johnson BD, DU LM, Desai D, Montgomery RR (2007). Lentivirus-mediated platelet-derived factor VIII gene therapy in murine haemophilia A. *J Thromb Haemost*; 5(2): 352-361. ISSN: 1538-7933

Shi Q, Wilcox DA, Fahs SA, Kroner PA, Montgomery RR (2003). Expression of human factor VIII under control of the platelet-specific alphaIIb promoter in megakaryocytic cell line as well as storage together with VWF. *Mol Genet Metab*; 7 9(1): 25-33. ISSN: 1096-7192

Song KS, Lee CH, Chung CS, Lee K, Yang YH, Kim KY (1993). The prevalence study on restriction fragment length polymorphism analysis for the detection of hemophilia A carrier. *Yonsei Med J*; 34(3): 239-242. ISSN: 0513-5796

Stephens JM, Joshi AV, Sumner M, Botteman MF (2007). Health economic review of recombinant activated factor VII for treatment of bleeding episodes in hemophilia patients with inhibitors. *Expert Opin Pharmacother*; 8(8): 1127-1136. ISSN: 1465-6566

Stites DP, Hershgold EJ, Perlman JD, Fudenberg HH (1971). Factor 8 detection by hemagglutination inhibition: hemophilia A and von Willebrand's disease. *Science*; 171(967): 196-197. ISSN 0036-8075

Surin VL, Zhukova EL, Krutov AA, Solov'ev GIa, Likhacheva EA, Pliushch OP, Grineva NI (1990). [Detection of hemophilia A carriers by testing polymorphic Bcl I and HINDIII sites using the PCR method with internal splitting control]. *Gematol Transfuziol*; 35(3): 3-6. ISSN: 0234-5730

Thompson AR (1986). Structure, function, and molecular defects of factor IX. *Blood*; 67: 565-572. ISSN 0006-4971

Tomokiyo K, Nakatomi Y, Araki T, Teshima K, Nakano H, Nakagaki T, Miyamoto S, Funatsu A, Iwanaga S (2003). A novel therapeutic approach combining human plasma-derived Factors VIIa and X for haemophiliacs with inhibitors: evidence of a higher thrombin generation rate in vitro and more sustained haemostatic activity in vivo than obtained with Factor VIIa alone. *Vox Sang*; 85(4): 290-299. ISSN 0042-9007

Toole JJ, Knopf JL, Wozney JM, Sultzman LA, Buecker JL, Pittman DD, Kaufman RJ, Brown E, Shoemaker C, Orr EC, et al. (1984). Molecular cloning of a cDNA encoding human antihaemophilic factor. *Nature* ; 312(5992): 342-347. ISSN : 0028-0836

Toschi V (2010). OBI-1, porcine recombinant Factor VIII for the potential treatment of patients with congenital hemophilia A and alloantibodies against human Factor VIII. *Curr Opin Mol Ther*; 12(5): 617-625. ISSN: 1464-8431

Toy L, Young EA, Longenecker JB (1983). Ascorbic acid, vitamin A, folic acid, and amino acids in blood of patients with hemophilia. *Blood*; 62(3): 532-537. ISSN 0006-4971

Van de Water NS, Williams R, Nelson J, Browett PJ (1995). Factor VIII gene inversions in severe hemophilia A patients. *Pathology*; 27(1): 83-85. ISSN:0031-3025

VandenDriessche T, Collen D, Chuah MK (2003). . Gene therapy for the hemophilias. *J Thromb Haemost*; 1(7): 1550-1558. ISSN: 1538-7933

von Auer Ch, Oldenburg J, von Depka M, Escuriola-Ettinghausen C, Kurnik K, Lenk H, Scharrer I (2005). Inhibitor development in patients with hemophilia A after continuous infusion of FVIII concentrates. *Ann N Y Acad Sci*; 1051: 498-505. ISSN: 0077-8923

Wacey AI, Kemball-Cook G, Kazazian HH, Antonarakis SE, Schwaab R, Lindley P, Tuddenham EG (19996) The haemophilia A mutation search test and resource site, home page of the factor VIII mutation database: HAMSTeRS. *Nucleic Acids Res;* 24(1): 100-102. ISSN: 0305-1048

Wadelius C, Blombäck M, Goonewardena P, Anvret M, Lindstedt M, Gustavson KH, Pettersson U (1991). Evaluation of DNA-based diagnosis for haemophilia A. *Scand J Clin Lab Invest* ; 51(7): 625-633. ISSN: 0036-5513

Wang L, Herzog RW (2005). AAV-mediated gene transfer for treatment of hemophilia. *Curr Gene Ther.* 2005 Jun; 5(3): 349-360. ISSN: 1566-5232

Wehnert M, Shukova EL, Surin VL, Schröder W, Solovjev GYa, Herrmann FH (1990a). Prenatal diagnosis of haemophilia A by the polymerase chain reaction using the intragenic hind III polymorphism. *Prenat Diagn;* 10(8): 529-532. ISSN: 0197-3851

Wehnert M, Shukova EL, Surin VL, Schröder W, Solovjev GYa, Grinjeva NI, Herrmann FH (1990b). Genomic carrier detection and prenatal diagnosis of haemophilia A in families at risk using the polymerase chain reaction (PCR). *Folia Haematol Int Mag Klin Morphol Blutforsch;* 117(4): 617-622. ISSN: 0323-4347

White GC, Shoemaker CB. (1989). Factor VIII Gene and Hemophilia A. *Blood;* 73(10): 1-12. ISSN 0006-4971

Wiestner A, Cho HJ, Asch AS, Michelis MA, Zeller JA, Peerschke EI, Weksler BB, Schechter GP (2002). Rituximab in the treatment of acquired factor VIII inhibitors. *Blood;* 100(9): 3426-3428. ISSN 0006-4971

Wood WI, Capon DJ, Simonsen CC, Eaton DL, Gitschier J, Keyt B, Seeburg PH, Smith DH, Hollingshead P, Wion KL, et al. (1984). Expression of active human factor VIII from recombinant DNA clones. *Nature;* 312(5992): 330-337. ISSN : 0028-0836

Wu G (1991). Prenatal diagnosis of hemophilia A by DNA analysis. *Zhongguo Yi Xue Ke Xue Yuan Xue Bao;* 13(6): 428-434. ISSN: 0376-2491

Yoshioka A, Fukutake K, Takamatsu J, Shirahata A; Kogenate Post-Marketing Surveillance Study Group (2003). Clinical evaluation of a recombinant factor VIII preparation (Kogenate) in previously untreated patients with hemophilia A. *Int J Hematol;* 78(5): 467-474. ISSN: 0925-5710

Youssoufian H, Antonarakis SE, Aronis S, Tsiftis G, Phillips DG, Kazazian HH Jr (1987). Characterization of five partial deletions of the factor VIII gene. *Proc Natl Acad Sci U S A;* 84(11): 3772-3776. ISSN: 0027-8424.

Zatloukal K, Cotten M, Berger M, Schmidt W, Wagner E, Birnstiel ML (1994). In vivo production of human factor VII in mice after intrasplenic implantation of primary fibroblasts transfected by receptor-mediated, adenovirus-augmented gene delivery. *Proc Natl Acad Sci U S A;* 91(11): 5148-5152. ISSN: 0027-8424

Zhang WW, Josephs SF, Zhou J, Fang X, Alemany R, Balagué C, Dai Y, Ayares D, Prokopenko E, Lou YC, Sethi E, Hubert-Leslie D, Kennedy M, Ruiz L, Rockow-Magnone S (1999). Development and application of a minimal-adenoviral vector system for gene therapy of hemophilia A. *Thromb Haemost;* 82(2): 562-571. ISSN: 1538-7933

21

The Different Effects of TGF-β1, VEGF and PDGF on the Remodeling of Anterior Cruciate Ligament Graft

Changlong Yu, Lin Lin and Xuelei Wei
Institute of Sports Medicine, Peking University Third Hospital, No.49, North Garden Road, Haidian District, P.R.China

1. Introduction

Rupture of anterior cruciate ligament (ACL) is a common knee trauma which leads to anterior knee instability. The ACL has long been thought to have poor capacity for healing with suture repair. ACL reconstruction is the standard of care which can restore the knee stability of ACL deficit knee. Although ACL reconstruction is an excellent operation for restoring the sagittal plane stability of the knee, significant problems remain. Studies have demonstrated that remodeling of the graft usually takes longer than expected, and many patients develop arthritis after an ACL tear, even if they have a reconstruction, with rates as high as 78% reported at 14 years post-operatively (1).

In ACL reconstruction, inflammation and necrosis of the graft can occur immediately after transplantation. The graft then undergoes revascularization and cellular repopulation from an extrinsic origin, followed by a remodeling period. In the early phase, the properties of the grafted tendon are deteriorated and do not recover to physiological levels even at 18 months after surgery (2). Therefore, the main goals of ACL reconstruction are to prevent the deterioration of grafted tendon and accelerate mechanical restoration of the deteriorated graft. New solutions are needed to accelerate and improve remodeling of tendon grafts.

The ACL graft remodeling process is regulated by a complex growth factor network. Many growth factors have been evaluated for their ability to stimulate tendon and ligament healing in vitro and in vivo. In enhancing ligament repair, the most interesting candidates are insulin-like growth factor-I (IGF-I), transforming growth factor β1 (TGFβ1), vascular endothelial growth factor (VEGF), epidermal growth factor (EGF), platelet derived growth factor (PDGF), and basic fibroblast growth factor (bFGF). PDGF and VEGF appear in the early stage of reconstruction, during the stage of graft maturing, the granular tissue becomes ligament-like tissue and both PDGF and VEGF are not able to be detected gradually, as the replacement, TGFβ1and other cytokines are involving in the reconstruction process to mature the ligament. TGFβ1 is the main cytokine for the maturing of ligament. Studies have demonstrated improved cellular proliferation and migration as well as increased collagen production rates with the addition of growth factors.

2. VEGF

Angiogenesis is an essential step in the process of tendon healing and tendon graft remodeling, in which neovascularization prompts delivery of inflammatory cells, fibroblasts and growth factors to the wound site. VEGF plays an essential role in angiogenesis, regulating the activation, migration, and proliferation of endothelial cells in various pathological conditions. It is well-known that angiogenesis is an essential step in the healing process of tendon and tendon graft remodeling. Two studies found that VEGF therapy can enhance revascularization in the graft, as well as promoting the infiltration of fibroblasts after ACL reconstruction; however, it did not affect the mechanical properties of the in situ freeze-thawed ACL model (3). Furthermore, it decreased the stiffness of the grafted tendon with increased knee laxity, 12 weeks after ACL reconstruction in a sheep model (4). Yoshikawa et al. examined the effects of an application of VEGF to a hamstring graft in a sheep ACL reconstruction model and demonstrated that the linear stiffness of the VEGF-treated graft was significantly lower than that of the PBS-treated group at 12 weeks (4). In this study, the stiffness of the VEGF165 group was higher than those of the control group at 12 weeks, although there was no significant difference ($P > 0.05$). There are two possible reasons for this difference.
In our study, the stiffness of the VEGF165 group was higher than those of the control group at 12 weeks, although there was no significant difference (5). There are two possible reasons for this difference. One is the method of applying this factor. In our study, the method was transfer of the VEGF165 gene, rather than the gene products. The secretion time and quantity of VEGF165 may be suitable for ACL graft remolding. The other possible reason is the use of BMSCs in our experiment. BMSCs have the capacity to differentiate into various mesenchymal lineages, including ligament, tendon, muscle, bone, cartilage and adipose tissue. Kanaya et al. reported that the intra-articular injection of BMSCs could accelerate the healing of partially torn knee ACLs in a rat model (6). Our study also demonstrated that the application of BMSCs is effective in enhancing collagen deposition and changing certain structural properties for improving tendon allograft remodeling after ACL reconstruction in a rabbit model (7). The exact reasons for the better healing observed in injured ACLs using BMSCs are uncertain. One possibility is that BMSCs directly differentiated into ligament fibroblasts within the healing environment. Alternatively, another possibility is that injected mesenchymal stromal cells directly contribute as a cellular source for ligament healing. BMSCs may also secrete a variety of growth factors, which may contribute to the activation and recruitment of local fibroblast precursors or enhance extracellular matrix synthesis.

3. PDGF

Many studies have also attempted to determine the effects of PDGF-BB on a ligament engineering system. It has been demonstrated that it promoted fibroblast proliferation, matrix synthesis, neovascularization, and mechanical properties. In our studies in the gene-transfected group, more cells and blood vessels could be found at 3 weeks, and more collagen was synthesized in the ACL as compared with the control and MSCs group (7).

Similar to our findings were the results of a study by Nakamuraetal, which described an increased vascularity and enhanced collagen deposition in the wound of a patellar ligament afte rPDGF-B gene transfer in rats (8).
The mechanisms by which PDGF affects ligament healing are complex. Kuroda et al. studied immunohistochemically the presence and the level of bFGF, TGF-ß, PDGFAA and PDGF-BB expression in a model of ACL reconstruction using a free patellar tendon autograft (9). They found that all tested growth factors were upregulated with a maximum expression at 3 weeks and up to 60% of all cells were stained PDGF positive. PDGF is one of the most effective growth factors during tendon graft remodeling.
Tendon grafts are exposed to the reduced PO2 of the intra-articular environment, Petersen et al. (10) showed that PDGF as well as hypoxia strongly enhanced VEGF secretion from tenocytes. Besides this VEGF-mediated angiogenetic effect, PDGF further more induces the synthesis of other growth factors, including IGF, and regulates the presence of other receptors (11). Therefore, it could be concluded that the expression of PDGF-BB by the small number of transfected cells may activate a cascade of PDGF-BB throughout the wound. Some researches (12) showed that there are some growth factors receptors such as PDGFR on the surface of MSCs. MSCs from bone marrow might have a better response to PDGF as compared with those from the ACL or MCL regarding proliferation and migration. Thus, it might be suggested that a tendon graft seeded with MSCs-PDGF-BB is more likely to promote MSCs or fibroblast proliferation and migration and accelerate graft tissue remodeling.
The observations of Kuroda et al. also imply that if a growth factor is administered to the tendon graft, its tissue concentration should be highest around the third week to enhance the effect of the other intrinsical growth factors (9). In our study at 3 weeks, we found significantly higher vascularity in the PDGF-transfected grafts. The concentration of PDGF-BB inarticular fluid from gene-transfected rabbit increased at 3 week, got to the highest point at 6 week and then dropped down. This rapid reduction in the level of their localization indicates that once the extrinsic cells infiltrate to the graft and revascularization is complete, these growth factors may have less significance for subsequent remodeling. Therefore, it is very important to find the appropriate time point for the administration of growth factors to promote healing.
In vivo study by Hildebrand et al. demonstrated that the improvements in the MCL structural properties were dose-dependent to PDGF-BB (13).That is, a higher dose of PDGF-BB improved more structural properties of the femur–MCL–tibia complex than a lower dose of PDGF-BB did. In both the MSCs group and gene-transfected group, although there are much more differences in morphology at the early stages, the structure of the ACL in the two groups have less significant differences at the later stages, especially at 12 weeks. For an ACL reconstruction model, we don't know if the dosage we used was appropriate to maximally enhance graft remodeling, or this indicates that the growth fact or PDGF may have early effect on the ACL reconstruction and have less significance for subsequent remodeling. It is essential to find an appropriate dosage for ACL reconstruction.

4. TGFβ1

Many studies indicate that TGFβ1 plays a key role in the healing process of ligaments. TGFβ1 increased both collagen and non-collagenous protein synthesis by the introduction of

ACL fibroblasts (14, 15). Furthermore, it has also been shown to increase ACL fibroblast proliferation. TGFβ1 enhanced graft remolding in ACL reconstruction by inhibiting mechanical deterioration (16).

In situ freeze-thawed ACL tissues, which were established as an autograft model, transfected with TGFβ1 and EGF, significantly reduced the increase in water content and cross-sectional area and reduced the deterioration of the ACL (17). However, the results were dose- and time-dependent, and of high cost. Furthermore, the clinical application of growth factors is hampered by delivery problems. Amiel et al. reported that a high dose of TGFβ1 inhibits proliferation of rabbit ACL fibroblasts (18). One study reported that an application of low-dose TGFβ1 mixed with fibrin sealant enhanced the remodeling process of the in situ freeze-thawed ACL, whereas a high dose of TGFβ1 had no effect (17). We demonstrated that TGFβ1 gene-modified BMSCs implanted within the Achilles allograft in ACL reconstruction significantly affects the biomechanical properties of the graft. Our results suggest that the transfer of the TGFβ1 gene, rather than the gene products, may be the most expeditious method of harnessing this factor for the purposes of accelerating ACL graft remolding (5).

Our results showed that the ultimate failure load and the stiffness of the grafted tendon were significantly increased in the TGFβ1 treatment group compared with the VEGF165 and control groups at 6, 12 and 24 weeks after surgery. Meanwhile toluidine blue staining of the grafts appeared positive only in the TGFβ1 group at 12 weeks. ACL has different histological characteristics from medical collateral ligament (MCL), which is more cartilage-like in nature. The normal ACL is positive to toluidine blue staining, so we hypothesized that TGFβ1 may promote early maturation of the graft. Histological examination and immunohistochemistry showed significantly enhanced cell infiltration and revascularization at 3, 6, and 12 weeks in the VEGF165 and the TGFβ1/VEGF165 groups. However, VEGF165 cDNA-transduced BMSCs exhibited no significant effects on the mechanical properties of the ACL graft, while TGFβ1/VEGF165 cDNA-transduced BMSCs showed the best biomechanical properties of the ACL graft at 24 weeks after surgery. This work shows that the use of TGFβ1 and the co-expression of TGFβ1/VEGF165 of gene therapy may be useful for accelerating the remolding of the graft after ACL reconstruction.

Previous study by Lee et al. demonstrated that VEGF and TGFβ1 were both expressed in ACL healing (18). We demonstrate here that the combination of TGFβ1 and VEGF165 gene has a synergistic effect on accelerating the remolding of the ACL graft, but few studies have defined the exact regulating mechanisms of these two growth factors during ligament healing. Several studies have demonstrated that together VEGF and TGFβ1 can enhance each the synthesis of one another (19, 20). These studies revealed that the mechanism of synergy is probably mediated through Smad3, HIF-1α/β, Smad3/4, PI3K/Akt or ERK1/2 signaling pathways.

5. The Effects of TGF-β1, VEGF165 transfer on achilles tendon healing

The Achilles tendon itself is a dense, regular connective tissue consisting primarily of type I collagen and interspersed specializedmesenchymal cells (tenocytes) responsible for the maintenance of collagen structure. With respect to reconstruction of the tendon, there are three key factors which must be addressed: the cell, the fiber, and their arrangement. The properties of the tendon matrix and its regulation by growth factors are largely uncharacterized. We examined the effects of implantation of BMSCs transduced with either the TGF-β1, VEGF165, or both on experimentally injured Achilles tendons in a rabbit model in vivo (21).

The maximum failure load, the tendon stiffness, and the elastic modular of the healing tendons were significantly increased in the TGF-β1 and the co-expression treatment groups compared with the other treatment groups at one, two, four, and eight weeks after surgery. Moreover, there was evidence of accelerated remodeling of the lesion in response to TGF-β1 and co-expression TGF-β1/VEGF165 treatment, while the size of the ruptured callus was increased in the presence of VEGF165. Histological examination showed a much more organized and homogeneous pattern of collagen fibers at all time points in the lesions of the TGF-β1 and the co-expression treatment groups. Both single fibrils and the collagen fibers had a greater diameter, with a higher degree of collagen crimp than the collagen of the other treatment groups. This was confirmed by Sirius red staining in conjunction with polarized light microscopy, which showed a higher shift of small yellow-green fibers to strong yellow-orange fibers after two, four, and eight weeks in the TGF-β1 and the co-expression treatment groups. Immunohistochemistry showed more vessels after one, two, four, and eight weeks in the VEGF165 treatment group, but only a few vessels in the co-expression treatment group. There was also an earlier shift from fibroblasts to fibrocytes within the healing tendon, with fewer fat cells present in the tendons of the TGF-β1 and the co-expression treatment groups compared with intact tendon. Thus treatment with TGF-β1 transduced BMSCs resulted in a promising acceleration and improvement of tendon healing, particularly influencing early tissue regeneration, leading to quicker recovery and improved biomechanical properties of the Achilles tendon. However, VEGF165 transduced BMSCs exhibited a negative role. The angiogenesis effects of VEGF165 were diminished by TGF-β1, while the collagen synthesis effects of TGF-β1 were only slightly affected by VEGF165. The TGF-β1 and VEGF165 synthesized of BMSCs with gene transfer were evaluated by ELISA. However, the stimulation effect is very weak with heterologous gene transfer in contrast with homologous gene transfer. In terms of the fibroblasts, the mRNA expression of Collagen type I, type III and Fibronectin were evaluated. All showed significant increasing under the stimulation of TGF-β1 or TGF-β1/VEGF165 co-existing. Nevertheless, the fibroblasts stimulated by VEGF165 showed no difference with control.

We demonstrated that gene modified BMSCs implanted within the tendon-repair site contributed to early tendon-healing following primary repair, and that growth factor signaling can regulate the mechanical properties of the tendon matrix by affecting tendon mass and architecture. These data provide a basis for future application of supplementary therapy of surgery for tendon and ligaments. Future studies determining the optimal growth factor(s), dose, and timing and site of administration are required, along with the interactions between different growth factors.

6. Summary

The effects of TGF-β1, VEGF and PDGF on the remodeling of anterior cruciate ligament graft are different. PDGF, VEGF and TGFβ1transfected MSCs accelerated cellular infiltration and enhanced collagen deposition in the graft. PDGF and VEGF promoted the angiogenesis of the graft, but did not show any improvement of the biomechanical nature of the graft. Only TGFβ1accerated the maturing of graft and improved the biomehchanical nature. TGFβ1 co-expression with VEGF165 in gene-transfected BMSCs could accelerate the remodeling of the reconstructed ligament. The cross-talk between TGFβ1 and VEGF165 has positive consequences, with TGFβ1/VEGF165-gene-transfected BMSCs could significantly promote angiogenesis of the reconstructed ligament, while achieving the best mechanical properties of the reconstructed ligament. However, the molecular mechanism that regulates these two growth factors during ligament healing still needs to be fully elucidated. The effects of other growth factors on the remodeling of ACL graft, such as IGF-1, bFGF, need further study.

7. References

[1] Von Porat A, Roos EM, Roos H. High prevalence of osteoarthritis 14 years after an anterior cruciate ligament tear in male soccer players: a study of radiographic and patient relevant outcomes .Br J Sports Med. 2004; 38: 263.

[2] Delay BS, McGrath BE, Mindell ER, Observation on a retrieved patellar tendon autograft used to reconstruct the anterior cruciate ligament. A case report. J Bone Joint Surg Am. 2002; 84: 1433-8.

[3] Ju YJ, Tohyama H, Kondo E, Yoshikawa T, Muneta T, Shinomiya K, Yasuda K, Effects of local administration of vascular endothelial growth factor on properties of the in situ frozen-thawed anterior cruciate ligament in rabbits, Am J Sports Med. 2006; 34:84-91.

[4] Yoshikawa T, Tohyama H, Katsura T, Kondo E, Kotani Y, Matsumoto H, Toyama Y, Yasuda K, Effects of local administration of vascular endothelial growth factor on mechanical characteristics of the semitendinosus tendon graft after anterior cruciate ligament reconstruction in sheep, Am J Sports Med. 2006;34 :1918-25.

[5] Xuelei Wei, Wei X, Mao Z, Hou Y, Lin L, Xue T, Chen L, Wang H, Yu C. Local administration of TGFβ-1/VEGF(165) gene-transduced bone mesenchymal stem cells for Achilles allograft replacement of the anterior cruciate ligament in rabbits. Biochem Biophys Res Commun.in press.

[6] Kanaya A, Deie M, Adachi N, Nishimori M, Yanada S, Ochi M, Intra-articular injection of mesenchymal stromal cells in partially torn anterior cruciate ligaments in a rat model.Arthroscopy. 2007; 23: 610-7.

[7] Li Feng, Hongti Jia, Changlong Yu. ACL reconstruction in a rabbit model using irradiated Achilles allograft seeded with mesenchymal stem cells or PDGF-B gene-transfected mesenchymal stem cells. Knee Surg Sports Traumatol Arthrosc. 2007;15(10):1219-27.

[8] Nakamura N, Shino K, Natsuume T, Horibe S, Matsumoto N, Kaneda Y, OchiT. Early biological effect of in vivo gene transfer of platelet-derived

growth factor (PDGF)-B into healing patellar ligament.GeneTher. 1998; 5:1165–70.

[9] Kuroda R, Kurosaka M, Yoshiya S, Mizuno K. Localization of growth factors in the reconstructed anterior cruciate ligament: immunohistological study in dogs .Knee Surg Sports Traumatol Arthrosc.2000; 8:120–6.

[10] Marui T, Niyibizi C, Georgescu HI, Cao M, Kavalkovich KW, Levine RE, Woo SL, Effect of growth factors on matrix synthesis by ligament fibroblasts. J Orthop Res. 1997; 15: 18-23.

[11] Petersen W, Pufe T, Zantop T, Tillmann B, Mentlein R. Hypoxia and PDGF have a synergistic effect that increases the expression of the angiogenetic peptide vascular endothelial growth factor in Achilles tendon fibroblasts. Arch Orthop Trauma Surg.2003;123:485–8.

[12] Yasuhiro Y, Abrahamson S. Dose-related effects of platelet-derived growth factor-BB vary by different rabbit tendons in vitro. Transactions of the 46th annual meeting of the Orthopaedic Research Society.2000.

[13] Minguell JJ, Erices A, Conget P. Mesenchymal stem cells. Exp Biol Med. 2003; 226:507–20.

[14] DesRosiers EA, Yahia L, Rivard CH. Proliferative and matrix synthesis response of canine anterior cruciate ligament fibroblasts submitted to combined growth factors. J Orthop Res. 1996;14: 200-8.

[15] Yamazaki S, Yasuda K, Tomita F, Tohyama H, Minami A. The effect of transforming growth factor-beta1 on intraosseous healing of flexor tendon autograft replacement of anterior cruciate ligament in dogs. Arthroscopy. 2005; 21: 1034-41.

[16] Azuma H, Yasuda K, Tohyama H, Sakai T, Majima T, Aoki Y, Minami A. Timing of administration of transforming growth factor-beta and epidermal growth factor influences the effect on material properties of the in situ frozen-thawed anterior cruciate ligament. J Biomech. 2003; 36:373-81.

[17] Amiel D, Nagineni CN, Choi SH, Lee J, Intrinsic properties of ACL and MCL cells and their responses to growth factors, Med Sci Sports Exerc. 1995; 27: 844-851.

[18] Lee J, Harwood FL, Akeson WH, Amiel D, Growth factor expression in healing rabbit medial collateral and anterior cruciate ligaments, Iowa Orthop J. 1998;18:19-25.

[19] Kobayashi T, Liu X, Wen FQ, Fang Q, Abe S, Wang XQ, Hashimoto M, Shen L, Kawasaki S, Kim HJ, Kohyama T, Rennard SI. Smad3 mediates TGF-beta1 induction of VEGF production in lung fibroblasts, Biochem Biophys Res Commun. 2005; 327: 393-8.

Li ZD, Bork JP, Krueger B, Patsenker E, Schulze-Krebs A, Hahn EG, Schuppan D.VEGF induces proliferation, migration, and TGF-beta1 expression in mouse glomerular endothelial cells via mitogen-activated protein kinase and phosphatidylinositol 3-kinase, Biochem Biophys Res Commun. 2005; 334:1049-60.

[20] Hou Y, Mao Z, Wei X, Lin L, Chen L, Wang H, Fu X, Zhang J, Yu C. Effects of transforming growth factor-beta1 and vascular endothelial growth factor 165 gene transfer on Achilles tendon healing. Matrix Biol. 2009;28(6): 324-35.

22

Different *ex Vivo* and Direct *in Vivo* DNA Administration Strategies for Growth Hormone Gene Therapy in Dwarf Animals

Cibele Nunes Peroni, Nélio Alessandro de Jesus Oliveira,
Claudia Regina Cecchi, Eliza Higuti and Paolo Bartolini
Biotechnology Department, National Nuclear Energy Commission (IPEN-CNEN), Cidade Universitária, São Paulo, Brazil

1.Introduction

Recombinant growth hormone (GH) was one of the first proteins to be synthesized via DNA recombinant techniques in the late seventies. It was also one of the first proteins to be used in studies of animal models for gene therapy, already in the eighties. This was due to the real therapeutic need for GH, combined with the fact that its detection by well-known immunoassay methods is facile and sensitive. Moreover, evident phenotypic effects can be observed and measured in several animal models (e.g., dwarf mice), some of which have GH deficiencies that closely resemble their human counterparts.

GH gene therapy has the potential advantage of circumventing laborious and expensive purification processes, quality control procedures and the repetitive injections that are required in the conventional treatment. The ideal situation would, of course, be to introduce the deficient protein into the circulation via a mechanism that resembles the natural process. These treatments have not yet reached the clinical stage for humans, the major challenge being to achieve a sustainable and regulated *in vivo* GH secretion. However, several interesting and promising *ex vivo* and direct *in vivo* DNA administration strategies for GH gene therapy have been developed and studied using animal models. These studies obviously open the way for the systemic delivery of other therapeutic proteins in addition to GH.

The various *ex vivo* models for GH gene therapy are based on the use of target cells, such as keratinocytes, fibroblasts, endothelial cells, peritoneal mesothelial cells, or skeletal myoblasts. These cells can also be encapsulated to prevent rejection when implanted in allogeneic hosts. The majority of the methodologies are carried out via cell isolation and *in vitro* cultivation, genetic modification by viral or non-viral vectors containing the GH gene and re-implantation of the secreting cells onto the animal.

Primary keratinocytes are one of the most attractive vehicles for gene transfer and gene therapy. They are among the most accessible cells in the body and can be serially propagated in culture; the procedure for their transplantation is already well established, e.g., for burn patients, and the therapy can be reversed by excision of the genetically modified tissue. Cutaneous gene therapy has already been demonstrated to be a powerful tool for the successful treatment of severe skin disorders such as epidermolysis bullosa [1]. Keratinocytes can also act as cellular bioreactors, secreting GH or other proteins systemically. When primary human keratinocytes were retrovirally transduced with the human (hGH) or mouse (mGH) growth hormone genes in our laboratory, they exhibited high and stable *in vitro* secretion. When these hGH-secreting keratinocytes were grafted onto immunodeficient dwarf mice (lit/scid), a significant body weight gain was obtained, despite low hGH serum levels. When the conventional epithelial sheet grafting methodology described by Ian Barrandon and coworkers in 1988 [2] was replaced by the implantation of an organotypic raft culture, peak values of up to 20 ng mGH/ml were observed in the circulation of lit/scid mice. However, this was followed by a rapid decline of the levels to a baseline value of ~2 ng/ml [3]. For comparison, the mGH serum concentration in heterozygous lit/+ mice is of the order of 6 ng/ml.

Among the various *ex vivo* methodologies for GH gene therapy, the implantation, by a Canadian research group [4], of encapsulated mGH-secreting myoblasts into the peritoneal cavity of Snell dwarf mice should be mentioned. Using this procedure, the recombinant allogeneic cells were protected from rejection and remained functional for at least 6 months. The animals showed a remarkable increase in body weight and the increase in body length doubled compared to the control group.

The GH gene therapy approach based on *in vivo* gene transfer via adenoviral injection developed by a Houston (TX) group led to a complete phenotypic correction of dwarfism in little mice (lit/lit) [5]. Nonetheless, this strategy suffers from several potentially serious problems that require more profound investigation prior to its adaptation to human therapy. One of these problems is the high expression of the transgene, mostly by hepatocytes, leading to continuously elevated GH and IGF-I circulating levels that may cause dysfunctions or cancer.

A much better option would appear to be the direct administration of naked plasmid DNA, a methodology that has been successfully adopted by several authors in the last decade. Analysis of growth parameters such as body weight, organ weight (quadriceps muscles, liver, kidneys, heart and spleen) and total (nose-to-tail) length of the animals have been used to study the endocrine and local (autocrine/paracrine) effects of hGH in greater depth after intramuscular DNA administration in immunodeficient dwarf mice (lit/scid) [6]. Although the majority of the strategies described for GH gene therapy are still limited by the absence of an appropriate mechanism for regulating *in vivo* hormone expression and secretion, a number of factors favor *in vivo* drug generation as the best alternative. In particular, this would avoid costly industrial productions, very expensive treatments and would improve the quality of life of patients (children and adults) suffering from GH deficiency (GHD).

In this chapter, we review the results reported in five studies from our laboratory, primarily involving *ex vivo* methodologies based on primary human keratinocyte retroviral transduction and direct plasmid DNA administration in immunodeficient (lit/scid) and immunocompetent (lit/lit) dwarf mice. We also analyze the data reported in nine studies by seven other research groups using *ex vivo* techniques based on transduced fibroblasts and myoblasts and *in vivo* methodologies based on direct adeno and adenoassociated viral vectors or on naked DNA administration. The animal models used by these authors include lit/lit, Snell dwarf mice, hypophysectomized rats and mice, growth hormone-releasing hormone knockout (GHRHKO) mice and growth-retarded swine.

2. *Ex vivo* strategies

In 1995, the Canadian group mentioned above reported that the growth defect of dwarf mice (Snell dwarf) could be partially corrected by implanting microencapsulated allogeneic myoblasts engineered to secrete mouse growth hormone. The encapsulation of these mouse myoblasts into GH-deficient Snell dwarf mice provided a completely homologous system [4]. The plasmid pKL-mGH, encoding mGH cDNA under the regulation of human β-actin promoter and also containing the neomycin resistance gene, was used to transfect the mouse myoblast cell line C2C12. G418 resistant clones were selected and screened for the level of mGH in the culture medium. Clone Myo-45, which secreted 147 ng of mGH/10^6 cells/day, was selected for encapsulation. Microcapsules were implanted via a 22G catheter into the peritoneal cavity and, by the end of the 3rd week, the body weight of the dwarf mice had increased about 1.6-fold and the increase in body length had doubled compared to the control group. There were also significant increases in the levels of non-esterified free fatty acids (a measure of the lipolytic effect of the capsule-delivered mGH), while peripheral organ weights and tibial growth plate thickness were also significantly greater. The authors hypothesized that most of the capsule-derived mGH was sequestered in the liver through the hepatic GH receptors, inducing the secretion of hepatic insulin-like growth factor I (IGF-I), which mediates most of the GH-dependent systemic metabolic effects. After 5 weeks, however, a lack of further growth in weight or length was evident in all of the mice. According to the authors, this was not due to the absence of mGH transgene expression by the encapsulated cells, but rather to the non-responsiveness of the mice to the hormone at this age (13-15 weeks). In fact, a second implantation of freshly-prepared capsules on day 42 did not result in any further growth enhancement. Moreover, encapsulated cells retrieved at the end of the experiment (178 days) continued to secrete *in vitro* >200 ng/10^6 cells/day of mGH. Interestingly, all the different groups of dwarf mice had low or undetectable GH levels in their plasma, i.e. 1.32-1.42 ng/ml at best, comparable to the detection limit of ≤ 0.62 ng/ml of the mGH RIA. The authors´ assumption was that the capsules probably delivered circulating levels of mGH below the detection limit of the assay. Nonetheless, this study demonstrated the clinical efficacy of this non-autologous system and its potential for widespread application in therapies requiring a continuous systemic supply of recombinant gene products.

Fibroblasts are also a potentially interesting cell type for *ex vivo* gene delivery because of their easy accessibility, facile culture *in vitro*, convenient re-implantation and their potential for delivering proteins to the circulation. In 1995 a research group at the Taiwan National University employed hypophysectomized rats as an animal model to explore the feasibility of using genetically engineered fibroblasts for growth hormone gene therapy [7]. A bicistronic retroviral vector controlled by the LTR promoter, which contained a porcine growth hormone (pGH) cDNA at the first cistron and a neomycin resistance gene at the second cistron, was used to infect primary rat embryo fibroblasts. The transduced cells exhibited an *in vitro* expression level of up to 1.18 μg pGH/10^6 cells/day and 5 x 10^6 cells/animal were injected directly into the peritoneum of hypophysectomized rats, leading to a significant growth of the tibia when tested at days 15 and 57 post-implantation. Alternatively, 1 x 10^6 cells were cast in collagen matrices (0.5 cm in diameter) and implanted underneath the skin on the back of the rats: a semi-quantitative RT-PCR confirmed that the pGH expression by these cells lasted up to 70 days. Unfortunately, a sensitive ELISA system was not available and pGH could not be detected in the sera of the animals. However, the tibia growth bioassay in hypophysectomized rats did provide clear evidence for the *in vivo* activity of pGH in a direct functional assay and confirmed that fibroblasts are indeed capable of persistently expressing foreign genes *in vivo*.

The same Chinese research group subsequently used primary porcine fetal fibroblasts, transduced with the same pGH-carrying vector described above, to enhance the weight gain of growth-retarded Tao-Yuan Swine, a local breed in Taiwan that is slow growing and fat, but palatable[8]. Immortalized fibroblasts were avoided because of their tumorigenic potential, even though they have been used quite successfully in several different studies in mice. The transduced primary cells were encapsulated with the same type of alginate-poly-L-lysine-alginate membranes used previously for mice myoblasts [4] and then implanted into the peritoneal cavity of the swine, resulting in a significant increase in weight gain already on day 16 post-implantation, even though no increase in serum pGH could be detected. The use of immunoprotective microcapsules thus constitutes a simple method of delivering recombinant genes *in vivo* and proved to be a valid approach for the improvement of the growth of these animals. Since the microcapsules obviate the need for patient-specific *ex vivo* preparations and are amenable to industrial-scale production and quality control, this approach is also potentially economically viable.

Our research group has focused its *ex vivo* activities mainly on the use of human primary keratinocytes that were retrovirally transduced with the human (hGH) or the mouse (mGH) GH genes, implanting them into immunodeficient dwarf (lit/scid) mice [3,9-11]. Epidermal keratinocytes were chosen as the target of our gene therapy methodology because they are among the most accessible cells in the body and can be serially propagated in culture, following the pioneering work of Rheinwald and Green [12]. When these cells were stably transduced with the hGH gene (under control of the retroviral LTR promoter), a high *in vitro* secretion of up to 7 μg hGH/10^6 cells/day was obtained [9]. Their grafting onto lit/scid mice led to circulating hGH serum levels of 0.2-0.3 ng/ml during a 12-day assay (peak value, 1.5 ng/ml at 4h). Grafted mice also showed an increase in body weight (0.060 g/animal/day), which was significantly higher ($P<0.01$) than that of the controls (0.023 g/animal/day). This was the first time that continuous *in vivo* secretion of the hormone and subsequent phenotypic alterations due to the grafting of transduced, hGH-secreting primary human keratinocytes had been demonstrated in lit/scid mice, an animal model known to be very sensitive to low concentrations of hGH [13].

Conventional epidermal sheets of these mGH-secreting keratinocytes, prepared by us using the classical technique of Barrandon et al.[2], showed a drop in secretion rates of >80% simply due to detachment of the epithelium from its substratum. Replacement of this conventional grafting methodology by organotypic raft cultures[14] completely overcame this problem. Employing a similar *ex vivo* strategy and this modification of the grafting resulted in a very high, stable *in vitro* secretion of up to 11 μg mGH/10^6 cells/day. Moreover, the amazing value of ~26 μg mGH/10^6 cells/day could be reached by clonal selection[11], performed by seeding the mGH-secreting keratinocytes at low densities (~500 cells/10 cm culture dish) and isolating colonies with a diameter of ~5 mm by the use of cloning cylinders. Cells were expanded four times by serial passage (approximately one passage/week), counted and the medium collected for mGH determination by radioimmunoassay. Clonal selection revealed that, after four serial passages (equivalent to > 30 cumulative cell doublings or > 10^7 cells), approximately 30% (7 out of 24) of the isolated clones maintained or presented increased mGH expression. This percentage represents the fraction of transduced keratinocyte stem cells present, a very important parameter for attaining the desired persistent gene therapeutic effect. The stable long-term grafting of such cultures onto *lit/scid* mice could be followed for more than 4 months, with a significant weight increase over the control group being observed in the first 40 days. Circulating mGH levels reached a peak of 21 ng/ml just 1h after grafting but, as already mentioned, these levels fell rapidly (in ~24 h) to baseline values [3]. Thus, in this study, an animal model for cutaneous gene therapy based on lit/scid mice and on the grafting of organotypic raft cultures was developed and the mGH-secreting primary human keratinocytes employed exhibited the highest *in vitro* secretion ever reported for any form of GH in these cells. However, the desired sustainability of the *in vivo* secretion of the transgene was not achieved.

Several hypotheses can be raised as the possible cause(s) of this immediate suppression or blocking of exogenous GH in the circulation of lit/scid mice after the grafting. These include: (i) a limited mGH circulatory half-life in lit/scid; (ii) a rapid clearance from the bloodstream due to a specific binding or selective transfer; (iii) impediments due to poor vascularization, to a fast inflammatory process or to an unidentified specific barrier; (iv) the occurrence of extremely efficient apoptotic events, transgene inactivation or promoter failure; (v) partial immune reactivity spontaneously developed by the immunodeficient mice, leading to some production of B and T cells (i.e., "leakiness"). Although several of these hypothetical mechanisms could be rationally or even experimentally excluded, so far we have been unable to positively prove the existence of any one of them. This led us think that comparative tests carried out by injecting mGH-expressing naked DNA, enhanced by *in vivo* electroporation, at approximately the same epidermal site as keratinocyte grafting, might prove to be informative. This resulted in studies from our laboratory of the *in vivo* administration of naked DNA to lit/lit and lit/scid mice, with the goal of comparing the circulating hormone levels obtained by this type of GH delivery with those obtained via implantation of GH-secreting cells.

3. *In vivo* approach

Adenovirus administration is an effective way of delivering therapeutic genes since they can be produced and purified in a concentrated form, which facilitates *in vivo* delivery. Another advantage is that potential oncogenic effects resulting from viral integration into critical chromosomal regions are unlikely because adenoviruses do not integrate into host chromosome DNA [5]. Since it is well-known that adenoviruses can elicit multiple innate immune responses after systemic administration, there are several approaches under investigation that attempt to overcome this limitation. These include modification of the adenoviral vector design, the use of tissue specific promoters and local administration routes and the utilization of immunosuppressive drugs or specific compounds to block important immune pathways known to be induced by adenovirus [15].

Concerning GH deficiency and dwarf animals, an adenoviral vector containing rat GH (rGH) cDNA was used in 1996 by the Houston group mentioned above to induce constitutive GH expression in hepatocytes of GH-deficient lit/lit mice [5]. When the recombinant adenoviral vector, controlled by the human elongation factor 1-α (EF1α) promoter, was administered via the tail vein of this animal at a dose of 10^8 pfu (plaque-forming units), high levels of GH were detected in the serum for at least 7 weeks. This viral dose led to an unbelievably high peak of the serum GH level of 1.9 μg/ml, which then decreased to ~125 ng/ml during the next 2 weeks, remaining at that level for the duration of the experiment (7 weeks). A viral dose of 10^9 pfu induced an even higher serum GH level of ~35 µg/ml, which then decreased to ~2.5 µg/ml over the next two weeks and stabilized at 1 µg/ml for the duration of the study. The authors attributed the decrease in GH expression in part to the ability of the host's immune system to recognize and subsequently eliminate the virally transduced cells. Little dwarf mice treated with 10^8 pfu of rGH adenovirus showed an increase in circulating IGF-I levels (from 61 to 238 ng/ml in 3 weeks). Although the serum GH levels increased dramatically, the serum IGF-I levels did not follow the same pattern. This may be due to the presence of reduced IGFBP-3 in GH-deficient humans and animals. A rapid weight gain, resulting in a body weight comparable to that of normal age-matched lit/+ animals, was achieved by 5 weeks of treatment. Total body length was also indistinguishable from that of lit/+ mice within 7 weeks of treatment and body composition was normal, with a reduction in the percentage of fat and increase in the water and protein contents. The animals treated with rGH adenoviruses exhibited slight, but significant, increases in liver and kidney sizes and a tendency to increase fasting blood glucose and insulin levels, which are known effects in response to prolonged exposure to high levels of GH. It was suggested, however, that the induced hepatic and renal hyperplasia warranted further investigation. According to the authors, the little mice dwarf phenotype could be corrected, with minimal side-effects, by constitutive GH expression achieved through *in vivo* recombinant adenoviral delivery. Because the correction of GH insufficiency by gene transfer may represent in the future an alternative to the conventional treatment, the importance of this work is undeniable since it was the first study to demonstrate a complete phenotypic correction of dwarfism. Nonetheless, a constitutive adenoviral-induced GH expression in hepatocytes producing extremely high GH serum concentrations, would meet serious obstacles to its application in humans.

In a subsequent study, carried out in 1999 by groups at the National Institute of Health (NIH, Bethesda, MD), an adenovirus encoding mGH cDNA was injected into the quadriceps muscle or submandibular ducts of mGH-deficient Snell dwarf mice to obtain a homologous system and thus avoid possible side effects resulting from species differences [16]. When the adenoviral vector was used *in vitro* to infect SMIE (submandibular immortalized ephitelial) cells, an epithelial cell line derived from the adult rat submandibular gland, the highest *in vitro* expression level obtained was ~184 ng mGH/ml at 72h post infection for cells infected at a MOI (multiplicity of infection) of 300. To test its *in vivo* efficacy, the virus was injected into the quadriceps muscle of Snell dwarf mice (5 x 10^9 pfu/animal), resulting in an average serum level of 42 ± 29.7 ng mGH/ml at 4 days post injection. Submandibular administration provided widely varying serum levels of 64.1, 3.4 and 11 ng mGH/ml in three individual animals. The intramuscular protocol was more efficient, providing an average 8% increase in body weight of the dwarf mice just 4 days post treatment and close to 100% by 30 days. This indicates that skeletal muscle gave a fairly stable transgene expression and suggests that it can be a highly useful tissue for the delivery of circulating proteins. To obtain enough serum to determine the various metabolic parameters, the adenoviral vector was also administered to young rats via the intravenous route. The main effects were an increase of ~ 35% in serum IGF-I levels, ~60% in cholesterol and ~40% in triglycerides, all changes that are consistent with systemic mGH action and anabolic effects. The mice and rats utilized in these studies received dexamethasone to limit the host immune response of these immunocompetent animals. The authors concluded that the adenoviral vector could be a valuable tool in preclinical mouse model studies. Even though administration via muscle is somewhat milder than via other tissues (e.g., the liver), we believe that most of the limitations related to adenoviral gene therapy are still present in this approach.

More recently, in 2008, a new generation of double-stranded adeno-associated viral vectors (dsAAV) encoding mGH cDNA driven by a universal promoter (CMV) were used by a group coordinated by Johns Hopkins University School of Medicine to prepare viral particles that were injected into GHRHKO mice, a model of isolated GH deficiency due to generalized ablation (knock-out, KO) of the GHRH gene [17,18]. These genetically modified dsAAV can infect dividing and non-dividing cells *in vitro* and *in vivo* with a long-term transgenic expression (up to 1 year) and elicit a lower toxicity and cellular immune response, therefore being generally considered to be safer than adenoviral vectors.

In an initial study, GHRHKO mice were injected intraperitoneally with either a single dose (low dose) or two doses (high dose) of 1×10^{11} viral particles at the 10th and 11th days of age and were followed up to the 6th or 24th week of life[17]. Body weight and length of both viral-treated groups became normal at 6 months of age and normal femoral and tibial lengths, body composition and weight of organs (liver, spleen, heart and kidney) were also obtained. At week 6, serum GH levels were higher in mice receiving both virus doses compared with controls, while they were normal at week 24. This is consistent with the results of previous studies showing that long-term expression by this type of viral vector is limited to the liver and skeletal and cardiac muscle. This was confirmed by the detection of GH mRNA in these same tissues of the GHRHKO mice. Nevertheless, serum IGF levels were significantly higher in both virus-treated groups compared to the control group at week 24, showing that the expressed GH is still functional in GH-deficient and immunocompetent mice and that no resistance to its effect was developed over time, since a species-specific GH cDNA was used. The use of a universal promoter is obviously a limitation for any clinical application of this approach because of the well-known long-term risks associated with excessive unregulated GH secretion. The authors concluded that, while the applicability of these findings is still very far from any possible clinical trial in humans, these new AAV vectors offer a good starting point for the development of novel regulated viral gene delivery systems for GH administration. Such systems could be based on the use of inducible promoters that can be regulated at will or of tissue-specific promoters, providing good systemic delivery together with limited local expression.

In a subsequent study, the same group utilized a dsAAV expressing mGH cDNA under the control of a muscle creatine kinase regulatory cassette in order to ensure adequate systemic delivery in conjunction with muscle-specific expression [18]. A low-dose (0.5×10^{11} pfu) and a high-dose (1×10^{11} pfu) of virus were injected into the right quadriceps muscle of GHRHKO mice at the age of day 10. Virus-injected GHD mice showed a significant ($P<0.05$) increase in body length and weight, however without becoming fully normal, and a significant ($P<0.05$) reduction in visceral fat at week 6 of age. Quantitative RT-PCR showed that GH mRNA expression in the quadriceps muscle of animals treated with the high-dose of virus was significantly higher than in the gastrocnemius and cardiac muscles or the kidney and liver of the same mice. At 6 weeks of age, serum GH and IGF-I levels in both treated groups were not significantly higher than those in the control mice. This study showed that, although the strategy of vector-mediated GH therapy is still not applicable at the clinical stage, systemic GH delivery to GHD animals is possible via a single injection of viral particles derived from dsAAV using an approach that limits GH expression to skeletal muscle. In fact, it is known that widespread gene expression can result in toxicity [19].

An alternative system for delivering genes *in vivo* is the administration of naked plasmid DNA. When carried out in certain tissues, particularly muscle, this is considered to be a practical method that can produce significant levels of gene expression, although lower than those achieved with viral vectors. The simplicity of this methodology has made it the most utilized non-viral system in clinical trials of gene therapy, representing as much as 18% of current trials [20].

A research group from a company in Texas has been a pioneer in GH naked DNA administration. They designed a muscle-specific gene medicine, composed of a hGH expression plasmid containing the chicken skeletal α-actin promoter complexed with a protective, interactive, non-condensing (PINC™) delivery system, to be administered intramuscularly in hypophysectomized rats [21]. This polymeric PINC gene delivery system consists of polyvinilpyrrolidone (PVP), which protects plasmids from extracellular nuclease degradation and facilitates the uptake of the plasmid by muscle cells. To test the *in vitro* hGH expression, C2C12 myoblasts were transfected with the muscle-specific hGH plasmid, showing a secretion rate of ~43 ng hGH/ml. The plasmid, formulated in saline or complexed to PVP, was then injected into the tibialis cranialis muscle of normal and hypophysectomized rats. The levels of hGH in normal rat muscle injected with 150 μg of hGH plasmid complexed with PVP were ~ 3 ng/gr muscle, i.e., approximately 10- to 15-fold higher than the control (plasmid in saline). Comparable hGH levels were detected in muscle extracts for up to 14 days, showing a decline 21 days after the injection. In hypophysectomized rats, a single but relatively high intramuscular dose (1.8 mg DNA/rat) of the hGH plasmid/PVP complex resulted in ~ 1.5 ng hGH/gr muscle (21 days post injection). The animals also showed a significant increase in growth, while serum IGF-I levels reached a value of 145.4 ± 77 ng/ml (vs. 34.7 ± 2.0 ng/ml before injection) at 21 days, declining thereafter. It is noteworthy that, after a single intra-muscular dose of this gene medicine, the increase in growth and the serum IGF-1 levels were comparable to those obtained with daily injections of recombinant hGH. Anti-hGH antibodies appeared in the serum at 14 days post injection, this antibody response being completely blocked by the administration of cyclosporine. hGH was not detectable in the sera of the injected animals, in spite of the increases in serum rat IGF-I levels and growth. This was attributed by the authors to the possibility that hGH levels were below the detection limit of the radioimmunoassay and/or that the human hormone was rapidly cleared from the circulation due to its short half-life in rodents. This gene medicine was shown to be effective over several weeks at a single intramuscular dose. Future work by the authors will be devoted to optimizing both the delivery system and the gene expression plasmid in order to produce the sustained levels of therapeutic protein necessary to permit the use of this specific gene-therapy approach in humans.

Another strategy used for *in vivo* GH delivery by a Danish group with which we are collaborating is hydrodynamic gene transfer. This transfer strategy is based on a rapid tail vein injection of naked plasmid DNA contained in a volume of buffer that corresponds to approximately 10% of the body weight of the animal. Although the exact mechanism is not clear, the rapid injection of a large amount of aqueous solution is likely to cause a transient right-side congestive heart failure with back-flow to the liver vessels. The liver is thus the target organ in this therapy, although the transfected vectors are mainly present as non-integrated episomes. This methodology was used to deliver hGH into hypophysectomized mice [22]. The entire plasmid pUC-UBI-hGH solution, containing the ubiquitin C promoter and the genomic hGH sequence, was injected (40-50 μg DNA/1.5-1.9 ml) within 3-9 seconds. High levels of hGH were obtained in the circulation of the mice, reaching a peak value of 67.1 ng/ml 13 days post injection and remaining stable at ~50 ng/ml throughout the study (68 days), with a concomitant normalization of circulating IGF-I (from a maximum of 599 ng/ml on day 13) and IGF-binding protein (IGFBP)-3 levels. Furthermore, longitudinal growth became normal in terms of tibia length and tail length, while body weight stabilized at a level 4-5 g below that of normal mice. Weights of the liver, spleen and lungs were normal, whereas that of the heart was only partially normal, with hGH mRNA being expressed exclusively in liver tissue. Although the hGH levels were ~20-fold higher than physiological baseline levels, the IGF-I and IGFBP-3 levels were comparable to those found in normal mice. The authors suggested that a modification of the hydrodynamic procedure, for example by using a catheter-mediated delivery to the isolated liver, could make the protocol feasible for future human applications. These data strongly suggest that non-viral hGH gene transfer could be a feasible alternative to daily hGH injections in GHD patients, but again there are serious obstacles that must be overcome before the procedure can be used clinically. Hydrodynamic transfer has been successfully applied in dogs [23], but, as pointed out by the authors, other routes for gene transfer can be more convenient for humans.

As already mentioned, our group started working with the administration of naked DNA and has described a strategy for *in vivo* GH gene therapy based on electroporation of hGH-coding plasmid in the quadriceps muscle of lit/lit and lit/scid mice [6]. Muscle was chosen for the establishment of the methodology since it has been demonstrated that gene delivery vectors can be stably maintained in postmitotic fibers after their injection and that this tissue is able to provide a long-term release of the therapeutic protein. The utilization of gene electrotransfer must also be emphasized because it is considered to be one of the most efficient, safest, most practical and less expensive non-viral methods of DNA delivery and also generally decreases the inter-individual variability. Using the pUC-UBI-hGH plasmid [22], we found the optimal electroporation conditions to be eight 50 V pulses of 20ms each at 0.5 s intervals. Employing these conditions, various amounts (12.5, 25, 50, 75 and 100 μg) of the purified plasmid were administered into the exposed right quadriceps muscle. Serum hGH levels, determined 3 days after DNA injection, provided a dose-response curve with a highly significant ($P<0.01$) linear correlation in the range of 0-50 μg of injected plasmid. Because 50 μg of DNA produced circulating hGH levels of 2-3 ng/ml for at least 12 days, a long-term body weight gain assay was carried out in lit/scid mice. After 60 days of continuous secretion of hGH, ranging from 1.5-3 ng/ml, the DNA-treated group increased from an average weight of 8.92 ± 1.29 g/mouse to 11.87 ± 0.53 g/mouse, corresponding to an average weight gain of 33.1% ($P<0.001$). In contrast, the control group (mice injected with saline followed by electroporation) decreased from 9.08 ± 0.95 g/mouse to 8.70 ±0.88 g/mouse, for a Statistically non-significant weight loss of 4.2%.

The DNA-injected quadriceps muscles presented a 48.1 % weight increase versus the saline-injected control ($P<0.001$), whereas the weight increase of non-injected quadriceps of treated animals was 31.0 % ($P<0.005$). DNA-injected quadriceps showed a 45.5 % increase compared to the non-injected quadriceps of the same treated mice ($P<0.001$). These data point to local (autocrine and/or paracrine) and systemic (endocrine) effects as a result of hGH DNA injection.

Another long-term experiment carried out with immunocompetent dwarf little mice (lit/lit), fail to produce the same degree of statistical significance. The body weight increase was somewhat lower (~21%) and the increase in body weight ceased after approximately one month. However, up to the 32nd day, the slope of the growth curve was 0.048 ± 0.038 g/mouse/day and the difference relative to the control curve (slope = 0.038 ± 0.016) was statistically significant ($P<0.01$).

This treatment with a single injection of 50 μg of pUC-UBI-hGH in lit/scid mice was also compared to regular injections of recombinant hGH (5 μg/twice a day/animal) during 30 days. The two different strategies provided a similar response in terms of weight variation, when comparing the body weight gain of 0.094 g/mouse/day for the naked DNA system and of 0.095 g/mouse/day for recombinant protein injected daily, while the slope for the control (saline injection followed by electroporation) was 0.22 g/mouse/day (manuscript in preparation)[8].

We have thus shown that intramuscular naked DNA hGH administration can be effective for promoting the growth of dwarf "little" mice, a model of human isolated growth hormone deficiency (IGHD). More must still be done, however, especially in terms of achieving long-lasting, sustained serum levels of the therapeutic protein.

4. Conclusions

As far as we know, the treatment of systemic protein deficiencies via gene therapy has not yet reached the stage of successful clinical applications, even for other diseases like hemophilia [24]. As shown here, however, total or partial correction of growth defects has been achieved in several animal models for GH gene therapy by the use of a variety of different *ex vivo* or *in vivo* methodologies, all of which have the potential for future developments. We believe that, among these, the intramuscular administration of hGH-coding naked DNA, followed by a properly adapted electroporation technique, is probably the most promising therapy for GH deficiency due to its simplicity, practicality and safety. The fact that the plasmid is maintained in an episomal state results in a lower expression, but at the same time it offers the possibility of avoiding dangerously high hormone levels and undesirable chromosomal integration. Obviously, more must still be done in the direction of obtaining a long-lasting *in vivo* expression of the transgene.

5. References

[1] Mavilio F, Pellegrini G, Ferrari S, et al. Correction of junctional epidermolysis bullosa by transplantation of genetically modified epidermal stem cells. *Nat Med* 2006; 12: 1397-1402.

[2] Barrandon Y, Li V, Green H. New techniques for the grafting of cultured human epidermal cells onto athymic animals. *J Invest Dermatol* 1988; 91: 315-318.

[3] Peroni CN, Cecchi CR, Rosauro CW, et al. Secretion of mouse growth hormone by transduced primary human keratinocytes: prospects for an animal model of cutaneous gene therapy. *J Gene Med* 2008; 10: 734-743.

[4] Al-Hendy A, Hortelano G, Tannenbaum GS, et al. Correction of the growth defect in dwarf mice with nonautologous microencapsulated myoblasts - an alternate approach to somatic gene therapy. *Hum Gene Ther* 2005; 6: 165-175.

[5] Hahn TM, Copeland KC, Woo SL. Phenotypic correction of dwarfism by constitutive expression of growth hormone. *Endocrinology* 1996; 137: 4988-4993.

[6] Oliveira NAJ, Cecchi CR, Higuti, E, et al. Long-term human growth hormone expression and partial phenotypic correction by plasmid-based gene therapy in an animal model of isolated growth hormone deficiency. *J Gene Med* 2010; 12: 580-585.

[7] Chen B.F., Chang W.C., Chen S.T., et al. Long-term expression of the biologically active growth hormone in genetically modified fibroblasts after implantation into a hypophysectomized rat. *Hum. Gene Ther.* 1995, 6: 917-926.

[8] Cheng W.T.K., Chen, B.C., Chiou, S.T., et al. Use of nonautologous microencapsulated fibroblasts in growth hormone gene therapy to improve growth of midget swine. *Hum. Gene Ther.* 1998, 9: 1995-2003.

[9] Bellini MH, Peroni CN, Bartolini P. Increases in weight of growth hormone-deficient and immunodeficient (lit/scid) dwarf mice after grafting of hGH-secreting, primary human keratinocytes. *FASEB J* 2003; 17: 2322-2324.

[10] Peroni CN, Gout PW, Bartolini P. Animal models for growth hormone gene therapy. *Curr Gene Ther* 2005; 5: 493-509.

[11] Peroni CN, Cecchi CR, Damiani R, et al. High-level secretion of growth hormone by retrovirally transduced primary human keratinocytes: prospects for an animal model of cutaneous gene therapy. *Mol Biotechnol* 2006; 34: 239-245.

[12] Rheinwald JG, Green H. Formation of a keratinizing epithelium in culture by a cloned cell line derived from a teratoma. *Cell* 1975; 6: 317-330.

[13] Bellini MH, Mathor MB, De Luca M, et al. Ultrasensitive in vivo bioassay detects bioactive human growth hormone in transduced primary human keratinocytes. *J Endocrinol Invest* 1998; 21: 1-6.

[14] Kolodka TM, Garlick J.A., Taichman, L. B. Evidence for keratinocyte stem *cells in vitro*: long term engraftment and persistence of transgene expression from retrovirus-transduced keratinocytes. *Proc Natl Acad Sci USA* 1998, 95: 4356-4361.

[15] Seregin SS, Amalfitano A. Improving adenovirus based gene transfer: strategies to accomplish immune evasion. *Viruses* 2010; 2: 2013-2036.

[16] Marmary Y, Parlow AF, Goldsmith CM, et al. Construction and *in vivo* efficacy of a replication-deficient recombinant adenovirus encoding murine growth hormone. *Endocrinology* 1999; 140: 260-265.

[17] Sagazio A, Xiao X, Wang Z, et al. A single injection of doubled-stranded adeno-associated viral vector expressing GH normalizes growth in GH-deficient mice. *J Endocrinol* 2008; 196: 79-88.

[18] Martari M, Sagazio A, Mohamadi A, et al. Partial rescue of growth failure in growth hormone (GH)-deficient mice by a single injection of a double-stranded adeno-associated viral vector expressing the GH gene driven by a muscle-specific regulatory cassette. *Hum Gene Ther* 2009; 20: 759-766.

[19] Wang CH, Liu DW, Tsao Y, et al. Can genes transduced by adeno-associated virus vectors elicit or evade an immune response? *Arch Virol* 2004; 149: 1-15.

[20] Edelstein ML, Abedi MR, Wixon J. Gene therapy clinical trials worldwide to 2007 - an update. *J Gene Med* 2007; 9: 833-842.

[21] Anwer K, Shi M, French MF, et al. Systemic effect of human growth hormone after intramuscular injection of a single dose of a muscle-specific gene medicine. *Hum Gene Ther* 1998; 9: 659-670.

[22] Sondergaard M, Dagnaes-Hansen F, Flyvbjerg A, et al. Normalization of growth in hypophysectomized mice using hydrodynamic transfer of the human growth hormone gene. *Am J Physiol Endocrinol Metab* 2003; 285: E427-E432.

[23] Zhang G, Vargo D, Budker V, et al. Expression of naked DNA injected into the afferent and efferent vessels of rodent and dog livers. *Hum Gene Ther* 1997; 8: 1763-1772.

[24] Doering CB, Spencer HT. Advancements in gene transfer-based therapy for hemophilia A. *Expert Rev Hematol* 2009; 2: 673-683.

23

Protection from Lethal Cell Death in Cecal Ligation and Puncture-Induced Sepsis Mouse Model by *In Vivo* Delivery of FADD siRNA

Yuichi Hattori and Naoyuki Matsuda
Department of Molecular and Medical Pharmacology, Graduate School of Medicine and Pharmaceutical Sciences, University of Toyama, and Department of Emergency and Critical Care Medicine, Nagoya University Graduate School of Medicine, Japan

1. Introduction

Sepsis is the leading cause of death in most intensive care units (Angus *et al.*, 2001; Martin *et al.*, 2003). Sepsis results from dysregulation of the normally protective anti-microbial host defense mechanism and represents a systemic inflammatory response that is associated with hypotension, insufficient tissue perfusion, uncontrolled bleeding, and multiple organ failure/dysfunction (Bone *et al.*, 1992; Natanson *et al.*, 1994). Accordingly, a major focus of sepsis research has been the development of anti-inflammatory strategies. In clinical trials, however, most of the therapies that may modify systemic inflammation have largely failed to reduce mortality in patients with severe sepsis (Zeni *et al.*, 1997; Natanson *et al.*, 1998; Marshall, 2000). These failed trials include administration of high-dose glucocorticoids; polyclonal and monoclonal antibodies against endotoxin and various inflammatory mediators such as tumor necrosis factor (TNF)-α; anti-inflammatories; nitric oxide (NO) inhibitors; anti-oxidants; and others. Hence, new understanding of the pathophysiological mechanisms underlying this complex disorder is needed to develop novel therapeutic strategies that will impact favorably on septic patient outcome.

Apoptosis is a second prominent feature of sepsis. This process is a mechanism of tightly regulated disassembly of cells caused by activation of certain specialized proteases called caspases. A number of laboratories have demonstrated that sepsis induces extensive lymphocyte apoptosis, which can impairment of immunoresponses, thereby predisposing patients to septic death (Ayala & Chaudry, 1996; Wesche *et al.*, 2005; Hotchkiss *et al.*, 2005; Lang & Matute-Bello, 2009; Matsuda *et al.*, 2010a). Parenchymal cells, including intestinal and lung epithelial cells, also have increased apoptotic cell death in animal models of sepsis (Coopersmith *et al.*, 2002a, 2002b; Perl *et al.*, 2007). An autopsy study comparing samples from multiple organ systems in 20 patients who died of sepsis with those from 16 critically ill, non-septic patients has shown that gut epithelial apoptosis is increased in septic patients (Hotchkiss *et al.*, 1999a). Moreover, it has been suggested that vascular endothelial cells may be undergoing apoptosis in sepsis (Hotchkiss *et al.*, 2002). In sepsis, endothelial cell apoptosis may be associated with microvascular dysfunction with reduced perfusion and oxygen, which could result in tissue hypoxia and, ultimately, in the development of organ failure (Matsuda & Hattori, 2007). This could explain partly the disappointment in a large number of sepsis trials conducted with interventions against individual steps in the inflammatory cascade, leading investigators to the question of whether death in septic patients stems from uncontrolled inflammation (Hattori *et al.*, 2010).

To reduce sepsis-induced apoptosis, caspase inhibitors have been examined in mice with cecal ligation and puncture (CLP)-induced sepsis. It has been reported that the pan-caspase inhibitor *N*-benzyloxycarbonyl-Val-Ala-Asp (*O*-methyl) fluoromethyl ketone (*z*-VAD) decreases lymphocyte apoptosis in the thymus and spleen, decreases blood bacterial counts, and improves survival in sepsis (Hotchkiss *et al.*, 1999b). In a similar study, the pan-caspase inhibitor L-826,920 (M-920) and the selective caspase-3 inhibitor L-826,791 (M-791) have shown a survival benefit being the result of the rescue of lymphocytes from apoptosis (Hotchkiss *et al.*, 2000). Furthermore, Kawasaki *et al.* (2000) have demonstrated that *z*-VAD decreases apoptosis on pulmonary endothelial cells and epithelial cells and prolongs the survival rate in a lipopolysaccharide (LPS)-induced acute lung injury (ALI) mouse model. However, successful anti-apoptotic therapy in sepsis with caspase inhibitors may be challenging, because caspase inhibitors themselves can have detrimental effects within the cell when large amounts of them must reach the cell cytosol to inhibit apoptosis that is initiated only by small amounts of caspases. In fact, survival in *z*-VAD high-dose group after CLP returns toward the level of the control (Hotchkiss *et al.*, 1999b), indicating that there appears to be close-limiting toxicity associated with the administration of *z*-VAD.

Small interfering RNA (siRNA) is another potential reversible inhibitor of the apoptotic death pathways. siRNA therapy may offer a unique alternative sepsis treatment to shorten the apoptotic arm of sepsis, revealing a number of targets within the apoptotic death pathways, which may be useful in designing stand-alone and/or adjuvant therapies that would have a significant impact on septic mortality. Although the causative agents of sepsis vary widely as do their traditional anti-microbial treatments, siRNA therapy targeted toward salvaging immune effector cells, vascular endothelial cells, and parenchymal cells from apoptosis has the potential to be beneficial in sepsis regardless of the source. We have generated synthetic double-stranded siRNA targeting Fas-associated death domain (FADD) and examined the therapeutic effect of systemic administration of the siRNA in the CLP mouse model, regarded as a highly clinically relevant animal model of polymicrobial sepsis. As described below, FADD is an essential component of the death-inducing signaling complex (DISC) for all death receptors (Thorburn, 2004; Lavrik *et al.*, 2005). Here we present that this RNA interference-mediated gene silencing *in vivo* is effective as gene therapy of the septic syndrome.

2. Apoptotic cell death pathways

Two major pathways are involved in the initiation of apoptotic cell death (Figure 1) (Roy & Nicholson, 2000). The first apoptotic pathway is mediated by specific ligands and surface receptors, which are capable of delivering a death signal from the microenvironment and can activate the execution of apoptosis in the cell cytoplasm and organelles (Herr & Debatin,

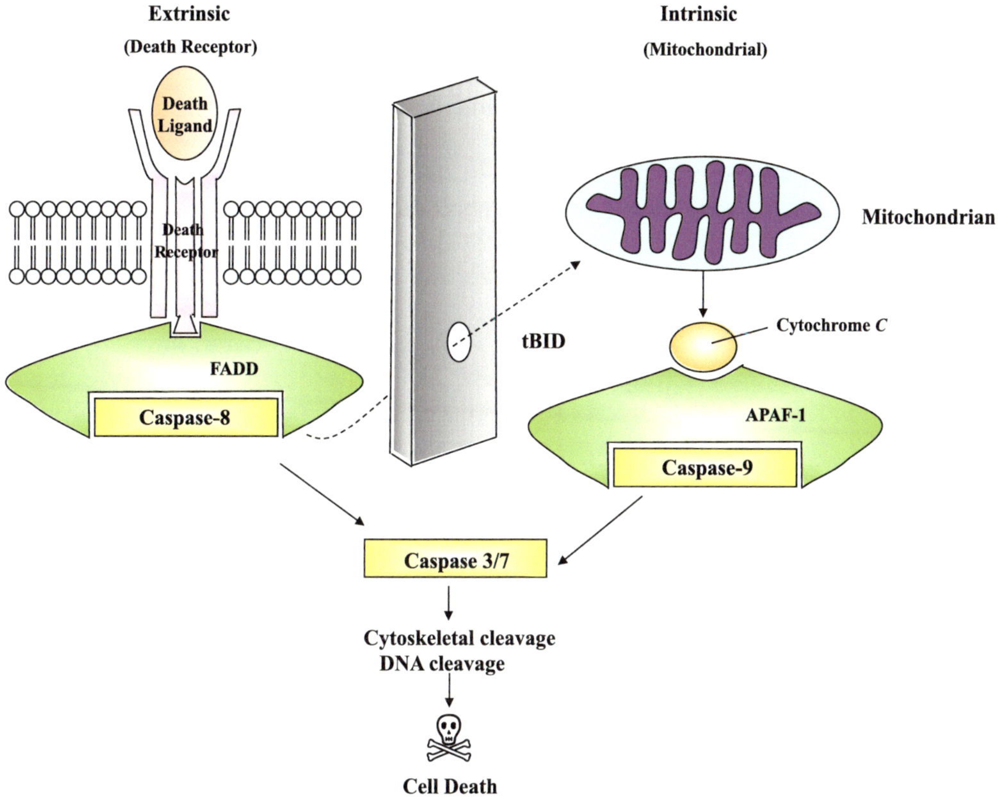

The extrinsic, death receptor-mediated apoptotic pathway involves the binding of TNF-α or FasL to its cell surface receptor, resulting in the activation of caspase-8 and, subsequently, caspase-3. FADD serves as a docking protein for caspase-8, tethering the enzyme to activated death receptor. The intrinsic, mitochondria-mediated apoptotic pathway results in the release of cytochrome *c*, which binds to APAF-1 and caspase-9, thus forming the apoptosome. This complex activates caspase-3, which is involved in the final common pathway of the cell death program. The interaction of these two cell death pathways *via* tBID are presented.

Fig. 1. Two major pathways involved in initiation of apoptosis.

2001). This pathway is termed the extrinsic pathway. The second apoptotic pathway called the intrinsic pathway is activated by mitochondrial injury (Korsmeyer, 1999). The two apoptotic signaling pathways ultimately converge into a common pathway causing the activation of effector enzymes termed caspases.

The extrinsic pathway involves activation of members of the TNF receptor (TNF-R) family with an intracellular death domain (DD), including TNF-R1, Fas, DR3, DR4, DR5, and DR6. These death receptors transmit apoptotic signals initiated by specific ligands such as TNF-α, Fas ligand (FasL), and TRAIL. Thus, once activated, death receptors recruit the adaptor molecule FADD (plus others in some cases) through the homophilic interaction of their own DD to the DD of the adaptor molecule. FADD can then recruit the apoptosis initiator enzyme procaspase-8 into the DISC as a consequence of the death effector domain-mediated homophilic interaction. Subsequently, procaspase-8 is activated proteolytically into caspase-8 and further activates the apoptosis effector enzymes caspase-3 and other executioner caspases (caspase-6 and caspase-7) (Thorburn, 2004; Lavrik *et al.*, 2005; Green & Kroemer, 2005).

The intrinsic pathway is initiated by stress signals through the release of apoptogenic factors such as cytochrome *c* from the mitochondrial intermembrane space. Upon release into the cell cytoplasm, cytochrome *c* promotes the formation of a complex between the caspase adaptor molecule APAF-1 and the apoptosis initiator enzyme termed procaspase-9 in a caspase-activating structure known as the apoptosome, and consequently triggers the apoptotic cascade by activating procaspase-9. Thus, the apoptosome, through newly activated caspase-9, activates the effector caspases along the common pathway of apoptosis (Korsmeyer, 1999).

In certain types of cells, there is extensive cross-talk that occurs between the extrinsic and intrinsic apoptotic pathways (Roy & Nicholson, 2000). Thus, the extrinsic and intrinsic apoptotic pathways are intimately connected. This appears to occur via the proteolysis of BID, which normally serves an anti-apoptotic role within the intrinsic mitochondrial-mediated pathway. BID is truncated to receptor pathway, whereupon tBID promotes activation of Bax and Bak and thereby induces cytochrome *c* release, leading to formation of the apoptosome (Esposti, 2002).

3. Impact of the FADD gene silencing with siRNA in sepsis therapy

3.1 Sepsis-induced up-regulation of death receptors

We initially verified the hypothesis that tissue expression of death receptors is up-regulated in sepsis. Polymicrobial sepsis was induced by CLP in BALB/c mice (Matsuda *et al.*, 2005). A middle abdominal incision was performed under anesthesia. The cecum was mobilized, ligated at 5 mm from its top, and then perforated in two locations with a 21-gauge needle, allowing expression of feces. The bowel was repositioned, and the abdomen was closed. Sham-operated animals underwent the same procedure except for ligation and puncture of the cecum. This model has high clinical relevance to humans, because it reproduces many hallmarks of sepsis that occur in patients (Hubbard *et al.*, 2005).

Immunoblot analysis showed that surface expression of the two death receptors TNF-R1 and Fas were up-regulated in lung tissues with time after CLP induction of sepsis (Figure 2A). Immunohistochemical studies indicated more abundant TNF-R1 expression in the inner wall of microvessels from septic mouse lungs (Figure 2B). Meanwhile, Fas was detected mainly in alveolar epithelial Type II cells (Matsuda *et al.*, 2009). Similar to these death receptors, DR4 and DR5, both of which mediate TRAIL-induced cell death, were up-regulated in septic mouse lungs (Matsuda *et al.*, 2009). We also found time-dependent increases in surface expression of TNF-R1 and Fas in mouse aortic tissues after CLP sepsis (Figure 3A). These death receptors are likely to be up-regulated mainly on endothelial cells, because the sepsis-induced up-regulation of TNF-R1 and Fas expression in aortic tissues was abolished when the tissues were denuded mechanically. Previous works from other laboratory have demonstrated that Fas expression is increased in hepatocytes and in selected gastrointestinal-associated lymphoid tissues (Chung *et al.*, 2001, 2003). Moreover, splenocytes harvested 24 hours after CLP and stimulated with the T cell mitogen concavalin A showed an increase in $CD4^+$ T-cell apoptosis as compared to sham controls, which was associated with an increase in Fas expression (Ayala *et al.*, 1999). Based on the findings of

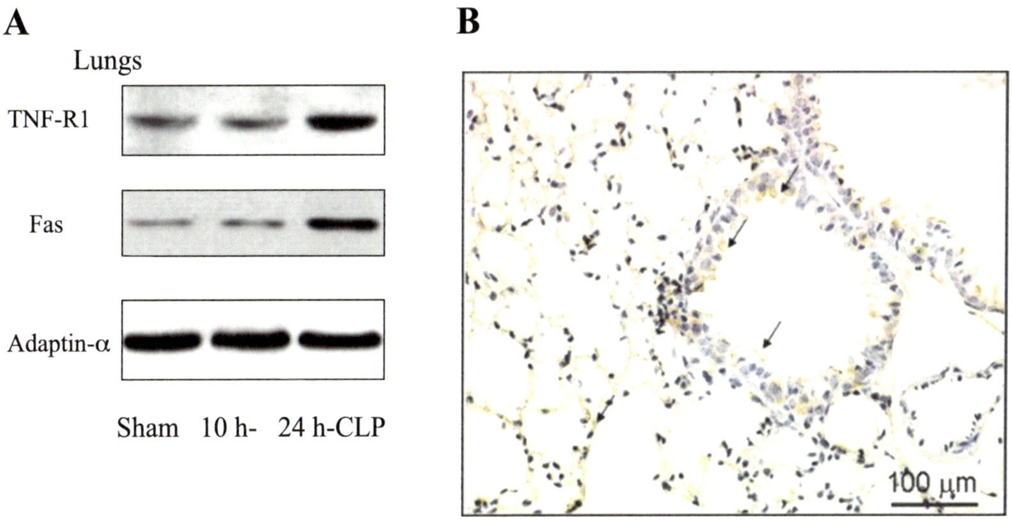

(A) Western blots of TNF-R1 and Fas in the membrane fractions of lung tissues from mice that were subjected to sham operation (control) and sepsis (10 and 24 hours after CLP). Adaptin-α served as loading control. (B) Immunohistochemical finding for TNF-R1 in the lung section from the mouse subjected to sepsis (24 hours after CLP). Positive staining is indicated by arrows.

Fig. 2. Increased death receptor expression in lung tissues of septic mice.

increased death receptor expression in tissues of septic mice, we suggest the importance of the extrinsic death receptor pathway in apoptotic cell death in sepsis, although a preeminent role for the intrinsic mitochondrial pathway has often been noted (Exline & Crouser, 2008). As presented in Figure 1, death receptors, after ligand binding, recruit the adaptor protein FADD through hemophilic interaction of their DD with the DD of FADD, and then FADD can recruit procaspase-8 to the DISC, thereby causing its activation (Thorburn, 2004; Lavrik et al., 2005). When FADD protein levels were assessed by Western blotting, induction of sepsis by CLP led to a time-dependent increase in FADD protein expression in aortic tissues (Figure 3B). This increase occurred on endothelial cells since FADD protein expression was not increased in endothelium-denuded aortic tissues from septic animals. For silencing of gene expression of FADD, siRNA oligonucleotides with the following sense and antisense sequences were designed: 5′-GCA GUC UUA UUC CUA Att-3′ and 5′-UUA GGA AUA AGA GGA GUA Ctt-3′ (Matsuda et al., 2009, 2010b). In vivo transfection of synthetic siRNAs via tail vein was performed at 10 hours after CLP with Lipofectamine RNAiMAX (Invitrogen). We used Opti-MEM I Reduced Serum Medium (Invitrogen) to dilute siRNAs and Lipofectamine RNAiMAX before complexing, by which 50 μg of FADD siRNA sequence was usually delivered. Systemic delivery of FADD siRNA nearly completely eliminated aortic protein expression of FADD (Figure 3B). We also confirmed that the increased levels of FADD mRNA and protein in lungs after CLP induction of sepsis were strongly suppressed by systemic application of FADD siRNA but not of scrambled siRNA (Matsuda et al., 2009). These findings suggested the successful efficacy of systemically administered siRNA for silencing tissue expression of FADD in septic mice.

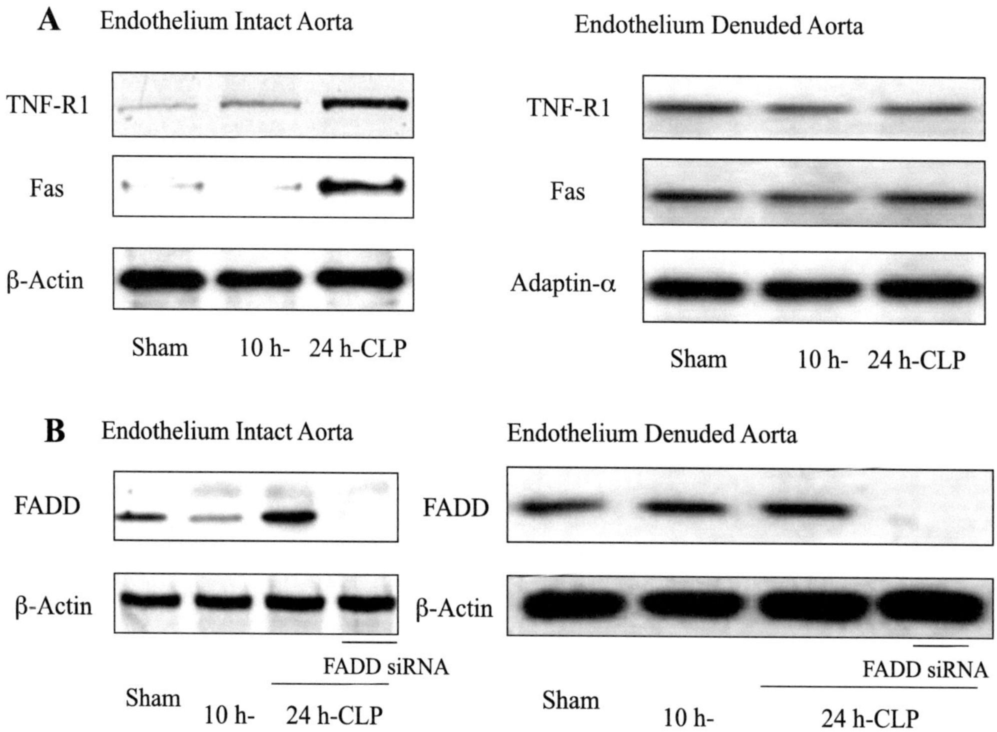

Western blots of TNF-R1 and Fas in the membrane fractions (A) and FADD in the total fractions (B) of aortic vessels from mice that were subjected to sham-operation (control) and sepsis (10 and 24 hours after CLP). β-Actin and adaptin-α served as loading control. In B, sepsis-induced up-regulation of FADD protein expression was eliminated by systemic delivery of FADD siRNA. Note that no increase in death receptors and FADD was observed when the endothelium was removed by gently rubbing the intimal surface.

Fig. 3. Endothelium-dependent increases in expression of death receptors and FADD in aortic vessels of septic mice.

3.2 Effect of FADD siRNA on cell apoptosis in sepsis

To assess whether FADD siRNA treatment has a beneficial effect on sepsis-induced apoptotic cell death in lungs, the tissue sections were labeled with an *in situ* TUNEL assay (Figure 4A). Apparently, no TUNEL-positive cells were observed in sham control mice. Induction of sepsis by CLP resulted in a striking appearance of TUNEL-positive cells. Apoptotic cells were identical morphologically to endothelial cells of capillary vessels in the alveolar septa and to epithelial type II cells (Matsuda *et al.*, 2009). In agreement with this finding, our recent immunofluorescence studies showed that the cleaved form of caspase-3 was present in cell types other than CD31-positive endothelial cells in lungs (Takano *et al.*, 2011). In lungs from CLP mice treated with FADD siRNA, but not with scrambled siRNA, TUNEL-positive cells were decreased sharply, providing a protective effect of FADD siRNA treatment on pulmonary cell apoptosis mediated by sepsis.

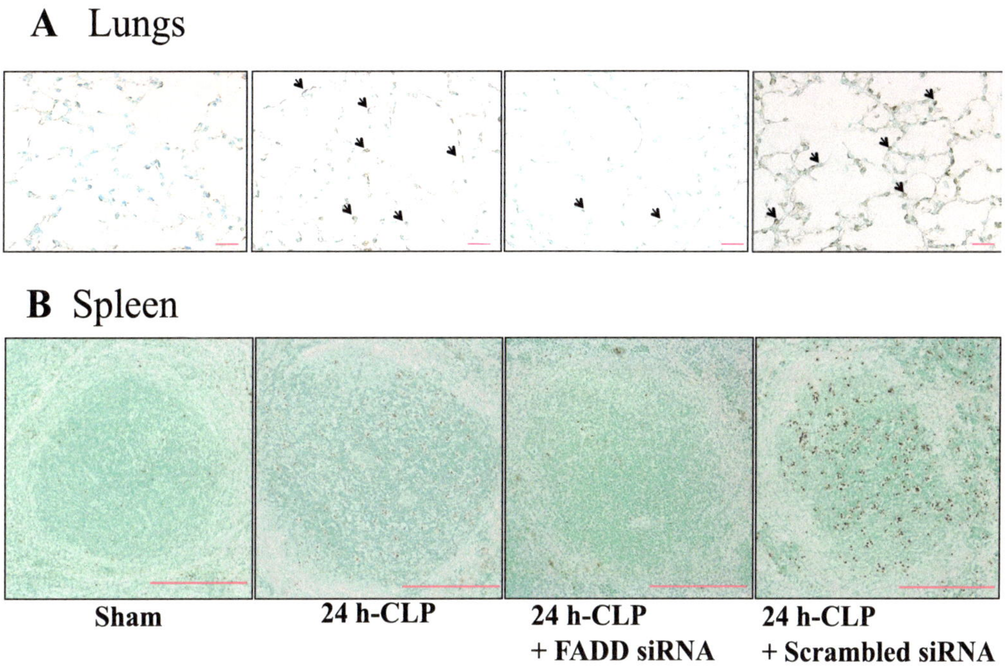

Sections of the lung (A) and spleen (B) were prepared from mice that were underwent sham procedure, CLP, CLP and FADD siRNA administration, or CLP and scrambled siRNA administration. Tissues were harvested 24 hours after surgery. In A, TUNEL-positive apoptotic cells are indicated by arrows. Scale bars = 20 μm (A) and 200 μm (B).

Fig. 4. Mouse lung and spleen tissue sections showing apoptotic cells by an *in situ* TUNEL assay.

Physiologic TUNEL-positive cells, morphologically identical to lymphocytes (Matsuda *et al.*, 2009, 2010a), were sporadically present in the spleen tissues from sham control mice (Figure 4B). In spleens 24 hours after septic insult, marked apoptosis of follicular lymphocytes were observed. Most apoptotic lymphocytes were located in the white pulp of the spleen. TUNEL-positive lymphocytes in spleen follicles were greatly reduced when FADD siRNA was systemically given after CLP. Administration of scrambled siRNA to septic mice showed more frequent TUNEL positivity than no treatment.

Light microscopic studies of aortic tissue sections from septic mice at 24 hours after CLP showed partial detachment of endothelial cells from the basal membrane (Matsuda *et al.*, 2007, 2010b). When the tissue sections were labeled with an *in situ* TUNEL assay, a significant number of apoptotic endothelial cells was found in aortas of septic mice (Matsuda *et al.*, 2007, 2010b). Furthermore, scanning electron microscopic analysis indicated that the structure of aortic endothelium displayed a remarkable morphological abnormality: most endothelial cells were badly swollen (Figure 5A). Such an endothelial histological injury was strikingly prevented by systemic treatment with FADD siRNA but not with scrambled siRNA.

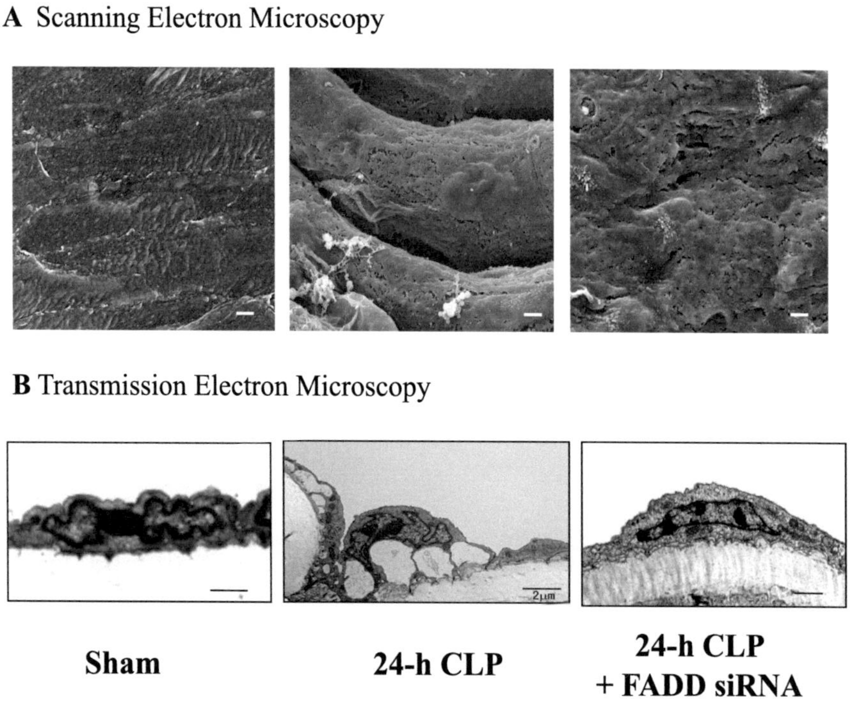

Mice were underwent sham procedure, CLP, or CLP and FADD siRNA administration. Aortic endothelial cells were evaluated by scanning electron microscopy (SEM, A) and by transmission electron microscopy (TEM, B) 24 hours after surgry. Septic mice showed anomalous swelling of cells (SEM) and autophagy-related vacuolation in the cytoplasm (TEM). These electron-microscopical changes were prevented by systemic treatment with FADD siRNA. Scale bars = 2 μm.

Fig. 5. Electron microscopic analysis of mouse aortic endothelial cells.

3.3 Effect of FADD siRNA on sepsis-induced autophagy in endothelial cells

A non-apoptotic and non-oncotic type of cell death has been recognized (Clarke, 1990). This type of cell death is characterized by the appearance of double- or multi-membrane cytoplasmic vesicles engulfing bulk cytoplasm and cytoplasmic organelles, such as mitochondria and endoplasmic reticulum, and their delivery to and subsequent degradation by the lysosomal system of the same cell (Gozuacik & Kimchi, 2004). This type of cell death is referred to as autophagic cell death, but it is still unsettled whether autophagy is the direct primary cause of cell death or a compensatory mechanism that tries to rescue a cell from dying. In starvation, autophagy provides an internal source of nutrients for energy generation, promoting cell survival. Defects in autophagy have been implicated in the pathophysiology of cancer and neurodegenerative diseases (Rabinowitz & White, 2010). On the other hand, systemic inflammatory response syndrome and multiple organ dysfunction syndrome are suggested to be accompanied by increased cell death, including autophagy, in the affected organs (Yasuhara *et al.*, 2007). A recent report has shown that LPS induces autophagy in human umbilical vein endothelial cells (Meng *et al.*, 2010). Moreover, LPS-induced systemic inflammation has been demonstrated to exert autophagy of hepatocytes in streptozotocin-induced diabetic rats (Hagiwara *et al.*, 2010).

Our ultrastructural analysis using transmission electron microscopy indicated the formation of autophagy-like vesicles in aortic endothelial cells of CLP septic mice (Figure 5B). Microtubule-associated protein 1A/1B-light chain 3 (LC3) is a soluble protein with a molecular mass of ~17 kDa that is distributed ubiquitously in mammalian tissues. Cleavage of LC3 at the carboxyterminus immediately following synthesis yields the cytosolic LC3-I form. LC3-I form is converted to LC3-II during autophagy. Thus, LC3-II is widely used as an indicator of autophagy (Kabeya *et al.*, 2000). Western blot analysis revealed significantly elevated aortic LC3-II levels in the CLP septic group (Figure 6). Very interestingly, these autophagy-related changes were prevented by systemic application of FADD siRNA (Figures 5B and 6).

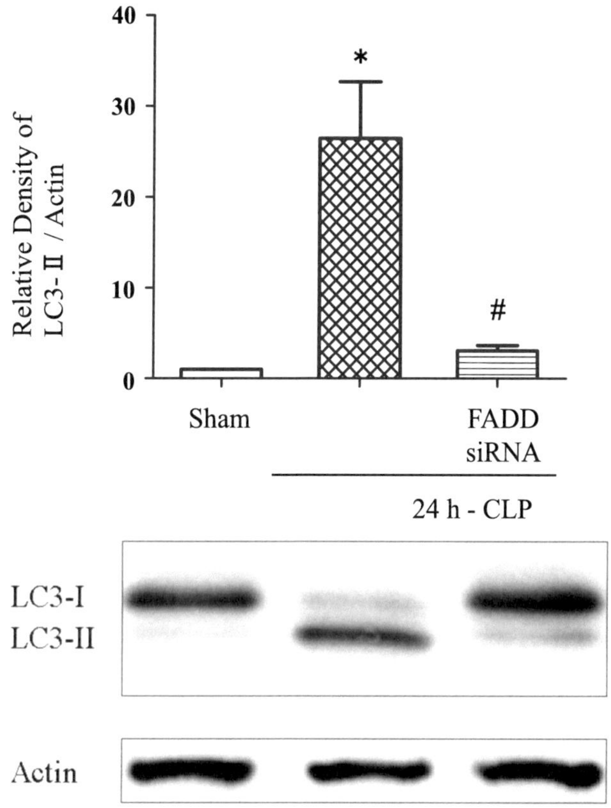

Immunoblotting of LC3 usually reveals two bands: the cytosolic form LC3-I and the membrane-bound form LC3-II. Sepsis (24 hours after CLP) resulted in a significant conversion of LC3-I to LC3-II. Tracking the conversion of LC3-I to LC3-II is indicative of autophagic activity. Systemic administration of FADD siRNA prevented this conversion. Summarized data are presented as the mean ± S.E. of five different experiments. **P*<0.05 vs. sham control. #*P*<0.05 vs. CLP alone.

Fig. 6. Immunoblot analysis of LC3 in mouse aortic vessels.

There are several lines of experimental evidence that apoptosis and autophagy may be interconnected in some settings, and in some cases even simultaneously regulated by the same trigger resulting in different cellular outcomes (Gozuacik & Kimchi, 2004). Previous data supporting the interconnection between the two types of cell death have come from gene expression profiles during steroid-triggered developmental cell death in the *Drosophila* system where several apoptosis-related genes are up-regulated together with autophagy-related genes (Gorski *et al.*, 2003; Lee *et al.*, 2003). In other cellular settings, autophagy may antagonize apoptosis and inhibition of autophagy may increase the sensitivity of the cells to apoptotic signals (Gozuacik & Kimchi, 2004). Moreover, apoptosis and autophagy may manifest themselves in a mutually exclusive manner. Inhibition of autophasic activity in cells may switch responses to death signals from autophagic to apoptotic cell death (Gozuacik & Kimchi, 2004). In addition, there are numerous reports showing a direct physical interaction between autophagy-inducing proteins and proteins involved in apoptosis, especially anti-apoptotic Bcl-2 family members (Liang *et al.*, 1998; Vande Velde *et al.*, 2000; Yanagisawa *et al.*, 2003).

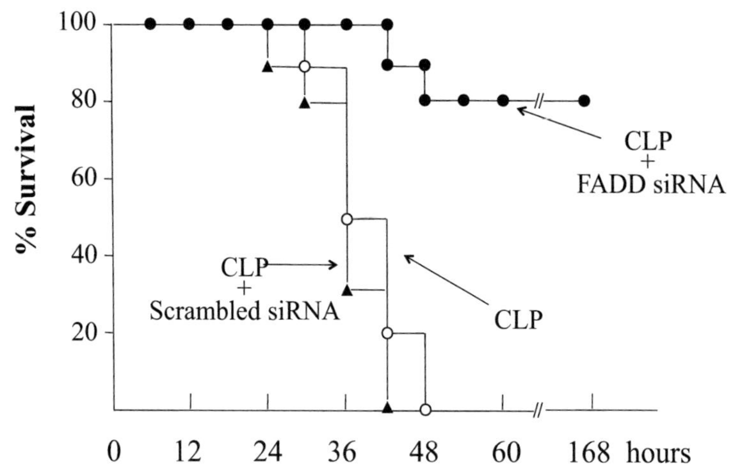

Mortality was monitored 4 times daily, and survival time was recorded for 7 days. Systemic delivery of FADD siRNA, but not scrambled siRNA, resulted in a significant survival benefit. Percentage survival of mice after CLP is plotted. Ten mice for each group underwent CLP.

Fig. 7. Kaplan-Meier survival curves after CLP in mice given FADD siRNA.

3.4 Effect of FADD siRNA on animal survival after CLP

To evaluate the impact of FADD siRNA on survival benefit in sepsis, we examined mortality in mice subjected to CLP (Figure 7). After CLP, mice exhibited signs of sepsis. Thus, they showed lack of interest in their environment, displayed piloerection, and had crusty exudates around their eyes. Finally, all animals subjected to CLP without treatment died within 2 days. Treatment of CLP mice with scrambled siRNA was without effect on survival. However, when FADD siRNA was administered to CLP mice, its survival advantage was very striking ($P<0.0001$; Log rank test). Even at the end of 7 days, a greater proportion of the animals given FADD siRNA survived CLP with 80%.

4. Conclusions

Despite recent advances in antibiotics and critical care therapy, sepsis treatment remains clinical conundrum, and its prognosis is still poor, especially when septic shock and/or multiple organ failure develop. Although a host of promising candidates for therapeutic intervention in sepsis have been propelled, almost all of these trials have failed to demonstrate a mortality benefit for patients suffering from sepsis. Ongoing research into this highly lethal disorder has shown that apoptosis is fully associated with an unfavorable outcome of sepsis and its inhibition may provide useful therapies for treatment of sepsis. Here we propose that FADD siRNA therapy may offer a unique alternative sepsis treatment to shorten the apoptotic arm of sepsis. This therapy salvaged immune effector cells, vascular endothelial cells, and parenchyma cells from apoptosis, which would arrest the development of complications arising from sepsis, including multiple organ failure, and ultimately have a beneficial impact on septic mortality. While appreciating that additional work is required to optimize preclinical and possibly clinical application, treatment with FADD siRNA will hopefully provide novel potential usefulness for gene therapy that could improve the survival of critically ill septic patients.

5. Acknowledgments

We thank Mieko Watanabe for her excellent secretarial assistance. We are grateful to Kengo Tomita for his expert help in creating the figures in this article. This work was supported by a Grant-in-Aid for Scientific Research from Ministry of Education, Culture, Sports, Science and Technology of Japan (18590233, 20590250) and by the Tamura Science Technology Foundation.

6. References

Angus, D.C.; Linde-Zwirble, W.T.; Lidicker, J.; Clermont, G.; Carcillo, J. & Pinsky, M.R. (2001). Epidemiology of severe sepsis in the United States: analysis of incidence, outcome, and associated costs of care. *Crit Care Med* 29, 1303-1310

Ayala, A. & Chaudry, I.H. (1996). Immune dysfunction in murine polymicrobial sepsis: mediators, macrophages, lymphocytes and apoptosis. *Shock* 6(Suppl 1), S27-S38

Ayala, A.; Chung, C.S.; Xu, Y.X.; Evans, T.A.; Redmond, K.M. & Chaudry, I.H. (1999). Increased inducible apoptosis in $CD4^+$ T lymphocytes during polymicrobial sepsis is mediated by Fas ligand and not endotoxin. *Immunology* 97, 45-55

Bone, R.C.; Balk, R.A.; Cerra, F.B.; Dellinger, R.P.; Fein, A.M.; Knaus, W.A.; Schein, R.M. & Sibbald, W.J. (1992). Definitions for sepsis and organ failure and guidelines for the use of innovative therapies in sepsis. The ACCP/SCCM Consensus Conference Committee. American College of Chest Physicians/Society of Critical Care Medicine. *Chest* 101, 1644-1655

Chung, C.S.; Song, G.Y.; Lomas. J.; Simms, H.H.; Chaudry, I.H. & Ayala, A. (2003). Inhibition of Fas/Fas ligand signaling improves septic survival: differential effects on macrophage apoptotic and functional capacity. *J Leukoc Biol* 74, 344-351

Chung, C.S.; Yang, S.; Song, G.Y.; Lomas, J.; Wang, P.; Simms, H.H.; Chaudry, I.H. & Ayala, A. (2001). Inhibition of Fas signaling prevents hepatic injury and improves organ blood flow during sepsis. *Surgery* 130, 339-345

Clarke P.G. (1990). Developmental cell death: Morphological diversity and multiple mechanisms. *Anat Embryol* 181, 195-213

Coopersmith, C.M.; Chang, K.C.; Swanson, P.E.; Tinsley, K.W.; Stromberg, P.E.; Buchman, T.G.; Karl, I.E. & Hotchkiss, R.S. (2002a). Overexpression of Bcl-2 in the intestinal epithelium improves survival in septic mice. *Crit Care Med* 30, 195-201

Coopersmith, C.M.; Stromberg, P.E.; Dunne, W.M.; Davis, C.G.; Amiot, D.M.; Buchman, T.G.; Karl, I.E. & Hotchkiss, R.S. (2002b). Inhibition of intestinal epithelial apoptosis and survival in a murine model of pneumonia-induced sepsis. *JAMA* 287, 1716-1721.

Esposti, M.D. (2002). The roles of Bid. *Apoptosis* 7, 433-440

Exline, M.C. & Crouser, E.D. (2008). Mitochondrial mechanisms of sepsis-induced organ failure. *Front Biosci* 13, 5030-5041

Gorski, S.M.; Chrittaranjan, S.; Pleasance, E.D.; Freeman, J.D.; Anderson, C.L.; Varhol, R.J.; Coughlin, S.M.; Zuyderduyn, S.D.; Jones, S.J. & Marra, M.A. (2003). A SAGE approach to discovery of genes involved in autophagic cell death. *Curr Biol* 13, 358-363

Gozuacik, D. & Kimchi, A. (2004). Autophagy as a cell death and tumor suppressor mechanism. *Oncogene* 23, 2891-2906

Green, D.R. & Kroemer, G. (2005). Pharmacological manipulation of cell death: clinical application in sight? *J Clin Invest* 115, 2610-2617

Hagiwara, S.; Iwasaka, H.; Koga, H.; Hasegawa, A.; Kudo, K.; Kusaka, J.; Oyama, Y. & Noguchi, T. (2010). Stimulation of autophagy in the liver by lipopolysaccharide-induced systemic inflammation in a rat model of diabetes mellitus. *Biomed Res* 31, 263-2671

Hattori, Y.; Takano, K.; Teramae, H.; Yamamoto, S.; Yokoo, H. & Matsuda, N. (2010). Insights into sepsis therapeutic design based on the apoptotic death pathway. *J Pharmacol Sci* 114, 354-365

Herr, I. & Debatin, K.M. (2001). Cellular stress response and apoptosis in cancer therapy. *Blood* 98, 2603-2614

Hotchkiss, R.S.; Chang, K.C.; Swanson, P.E,; Tinsley, K.W,; Hui, J.J.; Klender, P.; Xanthoudakis, S.; Roy, S.; Black, C.; Grimm, E.; Aspiotis, R.; Han, Y.; Nicholson, D.W. & Karl, I.E. (2000). Caspase inhibitors improve survival in sepsis: a critical role of the lymphocyte. *Nat Immunol* 1, 496-501.

Hotchkiss, R.S.; Coopersmith, C.M. & Karl, I.E. (2005). Prevention of lymphocyte apoptosis – a potential treatment of sepsis? *Clin Infect Dis* 41(Suppl 7), S465-S469

Hotchkiss, R.S.; Swanson, P.E.; Freeman, B.D.; Tinsley, K.W.; Cobb, J.P.; Matuschak, G.M.; Buchman, T.G. & Karl, I.E. (1999a). Apoptotic cell death in patients with sepsis, shock, and multiple organ dysfunction. *Crit Care Med* 27, 1230-1251

Hotchkiss, R.S.; Tinsley, K.W.; Swanson, P.E.; Chang, K.C.; Cobb, J.P.; Buchman, T.G.; Korsmeyer, S.J. & Karl, I.E. (1999b). Prevention of lymphocyte cell death in sepsis improves survival in mice. *Proc Natl Acad Sci USA* 96, 14541-14546

Hotchkiss, R.S.; Tinsley, K.W.; Swanson, P.E. & Karl, I.E. (2002). Endothelial cell apoptosis in sepsis. *Crit Care Med* 30(Suppl), S225-S228

Hubbard, W.J.; Choudhry, M.; Schwacha, M.G.; Kerby, J.D.; Rue, L.W.3rd; Bland, K.I. & Chaudry, I.H. (2005). Cecal ligation and puncture. *Shock* 24(Suppl 1), 52-57

Kabaya, Y.; Mizushima, N.; Ueno, T.; Yamamoto, A.; Kirisako, T.; Noda, T.; Kominami, E.; Ohsumi, Y. & Yoshimori, T. (2000). LC3, a mammalian homologue of yeast Apg8p, is localized in autophagosome membranes after processing. *EMBO J* 19, 5720-5728

Kawasaki, M.; Kuwano, K.; Hagimoto, N.; Matsuba, T.; Kunitake, R.; Tanaka, T.; Maeyama, T. & Hara, N. (2000). Protection from lethal apoptosis in lipopolysaccharide-induced acute lung injury in mice by a caspase inhibitor. *Am J Pathol* 157, 597-603

Korsmeyer, S.J. (1999). BCL-2 gene family and the regulation of programmed cell death. *Cancer Res* 59(Suppl 7), 1693s-1700s

Lang, J.D. & Matute-Bello, G. (2009). Lymphocytes, apoptosis and sepsis: making the jump from mice to humans. *Crit Care* 13, 109

Lavrik, L.; Golks, A. & Krammer, P.H. (2005). Death receptor signaling. *J Cell Sci* 118, 265-267

Lee, C.-Y.; Clough, E.A.; Yellon, P.; Teslovich, T.M.; Stephan, D.A. & Baehrecke, E.H. (2003). Genome-wide analyses of steroid- and radiation-triggered programmed cell death in *Drosophila*. *Curr Biol* 13, 350-357

Liang, X.H.; Kleeman, L.K.; Jiang, H.H.; Gordon, G.; Goldman, J.E.; Berry, G.; Herman, B. & Levine, B. (1998). Protection against fatal Sindbis virus encephalitis by beclin, a novel Bcl-2-interacting protein. *J Virol* 72, 8586-8596

Marshall, J.C. (2000). Clinical trials of mediator-directed therapy in sepsis: what have we learned? *Intensive Care Med* 26, S75-S83

Martin, G.S.; Mannino, D.M.; Eaton, S. & Moss, M. (2003). The epidemiology of sepsis in the United States from 1979 through 2000. *N Engl J Med* 348, 1546-1554

Matsuda, N. & Hattori, Y. (2007). Vascular biology in sepsis: pathophysiological and therapeutic significance of vascular dysfunction. *J Smooth Muscle Res* 43, 117-137

Matsuda, N.; Hattori, Y.; Jesmin, S. & Gando, S. (2005). Nuclear factor-κB decoy oligonucleotides prevent acute lung injury in mice with cecal ligation and puncture-induced sepsis. *Mol Pharmacol* 67, 1018-1025

Matsuda, N.; Takano, Y.; Kageyama, S.; Hatakeyama, N.; Shakunaga, K.; Kitajima, I.; Yamazaki, M. & Hattori, Y. (2007). Silencing of caspase-8 and caspase-3 by RNA interference prevents vascular endothelial cell injury in mice with endotoxic shock. *Cardiovasc Res* 76, 132-140

Matsuda, N.; Teramae, H.; Futatsugi, M.; Takano, K.; Yamamoto, S.; Tomita, K.; Suzuki, T.; Yokoo, H.; Koike, K. & Hattori, Y. (2010a). Up-regulation of histamine H_4 receptors contributes to splenic apoptosis in septic mice: Counteraction of the antiapoptotic action of nuclear factor-κB. *J Pharmacol Exp Ther* 332, 730-737

Matsuda, N.; Teramae, H.; Yamamoto, S.; Takano, K.; Takano, Y. & Hattori, Y. (2010b). Increased death receptor pathway of apoptotic signaling in septic mouse aorta: effect of systemic delivery of FADD siRNA. *Am J Physiol Heart Circ Physiol* 298, H92-H101

Matsuda, N.; Yamamoto, S.; Takano, K.; Kageyama, S.; Kurobe, Y.; Yoshihara, Y.; Takano, Y. & Hattori, Y. (2009). Silencing of Fas-associated death domain protects mice from septic lung inflammation and apoptosis. *Am J Respir Crit Care Med* 179, 806-815

Mwng, N.; Wu, L.; Gao, J.; Zhao, J.; Su, L.; Su, H.; Zhang, S. & Miao, J. (2010). Lipopolysaccharide induces autopsy through BIRC2 in human umbilical vein endothelial cells. *J Cell Physiol* 225, 174-179.

Natanson, C.; Esposito, C.J. & Banks, S.M. (1998). The sirens' songs of confirmatory sepsis trials: selection bias and sampling error. *Crit Care Med* 26, 1927-1931

Natanson, C.; Hoffman, W.D.; Suffredini, A.F.; Eichacker, P.Q. & Danner, R.L. (1994). Selected treatment strategies for septic shock based on proposed mechanisms of pathogenesis. *Ann Intern Med* 120, 771-783

Perl, M.; Chung, C.-S.; Perl, U.; Lomas-Neira, J.; de Paepe, M.; Cioffi, W.G. & Ayala, A. (2007). Fas-induced pulmonary apoptosis and inflammation during indirect acute lung injury. *Am J Respir Crit Care Med* 176, 591-601

Rabinowitz, J.D. & White, E. (2010). Autophagy and metabolism. *Science* 330, 1344-1348

Roy, S. & Nicholson, D.W. (2000). Cross-talk in cell death signaling. *J Exp Med* 192, F21-F25

Takano, K.; Yamamoto, S.; Tomita, K..; Takashina, M.; Yokoo, H.; Matsuda, N.; Takano, Y. & Hattori, Y. (2011). Successful treatment of acute lung injury with pitavastatin in septic mice: Potential role of glucocorticoid receptor expression in alveolar macrophages. *J Pharmacol Exp Ther* 336, 381-390

Thorburn, A. (2004). Death receptor-inducing cell killing. *Cell Signal* 16, 139-144

Vande Velde, C.; Cizeau, J.; Dubik, D.; Alimonti, J.; Brown, T.; Israels, S.; Hakem, R. & Greenberg, A.H. (2000). BNIP3 and genetic control of necrosis-like cell death through the mitochondrial permeability transition pore. *Mol Cell Biol* 15, 5454-5468

Wesche D.E.; Lomas-Neira, J.L.; Perl, M.; Chung, C.S. & Ayala, A. (2005). Leukocyte apoptosis and its significance in sepsis and shock. *J Leukoc Biol* 78, 325-337

Yanagisawa, H.; Miyashita, T.; Nakano, Y. & Yamamoto, D. (2003). HSpin1, a transmembrane protein interacting with Bcl-2/Bcl-x_L, induces a caspase-independent autophagic cell death. *Cell Death Differ* 10, 798-807

Yasuhara, S.; Asai, A.; Sahani, N.D. & Martyn, J.A.J. (2007). Mitochondria, endoplasmic reticulum, and alternative pathways of cell death in critical illness. *Crit Care Med* 35(Suppl), S488-S495

Zeni, F.; Freeman, B. & Natanson, C. (1997). Anti-inflammatory therapies to treat sepsis and septic shock: a reassessment. *Crit Care Med* 25, 1095-1100.

24

Muscle-Targeted Gene Therapy of Charcot Marie-Tooth Disease is Dependent on Muscle Activity

Stephan Klossner[1], Marie-Noëlle Giraud[2], Sara Sancho Oliver[3], David Vaughan[4] and Martin Flück[1,4]
[1]Institute of Anatomy, University of Berne, Berne,
[2]Department of Cardiovascular Surgery, Inselspital, Berne,
[3]Department of Medicine, University of Fribourg, Fribourg,
[4]Institute for Biomedical Research into Human Movement and Health, Manchester Metropolitan University, Manchester,
[1,2,3]Switzerland
[4]United Kingdom

1. Introduction

Charcot-Marie-Tooth disease (CMT) is the most common inherited neurologic disorder. Reportedly 10-28 cases exist per 100,000 in Western societies. CMT patients suffer from a variable degree of motor dysfunction which adversely affects locomotion and balance. These deficits explain by a slowing of impulse conduction in motor and sensory nerves. This affects the recruitment of muscle fibres for contraction whereby slow motor units are preferentially affected (Gale et al., 1982; Roy et al., 1996). This results in muscle weakness and wasting in the extremities of the body.

The inefficient propagation of excitatory signals in moto neurons towards peripheral muscle in CMT disease is caused by a myelination defect which has a genetic origin. Some 20 genes for axon proteins and myelin have been implicated in CMT, and allow the classification into specific subtypes of the disease. Frequently affected of these genes are peripheral myelin protein 22 (pmp22) and myelin protein zero (MPZ) which are mutated in a majority of cases (Braathen et al., 2011). CMT subtype 1A (CMT1A) is the most predominant disease type being associated with a duplication of the pmp22 gene (Wise et al., 1993; Magyar et al. 1996). The pmp22 gene encodes for a factor that is incorporated into the myelin sheet of neurons and is thought to control myelin thickness. The pathology on the CMT1A disease types is explained by slowed saltatory transduction in moto neurons due to the aberrant nerve insulation (Sereda & Griffiths, 1996).

Currently there is no cure for CMT. There are however a number of occupational interventions that can be used to effectively manage its symptoms (http://www.ninds.nih.gov/disorders/charcot_marie_tooth/detail_charcot_marie_tooth.htm). The most effective treatment consists of a rehabilitation programs with physical therapy as an active ingredient. This involves daily heel cord stretching exercises to prevent Achilles tendon shortening. Concomitantly, resistant training of CMT patients can lead to impressive

increases in maximal voluntary force (Lindeman et al., 1999). Exercise is thus encouraged within each individual patient's capability to condition motor performance in this neurological disease. Physical activity however only retards the irreversible degeneration and may have detrimental consequences if inappropriately administered (Vinci et al., 2003).
Gene transfer therapy is a promising route for future cures of muscular disorders. However major limitations appear regarding the treatment of neurological diseases such as CMT. In this case one would normally expect that the therapy must directly target moto neurons to initiate a compensatory mechanism that can correct the missing myelination. This is currently not feasible. In this regard the important positive influence of exercise on motor performance in CMT patients demands consideration as this may offers an indirect means to improve neuromuscular function. This relates to the well established feed forward control of the muscle phenotype by muscle use (Fluck & Hoppeler, 2003). It has been pointed out that the effects of increased muscle recruitment with exercise involve the promotion of the slow-oxidative expression program (Schmutz et al., 2010; Baumann et al., 1987). Recently, has been established that electrically imposed muscle recruitment can re-establish muscle functionality in denervated muscle of tetraplegic patients through the remodelling of the contractile and metabolic makeup (Boncompagni et al., 2007). The positive influence of exercise in CMT patients suggests that the use-dependent pathway importantly affects neuro-muscular function.
We reasoned that altered muscle use combined with gene therapy for focal adhesion kinase (FAK), an enzyme that regulates recruitment dependent slow oxidative gene expression, would be a suitable venue to promote pmp22 expression in skeletal muscle. Towards this end we investigated the use dependence of pmp22 expression in human skeletal muscle and assessed the nature of contractile defects in muscles of a mouse model for CMT at the molecular, cellular and functional level. Subsequently we tested whether overexpression of FAK can enhance pmp22 expression in skeletal muscle (Durieux et al., 2009).

2. Methods

Response to exercise in human muscle - A resting biopsy was collected with a conchotome from the non-exercising leg after an overnight fast and prior to exercise. Thereafter, each participant performed an acute single-legged endurance exercise bout at 60% of their Pmax on an Ergoline bicycle ergometer (Jaeger). There was an incremental warm-up period to reach their 60% Pmax, and after 20 minutes of cycling at 80 rpm, the resistance was increased by 5 W every 10 seconds until volitional exhaustion. A biopsy was collected with the ACECUT needle system (UK Surgical Ltd) from the exercised leg 8 hours after the bout of exercise. Biopsy position was standardized based on an ultra-sound measurement at 50% of femur length. This study was performed at Manchester Metropolitan University (United Kingdom) with permission of the institutional ethics Committee, in compliance with the Helsinki Convention for research on human subjects.
Model of altered muscle activity – Hindlimb suspension of rats was performed for 7 days as previously described (Fluck et al., 2005) at the Université Lyon 1 (France) and started 2 days after transfection. Subsequent reloading was provoked by allowing the animals to return to normal cage activity for 1 or 5 days.
Hindlimb suspension of mice was performed for 3 days as previously described at the University of Berne (Switzerland) (Dapp et al., 2004). This was achieved by attaching the tail via a swivel hook to a movable X-Y system; thereby preventing the mouse from touching the

ground with its hindlimbs while permitting free movement within the entire cage. Soleus muscles were extracted from anesthetized animals (5% isoflurane).

Animal model of CMT - Pmp22-tg mouse (pmp22tg) as CMT model (strain C3Hb6) were bred at the University of Fribourg. The original strain was a gift of U. Suter (University of Zurich). The pmp22-tg mice carry approximately 16 and 30 copies of the pmp22 gene and display a severe congenital hypomyelinating neuropathy due to the accumulation of overexpressed pmp22 in the Golgi compartment, and the concomitant interference with myelin assembly during Schwann cell differentiation (Niemann et al., 2000). This is characterized by an almost complete lack of myelin and marked slowing of nerve conductions (Magyar al., 1996). The animals entering the study were between 1.5- and 3-month of age.

Somatic transgenesis for FAK - Gene transfer of pCMV-FAK into soleus muscle of 3-month old male Wistar rats was essentially carried out as previously described (Durieux et al., 2009). In brief, soleus muscles of anaesthetized rats (60 mg of sodium pentobarbital per kg body) were surgically exposed. 70 microgram per 70 microliter of endotoxin-free plasmid in Tris-EDTA buffer (plasmidfactory, Bielefeld, Germany, www.plasmidfactory.de) was injected in the belly portion of the soleus muscle and three trains of 80-pulses of 100 microseconds duration, each at 100 mA, were delivered using needle electrodes with the GET42generator (Electronique et Informatique du Pilat, Jonzieux, France). The wound was closed with sutures and animals transferred to single cages. Right soleus muscles were injected with cytomegalovirus promoter-driven plasmids for the constitutive overexpression of chicken FAK (pCMV-FAK). The plasmid was a gift from Tony Parsons (University of Virginia, Charlottesville, USA). The (left) soleus muscles of the contralateral leg were injected with empty pCMV plasmid.

The experiments were performed at the Universities of Berne (Switzerland) and Lyon (France) with the permission of the local Animal Care Committee of the Canton of Berne (Switzerland) and following the recommendations provided by the European Convention for the protection of Vertebrate Animals used for Experimental and Scientific purposes (Strasbourg, 18.III.1986).

Muscle sampling – Collected muscles were frozen in nitrogen cooled isopentane and stored in sealed cryotubes at -80°C until use.

Transcript profiling – Transcript levels were assessed with microarray in total RNA. In brief, 25 micrometer cross-sections were prepared for 10 mm3 of muscle volume and total RNA extracted with the RNeasy mini-protocol (Qiagen, Basel, Switzerland) for skeletal muscle as described (Fluck, Schmutz et al. 2005). Integrity of the RNA was checked with denaturing agarose gel electrophoresis, and the concentration was quantified against ribosomal standard using the RiboGreen RNA quantification kit (Molecular Probes, Eugene, OR).

Subsequently RNA was labelled during reverse-transcription and hybridized to different platforms dependent on the species:

For human samples this involved the use of a full human genome Affimetrix platform through a commercial provider (DNA vision, Gosselies, Belgium). For statistical analysis raw signals were normalized to total mRNA signal on the array and assessed with statistical analysis of microarrays between pre and 8-hours post samples with T-tests (SAM).

For studies with rat and mouse soleus muscle, 3 micrograms of total RNA were reverse transcribed with SuperScript II (Life Technologies, Basel, Switzerland) using [α-32P]dATP and gene-specific primers. Radio-labelled target cDNA was hybridised in ExpressHyb solution overnight at 68°C to nylon membranes which spotted cDNA probes (BD

Biosciences, Allschwil, Switzerland). The membranes were washed (four times for 1 h in 2x SSC (0.3 M sodium chloride, 0.03 M sodium citrate), 1% SDS and once for 30 min in 0.1x SSC, 0.5% SDS at 68°C and exposed for 5 days to a phosphoimager (Molecular Dynamics, Sunnyvale, CA) for quantification with AIDA Array Easy software (Raytest Schweiz, Urdorf, Switzerland).

For the rat experiment cDNA microarrays (Atlas Rat 1.2, no. 7854; Clontech Laboratories, Ozyme, France) were used. More details to this cDNA array can be found on Gene Expression Omnibus (GEO, http://www.ncbi.nlm.nih.gov/geo/) under GPL153. Data sets have been deposited under sample codes GSM10045-GSM10062, and GSM17357-GSM17361. For statistical analysis, raw signals were normalized to beta actin signal on the array and assessed with T-tests.

For the mouse experiment custom-designed low-density Atlas cDNA expression arrays with 229 double-spotted probes of mouse cDNAs associated with skeletal muscle form and function were employed. More details to this cDNA array can be found on GEO under GPL1097. For statistical analysis raw signals were normalized to total mRNA signal on the array and assessed with SAM.

Microscopy - Fibre type analysis of mouse muscle was carried out on cryosections with specific antibodies using a two-step detection protocol as described (Fluck et al., 2002). In brief, 12 micrometer cryosections were prepared, fixed in cold acetone and wetted in phosphate-buffered saline (PBS). Tissue peroxidase activity was then quenched (10 min, 3% H2O2 in methanol), sections were washed in PBS and blocked with 3% BSA in PBS for 0.5 h. Subsequently the sections were incubated for 1 h at room temperature (20 °C) with 1:100 of a monoclonal antibody in 0.3 % BSA/PBS against slow (Chemikon Juro, Lucerne, Switzerland) or fast type myosin heavy chain (Sigma Chemicals, (Buchs, Switzerland), respectively. Following, 3 brief washing in PBS, the section was reacted for 30 min with peroxidase-conjugated goat anti-rabbit IgG (diluted 1:2000 in 0.3 % BSA/PBS; Jackson Laboratories, West Grove, PA, USA) and again washed with PBS. Immunoreactivity was detected with 3-amino-9-ethylcarbazole substrate (Sigma Chemicals, Buchs, Switzerland); the nuclei were counterstained with haematoxylin, and the sections were embedded in Aquamount (BDH Laboratory Supplies Poole, UK). The stain was visualised on film (Ektachrome 64T, Kodak) using a microscope/photograph system (Vanox-S, Olympus).

Micrographs were taken from corresponding fields and the fibre types were classified. Slow and fast type fibres were differentiated on the basis of the presence of immunoreactivity for either type I or type II myosin heavy chain isoforms. Subsequently the percentages of each fiber population were counted.

The overexpression of FAK in muscle fibres was detected out with a Leica TCS SP5 confocal microscope on a DMI6000 stage powered by Argon laser and He-Ne lasers (Leica Microsystem CMS, Mylton Keynes, UK). In brief, 12 micometer cryosections were reacted with a 1 : 100 dilution of rabbit FAK antibody A-17 (Santa Cruz) and MHC2 antibody in 0.3% BSA in phosphate-buffered saline (PBS) and reacted with fluorescent-labelled secondary antibodies (Alexa488-conjugated anti-rabbit IgG, and Alexa555-conjugated anti-mouse IgG, Molecular Probes/Invitrogen). Sections were embedded in fluorescence-compatible mounting medium (DAKO, Denmark). Signal for FAK and the co-detected myosin protein was inspected with fluorescence after excitation at 458 nm, 476 nm and 488 nm with sampling in channels between 510-533 nm (Alexa 488) and 593-614 nm (Alexa 555).

Myography - Soleus muscles were harvested from anesthetized animals (pentobarbital, 50 microgram/gram body weight) and equilibrated in Tyrod solution (mM/l: 118.0 NaCl, 4.7 KCl, 2.0 CaCl2, 1.2 MgSO4, 1.1 KH2PO4, 24.0 NaHCO3, 4.5 glucose, pH 7.3-7.4; 5% CO2 / 95% O2 @ 25°C). Muscles were transferred to Tyrod solution in the contraction chamber, connected to the force transducer (KG7; Muscle tester ORG (SI-Heidelberg, Germany) and equilibrated for 5-10 minutes by gazing with 5% CO_2 / 95% O_2 @ 25°C. Contractions were initiated by point stimulation via an Ion Optix myopacer. Signals were recorded using a Powerlab system (AD instruments, Germany) and using Chart 5 software. Measurement of single twitch, tetanus and fatigue were carried out: First the length of the inserted muscle was optimized for maximal force at a stimulation of 1 Hz, 10 V, 0.4 ms. For single twitch contractions, the muscle was stimulated at 1 Hz, 10 V, 0.4 ms. For the assessment of fatigue, a repeated 3-minute tetanic contraction protocol was used (55/60 Hz, 10 V, 0.4 ms in trains of 4 seconds on and off). Fatigue was defined as the contraction cycle when force dropped below 50% of original force. Before each measurement the Tyrod solution was exchanged. The measured muscles were frozen in liquid nitrogen-cooled isopentane to determine fiber size and distribution. Twitch parameters (latency, twitch-time to peak, t1/2 relaxation, maximal force) were determined from the digital recording. Measures from contralateral muscles were considered as separate biological replica. Statistical analysis was carried out with an unpaired t-test (Statistica 6.1).

2.1 Results

2.1.1 Regulation of myelin-specific transcripts by muscle activity

Muscle fibres of anti-gravitational muscles are active for a considerable duration during free movement and quiet standing (Hennig & Lomo, 1985). We wished to investigate transcript regulation of factors of the myelin sheet by muscle activity. Towards this end we carried out an exploratory microarray analysis with the slow oxidative soleus muscle of rats that was subjected to changes in muscle activity by hindlimb suspension. The model allows reducing load bearing activity to slow oxidative soleus muscle by non-invasive means with the suspension of hindlimbs with the option to increase muscle activity with subsequent reloading (Morey Holten model as referred by Dapp et al., 2004).

Transcript profiling of rat soleus muscle showed lowered expression of the myelin-specific transcripts, peripheral myelin protein 22 (pmp22), myelin protein zero (MPZ), myelin basic protein (mbp) as well as myelin proteolipid protein and myelin-associated glycoprotein with reduced muscle activity (Fig. 1). With reloading the abundance of all of these transcripts were sizably increased.

We assessed the response of myelin-specific factors in human knee extensor muscle to exhaustive exercise. It has been pointed out before that this exercise stress induces a compensatory expression response during the first 24 hours of recovery from exercise (Pilegaard et al., 2000; Fluck, 2006). The analysis in the mixed *vastus lateralis* muscle consolidated the observation on the regulation of myelin-specific transcripts by muscle use. Pmp22, mpz and mbp transcript levels were increased by 1.2 to 1.8-fold (table 1).

gene	abbr	mean	SE	p-value
myelin basic protein	MBP	1.7	0.3	2%
myelin expression factor 2	MYEF2	1.4	0.2	3%
peripheral myelin protein 22	PMP22	1.8	0.4	5%
myelin associated glycoprotein	MAG	1.1	0.1	5%
myelin protein zero	MPZ	1.2	0.1	21%
myelin oligodendrocyte glycoprotein	MOG	1.2	0.1	25%

Table 1. Expressional alterations in myelin-specific transcripts in human *vastus lateralis* muscle after endurance exercise.

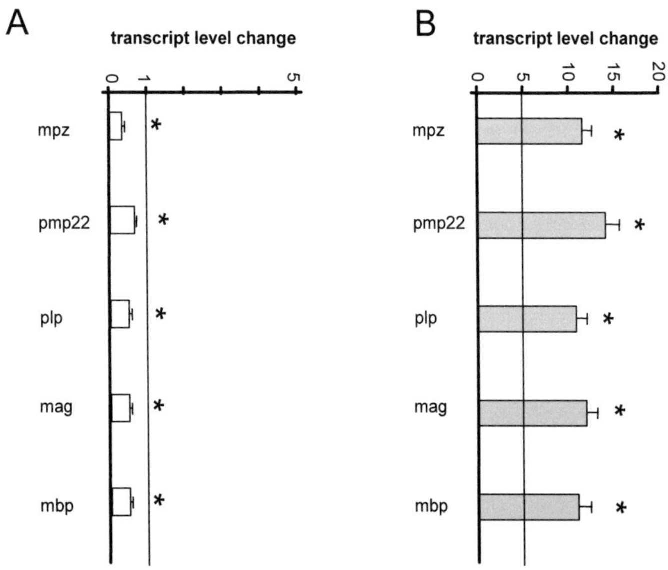

Fig. 1. Expression of myelin-specific transcripts depends on muscle activity. Bar graphs indicating mean ± standard error (SE) of level changes of five transcripts (per beta actin) in rat m. soleus with 7 days of hindlimb suspension vs. cage controls (A) and one day of reloading vs. hindlimb suspension (B). Asterisks denote significant effect based on a T-test. n=6. The line of identity is given. Abbreviations: mpz, myelin protein zero; pmp22, peripheral myelin protein 22; plp, myelin proteolipid protein; mag, myelin-associated glycoprotein; mbp, myelin basic protein.

2.2 Contractile defects in a mouse model of pmp22-dependent CMT

Pmp22-tg mice show reduced pmp22 protein expression, lack myelination, and demonstrate neurogenic muscle atrophy (Magyar et al., 1996).

We compared the muscles of pmp22-tg mice vs. strain matched controls to identify contractile defects with pmp22-dependent moto neuron aberration. Soleus muscle of pmp22-tg mice demonstrated a shift towards an atrophic, slow phenotype. This was indicated by the reduced muscle weight (Fig. 2D) and elevated percentage of slow type muscle fibres (Fig. 2A-C). This became manifest in prolonged time-to-peak and half time of muscle relaxation (Fig. 2D). The aberrations resulted in a reduction in RNA messengers for the slow oxidative expression program concomitantly with the elevated abundance of gene transcripts for fast type myogenesis (Fig. 3). The only exceptions were GAPDH and CA3 being involved in pH regulation of slow type muscle fibres.

2.3 Aberrant muscle plasticity in CMT mice with altered muscle use

Towards understanding the functional implication of motor unit recruitment for control of muscle gene expression we subjected pmp22-tg mice to 3 days of hindlimb suspension. Microarray experiments identified important alterations in transcript expression in *soleus* muscles with 3 days of reduced muscle activity (Fig. 4). The differences between suspended and cage control muscle distinguished between wildtype and pmp22-tg mice. This concerned gene ontologies defining the contractile and metabolic muscle phenotype of

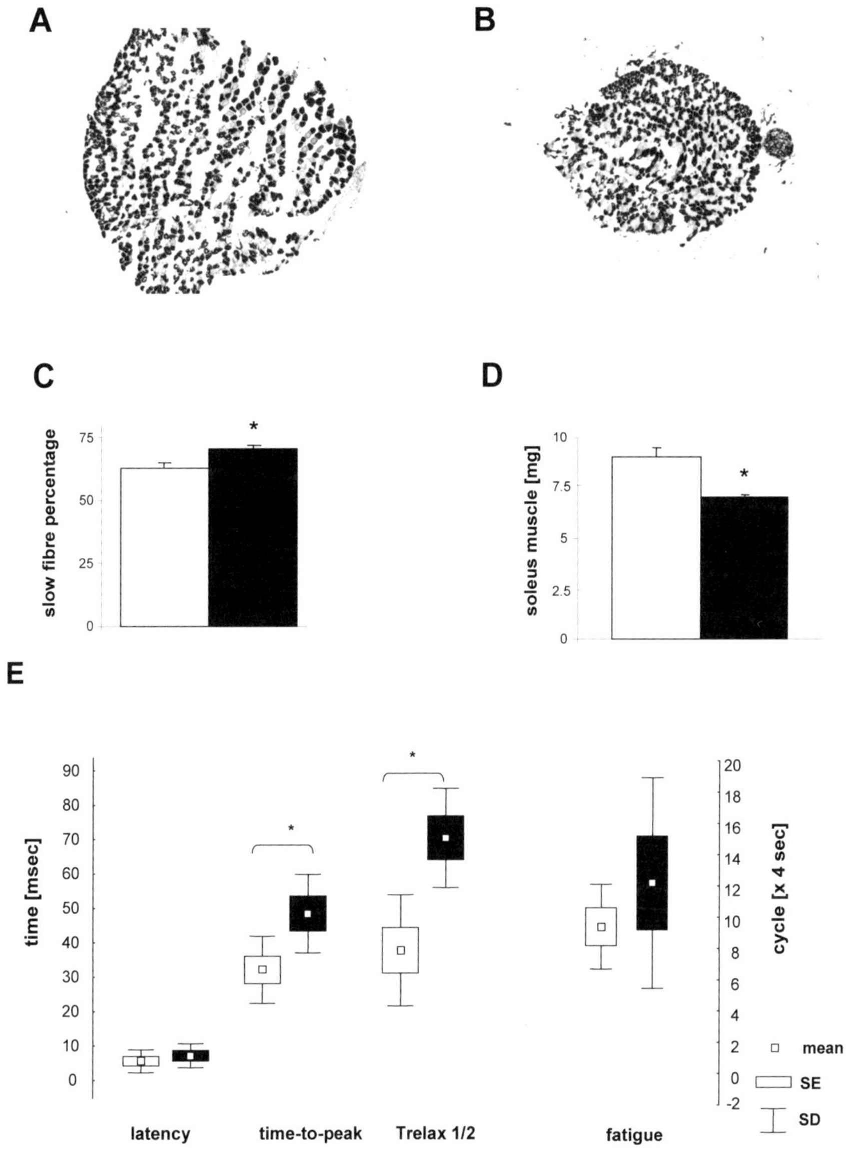

Fig. 2. Contractile aberrations in anti-gravitational muscle of pmp22-transgenic mice. A, B) Micrographs visualizing cross sections of soleus muscle from a wildtype (A) and pmp22-tg mouse (B) after staining for slow type myosin heavy chain. C, D) Bar graphs indicating mean ± SE of percentage of slow type muscle fibres (C) in soleus muscle and weight (D) of wildtype (white bar, n=5) and pmp22-transgenic mice (black bar, n=6). E) Mean ± SE and standard deviation (SD) of contractile parameters in soleus muscles of wildtype (n=6) and pmp22-transgenic mice (n=5). Asterisks denote significant effect based on a T-test.

skeletal muscle. Thereby transcript levels of factors of myogenesis, fast contraction, glycolysis and oxidative metabolism altered in opposite ways between wildtype and pmp22-tg muscle.

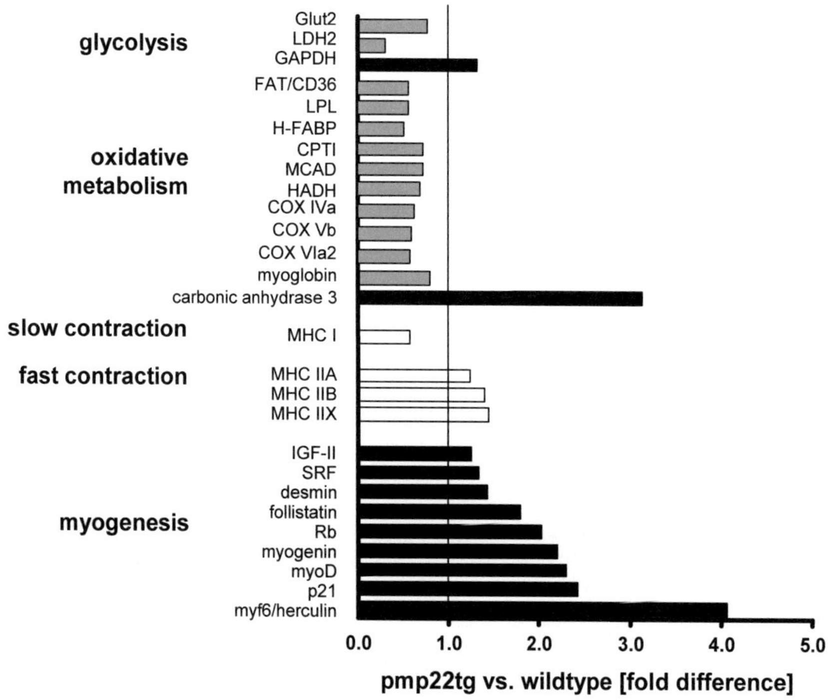

Fig. 3. Aberrant transcript expression in pmp22-transgenic mice. Bar graphs representing the mean fold difference in transcript levels between pmp22tg and wildtype mice for gene ontologies which set the phenotype of soleus muscle. Data were generated with custom mircrarrays for 229 selected factors, normalized to total mRNA and assessed with unpaired test using SAM (n=4). Black and grey bars denote significantly up-regulated and significantly down-regulated transcripts, respectively. Transcripts reflected by white bars were not significant altered. The line of identity is given. Abbreviations: Glut2, facilitative glucose transporter member 2; LDH2, lactate dehydrogenase 2; GAPDH; glyceraldehyde-3-phosphate dehydrogenase; COX IVa, cytochrome c oxidase subunit 4 isoform 1; COX Vb, cytochrome c oxidase subunit 5B; COX VIa2; cytochrome c oxidase subunit 6a2; CPTI, carnitine O-palmitoyltransferase 1; FAT/CD36, cluster of Differentiation 36/Fatty acid transport protein; HADH, 3-hydroxyacyl-CoA dehydrogenase; H-FABP; fatty acid binding protein of the heart; LPL, lipoprotein lipase; MCAD, medium-chain specific acyl-CoA dehydrogenase; MHC I; myosin heavy chain type I; MHC IIA; myosin heavy chain type IIA; MHC IIB; myosin heavy chain type IIB; MHC IIX, myosin heavy chain type IIX; IGF-I, Insulin-like growth factor I; SRF, serum response factor; Rb, retinoblastoma-associated protein; myoD, Myoblast determination protein 1; p21, cyclin-dependent kinase inhibitor 1; myf6/herculin; myogenic factor 6.

2.4 Muscle-targeted overexpression of the mechano-sensor FAK elevates myelin factor expression

We assessed whether overexpression of the governor of slow-oxidative gene expression, focal adhesion kinase (FAK), can control myelin factor expression and pmp22-dependent gene transcripts. Using gene electro transfer we introduced a constitutively active expression plasmid for FAK, pCMV-FAK, in soleus muscle of the right leg of Wistar rats.

Transfection of the contralateral muscle with empty pCMV plasmid served as intra-animal control. Immunofluorescence experiments showed that overexpression of FAK was confined to muscle fibres but was not observed in contralateral controls (Fig. 5). Microarray analysis demonstrated that FAK overexpression increased transcript levels of pmp22 along with the one of MBP in soleus muscle of active rats. Concurrently the expression of a battery of slow oxidative genes was increased (Durieux et al., 2009).

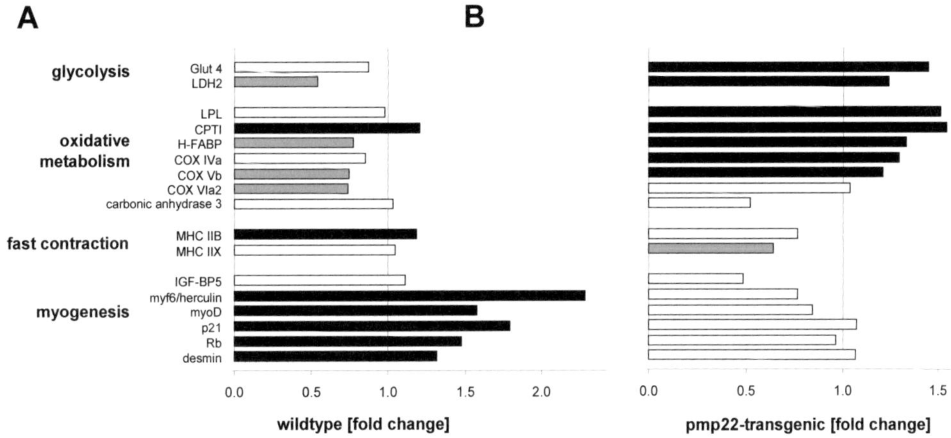

Fig. 4. Anomalous expression response of pmp22-transgenic mice to reduced muscle activity. Bar graph representing the mean fold difference in transcript levels in soleus muscle between wildtype mice (A, n=8) and pmp22tg (A, n=4) with 3 days of reduced load bearing (suspension) vs. cage controls. Data were generated with custom microarrays for 229 selected factors, normalized to total mRNA and assessed with a paired test between values from suspended and cage control muscle using SAM. Black and grey bars denote significantly up-regulated and significantly down-regulated transcripts, respectively. Transcripts reflected by white bars were not significant altered. The line of identity is given.

Abbreviations: Glut 4, facilitative glucose transporter member 4; IGF-BP5, Insulin-like growth factor binding protein 5. For others consult legend to figure 3.

2.5 FAK dependent elevation of pmp22 expression is use dependent

FAK signals mechanical stimuli in muscle to gene expression and protein synthesis (Durieux et al. 2009; Klossner et al., 2009). We subjected the FAK-transfected soleus muscles to 7 days of hindlimb suspension and subsequent one day of reloading to assess the interaction of muscle activity with gene therapy. Pmp22 transcript expression was little affected by reduced load bearing. With subsequent reloading however pmp22 levels were reduced. This effect was transient and was gone 5 days after reloading

3. Discussion

Skeletal muscle is the largest tissue of vertebrate species and most muscle groups rely on muscle activity to maintain their phenotype (Booth & Thomason, 1991). This is most pronounced in slow oxidative muscle types which are typically involved in control of gait and posture (Roy et al., 1996). This resembles the preferential affection of oxidative muscles

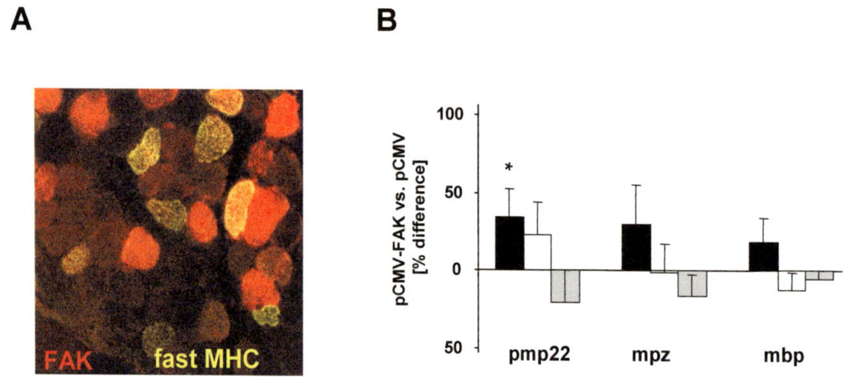

Fig. 5. FAK driven expression of myelination factors is dependent on muscle activity. A) Representative micrograph from a cryosections of a pCMV-FAK transfected soleus muscle of a rat after double staining for FAK (red) and fast type myosin heavy chain (MHC, yellow) as recorded with a confocal microscope. B) Bar graph representing the mean difference + SE of transcripts for three myelination factors pmp22, mpz and mbp between pCMV-FAK vs. empty (pCMV) transfected soleus muscle. Black, white and grey bars reflect data from cage controls, 7 days suspended and one day reloaded mice. Asterisks denote significant effect based on a T-test.

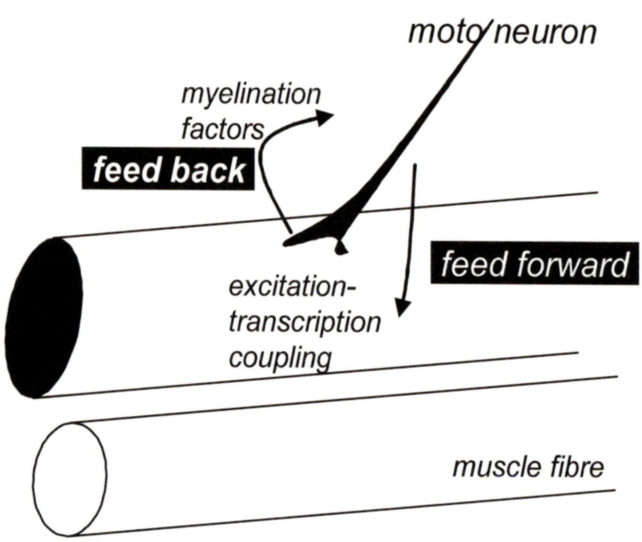

Fig. 6. Implication of excitation-transcription coupling in muscle control. Sketch summarizes a concept whereby moto neuron excitation (feed forward) with muscle use triggers the expression of myelination factors which exert feedback control on the muscle-nerve interaction.

in the trembler model of CMT disease (Gale et al., 1982). This use-dependent control of gene expression and protein synthesis (Fluck & Hoppeler, 2003; Wilkinson et al., 2008) is not taken into consideration in current gene therapy of neurological muscle disorders.

Here we prove the concept that muscle fibre targeted somatic transgenesis can affect nerve-related gene expression. The results point out that muscle activity importantly modifies the pre-translational effects of the somatic overexpression of the governor of the slow oxidative muscle program, FAK, on the expression of myelin-specific transcripts. This was shown by a similar regulation of pmp22, MPZ and MBP transcripts by muscle disuse with reduced load-bearing (down-regulation) in rats, increased load-bearing muscle activity in rats and with endurance exercise (up-regulation) in man (table 1, Fig. 1). The direction of the transcript levels points out that that myelin-specific transcript expression is related to fibre recruitment. Such a mutual control of the muscle-nerve interaction is known from the action of neurotrophic factors during normal development of the slow muscle fiber phenotype (Carrasco & English, 2003). These findings support the novel concept that in addition to feed forward control of muscle gene expression by muscle use (Calvo et al., 2001) a feedback mechanism exists whereby muscle activity in return regulates moto neurons (Fig. 6).

The functional consequences of use dependent expressional alterations in myelin sheet-specific factors in skeletal muscle remain to be explored. Pmp22 is a major component of myelin expressed in the compact portion of essentially all myelinated fibres in the peripheral nervous system and is produced predominantly by Schwann cells. Pmp22 is expressed in cranial nerves but not in the mature central nervous system. Studies in injured nerve suggested a role during Schwann cell growth and differentiation and maturation of the neuromuscular junction (Spreyer et al., 1991; Patel et al., 1992; Magyar et al., 1996). Interestingly the identified transcript level changes in our study are in line with the degeneration of NMJ with disuse (Deschenes et al., 2001) and neurological adaptation which improves fibre recruitment early with exercise (Roy et al., 1996). This supports a hypothesis whereby elevated myelin-specific transcript expression may allow the preservation and improvement of neuromuscular control of muscle fibres.

Previous examinations of soleus and EDL muscle in the trembler mouse model of CMT revealed that the deep/oxidative and soleus muscles are particularly affected by CMT but fibre type differences were not described (Gale et al., 1982). Our measures in the pmp22-tg model of CMT emphasize that in addition to altered muscle contractility, slow fibre size and transcript expression in the anti-gravitational muscle, m. soleus, is anomalous. The reduction in RNA messengers for the slow oxidative expression program (Fig. 3) is possibly explained by volumetric alterations in fibre size as suggested by visually larger CSA ratio between fast and slow type fibres reflecting atrophy of slow type fibres. Smaller type I fibres in animal models for pmp22-dependent motor and sensory neuropathy type has been noted before (Schuierer et al., 2005). This would increase the contribution of transcripts in fast type muscle fibres. The concomitantly elevated abundance of transcripts for fast type myogenesis between pmp22-tg and wildtype mice likely reflects altered regulation in fast muscle fibres (Deschenes et al., 2001).

A main finding of our investigation was that differences between pmp22 and wildtype mice were preserved in an 'opposite' transcript response of soleus muscle to reduced load-bearing. Altered transcript expression is a potentially important indicator of pathological changes with reduced muscle activity (Bey et al. 2003; Chen et al., 2007). In this regard it is important that the response of soleus muscle from wildtype mice to 3 days of unloading reproduced the changes reported in a different mouse strain after 7 days of reduced load-bearing (Dapp, Schmutz et al. 2004). This overlap concerned contractile (MHCIIB) and metabolic factors (COXVb, COXVIa2, LDH2). Exceptions concerned those involved in myogenesis which were not altered after 3 days in this study. Strikingly, the transcript response of soleus muscle of pmp22-tg mice to suspension "mirrored" the differences seen between the pmp22-tg mice and wildtype mice at baseline. These observations imply the existence of use-dependent mechanism that "inverts" expression responses in model of CMT.

This observation relates to the effects of current occupational therapy by exercise. We have shown before that FAK overexpression controls contractile performance of soleus muscle in a activity-dependent manner via the regulation of transcript expression (Durieux et al., 2009). Intriguingly with FAK overexpression and the resumption of loading bearing muscle activity, the transcript level of myelination factors were reduced compared to controls (Fig. 5). Our previous findings in the suspension model show that reduced myogenic factor RNA expression after 24 hours of the reloading stimulus is related to a concomitant increase is the encoded protein (Fluck et al., 2008). This relates to the observation that FAK acts as a molecular switch for transition between anabolic and catabolic reactions in skeletal muscle and controls the protein synthetic pathway via p70S6K (Durieux et al., 2009; Klossner et al., 2009) . This suggests that transcript level changes in the early phase of reloading may reflect inverse alterations in protein synthesis. These relationships imply that the 'muscle activity' is a confounding variable which would be valuable to be considered in somatic gene therapy of skeletal muscle. The fact that activity dependent gene regulation is reflected by the mechano-regulation of FAK activity by pTyr-397 phosphorylation (Durieux et al., 2009) indicates possible venues to stimulate this directly in situations where muscle activity is not an option.

The extent to which differences between slow and fast motor neurons are involved in the coupling between muscle excitation and gene expression (excitation-transcription coupling) is currently not well understood (Schiaffino & Serrano, 2002; Wakeling & Syme, 2002). Based on a preferential atrophy of slow type muscle fibres (Roy et al., 1996; Dapp et al., 2004), hindlimb suspension is expected to affect slow motor units more that fast type units. Our findings on the distinction of basal and disuse-induced transcript expression with slowed signal propagation down the motoneuron (Magyar et al., 1996) highlight the importance of correct excitation for control of gene expression (Calvo et al., 2001).

4. Conclusion

Our observations indicate that muscle dysfunction with Charcot-Marie-Tooth (CMT) is not due to a single, central mechanism. A novel, contraction-dependent feedback mechanism is identified that controls myelin-specific transcripts via a muscle fibre-related pathway. Somatic transfection of muscle fibres with the mechanosensor FAK prove the concept that pmp22 expression which is lowered in CMT can be stimulated when combined with skeletal muscle use. This indicates that muscle activity is a confounding variable that warrants exploration in future gene therapeutic strategies to treat and manage neuromuscular disease.

5. Acknowledgment

The study was financially supported by grants from the Région Rhône-Alpes, the Association Française contre les myopathies, and the Swiss National Science Foundation. The experiments were performed at the University of Berne (Switzerland), the University of Lyon (France), and Manchester Metropolitan University. The assistance of Dominique

Desplanches, Anne-Cécile Durieux, Damien Freyssenet and Prof. Hans Hoppeler during the suspension experiments is greatly acknowledged.

6. References

Baumann, H.; Jaggi, M.; Soland, F.; Howald, H. & Schaub, M. C. (1987). Exercise training induces transitions of myosin isoform subunits within histochemically typed human muscle fibres. *Pflugers Arch* 409(4-5): 349-60.

Bey, L.; Akunuri, N.; Zhao, P.; Hoffman, E. P.; Hamilton, D. G. & Hamilton, M. T. (2003). Patterns of global gene expression in rat skeletal muscle during unloading and low-intensity ambulatory activity. *Physiol Genomics* 13(2): 157-67.

Boncompagni, S.; Kern, H.; Rossini, K.; Hofer, C.; Mayr, W.; Carraro, U. & Protasi, F. (2007). Structural differentiation of skeletal muscle fibers in the absence of innervation in humans. *Proc Natl Acad Sci U S A* 104(49): 19339-44.

Booth, F. W. & Thomason, D. B. (1991). Molecular and cellular adaptation of muscle in response to exercise: perspectives of various models. *Physiol Rev* 71(2): 541-85.

Braathen, G. J.; Sand, J. C.; Lobato, A.; Hoyer, H. & Russell, M. B. (2011). Genetic epidemiology of Charcot-Marie-Tooth in the general population. *Eur J Neurol* 18(1): 39-48.

Calvo, S.; Vullhorst, D.; Venepally, P.; Cheng, J.; Karavanova, I. & Buonanno, A. (2001). Molecular dissection of DNA sequences and factors involved in slow muscle-specific transcription. *Mol Cell Biol* 21(24): 8490-503.

Carrasco, D. I. & English, A. W. (2003). Neurotrophin 4/5 is required for the normal development of the slow muscle fiber phenotype in the rat soleus. *J Exp Biol* 206(Pt 13): 2191-200.

Chen, Y. W.; Gregory, C. M.; Scarborough, M. T.; Shi, R.; Walter, G. A. & Vandenborne, K. (2007). Transcriptional pathways associated with skeletal muscle disuse atrophy in humans. *Physiol Genomics* 31(3): 510-20.

Dapp, C.; Schmutz, S.; Hoppeler, H. & Fluck, M. (2004). Transcriptional reprogramming and ultrastructure during atrophy and recovery of mouse soleus muscle. *Physiol Genomics* 20(1): 97-107.

Deschenes, M. R.; Britt, A. A.; Gomes, R. R.; Booth, F. W. & Gordon, S. E. (2001). Recovery of neuromuscular junction morphology following 16 days of spaceflight. *Synapse* 42(3): 177-84.

Durieux, A. C.; D'Antona, G.; Desplanches, D.; Freyssenet, D.; Klossner, S.; Bottinelli, R. & Fluck, M. (2009). Focal adhesion kinase is a load-dependent governor of the slow contractile and oxidative muscle phenotype. *J Physiol* 587(Pt 14): 3703-17.

Fluck, M. (2006). Functional, structural and molecular plasticity of mammalian skeletal muscle in response to exercise stimuli. *J Exp Biol* 209(Pt 12): 2239-48.

Fluck, M. & Hoppeler, H. (2003). Molecular basis of skeletal muscle plasticity--from gene to form and function. *Rev Physiol Biochem Pharmacol* 146: 159-216.

Fluck, M.; Mund, S. I.; Schittny, J. C.; Klossner, S.; Durieux, A. C. & Giraud, M. N. (2008). Mechano-regulated tenascin-C orchestrates muscle repair. *Proc Natl Acad Sci U S A* 105(36): 13662-7.

Fluck, M.; Schmutz, S.; Wittwer, M.; Hoppeler, H. & Desplanches, D. (2005). Transcriptional reprogramming during reloading of atrophied rat soleus muscle. *Am J Physiol Regul Integr Comp Physiol* 289(1): R4-14.

Fluck, M.; Ziemiecki, A.; Billeter, R. & Muntener, M. (2002). Fibre-type specific concentration of focal adhesion kinase at the sarcolemma: influence of fibre innervation and regeneration. *J Exp Biol* 205(Pt 16): 2337-48.

Gale, A. N.; Gomez, S. & Duchen, L. W. (1982). Changes produced by a hypomyelinating neuropathy in muscle and its innervation. Morphological and physiological studies in the Trembler mouse. *Brain* 105(Pt 2): 373-93.

Hennig, R. & Lomo, T. (1985). Firing patterns of motor units in normal rats. *Nature* 314(6007): 164-6.

Klossner, S.; Durieux, A. C.; Freyssenet, D. & Flueck, M. (2009). Mechano-transduction to muscle protein synthesis is modulated by FAK. *Eur J Appl Physiol* 106(3): 389-98.

Lindeman, E.; Spaans, F.; Reulen, J.; Leffers, P. & Drukker, J. (1999). Progressive resistance training in neuromuscular patients. Effects on force and surface EMG. *J Electromyogr Kinesiol* 9(6): 379-84.

Magyar, J. P.; Martini, R.; Ruelicke, T.; Aguzzi, A.; Adlkofer, K.; Dembic, Z.; Zielasek, J.; Toyka, K. V. & Suter, U. (1996). Impaired differentiation of Schwann cells in transgenic mice with increased PMP22 gene dosage. *J Neurosci* 16(17): 5351-60.

Niemann, S.; Sereda, M. W.; Suter, U.; Griffiths, I. R. & Nave, K. A. (2000). Uncoupling of myelin assembly and schwann cell differentiation by transgenic overexpression of peripheral myelin protein 22. *J Neurosci* 20(11): 4120-8.

Patel, P. I.; Roa, B. B.; Welcher, A. A.; Schoener-Scott, R.; Trask, B. J.; Pentao, L.; Snipes, G. J.; Garcia, C. A.; Francke, U.; Shooter, E. M.; Lupski, J. R. & Suter, U. (1992). The gene for the peripheral myelin protein PMP-22 is a candidate for Charcot-Marie-Tooth disease type 1A. *Nat Genet* 1(3): 159-65.

Pilegaard, H.; Ordway, G. A.; Saltin, B. & Neufer, P. D. (2000). Transcriptional regulation of gene expression in human skeletal muscle during recovery from exercise. *Am J Physiol Endocrinol Metab* 279(4): E806-14.

Roy, R. R.; Baldwin, K. M. & Edgerton, V. R. (1996). Response of the neuromuscular unit to spaceflight: what has been learned from the rat model. *Exerc Sport Sci Rev* 24: 399-425.

Schiaffino, S. & Serrano, A. (2002). Calcineurin signaling and neural control of skeletal muscle fiber type and size. *Trends Pharmacol Sci* 23(12): 569-75.

Schmutz, S.; Dapp, C.; Wittwer, M.; Durieux, A. C.; Mueller, M.; Weinstein, F.; Vogt, M.; Hoppeler, H. & Fluck, M. (2010). A hypoxia complement differentiates the muscle response to endurance exercise. *Exp Physiol* 95(6): 723-35.

Schuierer, M. M.; Mann, C. J.; Bildsoe, H.; Huxley, C. & Hughes, S. M. (2005). Analyses of the differentiation potential of satellite cells from myoD-/-, mdx, and PMP22 C22 mice. *BMC Musculoskelet Disord* 6: 15.

Spreyer, P.; Kuhn, G.; Hanemann, C. O.; Gillen, C.; Schaal, H.; Kuhn, R.; Lemke, G. & Muller, H. W. (1991). Axon-regulated expression of a Schwann cell transcript that is homologous to a 'growth arrest-specific' gene. *Embo J* 10(12): 3661-8.

Vinci, P.; Esposito, C.; Perelli, S. L.; Antenor, J. A. & Thomas, F. P. (2003). Overwork weakness in Charcot-Marie-Tooth disease. *Arch Phys Med Rehabil* 84(6): 825-7.

Wakeling, J. M. & Syme, D. A. (2002). Wave properties of action potentials from fast and slow motor units of rats. *Muscle Nerve* 26(5): 659-68.

Wilkinson, S. B.; Phillips, S. M.; Atherton, P. J.; Patel, R.; Yarasheski, K. E.; Tarnopolsky, M. A. & Rennie, M. J. (2008). Differential effects of resistance and endurance exercise in the fed state on signalling molecule phosphorylation and protein synthesis in human muscle. *J Physiol* 586(Pt 15): 3701-17.

Wise, C. A.; Garcia, C. A.; Davis, S. N.; Heju, Z.; Pentao, L.; Patel, P. I. & Lupski, J. R. (1993). Molecular analyses of unrelated Charcot-Marie-Tooth (CMT) disease patients suggest a high frequency of the CMTIA duplication. *Am J Hum Genet* 53(4): 853-63.